James B. Stiehl

Werner H. Konermann

Rolf G. Haaker

Navigation and Robotics in Total Joint and Spine Surgery

Springer

Berlin
Heidelberg
New York
Hongkong
London
Milano
Paris
Tokyo

James B. Stiehl

Werner H. Konermann

Rolf G. Haaker

Navigation and Robotics in Total Joint and Spine Surgery

With 460 Figures, 355 in Colors
and 31 Tables

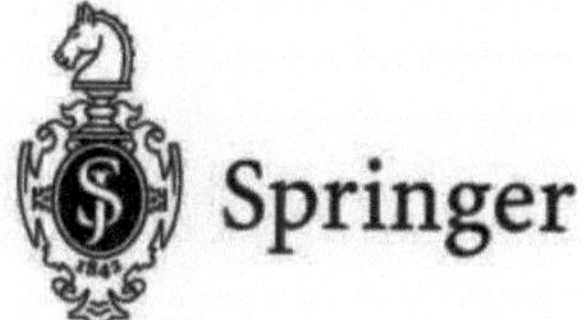

Springer

Stiehl, James B., Associate Professor, M.D.
Orthopaedic Hospital of Wisconsin
575 West Riverwood, Parkway, Suite 204
Milwaukee 53212, USA

Konermann, Werner H., Professor, M.D.
Orthopaedic Hospital
Am Mühlenberg, 37235 Hessisch-Lichtenau,
Germany

Haaker, Rolf G., Associate Professor, M.D.
Orthopaedic Hospital, St. Vincenz-Hospital
Danziger Straße 17, 33034 Brakel,
Germany

ISBN-13:978-3-642-63922-7   e-ISBN-13:978-3-642-59290-4
DOI: 10.1007/978-3-642-59290-4

Cataloging-in Publication Data applied for

Bibliographic information published by Die Deutsche Bibliothek
Die Deutsche Bibliothek lists this publication in the Deutsche Nationalbibliografie; detailed bibliographic data is available in the Internet at <http://dnb.ddb.de>

Springer-Verlag Berlin Heidelberg New York
a member of BertelsmannSpringer Science+Business Media GmbH
http://www.springer.de
© Springer-Verlag Berlin Heidelberg 2004
Softcover reprint of the hardcover 1st edition 2004

Editorial: Thomas Günther, Heidelberg
Production: Rainer Kusche, Sinzheim
Cover design: Design & Production, Heidelberg
Typesetting: Goldener Schnitt, Sinzheim

Printed on acid-free paper   18/3130 – 5 4 3 2 1 0   10 8 89 375

Foreword

Orthopaedic surgery is currently just a few moments past the sunrise of computer implementation for the performance of surgery itself. Our specialty has always seemed to have a nearly unique, over arching characteristic – it deals almost exclusively with alteration, typically rebuilding or reconstituting, structure. What we do has more of a structural impact than a physiologic one, even when compared to the structural alterations introduced by vascular and cardiac surgery. This structural reconstitution contrasts strongly with the largely excisional characteristic of most other surgical fields.

The relevance of this feature is that our specialty, as much as any, and more than most, needs precision of cutting, alignment, and replacement. As we contrast the rudimentary tools, we use in our operating rooms with the sophisticated robotic, computerized, and more extensively mechanized equipment of industry, we seem very far behind. We are almost ancient considering the pace of development and change over the last fifty years.

Many question the need, practicality, expense and therefore ultimate acceptance of these methods into orthopaedics. However, the quality I mention above, leads me to believe that eventually, hi-tech involving computer assistance and including robotic tools, will almost take over. The current era is and will be appreciated as a beginning – a time when new equipment and techniques are introduced, bugs worked out, and valuable tools refined, nearly perfected, with costs lowered.

Today every country feels the constraint of cost containment in health care. The social, economic environment seems, in the minds of many, to prohibit substantial incorporation of this methodology. This writer has confidence that real improvements from the incorporation of hi-technology will be recognized. And, considering the importance to each individual patient of the life-event that is his or her orthopaedic surgery, demand for best practice not cheapest will sustain. Along with social order there is perhaps nothing more important to an individual than health and therefore, healthcare. The dollars will be found. The choices made.

In this marvelous volume compiled by Doctors Stiehl, Konermann, and Haaker we are treated to the early logbook for a worldwide advance into this new age of high technology orthopaedics. The field is covered both widely and in depth. Contributions are from the pioneers and developers of these methods.

Kenneth A. Krackow
Buffalo, New York, USA
October 2003

Short Biography of the Editors

Stiehl, James B., Associate Professor, M.D.
Orthopaedic Hospital of Wisconsin
575 West Riverwood Parkway, Suite 204
Milwaukee 53212, USA
About the Editor:
Born in 1949, Adult Reconstructive Orthopaedic Surgeon. Residency at the University of Texas Health Science Center in San Antonio Texas under Drs. Charles Rockwood and David Green, and Fellowships at the Princess Margaret Rose Hospital, Edinburgh and Swiss AO Fellowship, Zurich. He is in private practice at Columbia St Mary's Hospital in Milwaukee, Wisconsin, USA. His main interests are in total joint arthroplasty and adult reconstructive surgery and he has a longstanding interest in biomechanical research in orthopaedics.

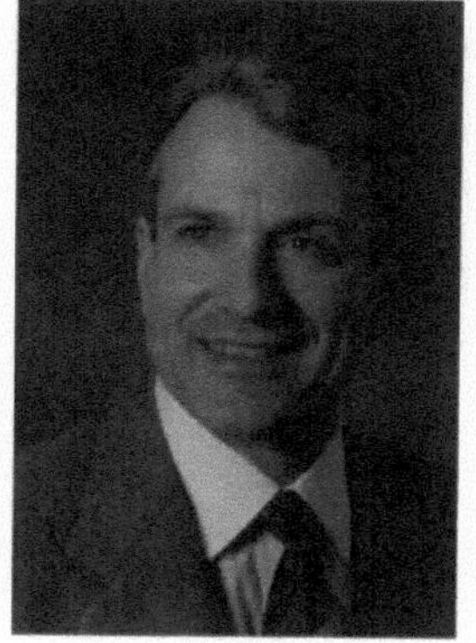

Konermann, Werner H., Professor, M.D.
Hospital of Orthopaedics and Traumatology
Am Mühlenberg 3, D-37235 Hessisch-Lichtenau, Germany
About the Editor:
Born in 1959, Specialist Orthopaedic Surgeon and Rheumatologist. Residencies in three German Universities at Tübingen, Münster and Mannheim. His thesis was done in biomechanics of the lumbar spine. He is now a Consultant Orthopaedic Surgeon for orthopaedics and traumatology in Hessisch Lichtenau, Germany. His main interest is in knee and hip arthroplasty and computer-assisted surgery.

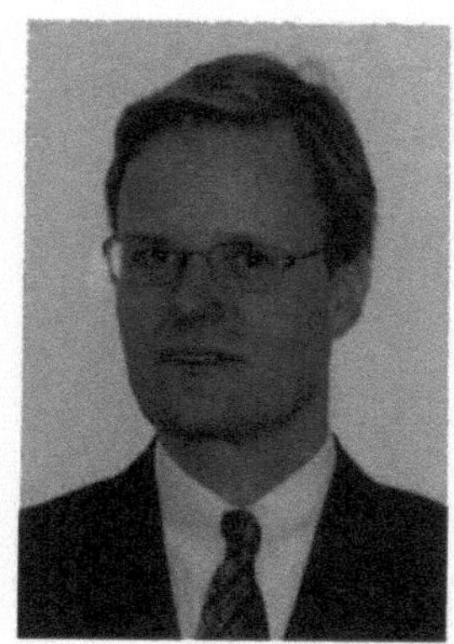

Haaker, Rolf G., Associate Professor, M.D.
Hospital for Orthopaedics and Rheumatology
St. Vincenz-Hospital, Danziger Str. 17, 33034 Brakel, Germany
About the Editor:
Born in 1959, Specialist Orthopaedic Surgeon and Rheumatologist. Residencies at the Sportsmedical Devision, Military Hospital in Warendorf and Koblenz followed by a recidency at the University in Bochum, Germany. His thesis was done in biomechanics of the multilevel lumbar spinal fusion. He is now a Chief Consultant Orthopaedic Surgeon in Bad Driburg-Brakel, Germany. He has a main interests in revision surgery of hip and knee arthroplasty, spine surgery and computer assisted surgery.

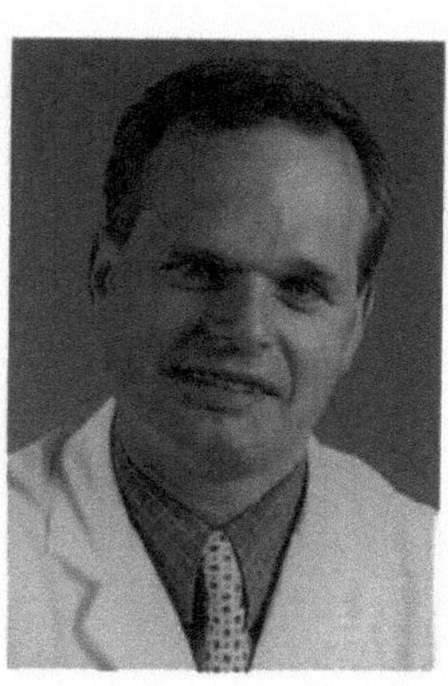

» The current discoveries teach us that whatever we thought is true actually was wrong. It appears to me that the only knowledge we can still trust is the fact that light speed is the fastest thing on earth. Possibly. «

EDWARD TELLER

Preface

With the advance of the technology age, the known body of knowledge composing medical science has tripled since 1960. Many important new treatments and methods have envolved during this period. For example, total joint arthroplasty, a recent innovation, has benefited millions of patients and is now one of the most common surgical procedures in medical practice. Yet, despite this success, basic issues such as component alignment and positioning are not always ideal, and may lead to unsatisfactory clinical results with early loosening or failure of the implants.

Computer navigation and robotics are considered to be controversial tools, but recent experience has revealed promising applications in hip and knee arthroplasty, spine surgery, ACL reconstruction and other operations.

At the first symposium for computer navigation and robotics in Bochum, Germany, an international faculty consisting of orthopaedic, trauma, and neurosurgeons as well as engineers, reported a wide range of applications for this technology and its current practical use. A state of the art publication resulted which also included the current technology development of several commercial interests. This groundwork leads to an overview of the current practical use of navigation and robotics.

In this book, an important premise was that the contributing authors reported honestly on their personal experiences, including both success and failures. Because the basic technologies of computer navigation and robotics have many applications, we felt compelled to combine the experiences in many surgical disciplines. Finally, we recognize the swift evolution of computer software and technology in this field, and we have attempted to highlight the evolutionary improvements to time-tested surgical methods as well as to offer new vistas in advanced surgical technique.

We are at the beginning of a new and revolutionary development in medicine, which will not replace the surgeon, but will help to improve accuracy and consistency of high precision in standard operations. In America, great enthusiasm has arisen for minimally invasive techniques especially in total joint replacement. Many opinions find navigation a critical element to the efficacy of the approach which can be found in this book. We consider this book a guideline and reference for navigational and robotic surgical tools as well as help for medicolegal concerns regarding minimizing risks, quality control and documentation.

We would like to express our sincere thanks to all authors who have generously contributed to this project. It is only through their efforts and dedication to advancing medical science that this book is possible.

We would like to thank our colleague Jens Boldt, St.-Vincent Hospital, Düsseldorf, for his tireless effort in translating many of the enclosed chapters from the original book published in the German language.

We are also very grateful to the publisher Springer-Verlag, Heidelberg, Germany, with special thanks to the editor, Thomas Günther, for expediting the production of this book.

James B. Stiehl
October 2003

Werner H. Konermann

Rolf G. Haaker

Sections

Contents

VI   Navigation: Spinal Surgery

VII   Visions of Surgeons

VIII   Visions of the Industry

Editors

Stiehl, James B.,
Associate Professor, M.D.
Orthopaedic Hospital
of Wisconsin
575 West Riverwood
Parkway, Suite 204
Milwaukee 53212, USA

Konermann, Werner H.,
Professor, M.D.
Orthopaedic Hospital
Am Mühlenberg 3
37235 Hessisch-Lichtenau,
Germany

Haaker, Rolf G.,
Associate Professor, M.D.
Orthopaedic Hospital
St. Vincenz-Hospital
Danziger Straße 17
33034 Brakel, Germany

List of Contributors

Arand, M.
Dept. f. Orthopaedic Surgery,
Hand- und Reconstructive
Surgery
University Hospital Ulm
Steinhövelstraße 9
89075 Ulm/Donau, Germany

Argenson, J.-N.
Hôpital Sainte Marguerite
Service de Chirurgie
Orthopédique et de
Traumatologie
BP 29,
13274 Marseille Cedex 09,
France

Aubaniac, J.-M.
Hôpital Sainte Marguerite
Service de Chirurgie
Orthopédique et de
Traumatologie
BP 29
13274 Marseille Cedex 09,
France

Babisch, J.
Orthopaedic Hospital
Friedrich-Schiller University
Jena
Waldkrankenhaus »Rudolf Elle«
Klosterlausnitzer Straße 81
07607 Eisenberg, Germany

Bäthis, H.
Department of Orthopaedic
Surgery
University Hospital Regensburg
Kaiser-Karl-V.-Allee 3
93077 Bad Abbach, Germany

Bale, R.J.
Department of Orthopaedic
Surgery
University Hospital Innsbruck
Anichstraße 35
6020 Innsbruck, Austria

Bargar, W.
1020 29th Street, Suite 450
Sacramento, CA 95816, USA

Begoc, N.
Praxim
4, Avenue de l'Obiou
Le Grand Sablon
38700 La Tronche, France

Berlemann, U.
Department of Traumatology
Surgery
Hannover Medical School
Carl-Neuberg-Straße 1
30625 Hannover, Germany

Bernsmann, K.
Orthopaedic Department
Girardet Clinic Essen
Girardet Straße 2–38
45131 Essen, Germany

Bertrand, F.
Praxim
4, Avenue de l'Obiou
Le Grand Sablon
38700 La Tronche, France

Birnbaum, K.
Department of Orthopaedic
Surgery
University Hospital RWTH
Aachen
Pauwelstraße 30
52074 Aachen, Germany

Boeri, C.
Chirurgie Orthopédique
et Traumatologique
Centre de Traumatologie
et d'Orthopédie
10, Avenue Baumann
67400 Illkirch Graffenstaden,
France

Böhling, U.
Auguste-Victoria Haspital
Orthopaedic Department
Rubenstr. 12, 512157 Berlin,
Germany

Boldt, J.
St. Vincent-Hospital
Orthopaedic Department
Schlossstraße 85
40477 Düsseldorf, Germany

Börner M.
Berufsgenossenschaftliche
Unfallklinik
Frankfurt am Main
Friedberger Landstraße 430
60389 Frankfurt am Main,
Germany

Breysse, M.
DePuy France
Z, Allé Irène Joliot
BP 256
69801 Saint Priest Cedex,
France

Briard, J.-L.
Clinique de Cédre
Bois Guilleaume
76235 Rouen-Cedex, France

Buechel, F.
Biomedical Engineering Trust
South Mountain Orthopaedic
61st Street
South Orange, New Jersey
07079, USA

Chiu P.
Division of Joint Replacement
Surgery
Department of Orthopaedic
Surgery
The University of Hong Kong
Room 509, 5th Floor,
Professorial Block
Queen Mary Hospital
Pokfulam, Hong Kong, China

Christ, R.M.
Orthopaedic Hospital
Auguste-Viktoria
Am Kokturkanal 2
32545 Bad Oeynhausen,
Germany

Christmann, S.
Brain LAB AG
Ammerthalstr. 8,
85551 Heimstetten, Germany

Clemens, U.
Orthopaedic Center and Center
for Rheumatology of Northern
Germany
St. Josef-Stift
Westtor 7
48324 Sendenhorst, Germany

Decker, N.
Department of Orthopaedic
Surgery
University Hospital RWTH
Aachen
Pauwelstraße 30
52074 Aachen, Germany

De Rycke, J.
Elisabeth Zuikenhuis
Department of Orthopaedic
Surgery
Gentse Steenweg 132
8340 Sjisele-Damme, Belgium

DiGioia, A.M.
ICAOS (Institute for Computer
Assisted Orthopaedic Surgery)
The Western Pennsylvania
Hospital
4815 Liberty Avenue
Mellon Pavilion, Suite 242
Pittsburgh, PA 15224, USA

Ditzen, W.
Berufsgenossenschaftliche
Unfallklinik Frankfurt/Main
Friedberger Landstraße 430
60389 Frankfurt am Main,
Germany

Dubrana, F.
Service de Chirurgie
Orthopédique
Traumatologique et Réparatrice
Chu de Brest
Hôpital de la Cavale Blanche
Boulevard Tanguy Prigent
29609 Brest-Cedex, France

Eichhorn, J.
Orthopaedic Praxis Clinic
Hebbelstraße 14a
94315 Straubing, Germany

Ellermann, A.
Arcus Sport Clinic
Wilhelm-Becker-Straße 15
75179 Pforzheim, Germany

Fink, C.
Department of Orthopaedic
Surgery
University Hospital Innsbruck
Anichstraße 35
6020 Innsbruck, Austria

Flecher, X.
Hôpital Sainte Marguerite
Service de Chirurgie
Orthopédique et de
Traumatologie
BP 29
13274 Marseille Cedex 09,
France

Frericks, B.
Medical University Hannover
Department of Orthopaedic
Surgery
Carl-Neuberg-Straße 1
30625 Hannover, Germany

Fritsch, E.
Orthopaedic University
Hospital, Homburg/Saar
Kirrberger Straße
66421 Homburg/Saar,
Germany

Fu, F. H.
David Silver Professor
and Chairman
Head Team Physician,
Univ. of Pittsburgh
Kaufmann Building, Suite 1011
3471 Fifth Avenue
Pittsburgh, PA 15213-3221, USA

Fuiko, R.
Department of Orthopaedic
Surgery
Orthopaedic Hospital the City
of Vienna – Gersthof
Wielemansgasse 28
1180 Vienna, Austria

Galad, D.D.
The Ohio State University
College of Medicine
Department of Orthopaedic
Surgery
2050 Kenny Road, Suite 3300
Columbus, OH 43221, USA

Gebhard, F.
Dept. for Orthopaedic Surgery,
Hand- und Reconstructive
Surgery
University Hospital Ulm
Steinhövelstraße 9
89075 Ulm/Donau, Germany

Geerling, J.
Department of Traumatology
Surgery
Hannover Medical School
Carl-Neuberg-Straße 1
30625 Hannover, Germany

Goesling, T.
Department of Traumatology
Surgery
Hannover Medical School
Carl-Neuberg-Straße 1
30625 Hannover, Germany

Gossé, F.
Medical University Hannover
Orthopaedic Surgery
Anna-von-Borries-Straße 1-7
30625 Hannover, Germany

Gotzen, L.
Trauma, Reconstructional and
Hand Surgery Department
Philipps University Medical
School, Marburg
Baldinger Straße
35033 Marburg, Germany

Grifka, J.
Department of Orthopaedic
Surgery
University Hospital Regensburg
Kaiser-Karl-V.-Allee 3
93077 Bad Abbach, Germany

Gruber, G.
ATOS-Praxis Clinic Heidelberg
Bismarckplatz 9–15
69115 Heidelberg, Germany

Grundei, H.
ESKA-Implants
Grapengeißerstraße 34
235565 Lübeck, Germany

Grützner, P.A.
Berufsgenossenschaftliche
Unfallklinik Ludwigshafen
Trauma Center, University of
Heidelberg
Ludwig-Guttmannstraße 13
67071 Ludwigshafen, Germany

Haaker, R.G.
Orthopaedic Hospital
St. Vincenz-Hospital
Danziger Straße 17
33034 Brakel, Germany

Hackbart, M.
Orthopaedic Hospital
Auguste-Viktoria
Am Kokturkanal 2
32545 Bad Oeynhausen,
Germany

Hagena, F.-W.
Orthopaedic Hospital
Auguste-Viktoria
Am Kokturkanal 2
32545 Bad Oeynhausen,
Germany

Hassenpflug, J.
Orthopaedic Department
Christian-Albrechts-University
Kiel
Michaelisstraße 1
24105 Kiel, Germany

Hebecker, A.
Siemens AG, Medical Solutions
SPC
Hartmannstraße 48
91052 Erlangen, Germany

Hey, J.
Siemens AG, Medical Solutions
SPC
Henkestraße 127
91050 Erlangen, Germany

Hille, E.
General Hospital Eilbeck
Department of Orthopaedic
Surgery
Friedrichsberger Str. 60
22081 Hamburg, Germany

Honscha, M.
Orthopaedic Clinic
Kreiskrankenhaus Marienhöhe
Mauerfeldchen 25
52146 Würselen, Germany

Hoser, C.
Department of Orthopaedic
Surgery
University Hospital Innsbruck
Anichstraße 35
6020 Innsbruck, Austria

Hüfner, T.
Department of Traumatology
Surgery
Hannover Medical School
Carl-Neuberg-Straße 1
30625 Hannover, Germany

Hurschler, C.
Medical University Hannover
Orthopaedic Surgery
Anna-von-Borries-Straße 1-7
30625 Hannover, Germany

Jaramaz, B.
Institute for Computer Assisted
Orthopaedic Surgery
The Western Pennsylvania
Hospital
4815 Liberty Avenue
Mellon Pavilion, Suite 242
Pittsburgh, PA 15224, USA

Jenny, J.-Y.
Chirurgie Orthopédique
et Traumatologique
Centre de Traumatologie
et d'Orthopédie
10, Avenue Baumann
67400 Illkirch Graffenstaden,
France

Julliard, R.
Clinique Mutualiste des Eaux
Claires
Rue Dr. Calmette
38000 Grenoble, France

Keil, C.
Berufsgenossenschaftliche
Unfallklinik Ludwigshafen
Trauma Center, University
of Heidelberg
Ludwig-Guttmannstraße 13
67071 Ludwigshafen, Germany

Kerschbaumer, F.
Department of Orthopaedic
Surgery and Rheumaortho-
paedics
University Hospital
Marienburgstraße 2
60528 Frankfurt a.M., Germany

Kettrukat, M.
Orthopaedic Hospital
Auguste-Viktoria
Am Kokturkanal 2
32545 Bad Oeynhausen,
Germany

Kfuri, M.
Medical University Hannover
Department of Orthopaedic
Surgery
Carl-Neuberg-Straße 1
30625 Hannover, Germany

Kiefer, H.
Department of Orthopaedic
and Trauma Surgery
Lukas-Hospital
Hindenburgstraße 56
32257 Buende, Germany

Kistner, S.
Orthopaedic Hospital
Am Mühlenberg
33735 Hessisch-Lichtenau,
Germany

Klapper, U.
Orthopaedic Clinic
Genaral Hospital Marienhöhe
Mauerfeldchen 25
52146 Würselen, Germany

Kluge, W.H.
Orthopaedic Hospital
Friedrich-Schiller University
Jena
Waldkrankenhaus »Rudolf Elle«
Klosterlausnitzer Straße 81
07607 Eisenberg, Germany

Kohn, S.
Orthopaedic University Hospital
Kirrberger Straße, Geb. 37
66421 Homburg/Saar, Germany

Knabe, K.
Medical University Hannover
Orthopaedic Surgery
Anna-von-Borries-Straße 1-7
30625 Hannover, Germany

Kohler, S.
Helios Clinic for Orthopaedic
Surgery
Barbara-Straße 11-12
99752 Bleicherode, Germany

Komistek, R.D.
Department of Biomedical
Engineering
University of Tennesse;
Knoxville
313 Perkins Hall
Knoxville, Tennessee, USA

Konermann, W.H.
Orthopaedic Hospital
Am Mühlenberg 3
37235 Hessisch-Lichtenau,
Germany

Kotten, B.
Axios 3 D Services GmbH
Marienstraße 16
26121 Oldenburg, Germany

Krackow, K.A.
Dept. of Orthopaedic Surgery
The State University of New
York at Buffalo
Orthopaedic Surgery B 2
Buffalo General Hospital
100 High Street, B-2
Buffalo, New York 14203-1126,
USA

Krämer, J.
University Hospital for Ortho-
paedic and Trauma Surgery
St. Josef-Hospital Bochum
Gudrunstraße 56
44791 Bochum, Germany

Krettek, C.
Medical University Hannover
Department of Orthopaedic
Surgery
Carl-Neuberg-Straße 1
30625 Hannover, Germany

Krismer, M.
Department of Orthopaedic
Surgery
University Hospital Innsbruck
Anichstraße 35
6020 Innsbruck, Austria

Kubiak-Langer, M.
Maurice E.-Mueller Research
Center for Orthopaedic Surgery
Inst. f. Surgical Therapy and
Biomechanics
University of Bern
Murtenstraße 35
3001 Bern, Switzerland

Kuenzler, S.
Department of Orthopaedic
Surgery and
Rheumaorthopaedics
University Hospital
Marienburgstraße 2
60528 Frankfurt a.M., Germany

Lampe, F.
General Hospital Eilbeck
Department of Orthopaedic
Surgery
Friedrichsberger Str. 60
22081 Hamburg, Germany

Langlotz, F.
Maurice E.-Mueller Research
Center for Orthopaedic Surgery
Institute for Surgical Therapy
and Biomechanics
University of Bern
Murtenstraße 35
3001 Bern, Switzerland

Langlotz, U.
Medivision
Eimattstraße 3
4436 Oberdorf, Switzerland

Lavallée, S.
Praxim
4, Avenue de l'Obiou
Le Grand Sablon
38700 La Tronche, France

Layher, F.
Orthopaedic Hospital
Friedrich-Schiller University
Jena
Waldkrankenhaus »Rudolf Elle«
Klosterlausnitzer Straße 81
07607 Eisenberg, Germany

Lefevre, C.
Service de Chirurgie
Orthopédique
Traumatologique et Réparatrice
Chu de Brest
Hôpital de la Cavale Blanche
Boulevard Tanguy Prigent
29609 Brest-Cedex, France

Lörke, C.
Department of Orthopaedic
Surgery
University Hospital Kassel
Wilhelmshöher Allee 345
34131 Kassel, Germany

Lüring, C.
Department of Orthopaedic
Surgery
University Hospital Regensburg
Kaiser-Karl-V.-Allee 3
93077 Bad Abbach, Germany

Machacek, F., jun.
Department of Orthopaedic
Surgery
Orthopaedic Hospital the City
of Vienna – Gersthof
Wielemansgasse 28
1180 Vienna, Austria

Mai, S.
Department of Orthopaedic
Surgery
University Hospital Kassel
Wilhelmshöher Allee 345
34131 Kassel, Germany

Malckowski, D.
Stryker Instruments
4100 East Milham Avenue
49001 Kalamazoo
Michigan, USA

Marx, A.
Orthopaedic Clinic
University of Essen
Pattbergstraße 1–3
45239 Essen-Werden,
Germany

Mattes, T.
Department of Orthopaedic
Surgery
University Hospital Ulm
Oberer Eselsberg 45
89081 Ulm, Germany

Merloz, P.
Centre Hospitalier
Universitaire de Grenoble
Hôpital Michallon
38000 Grenoble, France

Miehlke, R.
Orthopaedic Center and
Center for Rheumatology
of Northern Germany
St. Josef-Stift
Westtor 7
48324 Sendenhorst, Germany

Moctezuma de la Barrera, J.L.
Stryker Navigation
Bötzinger Straße 41
79111 Freiburg, Germany

Mortier, J.A.
Department of Orthopaedic
Surgery
Foundation Friedrichsheim
University Frankfurt/Main
Marienburgstraße 2
60528 Frankfurt/Main,
Germany

Moser, W.
PI (Presition Implant Systems)
Schachenallee 29
CH-5001 Aarau, Switzerland

Musahl, V.
David Silver Professor and
Chairman
Head Team Physician, Univ. of
Pittsburgh
Kaufmann Building, Suite 1011
3471 Fifth Avenue
Pittsburgh, PA 15213-3221, USA

Nassutt, R.
ESKA-Implants
Grapengießerstraße 34
23556 Lübeck, Germany

Nogler, M.
Department of Orthopaedic
Surgery
University Hospital Innsbruck
Anichstraße 35
6020 Innsbruck, Austria

Nolte, L.-P.
M.E. Mueller Institute
for Biomechanics
University of Bern
Murtenstraße 35
3010 Bern, Switzerland

Ohnsorge, J.A.K.
Department of Orthopaedic
Surgery
University Hospital RWTH
Aachen
Pauwelstraße 30
52074 Aachen, Germany

Ostermeier, S.
Medical University Hannover
Orthopaedic Surgery
Anna-von-Borries-Straße 1-7
30625 Hannover, Germany

Pashmineh-Azar, A.
Trauma, Reconstructional and
Hand Surgery Department
Philipps University Medical
School, Marburg
Baldinger Straße
35033 Marburg, Germany

Perlick, L.
Department of Orthopaedic
Surgery
University Hospital Regensburg
Kaiser-Karl-V.-Allee 3
93077 Bad Abbach, Germany

Picard, F.
Hôpital Sud
Orthopédie – Traumatologie
C.H.U. de Grenoble
38130 Échirolles, France

Plakseychuk, A.
ICAOS (Institute for Computer
Assisted Orthopaedic Surgery)
The Western Pennsylvania
Hospital
4815 Liberty Avenue
Mellon Pavilion, Suite 242
Pittsburgh, PA 15224, USA

Plaweski, S.
Centre Hospitalier et Universitaire de Grenoble
Hôpital Michallon
38000 Grenoble, France

Pohlemann, T.
Department of Traumatology
Surgery
Hannover Medical School
Carl-Neuberg-Straße 1
30625 Hannover, Germany

Portheine, F.
Helmholtz-Institut for
Biomedical Technology
University Hospital RWTH
Aachen
Pauwelstraße 20
52074 Aachen, Germany

Prymka, M.
Orthopaedic Department
Christian-Albrechts-University
Kiel
Michaelisstraße 1
24105 Kiel, Germany

Puhl, W.
Department of Orthopaedic
Surgery
University Hospital Ulm
Oberer Eselsberg 45
89081 Ulm, Germany

Radermacher, K.
Surgical Technology Lab
Helmholtz-Institut
for Biomedical Technology
University Hospital RWTH
Aachen
Pauwelstraße 20
52074 Aachen, Germany

Rao, R.
Spine Research
Department of Orthopaedic
Surgery
Medical College of Wisconsin
9200 West Wisconsin Avenue
Milwaukee, 53226, USA

Ritschl, P.
Department of Orthopaedic
Surgery
Orthopaedic Hospital
the City of Vienna – Gersthof
Wielemansgasse 28
1180 Vienna, Austria

Rosenberger, R.E.
Department of Orthopaedic
Surgery
University Hospital Innsbruck
Anichstraße 35
6020 Innsbruck, Austria

Rosenthal, A.
Orthopaedic Department
Girardet Clinic Essen
Girardet-Straße 2-38
45131 Essen, Germany

Rupp, S.
Clinic Karlsbad-Langen-
steinbach
Guttmannstraße 1
76307 Karlsbad, Germany

Rüther, W.
Orthopaedic Clinic
University Hospital Hamburg
Eppendorf (UKE)
Martinistraße 52
20246 Hamburg, Germany

Saragaglia, D.
Hôpital Sud
Orthopédie - Traumatologie
C.H.U. de Grenoble
38130 Échirolles, France

Saur, M.A.
Orthopaedic Hospital
Am Mühlenberg
37235 Hessisch-Lichtenau,
Germany

Schkommodau, E.
Institute for
Biomedical Technology
University Hospital RWTH
Aachen
Helmholtz-Institut, Dept. of
Surgical Therapy Technology
Pauwelstraße 20
52074 Aachen, Germany

Schmidt, K.
Catholic Hospital
Dortmund West
Orthopaedic Department
Zollernstraße 40
44379 Dortmund, Germany

Scholz, J.
Auguste-Victoria Hospital
Orthopaedic Department
Rubenstr. 125
12157 Berlin, Germany

Siebert, W.
Department of Orthopaedic
Surgery
University Hospital Kassel
Wilhelmshöher Allee 345
34131 Kassel, Germany

Siebold, R.
Arcus Sport Clinic
Wilhelm-Becker-Straße 15
75179 Pforzheim, Germany

Singrakhia, M.
Spine Research
Department of Orthopaedic
Surgery
Medical College of Wisconsin
9200 West Wisconsin Avenue
Milwaukee, 53226, USA

Solodky, P.
DePuy France
Z, Allé Irène Joliot
BP 256
69801 Saint Priest Cedex, France

Sott, A.
Department of Traumatology
Surgery
Hannover Medical School
Carl-Neuberg-Straße 1
30625 Hannover, Germany

Sparmann, M.
Department of Orthopaedic
Surgery
Immanuel Hospital
Königsstraße 63
14109 Berlin, Germany

Staudte, H.-W
Orthopaedic Clinic
General Hospital Marienhöhe
Mauerfeldchen 25
52146 Würselen, Germany

Steiner, A.
Siemens AG, Medical Solutions
SPC
Henkestraße 127
91050 Erlangen, Germany

Stiehl, J.B.,
Orthopaedic Hospital
of Wisconsin
575 West Riverwood
Parkway, Suite 204
Milwaukee 53212, USA

Stindel, E.
Service de Chirurgie
Orthopédique
Traumatologique et Réparatrice
Chu de Brest
Hôpital de la Cavale Blanche
Boulevard Tanguy Prigent
29609 Brest-Cedex, France

Stockheim, M.
University Hospital for
Orthopaedic and Trauma
Surgery
St. Josef-Hospital Bochum
Gudrunstraße 56
44791 Bochum, Germany

Strauss, J.M.
Orthopaedic Clinic
University Hospital Hamburg
Eppendorf (UKE)
Martinistraße 52
20246 Hamburg, Germany

Stukenborg-Colsman, C.
Medical University Hannover
Orthopaedic Surgery
Anna-von-Borries-Straße 1-7
30625 Hannover, Germany

Stulberg, D.S.
Northwestern Orthopaedic
Institute
Joint Replacement and Arthritis
Surgery
680 N. Lake Shore Drive
Suite 1028
Chicago, Illinois 60611, USA

Thomas, B.
UCLA Medical Center
10833 LeConte Ave # 76-134
Los Angeles, CA 99095, USA

Thomsen, M.
Foundation of Orthopaedic
University Hospital
Schlierbacher Landstraße 200a
69118 Heidelberg, Germany

Tingart, M.
Department of Orthopaedic
Surgery
University Hospital Regensburg
Kaiser-Karl-V.-Allee 3
93077 Bad Abbach, Germany

Troccaz, J.
TIMC Laboratory
Grenoble University
38000 Grenoble, France

Tümmler, H.-P.
Aesculap & Co. KG
Am Aesculap-Platz
78532 Tuttlingen, Germany

Venbrocks, R.-A.
Orthopaedic Hospital
Friedrich-Schiller University
Jena
Waldkrankenhaus »Rudolf Elle«
Klosterlausnitzer Straße 81
07607 Eisenberg, Germany

Vinel, H.
Hôpital Sainte Marguerite
Servie de Chirurgie
Orthopédique et de
Traumatolgie
BP 29, 13274 Marseille Cedex 09,
France

Vock, B.
Berufsgenossensch. Unfallklinik
Ludwigshafen
Trauma Center,
University of Heidelberg
Ludwig-Guttmannstraße 13
67071 Ludwigshafen,
Germany

Wahrburg, J.
Department of Orthopaedic
Surgery and
Rheumaorthopaedics
University Hospital
Marienburgstraße 2
60528 Frankfurt a.M.,
Germany

Wasielewski, R.C.
The Ohio State University
College of Medicine
Department of Orthopaedic
Surgery
2050 Kenny Road, Suite 3300
Columbus, OH 43221, USA

Weidner, A.
Spine Center
Lengericher Landstr. 19b
49078 Osnabrück, Germany

Wentzensen, A.
Berufsgenossensch. Unfallklinik
Ludwigshafen
Trauma Center, University
of Heidelberg
Ludwig-Guttmannstraße 13
67071 Ludwigshafen,
Germany

Wiese, M.
University Hospital for Ortho-
paedic Surgery
St. Josef-Hospital Bochum
Gudrunstraße 56
44791 Bochum, Germany

Wiesel, U.
Berufsgenossenschaftliche
Unfallklinik
Frankfurt am Main
Friedberger Landstraße 430
60389 Frankfurt am Main,
Germany

Windhagen, H.
Medical University Hannover
Orthopaedic Surgery
Anna-von-Borries-Straße 1-7
30625 Hannover, Germany

Willburger, R. E.
University Hospital
for Orthopaedic Surgery
St. Josef-Hospital Bochum
Gudrunstraße 56
44791 Bochum, Germany

Wixson, R.L.
Clinical Orthopaedic Surgery
Northwestern University
Feinberg School of Medicine
Northwestern Center for
Orthopaedics
676 North St. Clare, Suite 450
Chicago, IL 60611, USA

Wolke, B.
Department of Orthopaedic
Surgery
Immanuel Hospital
Königsstraße 63
14109 Berlin, Germany

Zettl, R.
Department of Orthopaedic
Surgery
Orthopaedic Hospital the City
of Vienna – Gersthof
Wielemansgasse 28
1180 Vienna, Austria

Zheng, G.
M.E. Mueller Institute
for Biomechanics
University of Bern
Murtenstraße 35
3010 Bern, Switzerland

Zichner, L.
Department of Orthopaedic
Surgery
Foundation Friedrichsheim
University Frankfurt/Main
Marienburgstraße 2
60528 Frankfurt/Main,
Germany

Ziring, E.
Trauma, Reconstructional and
Hand Surgery Department
Philipps University Medical
School, Marburg
Baldinger Straße
35033 Marburg, Germany

I Computer-Assisted Orthopaedic Surgery

1 Basics of Computer-Assisted Orthopadic Surgery (CAOS)

L.-P. Nolte, F. Langlotz

Introduction

When surgeons started dissection of cadavers in order to broaden their knowledge on the interior of their patients' bodies, they could better understand and treat pathologies that were invisible from the exterior. More and more complex interventions could be carried out with increasing experience, in particular after the introduction of anesthesia by Horace Wells in 1844.

To minimize the damage to the surrounding tissue that is caused by an operation, tools were soon developed to realize a preoperative planning as precisely as possible. Neurosurgery took on a leading role in this development, which is no wonder considering the sensitivity of the anatomical structures with which this discipline usually

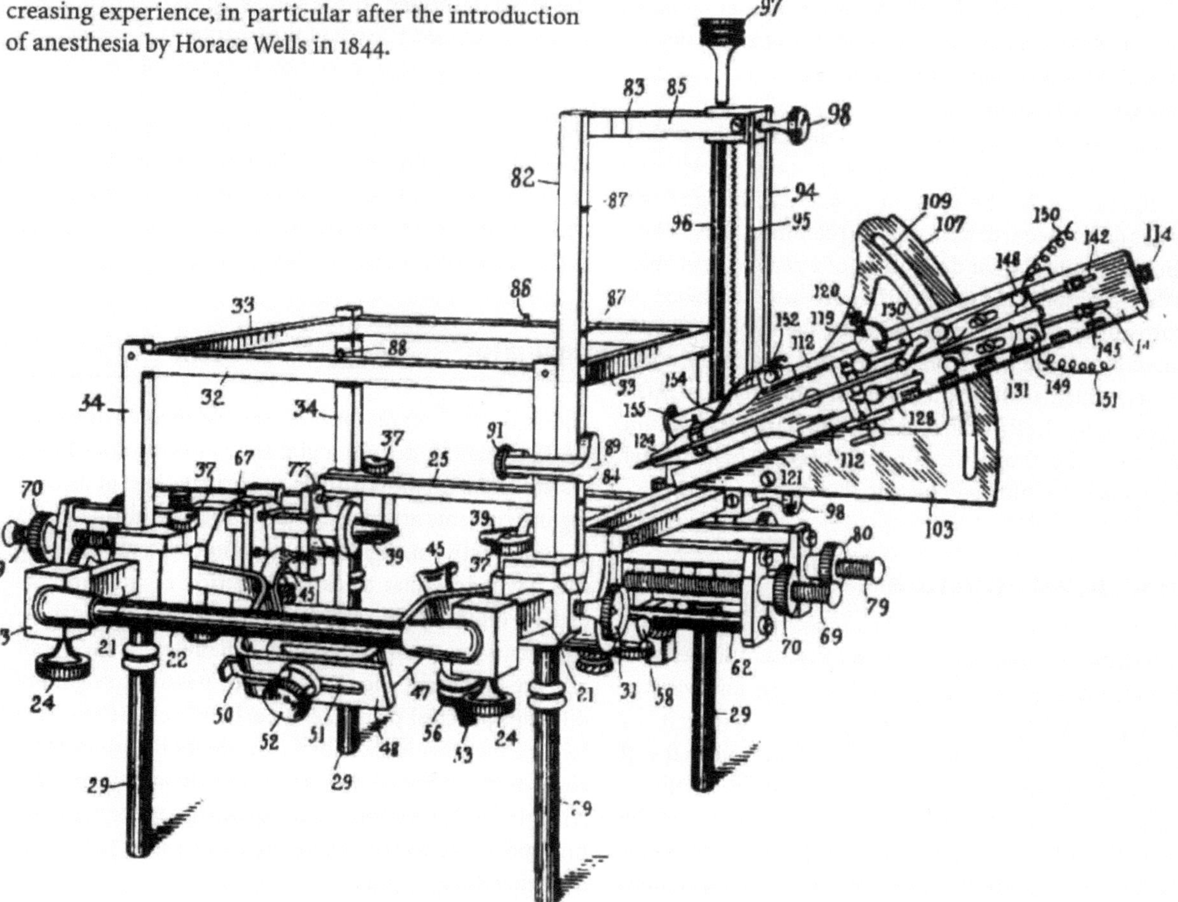

☐ **Fig. 1-1.** »Stereotactic apparatus« as presented by Clarke and Horsley in 1906

deals. Clarke and Horsley presented a »stereotactic apparatus« (Fig. 1-1) as early as the beginning of the last century. The device should allow location of a target within the brain that had previously been marked in an anatomical atlas [5]. Stereotactic frames are nowadays common instruments during neurosurgical interventions [9]. They are based on the same principles that were the foundation of Clarke and Horseley's construction. For a long time orthopaedics declined the use of comparable systems, because frame-based surgery is obviously impractical in most cases. Only in the last 10 years were devices developed that enable the orthopaedic surgeon to realize a preoperative plan accurately during an operation.

Two classes of apparatuses may be distinguished: Surgical navigation systems – precisely: surgical free-hand navigation systems – determine the spatial loca- tion of conventional instruments held in the surgeon's hand, and they provide positional feedback on a computer monitor in real-time [1, 6, 13, 16]. Such a system is a passive device that is used as an orientation aid, similar to a GPS satellite navigation system.

The second class consists of medical robots that autonomously carry out one step of an operation without any interaction by the surgeon [3, 8, 17]. Although both classes do not seem to have much in common, they in fact represent quite similar derivatives of a general principle. Both are based on concepts that are also the heart of neurosurgery's frame systems. Even the apparatus presented by Clarke and Horsley fits into this framework. Consequently, this chapter will use the term »CAOS systems« for both orthopaedic free-hand navigation systems and orthopaedic surgical robots. Their mutual conceptual structure will be elucidated.

Conceptual Structure

Each clinically used CAOS system consists of three components that are related to each other in a certain way [4]. The type of relation differs depending on whether it is a surgical robot or one of the navigation systems that will be described below. In any case, each of the three components is required to guarantee proper functioning of the entire setup. From a mathematical standpoint, the components are regarded as non-deformable rigid bodies, each of them featuring a three-dimensional coordinate system. Geometric entities such as points, angles, planes, axes, or volumes are defined with respect to these local frames of reference.

Therapeutic Object

The therapeutic object represents the target of the surgical intervention. In the domain of orthopaedic applications, the therapeutic objects are usually bony structures. However, the target may also be an implant, e.g., when a locking screw is supposed to be placed through the distal hole of an intra-medullary nail that has been implanted to stabilize a femoral fracture. In a few cases, the aforementioned rigid body principle is violated. For unstance, in traumatology the individual fragments of an unstable fracture have to be treated as separate therapeutic objects. The steps described in the following paragraphs then have to be applied to each of the fragments.

Pure soft tissue surgery, however, cannot be supported by the principles described in this chapter. Only if the tissue in question is very close to some bony structure is it a valid assumption to regard both as one rigid body. For example, nucleotomies could be supported by a CAOS system if one of the vertebrae, which are linked by the treated disk, was defined as therapeutic object.

Navigator

The navigator represents the central element in each CAOS system. It defines a global or »world« coordinate system, in which the positions and orientations of the acting instruments are given. While a robot is also referred to as an »active navigator«, navigation systems use passive navigators that track the position of instruments usually remotely. During active navigation surgical instruments are mounted onto the actuator of the robot and are guided by the machine. For passive navigation, different physical principles to achieve remote position sensing have been described [1, 2, 18], but neither ultrasonic determination [18] nor the use of magnetic trackers [1] proved to be successful techniques. The former measurement principle is very sensitive to temperature variations and therefore requires accurate calibration prior to each usage. Moreover, no commercial ultrasound-based tracking product is currently available, on which a surgical navigation system could be based. Wallny et al. used a custom-made ultrasonic tracker in their setup. Electromagnetic tracking systems use a coil to generate a magnetic field and then measure the characteristics of that field. Although this is the only technique not relying upon a direct line-of-sight between the measuring device and the object of interest, electromagnetic tracking suffers from a severe disadvantage. The field characteristics are very vulnerable to the presence of metallic and even non-metallic objects. Neither the qualitative nor the quantitative nature of this undesired influence and the resulting measurement errors can be predicted. Consequently, it is also not possible to compensate for them.

Optoelectronic tracking of surgical instruments shall be described in more detail in the following section. This technology is nowadays used within free-hand navigation systems. In order to determine the spatial position of any rigid surgical instrument, it is sufficient to acquire the exact location of at least three non-collinear points on this object. These points are created by actively infrared light emitting diodes (LEDs), or by passively infrared light reflecting spheres with a specially coated surface (see Fig. 1-2). Using light at infrared wave lengths guarantees an OR-compatible set-up. Moreover, the influence of other light sources on the measurement device is minimized. In the following, LEDs and spheres are referred to as »markers«. They are mounted onto the instruments to be tracked in sets of three, four, or even larger quantities. Camera systems that consist of two or three single CCD (charged coupled device) cameras then observe the signals coming from the markers. Using larger numbers of markers creates redundancy and allows for the determination of an instrument's position at an arbitrary spatial orientation, even when one or more markers are currently not facing the camera system. When LEDs are used, they are flashed in a fast sequence one after the other. For the cameras, only one light flash is visible at a time, and it can be assigned to one particular LED, allowing easy identification of a large number of different, simultaneously used instruments. Passive markers are illuminated by flashes of infrared light originating from a light source on the camera system. They reflect patterns of single light points. Analyzing consecutive image frames enables the system to recognize marker signals that move

synchronously and thus must represent one rigid body. In order to unambiguously distinguish several instruments within a set, different sphere arrangements are chosen for different rigid bodies. Both tracking approaches have their advantages and disadvantages. The most obvious difference is the presence of cables that almost every active marker system requires in order to control the LEDs. They demand a certain discipline and tidiness at the operating table, especially when large instrument sets are used. Passive marker systems, on the other side, contribute considerably to the per-case costs, because the spheres should be regarded as disposables. Moreover, the accuracy by which the center of reflection is determined decreases if the sphere is partly covered, e.g., by a blood splash.

Referencing

The so-called referencing is essential for navigation systems as well as robots. It allows expressing of an instrument's position relative to the therapeutic object. Referencing establishes a local frame of reference on this object and thus integrates it into the coordinate space of

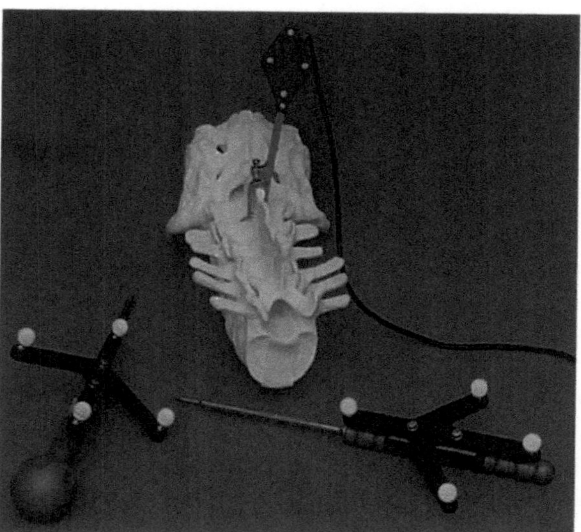

Fig. 1-2. A dynamic reference base with active markers (LEDs) is visible in the background. The two instruments in the front are equipped with passive markers. A tracking system can distinguish between both instruments, because the two sphere sets are arranged in geometrically different quadrangles

the navigator. During active navigation the therapeutic object is rigidly connected to the robot, e.g., by means of a bone clamp or with a screw attachment. Surgical navigation requires a marker shield to be clamped or screwed (◘ Fig. 1-2) onto the therapeutic object as soon as surgical exposure allows it. The attached probe is known as a »dynamic reference base« (DRB), because it makes a loose coupling rather than a statically rigid connection to the navigator. In either case, a stable link to the bone is certainly mandatory during the entire time of CAOS usage.

Virtual Object

Last but not least, the virtual object represents an image of the therapeutic object. The first navigation systems were introduced when no medical imaging modalities were available. Anatomical atlases were used instead, and surgeons accepted that deviations from such »normalized anatomies« necessarily must lead to inaccuracies.

Nowadays, a wide variety of methods are available, permitting imaging of basically every structure within the human body [12]. However, this chapter focuses only on those methods that are of importance for the application of CAOS technology in orthopaedics and traumatology. To further organize the significant number of potential virtual objects, they are categorized according to the time and method of image generation.

Preoperative Imaging

Computed tomography (CT) is definitely the most important representative of preoperative imaging for orthopaedic surgery. A CT is a three-dimensional, geometrically precise data set that is well suited for the visualization of bone, because interior structures are displayed clearly and with a high bone-soft tissue contrast. Moreover, CT scans are created digitally, so post-processing within computer-based systems is easy. Magnetic resonance imaging (MRI) is also three-dimensional and digital, and furthermore does not expose the patient to any radiation. However, MRI scans so far are not regularly used in CAOS systems. Compared to CTs, geometric inaccuracies and a rather low bone-soft tissue contrast limit their broad usage as virtual objects.

Theoretically, the use of digital X-rays or scanned conventional X-rays would be possible. However, the missing third dimension in these projection images and the difficulties related to a precise calibration of X-ray machines make computed tomography superior in most cases.

Registration for Preoperative Imaging

The so-called registration [14], also referred to as »matching«, is a procedure that closes the gap between the virtual object on one side and the navigator, instruments, and the therapeutic object on the other side. In the case of free-hand navigation, registration allows displaying on a monitor the position of an instrument measured by the navigator in relation to the therapeutic object. In active navigation systems registration enables the robot to autonomously reproduce a plan on the therapeutic object that has been defined pre-operatively in the virtual object. It would be ideal if CAOS systems could use some kind of table that provides a one-by-one relationship assigning any 3D point in one of the objects to its counterpart in the other one. Obviously, the set-up of such a table is impossible for an infinite number of points in the working volume, but it is not necessary, either, since each involved object is a rigid body. For rigid bodies, the spatial relationship between their local coordinate systems may be expressed simply by a coordinate transformation, consisting of three translational and three rotational components, as well as a scaling factor. There are two common methods to determine these parameters: paired-points and surface registration. The former approach fills in parts of the aforementioned table. Prominent points are marked preoperatively in the CT scan and intraoperatively on the patient using a space digitizer (pointer). They act as representatives allowing estimation of the unknown transformation. Anatomical landmarks or artificial markers (fiducials) are used. If a paired-points registration is based on these fiducials, several screws, spheres, or pins [15] are implanted under local anesthesia prior to the planned intervention and the preoperative CT scan. These artificial objects are easily visible on the scanned images and intraoperatively on the patient. As a consequence, carrying out an exact matching between the rigid bodies is very easy or can even be automated. Surface registration is often used to refine the transformation that had been calcula-

Intraoperative Imaging

Preoperative imaging is the method of choice for a large number of navigation systems, and it is compulsory for the usage with orthopaedic surgical robots. Nevertheless, several disadvantages exist. The acquisition of a CT requires additional financial and logistic efforts. In many cases in which navigation is supposed to be applied, no diagnostic CT scan is available or it cannot be used, because it had, for instance, been created by an external facility and is retrievable as conventional film only, rather than as digital data. For the acquisition of a CT for a navigated intervention, the patient is usually required to come to hospital earlier, again causing additional costs. Last but not least, bony topology is often altered by the operation causing a mismatch between the intraoperative situation and the preoperative image. Examples are the reduction of complicated fractures or repositioning osteotomies.

As an alternative, C-arm imaging can be applied to create virtual objects intra-operatively [10, 11]. When compared to CT as imaging means, fluoroscopy suffers from the fact that a series of projection images serves as the navigation basis rather than a three-dimensional data set. These disadvantages are – at least partly – offset by a novel C-arm device that will be presented in chapter 3 (The intraoperative usage of ultrasonic and endoscopic equipment within orthopaedic navigation systems is still in its laboratory phase, and they will not be presented here. Interested readers are referred to chapter 71).

Registration for Intraoperative Imaging

In theory the projection model of a C-arm is that of a simple pinhole camera [7]. In this analogy, the position of the X-ray source is equivalent to the aperture of the camera. In reality, however, effects such as Earth's magnetic field considerably distort the images acquired with a fluoroscope. Would these adverse effects not be accounted for, they would prohibit precise navigation within C-arm images. To correct these errors, the image intensifier unit is equipped with a plate carrying a regular pattern of metal spheres or other markers. The precise location and relationship of one marker to another is well-known and allows for the adjustment of image distortions.

If a tracking system is observing both the fluoroscope and a DRB while such intrinsically calibrated images are acquired, the coordinate transformation between virtual

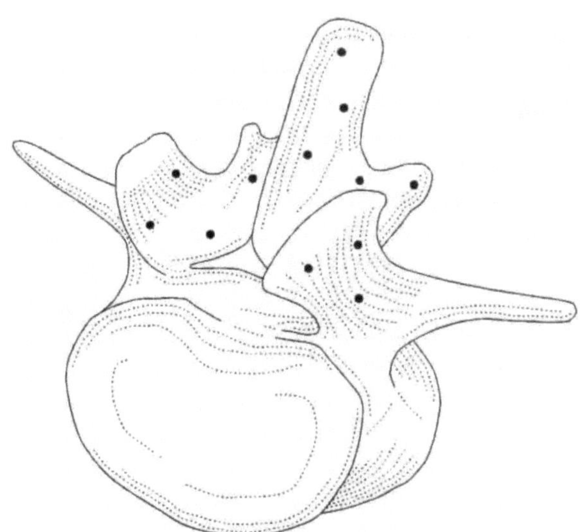

Fig. 1-3. The geometry of a vertebra can be described with sufficient accuracy using only a relatively small number of digitized points. For an acceptable surface registration result, points should be distributed widely over the intra-operatively accessible anatomy

ted by means of a preceding paired-points matching. The technique is based on the fact that a rather small number of points digitized on the accessible bone surface usually describe the surface contour very precisely (Fig. 1-3). Preoperative image processing allows for the extraction of the exact shape of the bony surface from CT data.

Verification

The registration of preoperative image data sets calculates a coordinate transformation using manually acquired data. Obviously, such data acquisition introduces measurement errors and consequently, the calculated result has to be verified. This step is mandatory for the safe intraoperative usage of a navigation system and to guarantee that the achieved accuracy is sufficient for the intended operation. Additional points on the bony anatomy are touched with the tracked pointer, and the surgeon checks whether the corresponding location in the virtual object is displayed correctly by the navigation system. Registration and verification are the most crucial steps in the application of intraoperative navigation, because here the surgeon influences or subjectively judges the operational accuracy of the system.

object and therapeutic object can be determined automatically without a manual paired-points or surface registration.

For this purpose, markers are attached to the image intensifier unit of a C-arm, allowing its spatial position to be determined during image acquisition. If the location of the X-ray source is known in addition, the aforementioned projection model can be applied to the measured instrument position, which eventually is displayed at its correct spot in the image. However, it must be noted that C-arms deform under their own weight. Consequently, the X-ray source location with respect to the measured intensifier position slightly varies from image acquisition to image acquisition. Sufficient accuracy can only be achieved if this negative effect is also considered. Two alternative solutions have been developed.

For the two-plates-method, a second marker plate is affixed in front of the image intensifier, parallel to the first one. The projection shadows of all the spheres can be detected automatically in the acquired images. They enable estimation of the unknown X-ray location by means of triangulation. In order to achieve as high an accuracy as possible, a large plate distance would be desirable. However, the second plate limits the volume of operation of the fluoroscope. Consequently, a compromise between precision and practicality has to be found.

With a one-plate-calibration, only the first described plate for image distortion correction is required intra-

operatively. During set-up of the C-arm for navigation use, the position of the X-ray source is determined once using the two-plate-method. In a subsequent calibration procedure, the tracking system measures the source's shift with respect to the intensifier location, as a function of the C's orientation. For this purpose, the X-ray source is temporarily equipped with markers, and the fluoroscope is moved through its full range of motion step by step. The acquired data are stored in a file for intra-operative usage. The advantage of this method is obvious. The pre-calibration is carried out extra-operatively. Therefore, an extremely large distance between both calibration plates may be chosen (■ Fig. 1-4) making this approach potentially more accurate.

Surgeon-Defined Anatomy

Another possibility for the intraoperative creation of virtual objects is the so-called »surgeon-defined anatomy« approach (see chapter 4). It completely abandons the use of any radiological images. Instead, after the attachment of a DRB and prior to the navigation the surgeon creates a virtual model of the situs by digitizing specific points, lines, surfaces, etc. with a navigated instrument. As an example of an alternative, the center of the hip may be defined by passively pivoting the femur through its range of motion and calculating the center of this rotation. In both cases, the system records the associated spatial data and step-by-step combines them into an abstract copy of the operation field. The resulting simplified model allows for planning and subsequent simulation of the intended surgical steps prior to execution. The technique is being used during knee ligament and total knee replacement. After recording of the anatomical situation it enables the simulation of alternative implant positions and postoperative results without resection of bone or the usage of trial implants.

Conclusion

This introduction has described various principles, concepts, and methods that the following chapters of this book will now elucidate more deeply. For a more thorough understanding of the material, readers are advised to consult the literature cited by the authors.

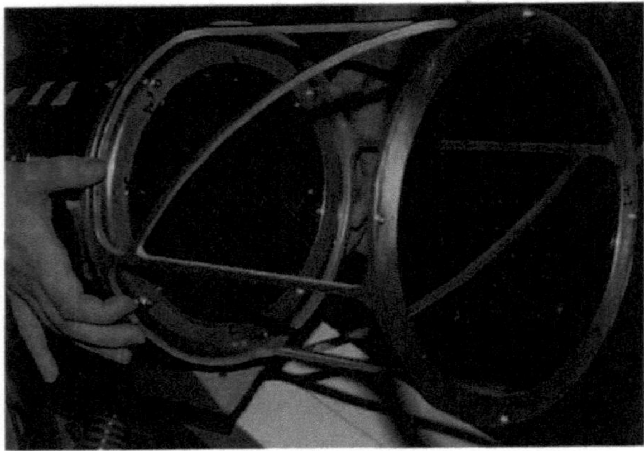

■ Fig. 1-4. This C-arm is pre-calibrated for the use within a navigation system with the help of a two-plate calibration cage. Both endplates of the cage contain metal markers that enable determination of the projection parameters of the fluoroscope for different orientations of the C. Intraoperatively, this data is used to enable navigation with only one marker plate

References

1. Amiot LP, Labelle H, DeGuise JA, Sati M, Brodeur P, Rivard CH (1995) Computer-assisted pedicle screw fixation – a feasibility study. Spine 20: 1208–1212

2. Berlemann U, Langlotz F, Langlotz U, Nolte L-P (1997) Computerassistierte Orthopädische Chirurgie (CAOS) – Von der Pedikelschraubeninsertion zu weiteren Applikationen. Orthopäde 26:463–469

3. Börner M, Bauer A, Lahmer A (1997) Computerunterstützter Robotereinsatz in der Hüftendoprothetik. Unfallchirurg 100:640–645

4. Bowersox JC, Bucholz RD, Delp SL et al. (1997) Excerpts from the Final Report for the Second International Workshop on Robotics and Computer Assisted Medical Interventions, June 23–26, 1996, Bristol, England. Comput Aided Surg 2:69–101

5. Clarke RH, Horsley V (1906) On a method of investigating the deep ganglia and tracts of the central nervous system (cerebellum). Br Med J 2:1799–1800

6. DiGioia AM, Jaramaz B, Blackwell M et al. (1998) Image guided navigation system to measure intraoperatively acetabular implant alignment. Clin Orthop 355:8–22

7. Gembran KD, Thorpe CE, Kanade T (1988) Geometric camera calibration using systems of linear equations. Proceedings of the IEEE Conference on Robotics and Automation, pp 562–567

8. Heeckt R, Rühl M, Buchhorn G et al. (1999) Computer Assisted Surgical Planning and Robotics mit dem CASPAR-System. In: Jerosch J, Nicol K, Peikenkamp K (Hrsg) Rechnergestützte Verfahren in Orthopädie und Unfallchirurgie. Steinkopff, Darmstadt, S 414–433

9. Heese O, Gliemroth J, Kehler U, Knopp U, Arnold H (1999) A new technique for attaching a stereotactic frame to the head. Minim Invasive Neurosurg 42:179–181

10. Hofstetter R, Slomczykowski M, Bourquin Y, Nolte L-P (1997) Fluoroscopy based surgical navigation: concept and clinical applications. In: Lemke HU, Vannier MW, Inamura K (eds) Computer assisted radiology and surgery. Elsevier, Amsterdam, pp 956–960

11. Joskowicz L, Milgrom C, Simkin A, Tockus L, Yaniv Z (1998) FRACAS: a system for computer-aided image-guided long bone fracture surgery. Comput Aided Surg 3:271–288

12. Langlotz F (2002) State-of-the-art in orthopaedic surgical navigation with a focus on medical image modalities. J Visual Comput Animat 13: 77–83

13. Lavallée S, Sautot P, Troccaz J, Cinquin P, Merloz P (1995) Computer-assisted spine surgery: a technique for accurate transpedicular screw fixation using CT data and a 3D optical localizer. J Image Guid Surg 1: 65–73

14. Lavallée S (1996) Registration for computer-integrated surgery: methodology, state of the art. In: Taylor RH, Lavallée S, Burdea GC, Mösges R (eds): Computer-integrated surgery. MIT Press, Cambridge, pp 77–97

15. Nogler M, Maurer H, Wimmer C, Gegenhuber C, Bach C, Krismer M (2001) Knee pain caused by a fiducial marker in the medial femoral condyle: a clinical and anatomic study of 20 cases. Acta Orthop Scand 72:477–480

16. Nolte LP, Zamorano LJ, Visarius H, Berlemann U, Langlotz F, Arm E, Schwarzenbach O (1995) Clinical evaluation of a system for precision enhancement in spine surgery. Clin Biomech 10:293–303

17. Taylor RH, Joskowicz L, Williamson B et al. (1999) Computer-integrated revision total hip replacement surgery: concept and preliminary results. Med Image Anal 3:301–319

18. Wallny T, Klose J, Steffny G, Schulze-Bertelsbeck D, Perlick L, Schumpe G (1999) Dreidimensionaler Ultraschall und intraoperative Navigation: Ein neuer Einsatz des Ultraschalltopometers bei Umstellungsosteotomie des proximalen Femurs. Ultraschall Med 20:158–160

2   CT-Based Navigation Systems

B. Jaramaz, A. M. DiGioia III

Introduction

Medical imaging modalities in diagnostic and clinical use today offer a wide range of possibilities for design and implementation of computer-assisted surgical systems. Among those modalities, computed tomography (CT) scan has a prominent role, since it provides three-dimensional images of relatively high accuracy. It is especially well suited for orthopaedics, since the bone separates from the rest of the tissue by its intensity, which makes the bone segmentation a relatively simple task.

CT scanners are large machines, typically housed in the hospital's radiology departments or at separate imaging facilities. Attempts to integrate CT scanners in the operating room, or to develop navigation systems integrated with CT scanners did not have much success so far, especially in orthopaedics. However, because bones don't change shape between the time of the scan and the time of the surgery, it was possible to design procedures in which the imaging, planning and image guided intervention could be done at different times, as three separate consecutive events. Most of the early surgical navigation procedures and all of the robotic procedures in orthopaedics have been designed this way – sometimes referred to as „canned reality" procedures.

This overview identifies the most important technical components of CT-based CAS systems, using the example of the HipNav system, developed by our team. HipNav (CASurgica, Inc.) is the surgical navigation system developed initially to address the problem of cup alignment in total hip replacement [3]. It has introduced several new concepts in the computer-assisted surgery, most notably the concept of patient-specific preoperative simulation for joint replacement procedures. Proper alignment of implant components is one of the most important factors that contribute to the joint stability; misalignment of

components reduces the safe range of motion and can lead to dislocation of the joint, or repeated impingement of components that can result in excessive wear and generation of wear debris. Especially sensitive is the alignment of the cup part, since the orientation of the cup is not restricted by the shape of the bone cavity. Currently used mechanical tools for positioning of the cup aligns the cup with respect to global body landmarks, often resulting in inadequate cup alignment. HipNav relies on the CT-scan image for planning, and both the cup and the femoral stem of the desired type and size are selected from the 3D model database and placed in the respective bones.

Image Segmentation, Preoperative Planning and Simulation

With CT technology, three-dimensional image is created by a mathematical reconstruction of the X-ray images acquired in a systematic and sequential order from a source-receiver assembly that rotates in a circular pattern. The image has characteristics of X-rays, and its relatively high accuracy and the image characteristics make it very suitable for surgical navigation, especially in orthopaedics. The bones can be easily distinguished from any other tissue, and can be easily segmented out. The bones are also the least deformable parts of the body, and therefore the most stable references for navigation, making it possible for different phases of surgical planning and execution to be performed well after the patient imaging.

Preoperative planning is typically done in three orthogonal cross-sectional views made through the CT scan. The target bone can also be visualized as three-dimensional object and rendered in the perspective view from an arbitrary viewpoint, which can be useful in some planning and navigation tasks (◨ Fig. 2-1). In order to create this kind of rendering, the organs and tissues of interest need to be segmented out from the rest of the image, and their boundaries have to be determined. Surface models are then built, which describe the surface of the bone of interest as a contiguous set of triangles fully encompassing the bone's volume.

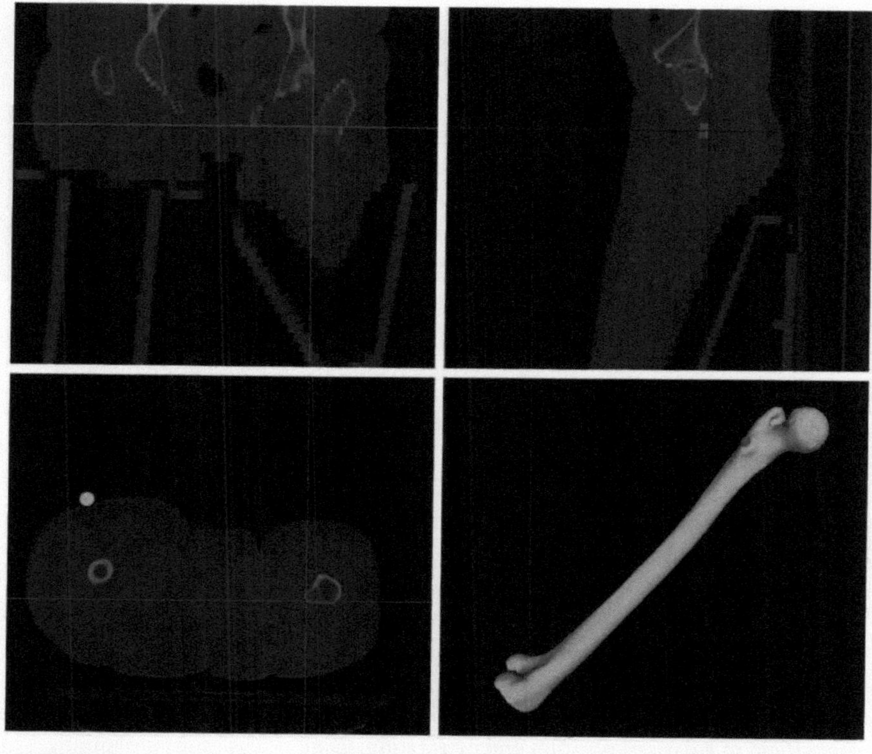

◨ **Fig. 2-1.** Cross sections through a CT scan and a surface model of the femur derived from the scan. The same point is identified with the cross hairs in the CT cross sections and with a small sphere in the surface model

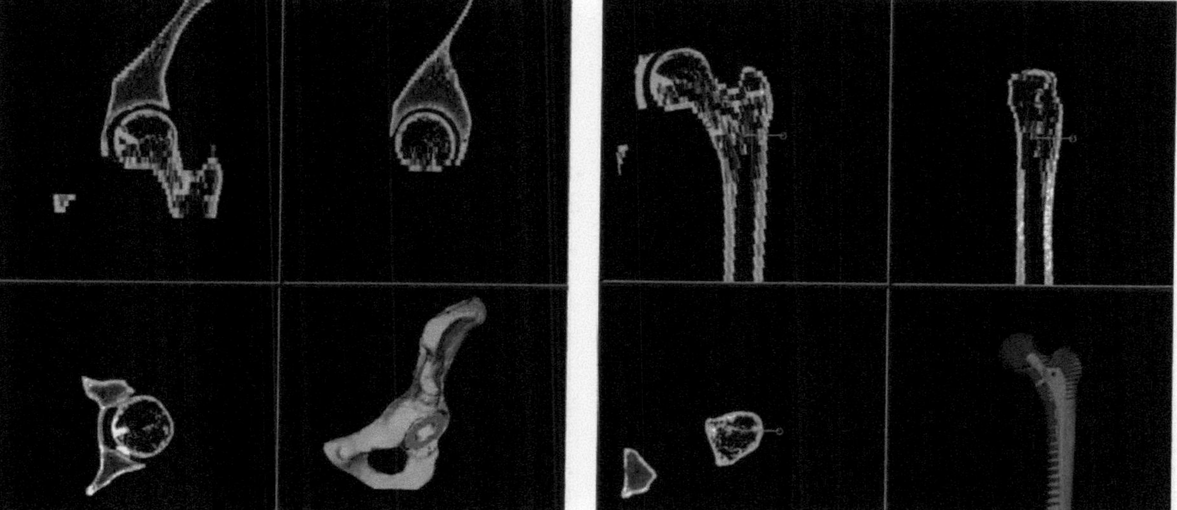

◨ **Fig. 2-2.** Surgical planning with HipNav: Planning of the cup implant; planning of the femoral implant (Copyright CASurgica, Inc.)

Early applications of image-guided surgery where the goal is to accurately and precisely reach the target and to choose the access trajectory so that the damage to the collateral tissue is minimized (such as tumor removal, fracture stabilization and biopsy tasks) are fairly simple from the planning point.

HipNav has introduced more a complex planner enhanced with a simulator, providing analytical capability that can aid the surgeon in making the critical preoperative planning decisions. As a 3D imaging modality, CT scan provides a basis for complex three-dimensional planning, which can greatly enhance the surgeon's capability to visualize the surgical task, examine the potential solution and explore the alternatives. HipNav planner incorporates a range of motion (ROM) simulator that can aid the surgeon in the optimal selection and orientation of implant components (◘ Fig. 2-2).

Planning is performed with respect to the anatomic coordinate systems derived from the anatomic landmarks. In the pelvis, the anterior pelvic plane is defined with the most anterior points – anterior iliac spines and the mid pubis symphysis point. In the femur the reference system is defined with the center of the femoral head and the plane defined by the lesser trochanter and the posterior condyles [4]. After the landmarks are automatically detected in the planner, the alignment of implant components can be uniquely defined. The surgeon selects the implant components from the database and places them in a desired position and orientation, using both cross-sectional CT views and 3D surface models. In the final stage, the virtual replacement joint is assembled and tested for the range of motion. The range of motion analysis is performed for any desired leg motion path, to test the impingement limits of that motion. Both prosthetic and bone impingement are detected. The effects of the change of any relevant parameter (orientation, size, position, pelvic flexion) on ROM and on component offset and leg length can be examined in real time, helping the surgeon in optimizing the plan (◘ Fig. 2-3). The implants then can be reoriented, or alternative components can be selected, so that the safe range of motion is maximized, and the leg length is properly planned. Once the surgical plan is developed, it becomes a blueprint for surgical intervention. Its surgical execution is typically dependent on several technical steps, in particular on tracking, registration, and navigation.

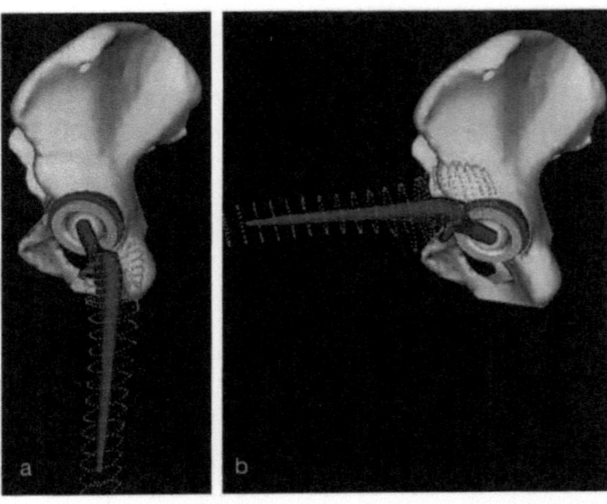

◘ **Fig. 2-3a, b.** Surgical planning with HipNav: Range of motion test: **a** neutral position, **b** internal rotation in flexion. *Red dot* indicates the impingement point (Copyright CASurgica, Inc.)

Intraoperative Steps

Tracking

The key component of surgical navigation is the ability to determine accurately and precisely at every step where the target bones and surgical tools are in space and how their position corresponds to the preoperative image that was used for planning. This is typically achieved by using tracking systems and by rigidly attaching tracking markers to bones of interest and to the surgical tools, and by tracking those markers using localizing devices (◘ Fig. 2-4).

The most commonly used tracking systems are the optical and electromagnetic ones. The optical localizers consist of two (Polaris, NDI, Ontario, Canada) or three (OptoTrak, NDI, Ontario) CCD cameras placed in the rigid enclosure that detect the position of infrared light emitting diode (LED) markers in space using triangulation. Typically four to six LEDs are placed on one target marker and lighted in sequence so that the position of each can be calculated separately. Knowing the relative position of LEDs on the marker it is possible to calculate the position of the marker in space. If these markers are then attached rigidly to another object such as medical instrument or bone, one can inherently track the position

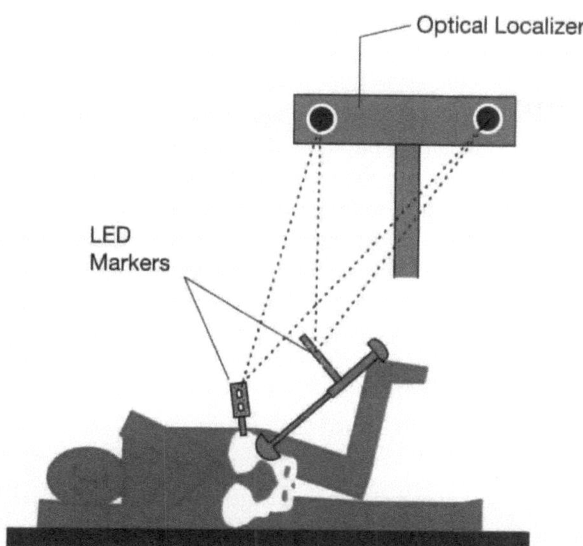

Fig. 2-4. Tracking with an optical system: Optical localizer tracks the positions of markers attached to a bone and a surgical tool

of those objects in space as well. The orientation of tools relative to the bone of interest can then be calculated and compared to the planned one. While the accuracy of optical tracking systems is currently the highest of all tracking systems, they require a line of sight to be maintained throughout the surgery, which sometimes represents a difficulty in the organization and ergonomics of the operating room. An alternative tracking modality is electromagnetic (EM) tracking. In EM tracking the emitting coil emits an electromagnetic field that induces the electricity current in the receiving coil. The position

of the receiving coil is detected by measuring the induced current and solving the EM field equation for spatial variables. This method does not require the line of sight between the localizer and its target and can therefore enable better OR ergonomics. While it approaches the accuracy of the lower-end optical trackers, it is susceptible to the presence of ferromagnetic objects and other disturbances in the EM field.

Registration

In order to implement the surgical plan, the position of the patient's bone in the operating room has to be correlated with the position of the same bode in the plan image. This involves finding the geometric transformation that would map the patient's intraoperative position to coincide with the position in the plan space. The calculation of this position is called registration. The simplest registration is the fiducial registration. It involves the insertion of fiducials (implanted physical markers) into the bone before the image (CT scan) is obtained, and keeping them inserted throughout the surgical procedure.

The markers are designed to be clearly and easily identified both in the image and during the surgery. Three such markers placed in predetermined anatomical areas are sufficient for registration. Although this type of registration is conceptually and computationally simple, it requires that additional screws are placed in bone for their attachment, typically several days before surgery, causing inconvenience and increasing the risk of in-

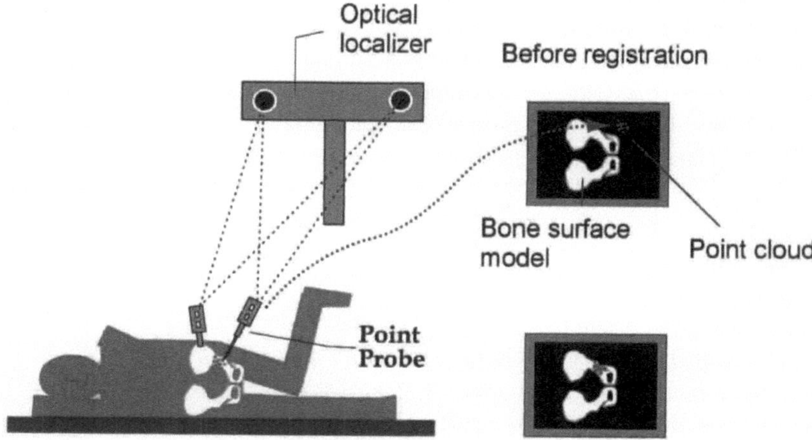

Fig. 2-5. Shape-based registration. Bone surface coordinates are measured using a point probe. The resulting point cloud is matched with the surface model

fection, and whenever possible this method is being replaced with alternative methods.

Shape based registration is one of the alternatives to fiducial registration, in which the shape of the part of the bone surface is measured intraoperatively and matched to the surface model developed from the CT scan. Intraoperative shape measurement of the bone surface can be done by a tracked pointing probe, an ultrasonic probe or a laser range scanner. If the pointing probe is used, coordinates of a discrete set of points (point cloud) on the bone surface are acquired. Registration is achieved by minimizing the distance between the perturbed point cloud and the surface model of the bone (☐ Fig. 2-5).

Ultrasound registration is based on measuring the bone surface profiles with an ultrasonic probe and is a promising alternative [1], especially for less and minimally invasive applications, where the bone surface exposure is not sufficient to acquire a widely distributed cloud of points. Some CAOS applications use intraoperative imaging for navigation, and when the tracking markers are inserted before the image is acquired, can avoid the need for the explicit registration.

Navigation

Once the tracking is established and the registration is performed, the surgeon can learn at any time what is the position of tracked surgical tools relative to the target bones, and how does it compare to the planned one. The computer interfaces enable the surgeon to then interactively reposition the tools to match the planned positions and trajectories and in effect assist them in navigating the patient's anatomy. Typical interfaces show the tools current position in the cross sections through the patient's image, or as a three-dimensional view from the chosen point of view. Simple interfaces similar to those used by airplane pilots guide the surgeon to desired tool alignment.

In HipNav surgery, one tracking marker is attached to the iliac wing of the pelvis through a small incision and the other markers are attached to the cup placement tool and the pointing probe, respectively. Shape-based registration is performed by collecting coordinates of 46 points through the incision and percutaneously at the iliac spine using the pointing probe and by matching those points to

the surface model of the pelvis. Once the registration is completed (typically 1–2 min), the pelvis can be tracked in real-time. The current orientation of the cup alignment tool is compared against the planned one and displayed as a simple cross hair interface, that allows the surgeon to interactively align the tool in accordance with the preoperatively planned alignment. ☐ Figure 2-6 shows the navigation interface for cup tool alignment in HipNav. Two circles with crosses represent the opposite ends of the tool axis. The cup guide is aligned in the preoperatively planned position when the circles' centers coincide.

Intraoperative Feedback

It is important to provide the surgeons with the feedback on their actions. In orthopaedic procedures, this providing updated images ranges from showing relative positions of tools and bones, to bone images modified for the cuts that are made. This also means that the relevant updates, such as updated range of motion or the measurements of stress in bone, can be provided. Some of this information is simply geometry updates and some require more elaborate and complex measurements.

The amount of information available to surgeons in the OR can already be overwhelming and is going to increase even more with increased sophistication and complexity of computer-assisted procedures. One of the goals of application developers is to make this information easier to comprehend. This is achieved by prioritizing and simplifying the information, by using visual means wherever possible, making it intuitive and logical and by not diverting the surgeons attention from the main task. With the increased emphasis on minimally invasive procedures, it is important to find the ways to replace direct vision with surrogates that enable confident navigation. Supplemental information can be brought into surgeon's field of view by using »hybrid reality« devices that can combine display information with the real view of the operating field. Head mounted display can provide surgeon with vital statistics, relevant patient preoperative information and images while they look at the operating field. The remaining problems with these devices are the additional weight that is carried on surgeon's head throughout the surgery and the need to focus at two different planes at the same time, which can

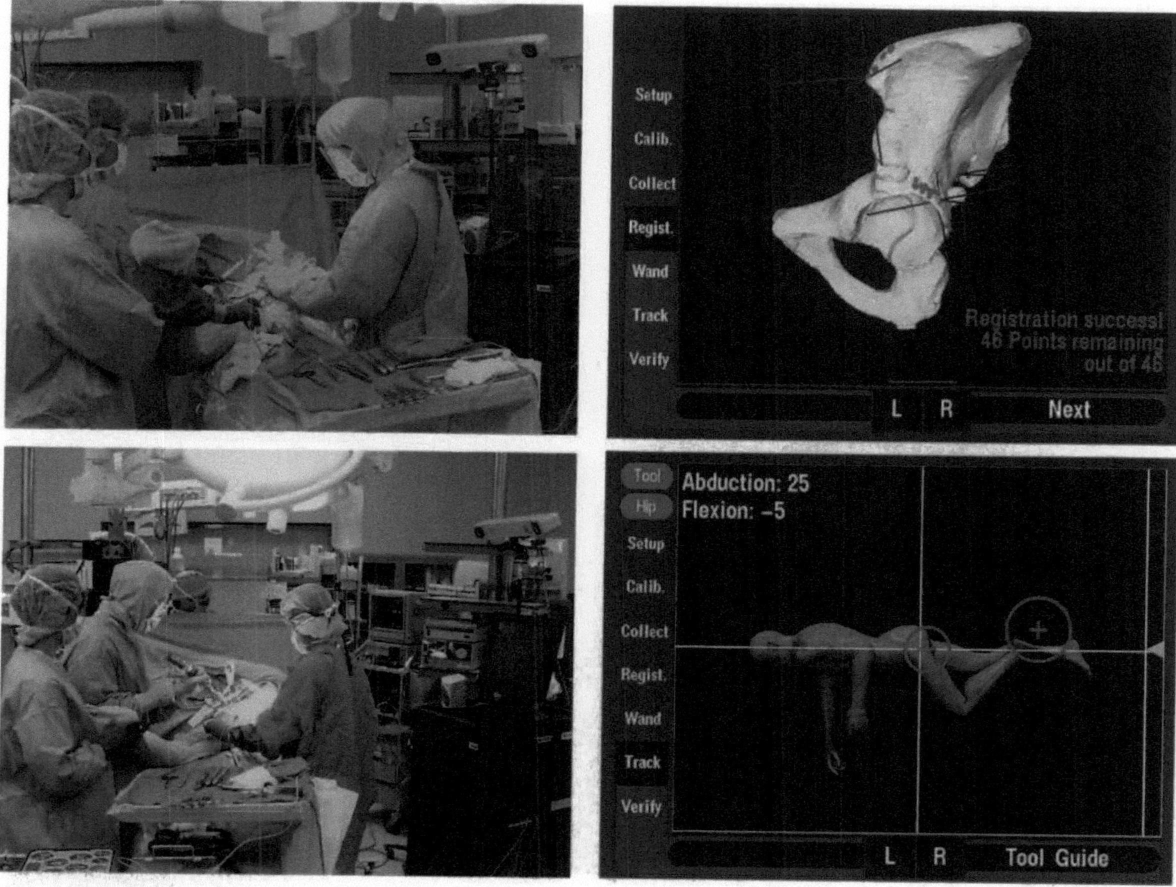

Fig. 2-6. Characteristic steps of HipNav surgery: Collection of registration points (optical localizer is in the top right), point cloud and a surface model of the pelvis after registration; the surgeon is inserting the acetabular cup implant; navigation interface during cup insertion (Copyright CASurgica, Inc.)

cause headache. Devices such as image overlay [2] can eliminate both concerns by independently supporting the display system and placing the virtual image in the same plane with the real image.

Discussion

CT-based navigation procedures can improve the ways surgery is planned and performed by increasing the accuracy and reducing the invasiveness of those procedures. They hold the promise to improve the patient outcomes and permanently change the way many surgical procedures are done today.

Because of the cost of CT scan, associated (in some cases) additional work for image segmentation and intraoperative registration, image-free (Aesculap AG, Tuttlingen, Germany) and fluoroscopic (Medivision, Oberdorf, Switzerland) procedures have been developed as alternative surgical navigation approaches. Recently, fluoroscopy has been used to create intraoperative 3D images similar to CT scans (Siremobil – Siemens Medical, Germany; FluoroCAT – VTI, Lawrence, Massachusetts, USA). This method combines the advantages of three-dimensional CT scan with the reduced cost of imaging and eliminated need for registration, since the images are acquired after the bone tracking is initiated.

However, new developments that eliminate the need of manual processing of the CT data, improvement in the imaging speed, and the overall trend in medical imaging to make CT scanners widely available and less expensive, combined with the superb performance, ability to provide the best guidance interface, amount of information and its performance in minimally invasive procedures will ensure that CT-based procedures will have a place it deserves in the CAOS family in the future.

References

1. Amin DV, Kanade T, DiGioia AM III, Jaramaz B, Nikou C, LaBarca RS (2001) Ultrasound based registration of the pelvic bone surface for surgical navigation. 1st Annual Meeting of the International Society for Computer Assisted Orthopaedic Surgery (CAOS-International), February 7–10. Davos, Switzerland

2. Blackwell M, Morgan F, DiGioia A (1998) Augmented reality and its future in orthopaedics. Clin Orthop Rel Res 345: 111–122

3. DiGioia AM III, Jaramaz B, Nikou C, LaBarca RS, Moody JE, Colgan B (2000) Surgical navigation for total hip replacement with the use of HipNav. Operative Techniques in Orthopaedics 10: 3–8

4. Nikou C, Jaramaz B, DiGioia AM III, Levison TJ (2000) Description of anatomic coordinate systems and rationale for use in an image-guided total hip replacement system. In: Delp SL, DiGioia AM, Jaramaz B (eds) Medical image computing and computer assisted intervention, MICAI 2000. Springer, Berlin Heidelberg New York Tokyo, pp 1188–1194

3 C-Arm-Based Navigation

A. Hebecker

Concepts of Image-Based Surgical Navigation

The common feature of CT- and C-arm-based surgical navigation is the coupling of the medical image and the surgical action: The surgeon sees the instrument displayed as a virtual instrument in the medical image in real time. This is achieved by using surgical instruments equipped with infrared (IR) LEDs (active markers) or with reflecting spheres (passive markers), enabling the instrument to be »seen« by a camera.

The terms **CT-** or **C-arm**-based navigation indicate the origin of the medical images and until now have been used as synonyms for navigation on **3D data records with manual registration** and on **2D projection images without manual registration**. However, in order to simplify differentiation between the concepts of image-based navigation after the introduction of the isocentric 3D C-arm SIREMOBIL Iso-C^{3D} (◼ Fig. 3-1) it is more helpful to refer only to **navigation with manual registration** as opposed to **navigation without manual registration** or **direct navigation** and then to differentiate between 2D and 3D navigation in that context (◼ Table 3-1).

These two concepts of image-based surgical navigation can be described as follows:

Navigation with Manual Registration. Navigation on 3D data records, for example on CT data recorded pre-operatively or on 3D data recorded intra-operatively by the SIREMOBIL Iso-C^{3D} C-arm. The individual steps in the workflow are as follows:

Step 1. (**Image transfer**): The medical images are loaded onto the navigation computer via a network or from portable data media.

Step 2. (**Tracking**): The surgical instruments are fitted with active or passive markers and are tracked by a camera.

Step 3. (**Referencing**): An active or passive reference marker is attached to the patient in the OR. This is to allow automatic recording of and compensation for relative movements of the patient and the camera.

Step 4. (**Registration**): Correlation between the patient and the image is established by defining certain

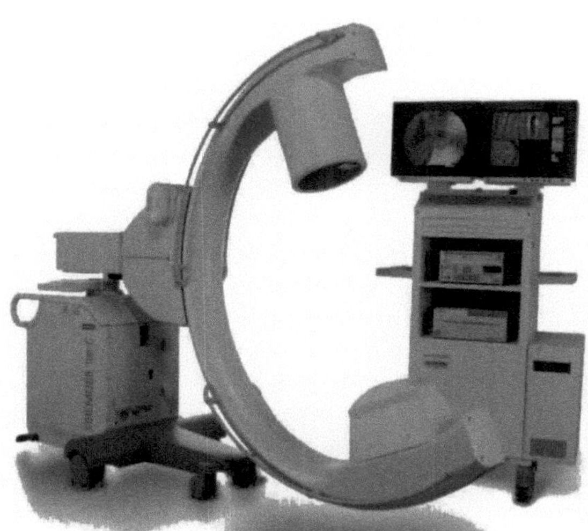

◼ **Fig. 3-1.** SIREMOBIL Iso-C^{3D}: an isocentric mobile C-arm for intra-operative two- and three-dimensional imaging

◼ **Table 3-1.** Overview of the concepts of image-based surgical navigation

	With manual registration	Without manual registration
2D navigation	—	Conventional C-arms, SIREMOBIL Iso-C^{3D}
3D navigation	CT, SIREMOBIL Iso-C^{3D}	SIREMOBIL Iso-C^{3D}

prominent points in the image and assigning them to points on the patient using a tracked device referred to as the pointer. There are two different methods: one is paired-point matching, involving a small number of correlation points, and the other is surface matching, which is more exact and involves a greater number of points. In paired-point matching the correlation points on the patient can either be unique anatomical points or markers applied either preoperatively or intra-operatively, known as fiducial markers. The registration procedure is simplified by using 3D/2D matching, which involves registration of a 3D data record with the help of two 2D C-arm X-ray images taken intra-operatively and enables the surgical intervention to be carried out as a minimally invasive procedure in spite of registration.

Step 5. (**Navigation**): The surgical instrument is displayed as a virtual instrument (as an animated object) in the medical images in real time.

Navigation Without Manual Registration. Navigation on one or more C-arm 2D projection images recorded intra-operatively or on 3D data from the SIREMOBIL Iso-C^{3D} C-arm recorded intra-operatively. This simplifies the workflow compared to navigation with manual registration, and the surgical intervention can be carried out as a minimally invasive procedure:

Step 1. (**Tracking**): The surgical instruments are fitted with active or passive markers and are tracked by a camera.

Step 2. (**Referencing**): A reference marker is attached to the patient in the OR. This is to allow automatic recording of and compensation for relative movements of the patient and the camera.

Step 3. (**Image acquisition and transfer**): Images are taken using the C-arm and loaded into the navigation computer. For this purpose the C-arm is equipped with active or passive markers and is tracked by the camera during image acquisition. This means that there is no need for manual registration.

Step 4. (**Navigation**): The surgical instrument is displayed as a virtual instrument (as an animated object) in the medical images in real time.

Direct Navigation in Two-Dimensional Projection Images

A common feature of both techniques of direct navigation, i.e. 2D and 3D navigation, is that the navigation system's camera tracks not only the surgical instrument but also the C-arm representing the imaging system.

In direct 2D-navigation a device with several functions is attached to the image intensifier of the C-arm (◻ Fig. 3-2):

1. Making the C-arm visible to the navigation system: The attachment is fitted with either active or passive markers. This enables the navigation system's camera to detect the position of the C-arm from which an X-ray image is being taken. Through the use of calibration, the location and the relative position of the projection image are therefore known.

2. Compensating for image distortion in the image intensifier: The earth's magnetic field causes images to be distorted in 2D projections. The magnitude of these distortions is determined using a ball plate in front of the input window of the image intensifier. Compensation is performed by software.

3. Online or offline calibration of the C-arm: Calibration is necessary because the C-arm is subject to mechanical twisting in different ways depending on its position. This intrinsic movement of the C-arm is measured either during image acquisition (online calibration) or once only during installation of the navigation system on the C-arm (offline calibration) and is taken

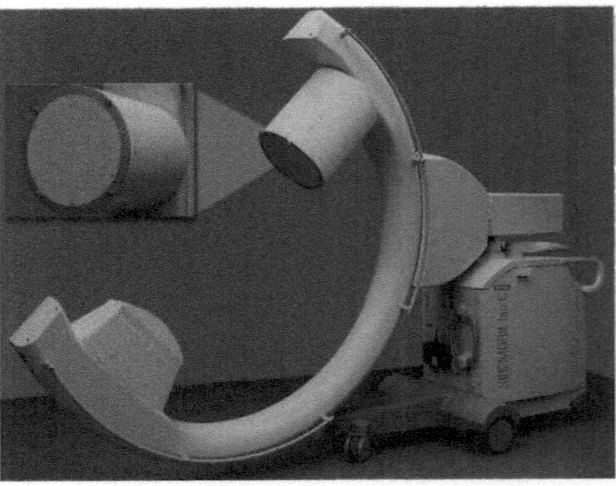

◻ **Fig. 3-2.** C-arm with navigation attachment for direct 2D navigation

into account in the software. The advantage of offline calibration is that the distance between the patient and the image intensifier is not reduced in practice. However, offline calibration during installation of the system involves more time and effort than online calibration.

Direct 2D navigation can be carried out with both isocentric and non-isocentric C-arms.

Direct Navigation in Three-Dimensional Image Data

Direct 3D navigation is based on intra-operative 3D imaging with an isocentric C-arm and on automatic recording of the correlation between the region of interest (ROI) in the patient and the corresponding 3D data record by the navigation system.

3D Imaging with an Isocentric Mobile C-Arm

SIREMOBIL Iso-C^{3D} makes 3D imaging possible as a result of its isocentric design and 190° orbital motion in

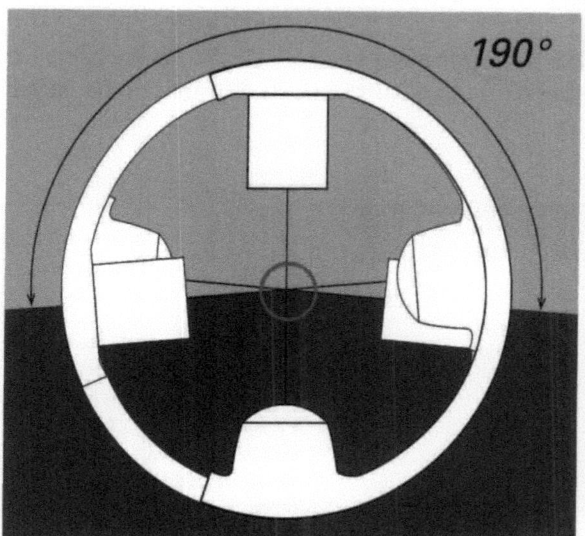

■ **Fig. 3-3.** The isocentric mobile C-arm SIREMOBIL Iso-C^{3D} is automatically rotated through 190° for intraoperative 3D image acquisition. The central beam always remains in the isocenter of the C-arm during the orbital movement

combination with its hidden cable routing. In contrast with non-isocentric C-arms, the central beam is always located in the center of rotation of the C-arm, irrespective of the orbital angle (■ Fig. 3-3). This means that the ROI always remains in the same position, regardless of the

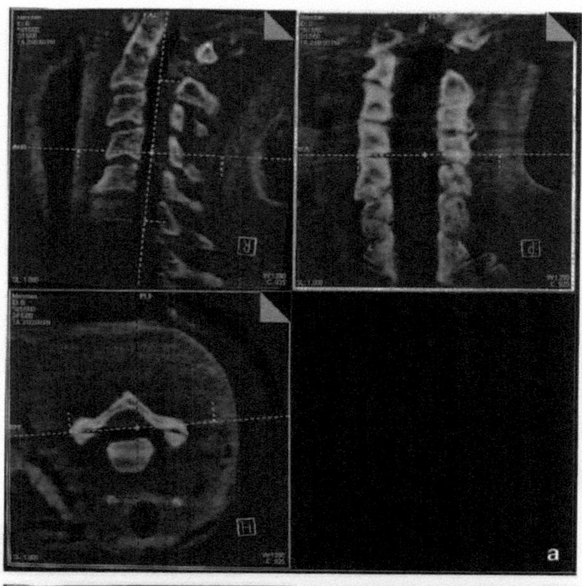

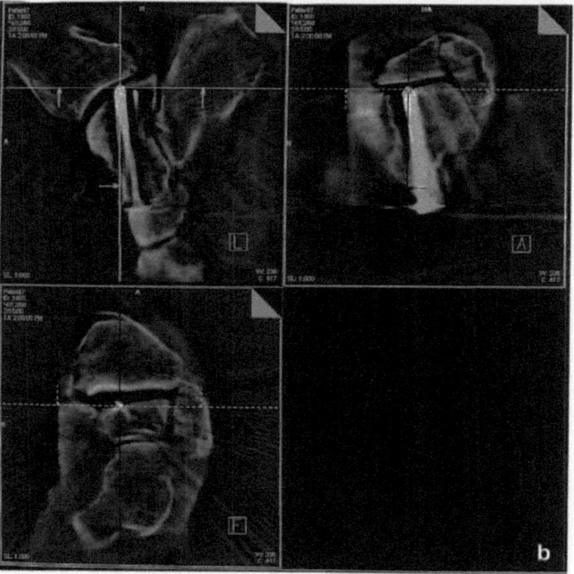

■ **Fig. 3-4a,b.** Example of the presentation of results from SIREMOBIL Iso-C^{3D}. **a** Cervical spine in three MPR scan planes. **b** Simulated screw osteosynthesis of the talus with no fracture. Representation of the incorrectly positioned screw tip in the joint cavity in three standard MPR planes

current projection angle, allowing a volume of data to be generated around the isocenter.

During 3D operation the orbital movement of the C-arm is motor-controlled. As a result, a defined number of fluoroscopic images can be acquired at fixed angular intervals during a continuous automated orbital rotation through 190°. Simultaneously, an isotropic 3D data cube with an edge length of approximately 12 cm, shown in high resolution in the submillimeter range, is calculated in the isocenter. As soon as the rotation is completed, this can be used to produce any required multiplanar reconstructions (MPR) in real time (◘ Fig. 3-4). The system is operated either directly at the operating table using a special mouse or at the monitor trolley.

The field of application for SIREMOBIL Iso-C^{3D} has so far been limited to high-contrast objects such as bones and joints because of the lack of soft tissue differentiation, as with CT.

Automatic Registration

During installation of the navigation system, the correlation between the 3D reconstruction volume and a special reference point on the C-arm is determined in an offline calibration procedure. The reference point can be located by the navigation system's camera because there is a fixed correlation between this point and the active or passive markers on a marker ring attached to the C-arm.

During the surgical procedure the navigation system's camera detects the position of the reference point with the aid of the marker ring. Because of the measurements taken during offline calibration, the navigation system's computer immediately knows the position and orientation of the 3D data record in the OR. The position of the surgical instrument – which is also tracked by the camera – can therefore be displayed automatically as a virtual object in the 3D image without manual registration (◘ Fig. 3-5).

The solution for automatic registration described here follows the approach of an open interface, which means that fundamentally it can be implemented by all manufacturers of navigation systems. Under simulated clinical conditions, i.e. if movements of the C-arm and the camera system are allowed, an overall accuracy of under 2 mm is achieved for the surgical intervention [13]. It must be pointed out, though, that the widely used but less accurate Polaris camera manufactured by Northern Digital was used for these measurements. If the more accurate Optotrak camera from the same manufacturer is used instead of the Polaris, it can be assumed that the accuracy of the system as a whole consisting of C-arm and navigation system will be higher.

Advantages of Direct Navigation

The great advantage of direct 2D and 3D navigation is that the surgical instrument is displayed in the image

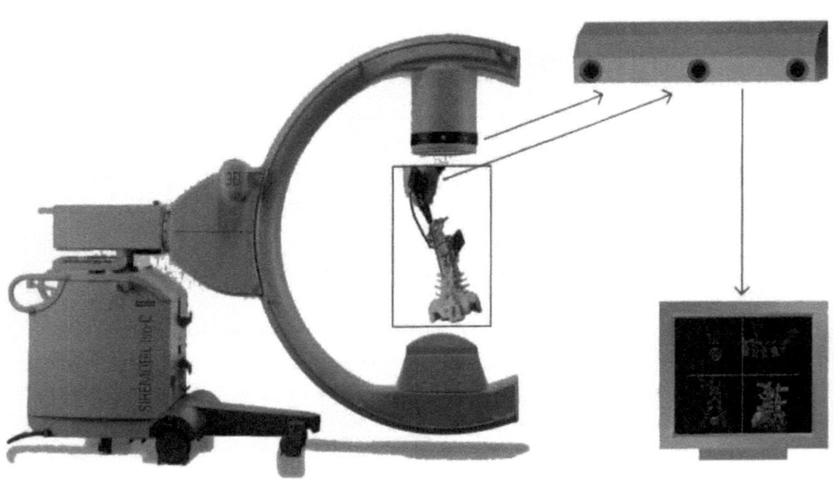

◘ **Fig. 3-5.** Schematic diagram of direct 3D navigation with SIREMO-BIL Iso-C^{3D}: The C-arm is fitted with a marker ring. The positions of the surgical instruments and of the C-arm are detected by the navigation system's camera. In the navigation computer the instrument is displayed in the 3 MPR scan planes and the SSD (surface shaded display) surface imaging of the object immediately after 3D image acquisition immediately, i.e. without the time-consuming manual registration procedure. The underlying principle can be expressed as »shoot and navigate«. It is impossible for errors to occur as a result of potentially incorrect manual registration. In addition, the large surgical incisions necessary for manual registration are avoided, which means that direct navigation supports minimally invasive surgery to a considerable extent.

As image-based direct navigation is always performed using the C-arm, the X-ray images can repeatedly be produced intra-operatively, in other words, at the same time as the surgical intervention with the patient in the final OR position.

For the sake of completeness it is worth mentioning some other advantages of navigation based on the use of the C-arm in the OR:

- Increased accuracy of the surgical intervention. 2D navigation achieves this by displaying the surgical instruments in several projection images at the same time (for example a.-p. and lateral), while 3D navigation does so by providing up-to-date 3D information during the operation without the registration errors that might otherwise occur. Any required sectional image can be freely selected from within the 3D data record for the purposes of navigation. In addition it is possible to display other views, such as axial images along the spine which cannot be generated using projection techniques.
- Removal of the C-arm after image acquisition. This allows better use of the available space and reduces the risk of the spread of infection during the surgical procedure.
- Continuous display of the surgical instrument in the stored image. Additional X-ray radiation from the C-arm can therefore be avoided.

Indications for Direct Navigation

The indications for which this navigation technique is predestined arise from its advantages. In general, direct navigation is always helpful in the positioning of guide wires, screws and implants accurately and quickly in a minimally invasive intervention. This is achieved by displaying images in different projections simultaneously (e.g. a.-p. and lateral) and also by generating 3D images

during the surgical procedure. It is also possible, however, to distinguish between typical indications for direct 2D navigation on the one hand and 3D navigation on the other, although the distinction proposed below will doubtlessly not apply in all cases. It follows the principle of always choosing the easiest way to acquire the required information. 2D navigation will always be sufficient in cases where only a small number of projections is needed to achieve spatial correlation.

Typical indications for direct 2D navigation:
- long bones: Insertion of intra-medullary nails including distal locking [15, 16],
- corrective osteotomy of long bones,
- hip endoprosthetics, especially acetabulum and shaft navigation,
- insertion of screws in the femoral neck [2].

Typical indications for direct 3D navigation:
- fractures which include the joint region: upper and lower limbs (elbow, distal radius, scaphoid bone, knee, distal tibia, calcaneus, talus, etc.) and acetabulum,
- spine: positioning of pedicle screws in the lumbar and thoracic spine, cervical spine fixation, e.g. from C_1 to C_2 [1, 9],
- pelvis: fractures, insertion of screws in the iliosacral region, osteotomies.

The use of navigation systems based on preoperatively produced CT data records has already resulted in a considerable reduction in the number of positioning errors occurring when inserting pedicle screws to stabilize fractures of the spine [11]. However, situations can arise where the position of the bones relative to each other during the surgical intervention is no longer the same as the position shown in the preoperative CT, for example as a result of repositioning of the patient on the operating table or because of the surgical procedure [6, 8]. Another important factor causing irregularities is the manual registration procedure. These problems can be avoided by using direct 2D navigation [12], albeit at the cost of a lack of 3D information. Only direct 3D navigation promises to become the real solution to these problems.

All navigation systems on the market today are confronted by an additional problem: In spinal surgery as well as in the reconstruction of joint fractures these systems do not allow for an accurate intra-operative assessment of the result of repositioning because the number and the types of the navigated bone fragments are presently limited to a few large fragments and because no intra-operative updating of the image data record is available. Especially when checking the position of dislocated fragments and of implants (for example bone plates and screws for osteosynthesis) and also during reconstruction of joint surfaces, simply using SIREMOBIL Iso-C^{3D} for intra-operative 3D imaging alone without navigation provides a considerable information gain and consequently results in higher quality and greater safety in the OR [4, 5, 10, 14]. One crucial factor for the OR workflow is the possibility of using SIREMOBIL Iso-C^{3D} both in conventional 2D mode and in 3D mode without reducing access to the patient, which would require additional logistical efforts. When performing a repositioning of bone fragments of this nature without navigation, the workflow can be outlined as follows [3]:

1. 2D mode: repositioning of bone fragments and preliminary fixation with Kirschner's wire,
2. 3D mode (»preliminary scan«): checking of position in the 3D reconstruction,
3. 2D mode: definitive osteosynthesis,
4. 3D mode (»definitive scan«): final 3D reconstruction. This avoids the need for a postoperative CT and avoids a follow-up operation in the event of fragments or implants being incorrectly positioned.

The use of intra-operative direct 3D navigation enables navigation to be carried out in a current 3D data record, for example in order to proceed with the osteosynthesis procedure after repositioning of the bone fragments is completed. It is feasible that the use of image segmentation will in future make it possible to apply 3D navigation to the repositioning of bone fragments as well.

Conclusion and Outlook

The use of direct 3D navigation with SIREMOBIL Iso-C^{3D} allows surgeons to move a vital step closer to their real aim, which is to perform minimally invasive interventions accurately and speedily with online visualization of their instruments in constantly updated 3D data volumes of the patient.

In contrast with CT-based navigation – which relies on 3D records obtained preoperatively, in other words »old« records – SIREMOBIL Iso-C^{3D} enables the 3D data record to be updated repeatedly during the operation, without manual registration and hence with the minimum of invasive intervention. While it is true that CT and MRI units have recently found their way into operating theaters, with the result that updated intra-operative images are also available for navigation from these devices, the effort and expenditure is much higher.

Until now, working without manual registration has only been possible when using C-arm-based 2D navigation on projection images – with the associated effect that the images have a relatively low information content.

In future the use of image fusion during the surgical intervention will lead to new application opportunities. New technologies, such as the use of flat-panel detectors, may widen the scope of use of mobile C-arms, especially with respect to the differentiation of soft tissue which will then be possible. A virtual intraoperative »view inside the bones and joints« [7] is finally entering the realm of the feasible.

References

1. Arand M, Hartwig E, Hebold D, Kinzl L, Gebhard F (2001) Präzisionsanalyse navigationsgestützt implantierter thorakaler und lumbaler Pedikelschrauben. Unfallchirurg 104: 1076–1081
2. Arand M, Schempf M, Kinzl L, Fleiter T, Pless D, Gebhard F (2001) Präzision standardisierter Iso-C-Arm-basierter navigierter Bohrungen am proximalen Femur. Unfallchirurg 104: 1150–1156
3. Euler E, Heining S, Fischer T, Pfeiffer KJ, Mutschler W (2002) Initial clinical experiences with the SIREMOBIL Iso-C3D. electromedica 70: 64–67
4. Euler E, Wirth S, Pfeifer KJ, Mutschler W, Hebecker A (2000) 3D-imaging with an isocentric mobile C-arm. electromedica 68: 122–126
5. Euler E, Wirth S, Linsenmaier U, Mutschler W, Pfeifer KJ, Hebecker A (2001) Vergleichende Untersuchung zur Qualität C-Bogen-basierter 3D-Bildgebung am Talus. Unfallchirurg 104: 839–846
6. Gebhard F, Kinzl L, Arand M (2000) Grenzen der CT-basierten Computernavigation in der Wirbelsäulenchirurgie. Unfallchirurg 103: 696–701
7. Gebhard F, Arand M, Fleiter T et al. (2001) Computer assistierte Chirurgie, Entwicklung und Perspektiven 2001. Orthopäde 30: 666–671
8. Grützner PA, Vock B, Köhler T, Wentzensen A (2002) Rechnergestütztes Arbeiten an der Wirbelsäule. OP Journal 17: 185–190
9. Kandziora F, Stöckle U, König B, Khodadadyan-Klostermann C, Mittlmeier Th, Haas NP (2001) C-Bogen-Navigation zur transoralen atlantoaxialen Schraubenplatzierung. Chirurg 72: 593–599
10. Kotsianos D, Rock C, Euler E et al. (2001) 3D-Bildgebung an einem mobilen chirurgischen Bildverstärker (Iso-C-3D): Erste Bildbeispiele zur

Frakturdiagnostik an peripheren Gelenken im Vergleich mit Spiral-CT und konventioneller Radiologie. Unfallchirurg 104: 834–838

11. Laine T, Lund T, Ylikoski M, Lohikoski J, Schlenzka D (2000) Accuracy of pedicle screw insertion with and without computer assistance: A randomised controlled clinical study in 100 consecutive patients. Eur Spine J 9: 235–240

12. Nolte LP, Slomczykowski MA, Berlemann U et al. (2000) A new approach to computer-aided spine surgery: fluoroscopy-based surgical navigation. EuroSpine J 9: 78–88

13. Ritter D, Mitschke M, Graumann R (2002) Markerless navigation with the intraoperative imaging modality SIREMOBIL Iso-C3D. electromedica 70: 47–52

14. Rock C, Linsenmaier U, Brandl R et al. (2001) Vorstellung eines neuen mobilen C-Bogen-/CT-Kombinationsgerätes (Iso-C-3D): Erste Ergebnisse der 3D-Schnittbildgebung. Unfallchirurg 104: 827–833

15. Suhm N (2001) Intraoperative accuracy evaluation of virtual fluoroscopy – a method for application in computer-assisted distal locking. Comp Aid Surg 6: 221–224

16. Suhm N, Jacob AL, Nolte LP, Regazzoni P, Messmer P (2000) Surgical navigation based on fluoroscopy – clinical application for computer-assisted distal locking of intramedullary implants. Comp Aid Surg 5: 391–400

4 CT-Free-Based Navigation Systems

S. D. Stulberg

Introduction

The success of total knee replacement surgery depends on several factors, including proper patient selection, appropriate implant design, correct surgical technique, and effective peri-operative care. The outcome of total knee replacement surgery is particularly sensitive to variations in surgical technique [1, 2, 8, 12, 13, 16–19, 35, 43, 45]. Incorrect positioning or orientation of implants and improper alignment of the limb can lead to accelerated implant wear and loosening and suboptimal functional performance. A number of studies have suggested that alignment errors of greater than three degrees are associated with more rapid failure and less satisfactory functional results of total knee arthroplasties [2, 3, 8, 9, 11, 14, 20, 24, 27, 30, 31, 36–38, 44, 46].

Mechanical alignment guides have improved the accuracy with which implants can be inserted. Although mechanical alignment systems are continually being refined, errors in implant and limb alignment continue to occur. It has been estimated that errors in tibial and femoral alignment of more than three degrees occur in at least ten percent of total knee arthroplasties, even when performed by experienced surgeons using mechanical alignment systems of modern design. Computer-based alignment systems have been developed to address the limitations inherent in mechanical total knee instrumentation [4–7, 10, 15, 22, 23, 25, 26, 32–34, 39–42]. Three types of computer-based TKA systems are currently in various stages of development:

- image-free navigation systems (also referred to as intra-operative models);
- image-based navigation systems; and
- robotic systems.

Image-free navigation systems utilize information that is acquired in the operating room, during the performance of the total knee replacement. An image-free navigation technique is described in this chapter. The technique that is described:

1. Uses commonly available, relatively inexpensive computer equipment (e.g. desk-top computer, low-end optical localizer)
2. Is currently available for clinical use.
3. Has available preliminary multi-center clinical results comparing the use of the system with mechanical devices [21, 28, 29, 32, 33, 40].

The goal of the image-free computer-assisted system is to increase the accuracy and reproducibility with which the objectives of a mechanical alignment system are achieved.

After describing the computer-assisted TKA surgical techniques, I will review the preliminary results that have been obtained with this approach. I will also compare these results with those obtained using conventional mechanical systems.

Surgical Technique

Preoperative Planning

Mechanical instrumentation differs significantly from computer-assisted TKA instrumentation in the role that preoperative planning plays in the performance of the procedure. Mechanical instrumentation systems that utilize intra-medullary femoral alignment guides require that the surgeon determines the desired anatomic alignment (femoral-tibial angle) on a full-length (including hip, knee and ankle joint) standing anterior-posterior (AP) radiograph. Some surgeons may also wish to determine the desired posterior slope of the tibial cut by using a lateral radiograph. In addition, many surgeons find it helpful to estimate the desired size of the femoral and tibial implants by holding scaled templates of these implants against AP and lateral radiographs of the knee joint.

The image-free navigation technique eliminates the need for these preoperative planning steps. The image-free technique locates the centers of the hip, knee and ankle joint during the surgical procedure. The pre-surgical medial-lateral and flexion-extension deformities are calculated from this information. Mechanical systems use the information obtained during preoperative templating to determine the appropriate setting on the fe-moral intra-medullary alignment guide (anatomic axis) that will correct the preoperative medial-lateral de-formity to a mechanical axis of zero. The image-free navigation system uses the information obtained during intra-operative registration to align the cutting blocks to correct the preoperative medial-lateral and anterior-posterior deformities to mechanical axes of zero. In ad-dition, the image-free navigation system allows the surgeon to determine intra-operatively the desired posterior slope of the tibia and correct sizes of the femoral and tibial implants. Image-free navigation systems eliminate the need to acquire this information preoperatively.

Patient Positioning and Surgical Exposure

Mechanical alignment and computer-assisted surgical techniques use similar approaches for patient positioning and surgical exposure. Leg holders and pneumatic tourni-quets, routinely used with mechanical instrumentation, can also be used for the computer-assisted technique.

No alterations in the surgical incision usually used for TKA surgery need to be made for the computer-as-sisted technique. Although this procedure will require the placement of screws to hold diode containing rigid bodies in the proximal tibia and distal femur, the sites for these screws can be reached through a conventional incision and exposure.

I prefer a straight midline skin incision and a medial para-patellar exposure of the knee. This exposure extends distally along the medial-most edge of the quadriceps tendon and patella to a point just medial and distal to the patellar tendon insertion on the tibial tubercle. The super-ficial and deep medial collateral ligament are elevated around the anterior medial half of the tibia. The ligamen-tum mucosum, infra-patellar fat pad, and anterior lateral capsule are elevated from the anterior-lateral surface of the tibia. The patellar is everted laterally, and the knee is placed in 90° of flexion. The anterior cruciate ligament is resected, the osteophytes are removed, and the fat pad trimmed to allow adequate exposure of the tibia.

Locating the Centers of the Hip, Knee and Ankle Joint

The initial step in the performance of a TKA using ima-ge-free navigation is the determination of the centers of the hip, knee and ankle joints. Equipment unique to com-puter-assisted surgery must be used to determine these joint centers. This equipment is also used to guide the po-sitioning of the cutting blocks during the performance of the TKA (❏ Fig. 4-1).

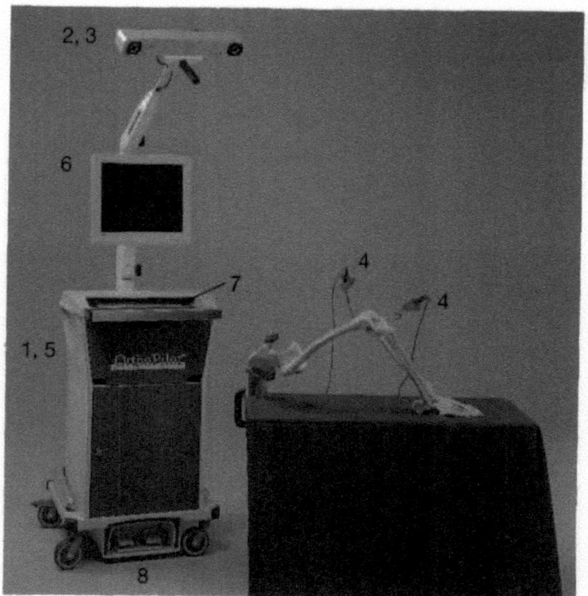

❏ **Fig. 4-1.** The image-free navigation system components: *1* Instrument stand with isolation transformer, *2–3* camera system and control unit, *4* infrared transmitters (rigid bodies), *5* workstation, *6* computer monitor, *7* keyboard and mouse, *8* foot control

The equipment includes:

- an optical localizer;
- rigid bodies containing diodes;
- 3.5-mm stainless steel bicortical screws specifically designed to hold one of the rigid bodies on the bone;
- a metal plate to hold a rigid body to the foot; and
- a computer, a monitor, and a foot control.

The localizer consists of cameras that detect the infrared radiation emitted by the diodes contained in the rigid bodies (see Fig. 4-3). The rigid bodies are securely affixed to the bones by using bicortical screws so that they do not move relative to the bones when the leg is flexed, extended, and rotated. The localizer is connected to the computer and the monitor. The position of the leg and bones can be seen on the computer screen when the surgeon activates the foot control. The optical localizer is positioned at the level of the knee joint on the side opposite to the extremity on which the TKA is to be performed.

The screws that hold the rigid bodies are inserted at the beginning of the surgical procedure. Femoral and tibial screws are placed immediately after making the skin incision and exposing the knee joint. The femoral screw is inserted into the medial cortex approximately four inches proximal to the knee joint. The tibial screw is inserted into the anterior-medial cortex approximately 8 cm below the tibial plateau (☐ Fig. 4-2). The heads of these screws have been specially designed to hold the rigid bodies.

The center of the femoral head is determined first using a kinematic registration technique. This requires that the femur be flexed, extended, abducted, adducted, and rotated. This movement generates a cloud of points on a sphere. The center of the sphere (i.e. the femoral head) that created this array of points can then be computed. The technique used to move the femur is important for accurately determining the center of the femoral head. Excessive hip motion will cause the pelvis to move. Inadequate motion will not generate adequate information to allow a calculation of the femoral head center. Therefore, visual cues are displayed upon the computer screen to guide the surgeon during the acquisition of the information (☐ Figs. 4-3 to 4-5). Once the registration

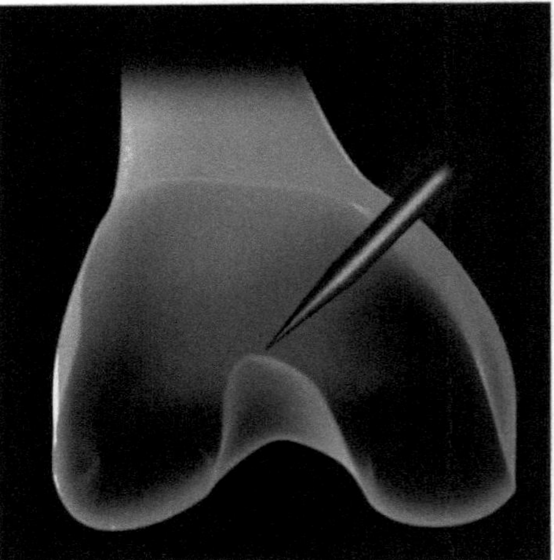

☐ **Fig. 4-3.** The anatomic center of the knee is palpated to determine the optimal motion for registering the center of the femoral head

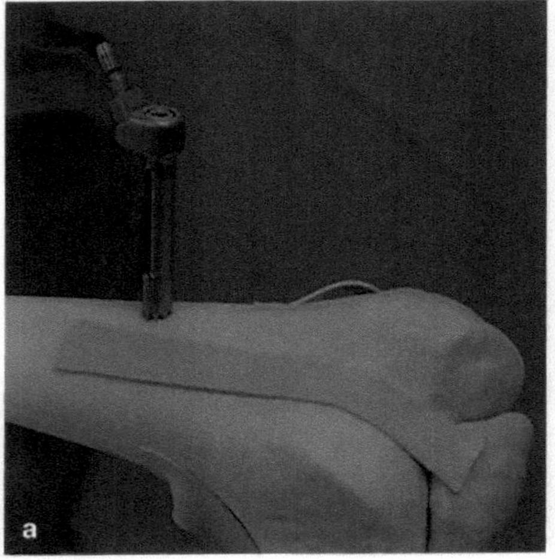

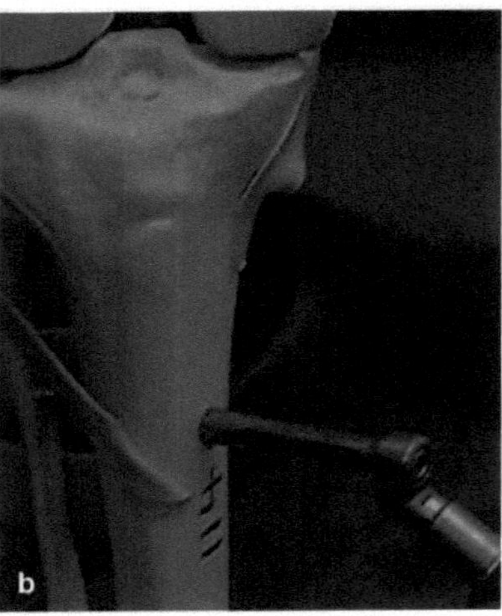

☐ **Fig. 4-2a, b.** Placement of screws and attachment of transmitters. 4.5 mm cortical screws are placed in the distal femur and proximal tibia with adapters that allow the infrared transmitters to be attached. The screws must be positioned so that the transmitters are visible to the camera. The screws must also be rigidly fixed to the bones so that they do not move during surgery

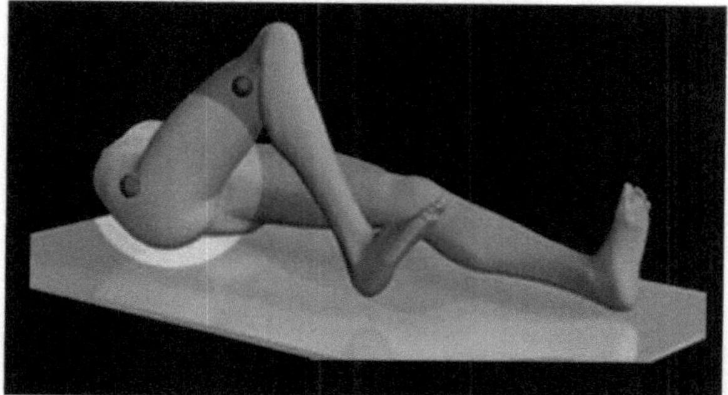

Fig. 4-4. Positioning the limb to determine the kinematic center of the femoral head. This screen shows the surgeon how to position the leg and confirms that the transmitter on the femur is visible to the camera

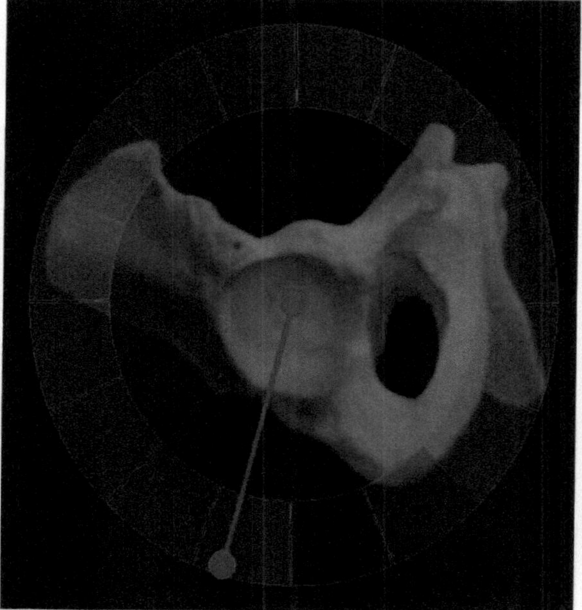

Fig. 4-5. Registering the center of the femoral head: The point on the screen guides the movement of the leg and assures that registration of the center of the femoral head is accurate.

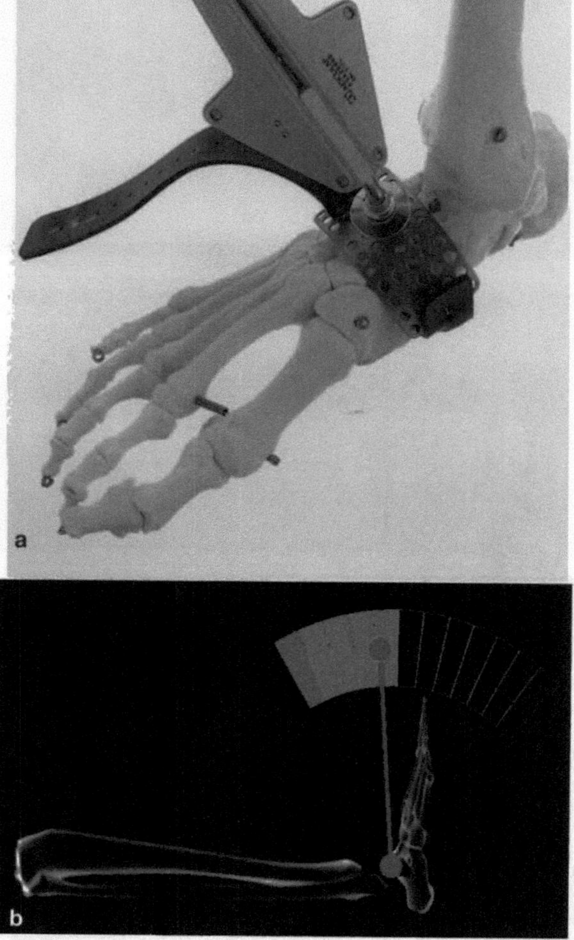

Fig. 4-6a, b. Kinematic registration of the center of the ankle joint. **a** The transmitter is mounted on the adapter to the foot in such a way that the diodes in the front of the transmitter point toward the camera. **b** The movement of the ankle joint is guided by the pointer to assure accurate registration of the center of the ankle joint

is completed, the surgeon is instructed to proceed to the next step, kinematic registration of the center of the ankle joint.

The center of the ankle joint is determined by attaching a metal plate containing an adapter to hold a rigid body to the foot with a rubber band. The rigid body is then attached to this plate. The ankle joint is then flexed and extended. Visual cues to guide the movement of the ankle joint during registration are displayed on the computer screen (Fig. 4-6). Once adequate information has been obtained to permit calculation of the center of the ankle joint, the surgeon is instructed to proceed to the next step, kinematic registration of the center of the knee joint.

The kinematic center of the knee joint is determined by slowly flexing and extending the knee from zero to 90°. As with hip and ankle joint registration, the surgeon is provided with visual cues on the computer screen.

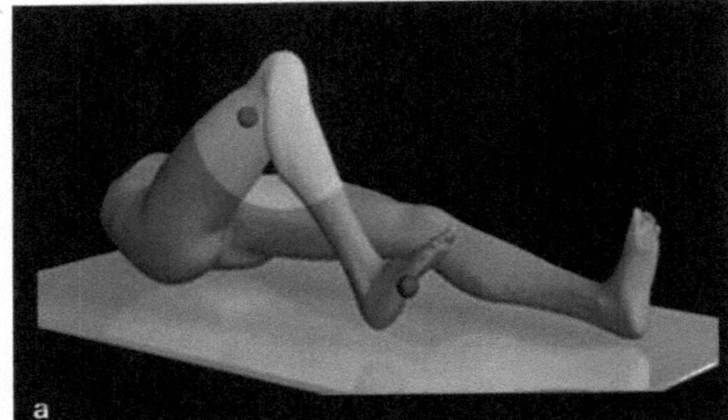

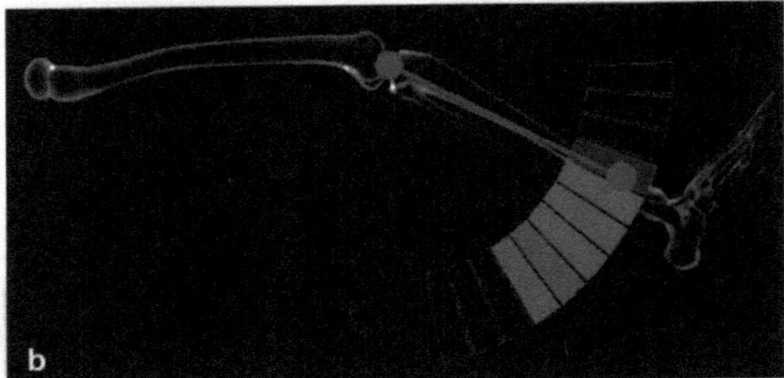

Fig. 4-7a, b. Kinematic registration of the center of the knee joint. **a** A video clip of the knee motion during registration guides the surgeon. **b** The pointer guides the movement of the knee joint to assure accurate registration

Although not essential, the accuracy of the registration may be increased by rotating the tibia on the femur with the knee flexed 90° (**Fig. 4-7**).

Kinematic registration of the hip, knee and ankle joints makes it possible to determine the mechanical axes of the extremity in the frontal and sagittal planes. However, in order to

- determine the level from the knee joint line of the femoral and tibial resections,
- calculate the size of the femoral component,
- place the femoral and tibial cutting blocks in correct medial/lateral position; and
- orient the femoral cutting block in proper rotation,

it is necessary to perform a surface registration of the knee and ankle joint. Surface registration of these joints also increases the accuracy of the calculation of the joint centers established initially using kinematic registration.

Establishing the Tibial and Femoral Reference Points

To determine the level of the tibial resection, a pointer to which a diode containing rigid body is attached, is placed on the point on the tibial plateau from which the depth of the tibial resection is to be measured. This is usually the deepest point on the least damaged side of the plateau (**Figs. 4-8 and 4-9**).

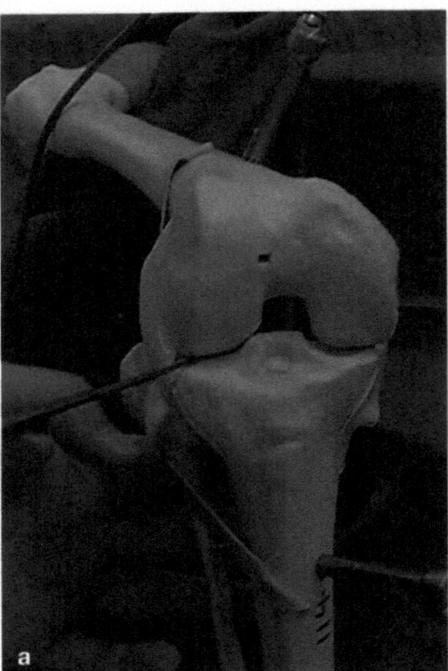

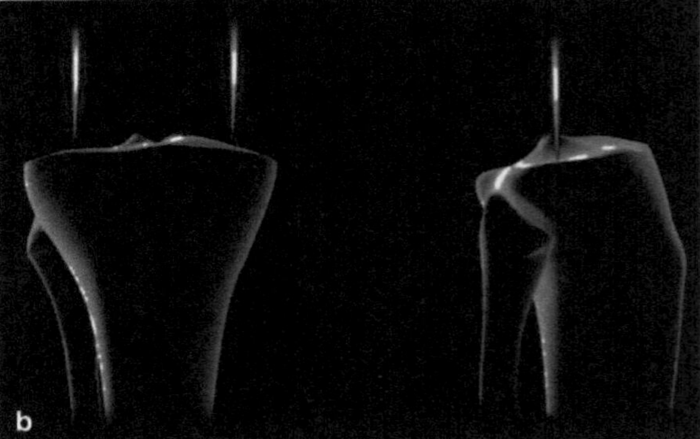

Fig. 4-8a, b. Establishing the level of tibia resection. **a** The tip of the pointer is placed on the point on the tibial plateau from which the depth of the tibial resection is to be measured. This is usually the deepest point on the least damaged side of the plateau. **b** The monitor directs the placement of the pointer on the plateau

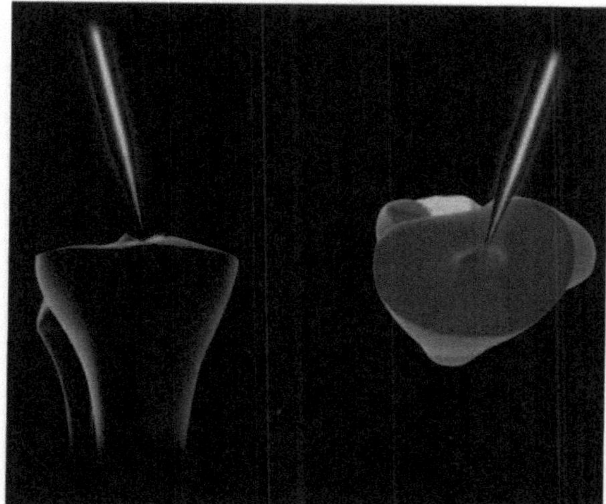

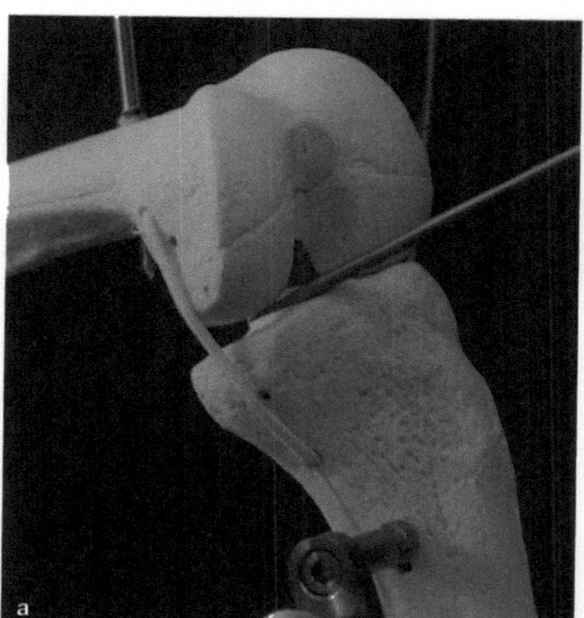

Fig. 4-9. Surface registration of the center of the intercondylar eminence of the tibia. This information is used with the kinematic information to optimize the determination of the center of the knee joint

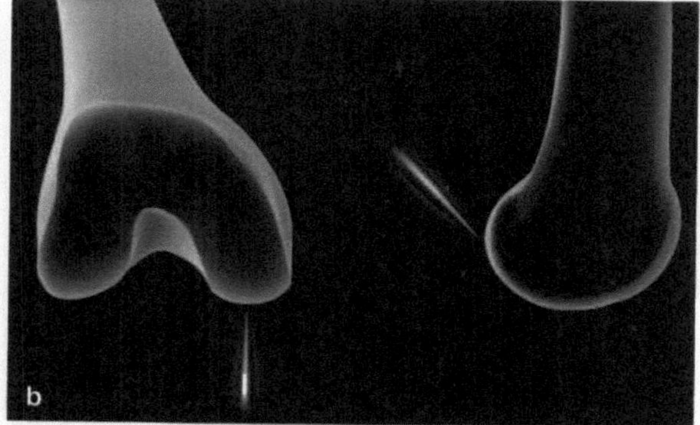

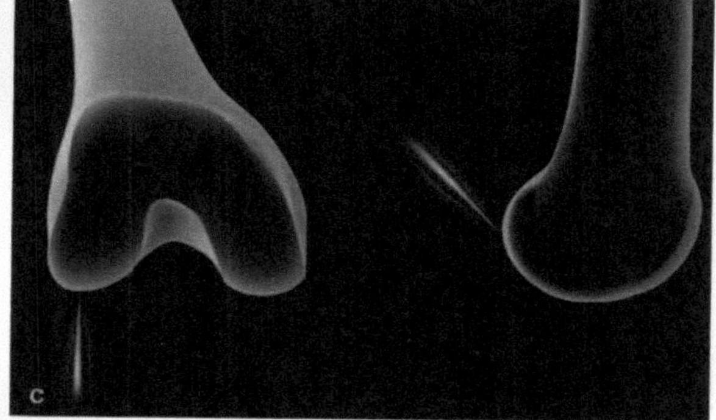

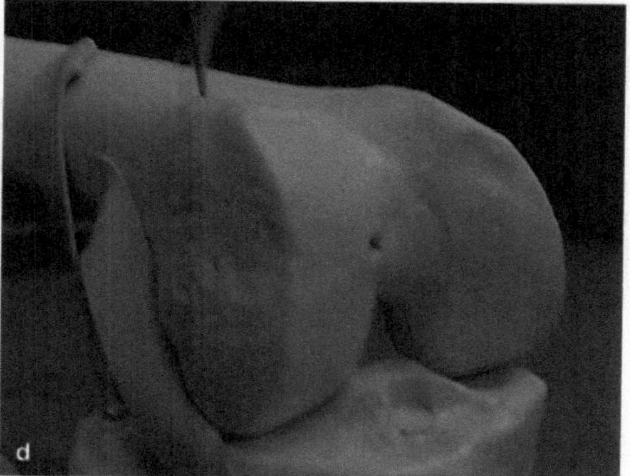

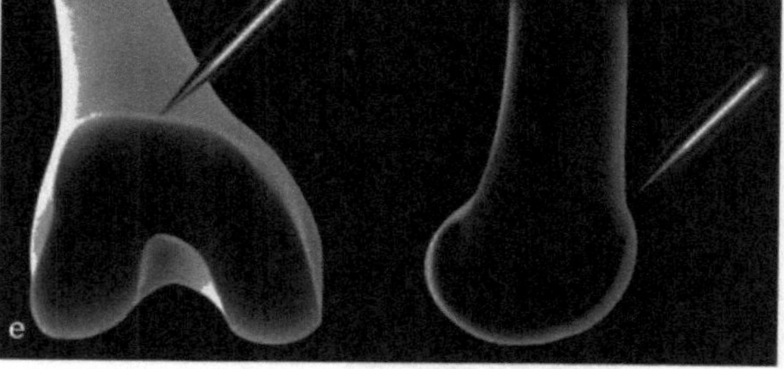

Fig. 4-10a-e. Surface registration of the femur: this step accomplishes 3 goals: 1. optimizing the center of the knee joint with the previously acquired kinematic data; 2. determining the size of the femoral component; 3. establishing the rotation of the femoral implant. **a–c** palpation of the dorsal midpoints of the medial and lateral femoral condyles; **d, e** palpation of the anterior cortical surface of the femur

To determine the size and rotation of the femoral component, the rigid body containing pointer is placed on the posterior-medial, and posterior-lateral femoral condyles at the points farthest from the anterior femoral cortex. The anterior femoral cortex is then palpated with the pointer directly above the center of the trochlea (◘ Fig. 4-10).

Although rotation of the femoral component is usually determined using the posterior condylar axis, it is also possible to use the epicondylar axis by using the pointer to locate the medial and lateral epiconcyles. This axis is compared to the measured posterior condylar axis using an orientation block that abuts against the distal and posterior condyles (◘ Fig. 4-11).

The palpation registration step is completed by using the pointer to locate the medial and lateral malleoli and midpoint of the ankle joint in the frontal plane. This information is used to confirm the determination of the center of the ankle joint originally calculated using kinematic registration (◘ Fig. 4-12).

In order to determine the correct level of distal femoral resection, the distal femoral condyles must be registered. This is done using a block placed against the distal femur positioned so that its mechanical axis is zero (◘ Fig. 4-13).

Once the registration process has been completed, it is possible to orientate the femoral and tibial cutting blocks and position them to guide the levels of resection. Prior to positioning the cutting blocks, however, the presurgical alignment in the frontal and sagittal planes, the medial-lateral stability in extension and the range of motion are measured and recorded (◘ Fig. 4-14).

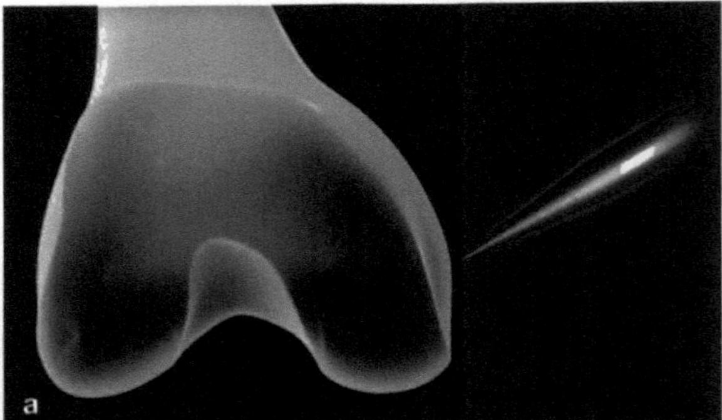
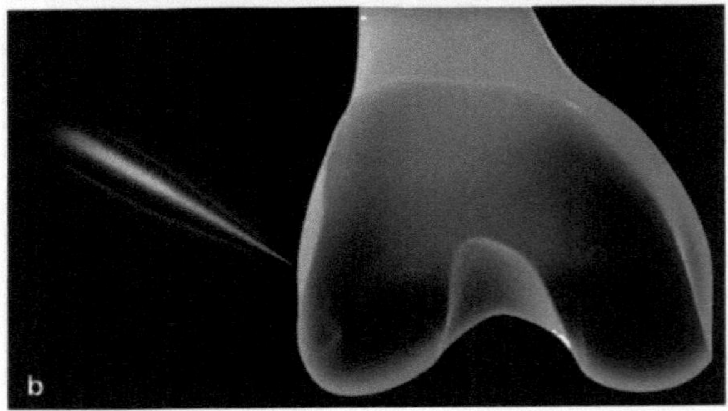

◘ **Fig. 4-11a, b.** Determination of the epicondylar axis: Palpation of the medial and lateral epicondyles with the pointer establishes the epicondylar axis. This information can be used to aid in the rotational positioning of the femoral component

Preparation of the Tibia

A rigid body is placed on the tibial cutting block, which is then attached to a tibial orientation instrument. This device is analogous to the external tibial alignment guide of conventional manual instruments. The orientation instrument is secured to the tibia with pins.

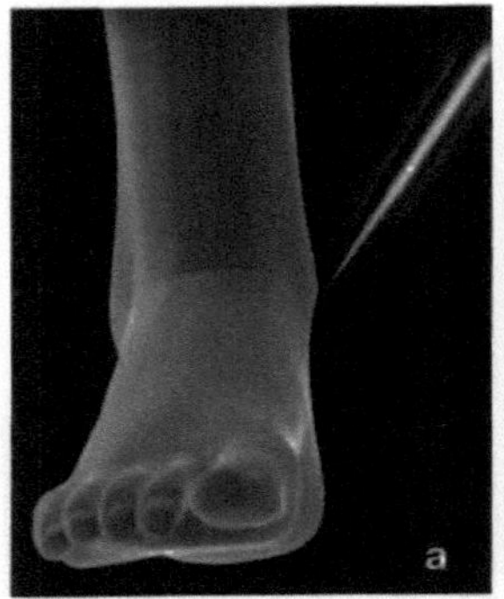
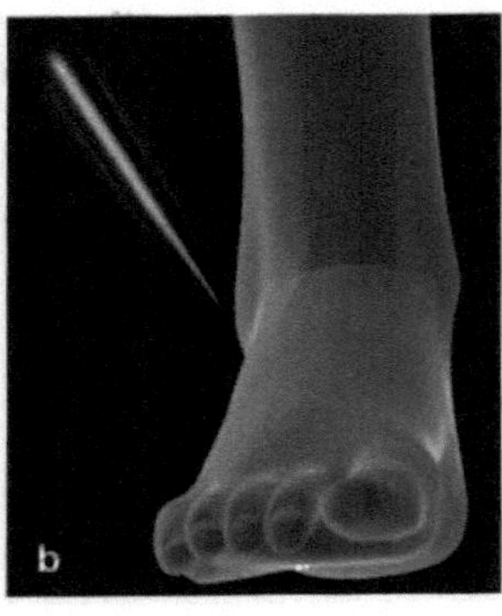
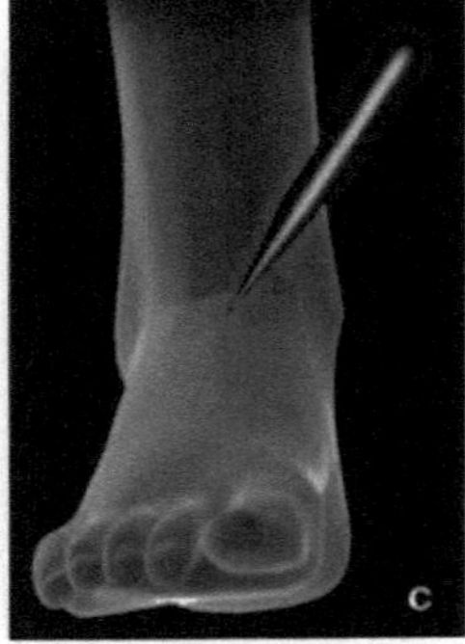

◘ **Fig. 4-12a-c.** The medial and lateral malleoli and the mid-point of the tibia in the frontal plane are palpitated to determine the center of the ankle joint. These data are integrated with the previously acquired kinematic data to optimize the registration of the ankle joint center

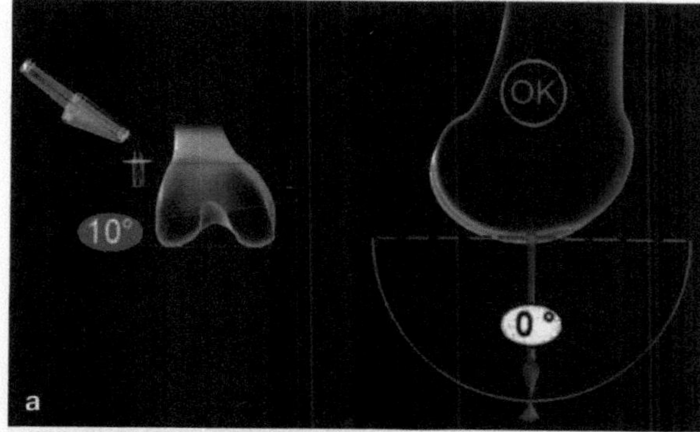

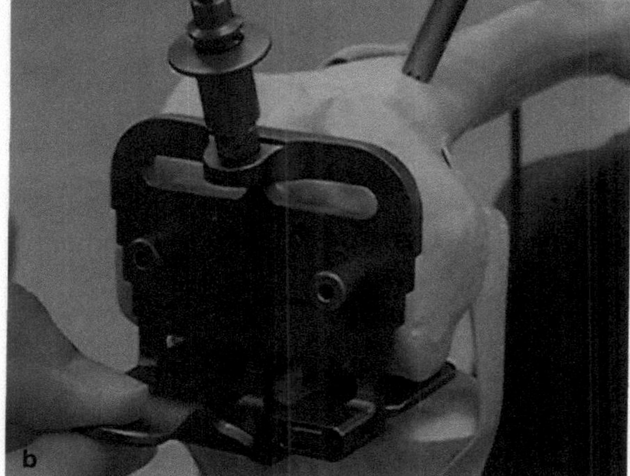

☐ Fig. 4-13a, b. Registration of the distal femoral condyles: The location of the distal femoral condyles is determined. This permits the measured resection of the distal femur

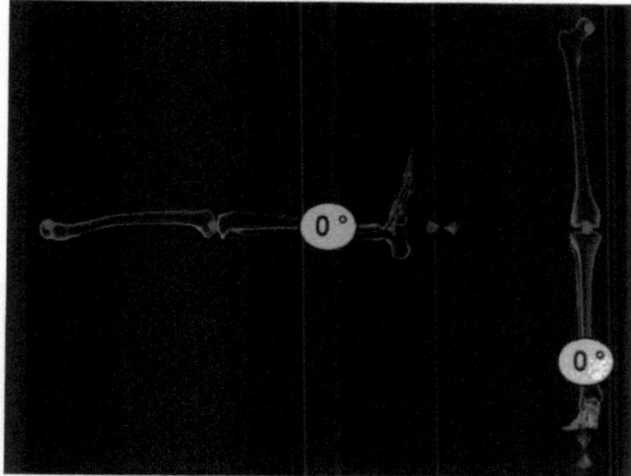

☐ Fig. 4-14. Determination of the preoperative alignment. Once the centers of the hip, knee and ankle joint are determined, the preoperative alignment of the leg, the range-of-motion of the knee and the preoperative stability of the knee joint can be measured and recorded

The frontal and sagittal orientation of the cutting block and the level of tibial resection are then determined. The location and orientation of the cutting block are displayed on the computer screen. The desired orientation of the tibial cutting block is exactly perpendicular to the frontal and sagittal mechanical axes of the tibia. The amount of tibial resection can be directly determined from the computer screen (☐ Fig. 4-15).

Once the tibial cutting block is in the desired position, it is fixed to the tibia with pins. The tibial orientation instrument is removed. The position of the cutting block is checked using the navigation equipment. The tibia resection is then performed.

Conventional manual tibial instrumentation is quite similar to the jig used with the navigation system. The manual instrumentation requires the surgeon to visually locate the center of the knee joint (tibial spine) and center of the ankle joint. The surgeon must also visually align the extra-medullary tibial rod parallel to the sagittal longitudinal axis of the tibia. The cutting block is then placed perpendicular to the visually determined frontal and sagittal axes of the tibia. The tibial manual instrumentation technique is analogous to using the palpation registration sequence in the computer-assisted technique. The level of tibial resection in the manual technique is determined using a stylus. The level in the computer technique is a direct measurement from the point at which a stylus would be placed. In both techniques, the tibial instrumentation is rotated until it points to the medial third of the tibial plateau.

Preparation of the Femur

A rigid body is attached to the femur cutting block. This block is attached to the femoral orientation guide and placed on the distal femur. The orientation and level of the block are then adjusted until the desired position as seen on the computer screen is obtained. The block is then fixed to the femur with pins and the orientation guide removed. The position of the cutting block is checked. The distal femur is then resected (☐ Fig. 4-16a, b).

The femoral orientation guide with a rigid body attached is then repositioned against the resected distal femoral surface. The posterior plates of the guide are placed against the posterior surfaces of the medial and

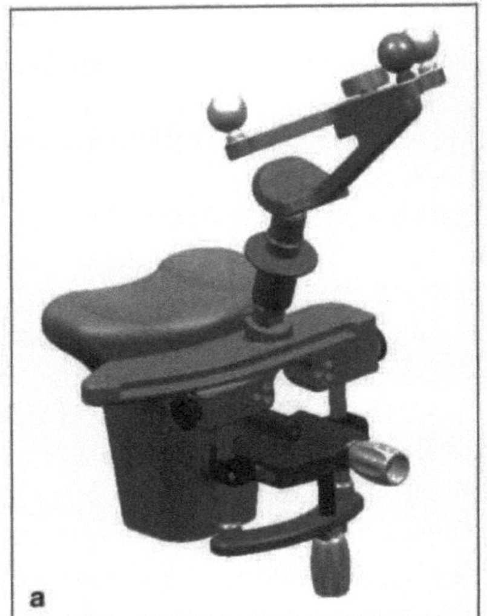
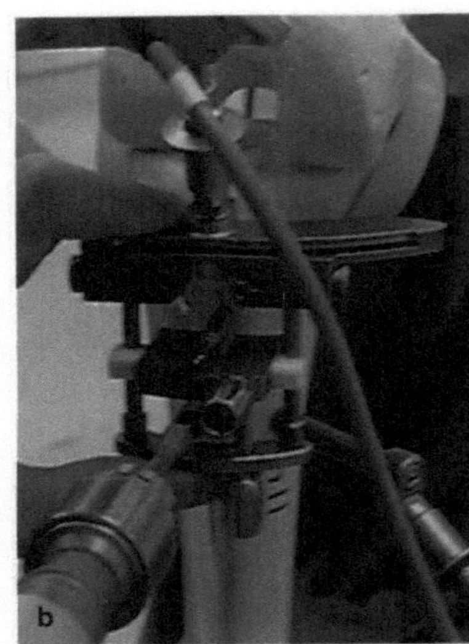
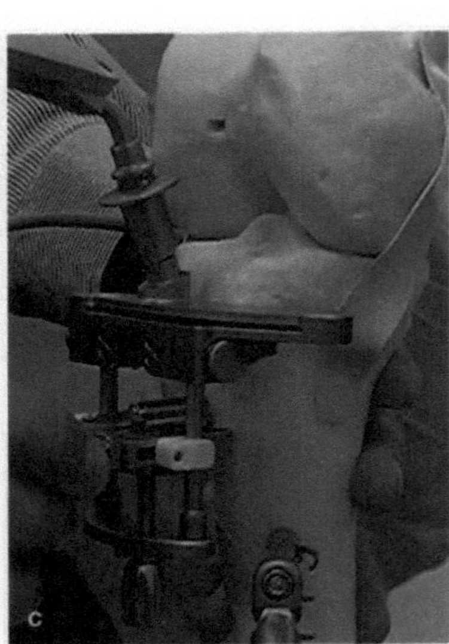
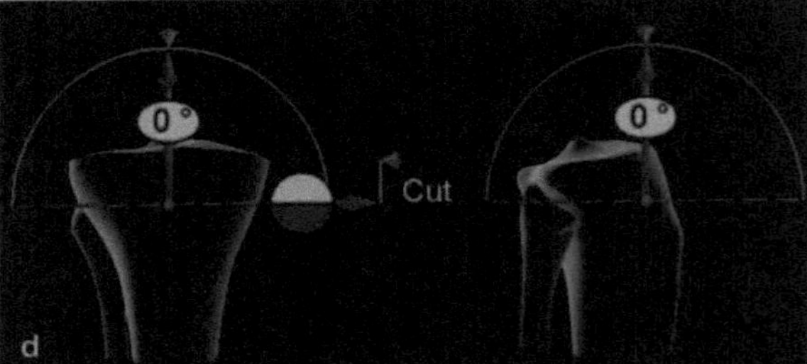

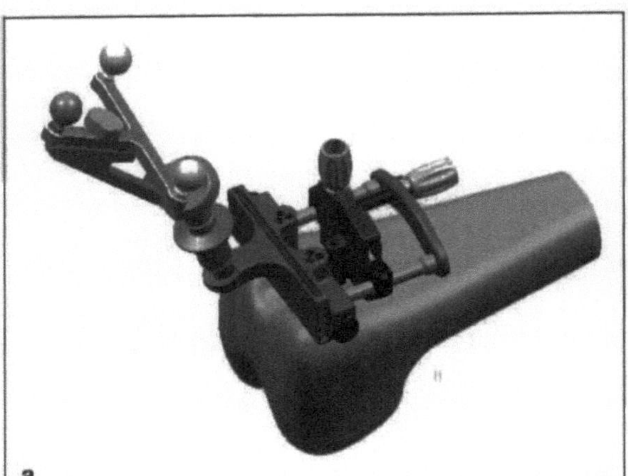
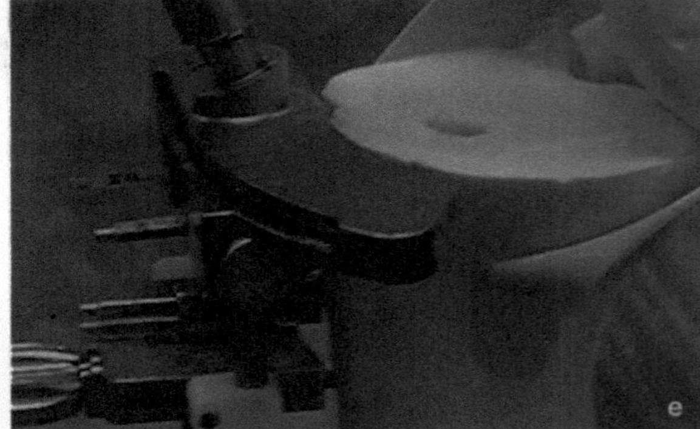
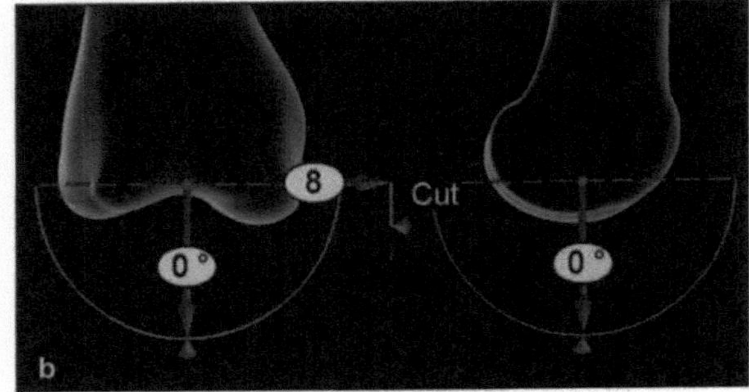

Fig. 4-15a–e. a–c The tibial instrumentation with attached transmitters is positioned on the tibia. **d–e** The depth and alignment of the tibial resection is displayed on the monitor

Fig. 4-16a, b. a The femoral orientation and cutting blocks with attached transmitters are placed on the distal femur. **b** The depth and alignment of the distal femoral resection is displayed on the monitor.

lateral femoral condyles. The rotation of the femoral component in relation to the posterior condyles can then be established. If desired, the epicondylar axis can also be used to determine the rotational positioning of the orientation

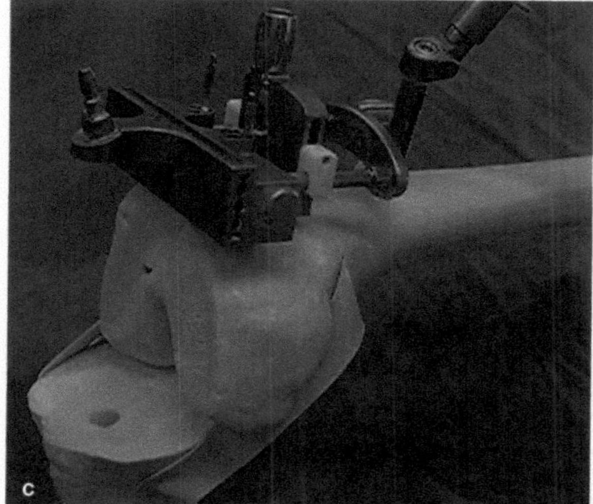

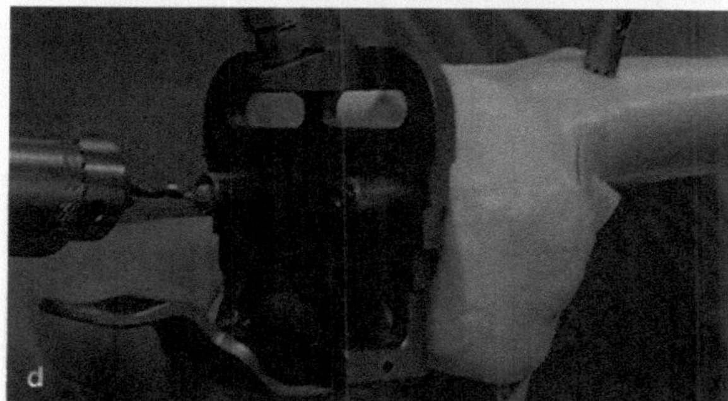

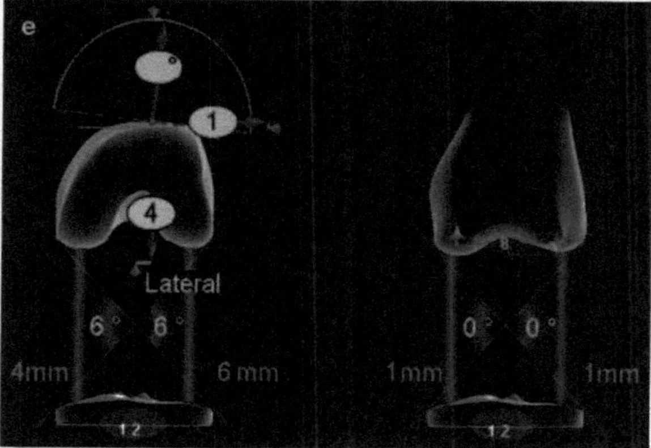

◻ Fig. 4-16c-e. c The distal cut is performed. **d–e** The rotation and anterior-posterior position of the cutting block is displayed on the monitor and guides the anterior and posterior femoral resectors

guide. Holes for the femoral cutting block are then drilled through the orientation guide. The cutting block for the femoral component whose size has been previously determined is then secured to the distal femur. The position of the block is checked and the anterior-posterior and chamfer resections are performed (◻ Fig. 4-16c).

Trial Reduction

Once the femoral and tibial resections are completed, a trial reduction is carried out. The polyethylene insert that best balances the knee in flexion and extension is selected. The navigation system is used to measure the final alignment of the extremity, the amount of medial-lateral laxity in extension and the final range of motion. The system can be used to guide the release of tight soft tissues medially, laterally and posteriorly.

Completion of the Procedure

The actual implants are then inserted. The navigation system is used to measure the final frontal and sagittal alignment of the extremity, the final medial-lateral stability and the final range of motion. These measurements are recorded in the computer.

The fixation screws for the rigid bodies are then removed. Closure is carried out in routine fashion.

Clinical Results

The OrthoPilot system described in this chapter has been used in more than 5000 total knee replacement cases. Most of these have been performed in France and Germany, the countries where the device was first introduced. Consequently, the results of the initial experience with the OrthoPilot have been published in French and German periodicals. Therefore, a summary of these reports (and the single American report currently available) is presented in ◻ Table 4-1.

These reports indicate that the navigation system is safe. There have been no reports of complications specifically associated with the use of the device. Moreover, clinical outcomes have not been adversely affected

□ Table 4-1. Accepted report of the use of the OrthoPilot System

Author	Clinic	Title	Study	n	Results	Original Title	Published in
M. Böhler, M. Messner, W. Glos, M. Riegler	Herz-Jesu-Krankenhaus Wien, Austria	Computer navigated implantation of total knee prostheses - A radiological study	Radiological follow-up evaluation	20	All patients femoro-tibial angles from 0-4°	Die computer-navigierte Implantation von Knietotalendo-prothesen – Eine radiologische Anwenderstudie	Acta Chir. Austria-ca, Vol.33, Supplement No. 175, 2001, p.63
S.L. Delp, S. D. Stulberg, B. Davies, F. Picard, F. Leitner	Northwestern University Chicago, USA; Imperial College London, U.K.; University of Grenoble, France	Computer Assisted Knee Replacement	Cadaver Study with OrthoPilot prototype of the femoral and tibial angle to the mechanical axis	7	Tibial angle in 90° to mechanical axis in all cases; femoral angle within 90° in 5 cases, within a deviation of +/- 3° in all cases	Computer Assisted Knee Replacement	Clinical Orthopae-dics, Volume 354, Lippincott-Raven Publishers, USA, September 1998, p.49-56
M. Janecek, P. Bucek, R. Hart	Urazova nemocnice Brno, Czech Republic	OrthoPilot (Aesculap) - Computer navigation of the prostheses of the knee joint	Comparative Study between 30 consecutive OrthoPilot cases with 30 randomly selected historic manual cases	60	0-2° varus or valgus: OrthoPilot 83%, manual 37%; 3-4° varus or valgus: OrthoPilot 17%, manual 46%; >4° varus or valgus: OrthoPilot 0%, manual 17%	OrthoPilot (Aesculap) - Computer-navigation der Endo-prothese des Kniegelenks	Acta Chir. Austria-ca, Vol.33, Supplement No. 175, 2001, p.51
JY. Jenny, C. Boeri	Centre de Trau-matologie et d'Orthopédie Strasbourg, France	Navigated implantation of total knee prostheses – A comparison with conventio-nal techniques	40 OrthoPilot cases were com-pared to a control group of 40 manual cases. Perfect alignment was defined as deviation of max. 3° for femorotibial, coronal and sagit-tal alignment of femoral and tibial components	80	0-3° varus or valgus: OrthoPilot 83%, manual 78% Perfect alignment in all criteria: OrthoPilot 65%, manual 30%	Navigiert-implantierte Knietotalendo-prothesen. Eine Vergleichs-studie mit konventionellem Instrumentatrium	Zeitschrift für Orthopädie und ihre Grenzgebiete, Band 139, März/April 2001, p.117-119
H. Kiefer, D. Lange-meyer, U. Schmer-witz	Lukas-Kranken-haus Bünde, Germany	Navigation total-knee-replacement	Prospective, controlled study comparing 100 OrthoPilot with 50 manual cases	150	0°: OrthoPilot 43%, manual 19%; 1-2° varus or valgus: OrthoPilot 32%, manual 26%; 3-4° varus or valgus: OrthoPilot 18%, manual 29%; >4° varus or valgus: OrthoPilot 7%, manual 26%	Computer-gestützte Navigation in der Knie-endoprothetik	European Journal of Trauma, 2001, E- Suppl. 1, Urban & Vogel, p.128-132

■ **Table 4-1.** Continued

Author	Clinic	Title	Study	n	Results	Original Title	Published in
W. Konermann, H. Reimers, F. J. Müller	Orthopädische Klinik Hessisch Lichtenau, Germany	Computer-controlled navigation in knee arthroplasty – First experiences with the OrthoPilot system	Follow-up of first 23 OrthoPilot patients	23	Mechanical axis within +/- 3° for all patients	Computergesteuerte Navigation in der Knieendoprothetik – Erste Erfahrungen mit dem OrthoPilot System	Zeitschrift für Orthopädie und ihre Grenzgebiete, Band 138, Sept/Okt 2000, DGOT Abstracts p.S61
R. K. Miehlke, U. Clemens, J.-H. Jens, S. Kershally	St. Josef-Stift Sendenhorst, Germany	Navigation in knee arthroplasty - Preliminary clinical experience and prospektive comparative study in comparison with conventional technique	Radiological follow-up of first 60 OrthoPilot patients	60	0-2° varus or valgus: 62%; 3-4° varus or valgus: 25% >4° varus or valgus: 3%	Navigation in der Knieendoprothetik - vorläufige klinische Erfahrungen und prospektiv vergleichende Studie gegenüber konventioneller Implantationstechnik	Zeitschrift für Orthopädie und ihre Grenzgebiete, Band 139, März/ April 2001, p.109-129
			Prospective comparison of the first 30 OrthoPilot cases with 30 manual cases	60	0-2° varus or valgus: OrthoPilot 63%, manual 57%; 3-4° varus or valgus: OrthoPilot 30%, manual 33%; >4° varus or valgus: OrthoPilot 7%, manual 10%		in the same paper
G. Pflüger, R. Kaar	Evangelisches Krankenhaus Wien-Währing, Austria	Experiences with the OrthoPilot - a computer assisted navigation system for implantation of total knee prostheses	Radiological follow-up evaluation	54	All patients within a deformation range of 3° varus or valgus	Erfahrungen mit dem OrthoPilot - ein computerunterstütztes Navigationssystem zur Implantation von Knieendoprothesen	Acta Chir. Austriaca, Vol.33, Supplement No. 175, 2001, p.51
D. Saragaglia, F. Picard, C. Chaussard, E. Montbarbon, F. Leitner, P. Cinquin	Hôpital Sud, CHU de Grenoble, France	Computer-assisted knee arthroplasty: comparison with a conventional procedure. Results of 50 cases in a prospective randomized study	Prospective, randomized study comparing 25 OrthoPilot with 25 manual cases	50	0-3° varus or valgus: OrthoPilot 100%, manual 84%	Mise en place des prothèses totales du genou assistée par ordinateur: comparaison avec la technique conventionnelle	Revue de chirurgie orthopedique et reparatrice de l' appareil moteur., 2001 Feb 1; 87(1): Masson-Periodiques, p.18-28
S. D. Stulberg, P. Loan, V. Sarin	Northestern University	Computer-assisted TKR surgery. A critical analysis of an initial experience with the OrthoPilot Navigation System	35 cases to evaluate safey, accuracy of system. Evaluate accuracy of manual instruments	35	OrthoPilot safe, noticeable variation in registering accuracy. Manual instruments most accurate in frontal plane, less accurate in sagital plane	Computer-assisted TKA surgery. A critical analysis of an initial experience with the OrthoPilot Navigation System	5th Annual North American CAOS Meeting, Pittsburg, PA

by the use of the OrthoPilot. The early versions of the OrthoPilot system required that a pin be placed in the rim of the ilium to allow monitoring of pelvic motion to registration of the hip joint. Many navigation systems still require this pin placement. No complications have been associated with the use of these pins.

The reports which compare the alignment results obtained with the OrthoPilot to results obtained using manual instrumentation indicate that overall limb alignment achieved with the navigation system is equal to or better than that achieved with manual instrumentation. If the alignment in all planes of the femoral and tibial components is compared, the OrthoPilot achieved perfect alignment much more frequently than manual instrumentation.

One of the goals of computer-assisted TKA systems is to increase the reliability and reproducibility of the procedure. The initial experience with the OrthoPilot indicates that this goal is being achieved. There are fewer alignment »outliers« when the navigation system is used.

Navigation systems also make it possible to determine the accuracy of evaluation tools that are currently being used to determine the outcome of total knee replacement. The OrthoPilot system has been used to demonstrate that pre- and postoperative radiographs are not accurate methods for determining implant and limb alignment. The system has also been used to determine pre- and postoperative medial-lateral ligament laxity and range of motion. It has been possible to correlate postoperative range of motion with postoperative medial lateral stability and establish that knees that are »tight« medial-laterally achieve the same degree of flexion as those which are less tight.

Finally, navigation systems, including the OrthoPilot, have been used to determine the accuracy and reproducibility of currently available manual instrumentation systems. It has been shown that manual intra-medullary systems are capable of producing accurate and reproducible alignment in the frontal plane. However, these systems are less reliable in reestablishing the mechanical axis in the sagittal plane. There is a tendency for the surgeon to leave a knee in slight flexion if a manual system and visual confirmation of final alignment are used.

Summary

Computer-assisted navigation systems have been developed for use in total knee replacement surgery to address the inherent limitations of mechanical instrumentation. Both image-free and image-based computer-assisted systems are now being used to implant total knees. As has been emphasized in this chapter, the alignment objectives which these computer-assisted systems attempt to optimize are the identical alignment goals that mechanical systems seek to achieve. It is anticipated that by improving the accuracy and reliability with which the frontal and sagittal axes are restored, the correct femoral and tibial implant rotation and size are achieved, and the correct medial-lateral and anterior-posterior ligament stability are established, the functional results of TKA will be improved, morbidity of TKA surgery will be decreased, and longevity of TKA will be increased. Longer term follow-up studies of TKA performed using computer-assisted techniques will have to become available before it can be determined whether these goals have been achieved.

There are other, perhaps equally important, potential benefits of using currently available computer-assisted total knee replacement systems. The designs of mechanical instruments can be improved with the information that is gathered by computer-based instrumentation systems. For example, it is clear from the initial use of computer-based systems that it is difficult for a surgeon to determine if the sagittal mechanical axis has been correctly restored. There is a tendency for surgeons to leave knees with slight flexion contractures. This tendency can be reduced if mechanical systems use pins in the femoral and tibial trials that are parallel when the knee is in full extension (assuming the implants are correctly aligned with the bones). The use of computer-assisted systems indicates that a number of relatively small changes in currently available mechanical instruments could improve the accuracy of these devices.

In addition, currently available computer-assisted systems are likely to influence the design of the next generation of total knee implants. The information obtained through the use of these systems is likely to influence the size distributions and dimensions of implants, the orientation of the patellar tracking mechanisms, and the location of the cam and post on posterior stabilized designs.

The use of currently available computer-assisted systems will also influence the ways in which total knee implants are inserted. For example, computer assisted systems allow a surgeon to determine how much medial-lateral laxity is present at the end of the TKA procedure. This laxity can be related to other outcomes, e.g. range of motion. Thus computer-assisted systems can help surgeons determine how to optimize the performance of TKA procedures using currently available implants.

Computer-assisted systems of the near future will have the capability of integrating information about human gait and knee function that is currently being obtained. This information can further increase the accuracy with which TKAs are performed and improve the quality of the outcome of those procedures.

References

1. Aglietti P, Buzzi R (1988) Posterior stabilized total condylar knee replacement. Three to eight year follow-up of 85 knees. J Bone Joint Surg 70B: 211–216
2. Aglietti P, Buzzi R, Gaudenzi A (1988) Patellofemoral functional results and complications with the posterior stabilized total condylar knee prosthesis. J Arthroplasty 3: 17–25
3. Berger RA, Rubash HE, Seel MJ, Thompson WH, Crossett LS (1993) Determining the rotational alignment of the femoral component in total knee arthroplasty using the epicondylar axis. Clin Orthop 286: 40–47
4. Besl PJ, McKay ND (1992) A method for registration of 3D shapes. IEEE Transaction on Pattern Analysis and Machine Intelligence 14: 239–256
5. Canny JA (1986) Computational approach to edge detection. IEEE Trans-actions on Pattern Analysis and Machine Intelligence PAMI 8: 679–698
6. Davies BL, Harris SJ, Lin WJ, Hibberd RD, Cobb JC (1997) Active compliance in robotic surgery –The use of force control as a dynamic constraint. J Eng Med Proc H IMechE 211: H4
7. Delp SL, Stulberg SD, Davies B et al. (1998) Computer assisted knee replacement. Clin Orthop 354: 49–56
8. Dorr LD, Boiardo RA (1997) Technical considerations in total knee arthroplasty. Clin Orthop 205: 5–11
9. Ecker ML, Lotke PA, Windsor RE et al. (1987) Long-term results after Total Condylar knee arthroplasty. Significance of radiolucent lines. Clin Orthop 216: 151–158
10. Fadda M, Bertelli, D, Martelli S et al. (1997) Computer-assisted planning for total knee arthroplasty. Proceedings of the First Joint Conference on Computer Vision, Virtual Reality and Robotics in Medicine and Medical Robotics and Computer Assisted Surgery, Grenoble, France. Springer, Berlin Heidelberg New York Tokyo, pp 619–628
11. Feng EL, Stulberg SD, Wixson RL (1994) Progressive subluxation and polyethylene wear in total knee replacements with flat articular surfaces. Clin Orthop 229: 60–71
12. Figgie HE, Goldberg VM, Heiple KG, Moller HS, Gordon NH (1986) The influence of tibial-pallellofemoral location on function of the knee in patients with posterior stabilized condylar knee prosthesis. J Bone Joint Surg 68A: 1035–1040
13. Freeman MAR, Todd RC, Bamert P et al. (1978) ICLH-Arthroplasty of the knee: 1968–1977. J Bone Joint Surg 60B: 339–344
14. Garg A, Walker PS (1990) Prediction of total knee motion using a three-dimensional computer-graphics model. J Biomech 23: 45–58
15. Glozman D, Shoham M, Fischer A (1999) Efficient registration of 3D objects in robotic-assisted surgery proceedings. Comput Aided Surg (in press) (Abstr)
16. Goodfellow JW, O'Connor JJ (1986) Clinical results of the Oxford knee. Clin Orthop 205: 21–42
17. Insall JN, Binazzi R, Soudry M et al. (1985) Total knee arthroplasty. Clin Orthop 192: 13–22
18. Insall JN, Ranawat CS, Aglietti P et al. (1976) A comparison of four models of total knee-replacement prostheses. J Bone Joint Surg Am 58: 754–765
19. Insall J, Scott WN, Ranawat CS (1979) The total Condylar prosthesis. A report of the hundred cases. J Bone Joint Surg Am 61: 173–179
20. Jeffery RS, Morris RW, Denham RA (1991) Coronal alignment after total knee replacement. J Bone Joint Surg Br 73: 709–714
21. Jenny JY, Boeri C (2000) Computer-assisted total knee prosthesis implantation without preoperative imaging: A comparison with classical instrumentation. Fourth Annual North American Program on Computer Assisted Orthopaedic Surgery, Pittsburgh, PA, pp 97–98
22. Kienzle TC, Stulberg SD, Peshkin M et al. (1996) A computer-assisted total knee replacement surgical system using a calibrated robot. In: Taylor RH, Lavallee S, Burdea GC, Mosges R (eds) Computer-integrated surgery: technology and applications. MIT Press, Cambridge, pp 409–416
23. Krackow KA, Bayers-Thering M, Phillips MJ, Mihalko WM (1999) A new technique for determining proper mechanical axis alignment during total knee arthroplasty: progress toward computer-assisted TKA. Orthopedics 22: 698–702
24. Laskin RS (1990) Total Condylar knee replacement in patients who have rheumatoid arthritis. A ten-year follow-up study. J Bone Joint Surg Am 72: 529–535
25. Leitner F, Picard F, Minfelde R et al. (1997) Computer assisted knee surgical total replacement. Proceedings of the First Joint Conference on Computer Vision, Virtual Reality and Robotics in Medicine and Medical Robotics and Computer Assisted Surgery, Grenoble, France. Springer, Berlin Heidelberg New York Tokyo, pp 630–638
26. Matsen III FA, Garbini JL, Sidles JA et al. (1993) Robotic assistance in orthopaedic surgery: A proof of principle using distal femoral arthroplasty. Clin Orthop 296: 178–186
27. Merkow RL, Soudry M, Insall JN (1985) Patellar dislocation following total knee replacement. J Bone Joint Surg 67A: 1321–1327
28. Miehlke RK, Clemens U, Kershally S (2000) Computer integrated instrumentation in knee arthroplasty: A comparative study of conventional and computerized technique. Fourth Annual North American Program on Computer Assisted Orthopaedic Surgery, Pittsburgh, PA, pp 93–96
29. OrthoPilot Users Meeting (2000) Tuttlingen, Germany
30. Oswald MH, Jacob RP, Schneider E, Hoogewoud H (1993) Radiological analysis of normal axial alignment of femur and tibia in view of total knee arthroplasty. J Arthroplasty 8: 419–426

31. Piazza SJ, Delp SL, Stulberg SD, Stern SH (1998) Posterior tilting of the tibial component decreases femoral rollback in posterior-substituting knee replacement. J Orthop Res 16: 264–270

32. Picard F, Leitner F, Raoult O, Saragaglia D, Cinquin P (1998) Clinical evaluation of computer-assisted total knee arthroplasty. Second Annual North American Program on Computer Assisted Orthopaedic Surgery, Pittsburgh, PA, pp 239–249

33. Picard F, Leitner F, Raoult O et al. (1999) Early clinical results with the Orthopilot System. Comput Aided Surg (Abstr)

34. Picard F, DiGioia AM, Sell D, Plakseychuk A, Moody IE, Jaramaz B, Nikoi C, LaBarca RS, Levinson T, Computer assisted measurement tool for total knee replacement. Evaluation of traditional instrumentation. Computer Aided Surgery (in press)

35. Ranawat CS, Adjei OB (1988) Survivorship analysis and results of total condylar knee arthroplasty. Clin Orthop 226: 6–13

36. Ritter MA, Faris PM, Keating EM, Meding JB (1994a) Postoperative alignment of total knee replacement: Its effect on survival. Clin Orthop 299: 153–156

37. Ritter MA, Herbst SA, Keating EM et al. (1994b) Radiolucency at the bone-cement interface in total knee replacement. J Bone Joint Surg AM 76: 60–65

38. Stern SH, Insall JN (1992) Posterior stabilized prosthesis: Results after follow-up of 9–12 years. J Bone Joint Surg 74A: 980–986

39. Stulberg SD, Picard F, Saragaglia D (2000) Computer-assisted total knee replacement arthroplasty. Operative Techniques in Orthopaedics 10: 25–39

40. Stulberg SD, Sarin V, Loan P (2001a) The use of computer-assisted navigation in TKR: results of an initial experience in 35 patients. Proceedings of the Fourth Annual American CAOS Meeting, Pittsburgh, PA

41. Stulberg SD, Sarin V (2001b) The use of a navigation system to assist ligament balancing in TKR. Proceedings of the Fourth Annual American CAOS Meeting, Pittsburgh, PA

42. Stulberg SD, Sarin V, Loan P (2001c) X-ray vs. computer assisted measurement techniques to determine pre and postoperative limb alignment in TKR surgery. Proceedings of the Fourth Annual American CAOS Meeting, Pittsburgh, PA

43. Teter KE, Bergman D, Colwell CW (1995) Accuracy of intramedullary versus extramedullary tibial alignment cutting systems in total knee arthroplasty. Clin Orthop 321: 106–110

44. Townley CD (1985) The anatomic total knee: instrumentation and alignment technique. The Knee: Papers of the First Scientific Meeting of the Knee Society. Baltimore, University Press, pp 39–54

45. Vince KG, Insall JN, Kelly MA (1989) The total condylar prosthesis: 10 to 12 year results of a cemented knee replacement. J Bone Joint Surg 71B: 793–797

46. Wasielewski RC, Galante JO, Leighty R, Natarajan RN, Rosenberg AG (1994) Wear patterns on retrieved polyethylene tibial inserts and their relationship to technical considerations during total knee arthroplasty. Clin Orthop 299: 31–43

5   Bone Morphing: 3D Reconstruction Without Pre- or Intraoperative Imaging – Concept and Applications

E. Stindel, J.-L. Briard, S. Lavallée, F. Dubrana, S. Plaweski, P. Merloz, C. Lefèvre, J. Troccaz

Introduction

Any computer-assisted procedure can be divided in three steps. The first one is called the **perception step**. During this stage, we have to build a specific model of the patient undergoing surgery. The second is the **reasoning step**, during which the surgeon plans the procedure based on the model built at the previous stage. Next, there is the **action step**. This takes place in the operating room, where the surgeon tries to perform, as accurately as possible, the procedure defined at step two. In practice, these steps are not linear, and are often merged into a computer-assisted surgical protocol (CASP) running on the surgetics system.

A complete description of these different steps has been published by the authors [7]. In this paper, we focus on the perception level. To develop a good guiding system, one needs a good model of the patient. It must be accurate and easy to obtain by the surgeon. The models vary and use different kinds of data, as a function of the type of surgery to be performed. If one wants to develop an intravascular guiding system for the treatment of atherosclerotic lesions, one would probably build the model from arteriographic images. If one wants to perform neurosurgery on some functional areas of the brain, one may include in the model functional information such as E.E.G. or fMRI data.

In orthopaedic surgery, models are built using different types of data depending on the procedure itself. We will distinguish between two classes of models:
- image-based models and
- non-image-based models.

In the first group, the model can be obtained preoperatively from radiographs or CT scans [2, 5, 9], or intraoperatively from fluoroscopic images [4]. In the second group, we will describe two subgroups: in the first one, called a geometric model, the data consist of several landmarks digitized on the patient [3, 6]. In the second group, the 3D shapes of the bones are built from data collected with a 3D optical localizer in relative coordinate systems attached to the bones using clouds of points and deformable models: this is the **bone morphing technology**, invented by PRAXIM (patents pending), after several years of research into deformable and statistical modeling performed at Grenoble University (TIMC Laboratory).

In common with any surgical procedure, orthopaedic surgery can be defined as a 3D action (the operation) in a 3D space (the operating room) on a 3D object (the patient). Therefore, there is an absolute need for 3D models and we think that every model based on 2D images is of little present-day interest, and without promise for the future. While geometric models, based on landmarks only, may be useful in some cases [6], they have several limitations and may not meet all the surgeon's requirement. Therefore, several applications based on 3D morphologic models have been developed and marketed; however, all these models used CT to provide the data. Building a 3D model from CT has some drawbacks:

- The high volume of orthopaedics procedures performed each day makes CT scans as routine preoperative procedures an unacceptably expensive exercise. Also, the radiation burden to the patients would be high.

■ Performing a CT scan takes 20 min per patient. To this has to be added the time it takes to transfer the data to the surgeon's computer or navigation system, and to initiate, check and validate the results of the segmentation/registration process.

This procedure, from the raw data to the 3D model, is time-consuming and sometimes cumbersome. Last but not least, because of complex phenomena of error propagation, including segmentation and registration, CT-based navigation is sometimes not as accurate as expected. If there is no alternative, CT is still the reference choice for navigation in orthopaedics; however, in 2000, PRAXIM achieved a breakthrough in orthopaedics by the introduction of bone morphing, which can outperform CT in some indications. In this paper, we describe the bone morphing technology, and demonstrate its applications in several indications when running the technology on the PRAXIM surgetics station.

Bone Morphing: 3D Morphologic Data Without Preoperative Imaging

In a non-image-based approach, building a 3D model which is specific to the patient's anatomy is quite challenging. This section describes how this goal is achieved in the PRAXIM surgetics method.

Acquisition of a Random Cloud of 1000 Points

The overall process can be divided into several technical steps. However, for the surgeon, there is only one action to perform: to digitize a cloud of random points on the surface of the bone. This step is achieved using a pointer with a 1-mm-radius spherical tip instead of using a sharp tip. This enables the surgeon to sweep the pointer quickly and smoothly over the bone and cartilage surfaces. The bone morphing algorithm will then compensate for the radius of the sphere to reconstruct the exact surface. This takes about one minute and thirty seconds for the entire surface of the distal femur, and around one minute for the proximal part of the tibia. If we add the patella (in a TKA procedure), the acquisition step takes only 3 min. There is

only one recommendation that must be borne in mind during the acquisition: the probe must stay in contact with the surface of the bone until the acquisition is complete. After these 3 min, there is nothing else that the surgeon needs to do. This is a fast and efficient procedure for the acquisition of the 3D data during surgery.

3D Statistical Shape Models from Point Data

The second step is to position and deform a statistical model of the bone in order to fit the cloud of points using the algorithm of Fleute et al. [1]. Intraoperatively we use a deformable model, rather than a library of bone models. This 3D deformable shape was built once, and is now used for every surgical procedure. Using the technique described below, PRAXIM have developed several models (acetabulum, tibia, femur, etc.) for use in different applications. However, inside each application there is only one deformable model that will fit small bones as well as very large shapes.

To obtain this 3D statistical shape, three steps are required:

1. acquisition of training shapes,
2. definition of a point-to-point correspondence with the training shape,
3. statistical analysis.

Step 1

A set of n dry human bones is digitized using the Optotrak 3D localizer (NDI, Waterloo, Canada), resulting in large n sets of non-organized points, randomly distributed on the bone surface. The value n must be sufficient to represent a good variability of the population. Each set of points represents the surface of one bone (femur, tibia, etc.). An additional bone is then digitized with a higher point density. The result of the reconstruction is a triangular mesh of vertices, which is considered as a mean template.

Step 2

Each of the n sets of points is matched to the template in such a way that each vertex of the template mesh is mapped to its anatomically corresponding point on the femur under study. This matching process is based on the result of octree-splines deformation published by Szeliski and Lavallée [8]. The result of this non-rigid 3D to 3D registration is a transformation function T, which maps every point P_i of the actual data space (the set of points) to a point M_i of the template in such a way that $M_i = T(P_i)$.

Step 3

After steps 1 and 2 we obtain a collection of n complete 3D reconstructions of the surfaces of the n femurs under study. Each training femur F is then represented by a vector m which describes the vertices of the mesh. The mean shape is then given by:

$$\overline{m} = \frac{1}{n} \sum m_i.$$

We then compute the deviations of each training shape from the mean shape using principal component analysis of the deformation field. The final shape is the one which minimizes the necessary deformation to match all the training bones.

Using the statistical process described above using a mean surface and the most significant statistical modes, a new instance of the mean shape is generated by adding a linear combination of the most significant variation vectors to the original mean shape for each bone of the training set. This is achieved by minimizing the residual errors between the reconstructed model and the cloud of random points. It provides the best statistical shape that corresponds to the patient.

Local Deformation to Compensate Pathology Using Octree-Splines

To compensate for deviation of any pathological shape from the statistical shapes, we deform again locally the statistical model adapted to the patient until it fits correctly and precisely the cloud of points using the Szeliski and Lavallée [8] octree-spline algorithm with hierarchical, locally adapted and regularized deformation. A volume embedding the 3D data is created. It is recursively divided into smaller and smaller cubes that create a non-uniform volumetric mesh (not a surface mesh), and

each coefficient of the basis functions applied to each point of the mesh is optimized to match the data, while the resulting global deformation has regularization properties that make it realistic and stable. This process is more stable and accurate than are simple affine registration methods.

Note that steps 2 and 3 are continuous and merged in a single process, so that the user only sees the points before bone morphing is applied at the end of the first step, and then, only two or three seconds later, the 3D model fitting on the points.

This elegant combination of different mathematical techniques makes the result unique. This patented PRAXIM technique is very robust and accurate, as well as extremely powerful in many applications of computer-assisted surgery. In 100% of the cases in which we have been able to test or use this algorithm, it has performed well, exactly as expected.

Clinical Applications of the Bone Morphing Technique on the Surgetics Station

Total Knee Arthroplasty (TKA)

Many computer-assisted protocols are now in use on the surgetics station to help surgeons during total knee replacement. A complete chapter of this book is dedicated to the surgetics LCS station. This chapter provides a complete description of the advantages of the bone morphing over other approaches, and of how it can be helpful during a TKA procedure.

ACL Replacement

A separated chapter of this book describes how bone morphing is also useful for surgetics ACL reconstruction.

Hip Replacement

During hip replacement procedures, bone morphing of the acetabulum can be used to

- check and guide reaming,
- give true 3D information on the thickness of the acteabular fossa as it is being reamed, and helps to determine the size of the acetabular reamer,
- perform a second acquisition peri-operatively (which is only possible with the bone morphing technique as CT-scan is no longer available!) to check the amount of bone removed by reaming, the sphericity of the acetabulum, and its size,
- help to optimize size choice, thus avoiding over-sizing then control the orientation of the cup.

Optionally, bone morphing can be used also on the femur to determine the anatomical pattern before surgery, and take this pattern into account during the intraoperative surgical planning.

High Tibial Osteotomy (HTO)

High tibial osteotomy is performed through very small incision. The major challenge in this procedure is to display the 3D anatomy of the upper part of the tibia without any preoperative imaging. Once again, the bone morphing technique helped us to achieve this goal. Most of points are acquired in the surgical incision, and a few others are collected transcutaneously on the opposite aspect of the tibia. With these two clouds of points, we are able to deform the model to obtain an accurate representation of the actual anatomy. This model is then used in the HTO computer-assisted surgical protocol to plan the cuts in 3 dimensions, thus respecting the constraints of the patient's 3D morphology whilst adjusting the varus and recurvatum angles to correct the deformity. This instantaneous planning is used to guide the saw to perform easy, accurate, and precise surgery.

Unicompartimental Knee Arthroplasty

The bone morphing can be used during an unicompartimental procedure in a way similar to total knee replacement. It helps to perform minimally invasive surgery providing a large amount of data with only small incision. Four areas are digitized through the small incision and several points are directly computed inside the model

such as the location of the most distal points of the posterior and distal condyle. An automatic determination of the femoral size component is performed using a by fitting a sphere to the model. On the tibial side, the ideal size is computed from the 3D data, and the component is automatically located by the system.

Future Perspectives

In the five cases described above, the data where acquired with the help of a probe located on the surface of the bones. However, in some cases it would be useful to have 3D data without any skin incision. The HTO procedure described above could benefit from such new techniques. It would be eminently useful if we could capture the entire 3D anatomy of the proximal part of the tibia, instead of the partial acquisition we are doing today. Therefore, some extensions to the actual technique have been developed and are progressively being realized by PRAXIM on the surgetics station.

Two new approaches are presented: echo-morphing and fluoro-morphing; in both cases, we use a deformable model. In the first case, this model is matched with 3D data obtained after automated segmentation of ultrasound images. In the second case, fluoroscopic images are used as input data.

Echo-Morphing

In minimally invasive surgery, surgeons are expecting tools that will provide complete 3D data with minimal access or without any skin incisions. The echo-morphing technique has been developed to meet this demand. In this technique, ultrasound images of the bone are acquired with a 2.5 US probe integrated in the surgetics station. Theses images are automatically segmented, and a 3D model of the bone is then matched to the points collected during the segmentation process. ◘ Figure 5-1 shows the result of the automatic segmentation of a femur. The segmentation is a fast process done in real time during surgery.

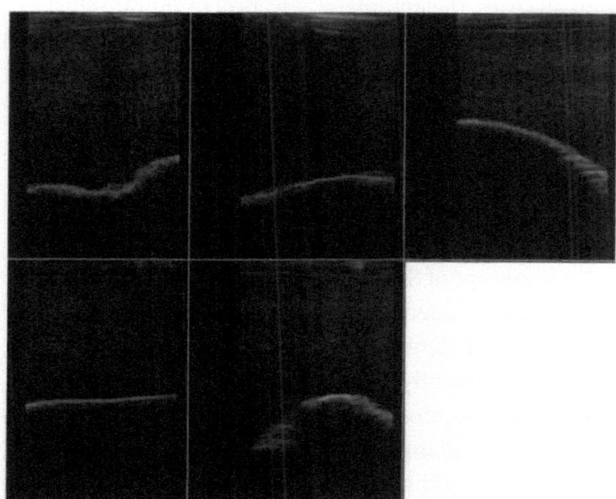

Fluoro-Morphing

Fluoro-morphing is a new technique developed by PRAXIM (patent pending), which is used for the reconstruction of bone from calibrated fluoroscopic data. Fluoroscopic images are first processed to extract the boundaries of the bone. A specific extended bone morphing process is used to deform a 3D statistical model in order to match the original images. ◻ Figure 5-2 shows the result of this registration step. This approach gives a true 3D specific model of the vertebra that is being operated on, using transcutaneous acquisition.

Conclusion

The bone morphing algorithm is a very accurate, fast and easy way to collect 3D shapes during surgery. It is now in routine use in many clinical applications, and will be followed by even more advanced techniques such as the echo- or fluoro-morphing for minimally invasive surgery.

These approaches have been developed to meet the surgeons' needs in various situations. The new technology appears to have several advantages over CT and over landmarks-based methods.

Advantages over CT:

1. It is possible to capture the true intraoperative 3D morphology of the bones. In some situations, the 3D preoperative morphology is of no interest. During a TKA, it is necessary to remove the osteophytes before

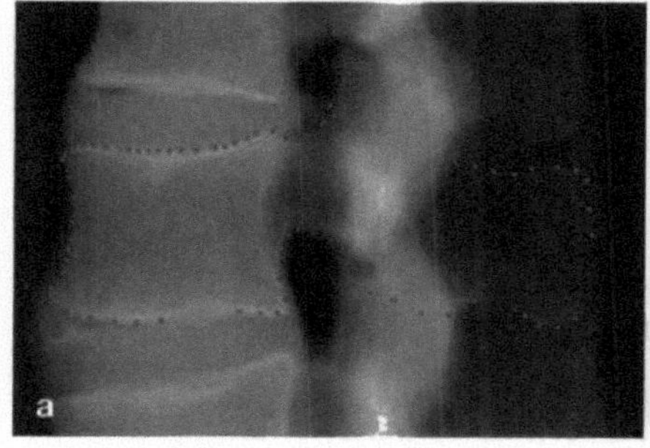

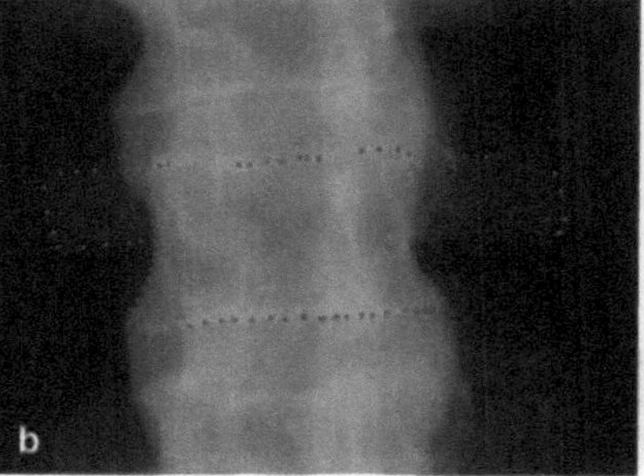

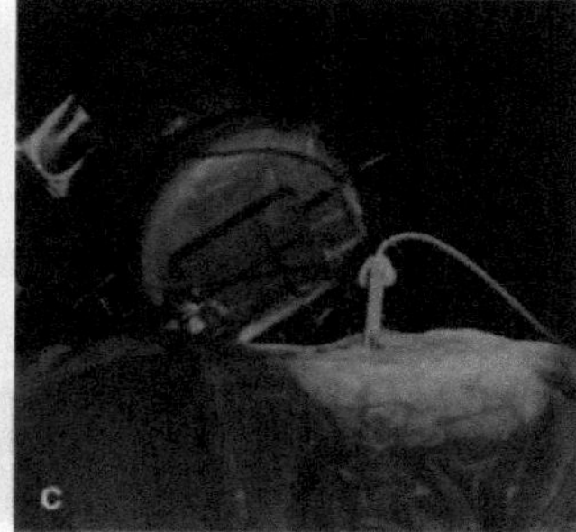

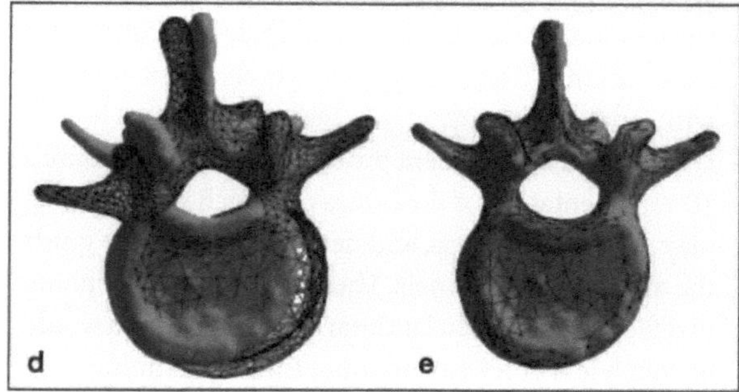

Fig. 5-2a-e. Fluoro-morphing. **a,b** Two calibrated images of the bone are acquired using a C-arm connected to a surgetics system (**c**); **d** shows the deformable model prior to fluoro-morphing compared to an image acquired with CT; **e** shows the result of 3D reconstruction with accurate matching to the reference image. No CT scan is required for this process; all that is needed are a few fluoroscopic images

doing the acquisition, and that is only possible if one can collect 3D shapes intraoperatively, or if one can perform a CT scan during the procedure. The situation is the same during an ACL replacement. In this case, we sometimes perform a notch plasty. Depending of the location and the size of the plasty, the potential anterior impingement pattern may change or disappear. Therefore, if one wants to plan an accurate graft position, one needs to have a model acquired after the notch plasty. None of this can be achieved with CT; all of this is made possible thanks to the bone morphing technique.

2. The time between the beginning of the acquisition and the final result is less than one minute thirty seconds, which is far faster than CT.

3. The issue of the accuracy of bone morphing was one of our major concerns when we began to use this algorithm. During the 10 first TKAs we performed with the system, we checked it and computed the root mean square error between the model and the set of points digitized by the surgeon. We only observed one measurement over one millimeter. This was the consequence of an error on the part of the surgeon in the acquisition of previous anatomical landmarks (not the bone morphing itself). After rejection, bone morphing was done again with an acceptable root mean square error of 0.506 mm for this patient. Therefore, we can state that bone morphing is as accurate as CT, and may be more accurate if we consider points 1 and 3 together.

Advantages over landmarks-based methods:
1. During total knee arthroplasty we need to have a 3D prosthesis center, and since all positioning parameters are linked together, we also want to have global planning. This is not possible if one only takes points into account. A visualization of the cuts prior to actual surgery makes it possible to anticipate difficulties and avoid them, prior to any cuts, which is not possible with landmarks only.

2. During ACL replacement procedures we want to have a 3D representation of the bones on which we could display anisometry maps, and determine targets to guide the drilling of the tunnels. There again, bone morphing meets our needs and a landmarks-based method would be much less efficient and more time-consuming.

3. In all cases, the automatic selection of points (such as the most distal point of the condyles) in the model itself is only possible if one has a 3D model of the bones. This decreases the variability of the measurements inherent in manual measurements made by the surgeon.

4. 3D imaging provides a user-friendly interface, and more importantly, a surgeon-friendly interface (SFI). This concept of SFI includes the idea that the friendly interface is based on a friendly surgical protocol. For fast and efficient surgery, a navigation system must provide instantly-comprehensible on-screen anatomical information to guide the surgeon.

5. During the planning stage, the surgeon can be provided with graphics data on the size of the cuts, the amount of bone that will be removed, the bone defect, and so on. None of this can be done if only geometric data are being used.

There is no doubt that making the 3D morphology of bones available to the surgeon during surgery is a real added value. Since intraoperative CT is not a technique in routine use, the only way to provide such information is the bone morphing technique described in this chapter. In June 2002, we presented bone morphing as a probable new standard in CAOS [7]. Six months later, we are convinced that what was »probable« has become »definite«.

References

1. Fleute M, Lavallée S, Julliard R (1999) Incorporating a statistically based shape model into a system for computer-assisted anterior cruciate ligament surgery. Medical Image Analysis 3: 209–222

2. Kienzle TC III, S Stulberg D, Peshkin M, Quaid A, Lea J, Goswami A, Wu CH (1996) A computer-assisted total knee replacement surgical system using a calibrated robot. In: Taylor R et al. (eds) Computer integrated surgery: technology and clinical applications. MIT Press, Cambridge, MA, pp 409–416

3. Kunz M, Strauss M, Langlotz F, Deuretzbacher G, Rüther W, Nolte LP (2001) A non-CT based total knee arthroplasty system featuring complete soft-tissue balancing. MICCAI, LNCS 2208, pp 409–415

4. Merloz P (2002) Chirurgie du rachis et visage pédiculaire: navigation à base TDM versus fluoronavigation virtuelle. In: Duparc J (ed) Chirurgie orthopédique assistée par ordinateur. Elsevier, Paris, pp 143–149

5. Nizard R (2001) First experience with the Navitrack system for total knee arthroplasty. In: Proceedings of the 21th Annual Meeting of the Israel Orthopaedic Association, Israel

6. Saragaglia D, Picard F, Chaussard C, Montbaron E, Leitner F, Cinquin P (2001) Mise en place des prothèses totales de genou assistée par ordinateur: comparaison avec la technique conventionnelle. Résultats d'une étude prospective randomisée de 50 cas. Revue de Chirurgie Orthopédique 87: 18–28

7. Stindel E, Briard JL, Merloz P, Plaweski S, Dubrana F, Lefevre C, Troccaz JL (2002) Bone morphing: 3D morphological data for total knee arthroplasty. Computer Aided Surgery 7: 156–168

8. Szelisky R, Lavallée S (1996) Matching 3-D anatomical surfaces with non-rigid deformations using octree-splines. Int J Comput Vision 18: 171–186

9. Taylor RH et al. (1996) An image-directed robotic system for precise orthopaedic surgery. In: Taylor RH et al. (eds) Computer integrated surgery: technology and clinical applications. MIT Press, Cambridge, MA, pp 379–396

II Total Hip Arthroplasty

6 Basics of Total Hip Replacement Surgery

B. J. Thomas, J. B. Stiehl

Total hip replacement has emerged as one of the most successful treatments available in modern medicine, with extraordinary gains in pain relief, quality of life, and return to normal function. A large body of knowledge has developed regarding the implants, surgical techniques, and the general outcomes. This review will cover recent concepts in the basic approach but will not deal with special conditions or treatment of complications.

Prosthetic Implants: State of the Art

Cemented Acetabular Components

Long-term data on cemented total hips continue to show that acetabular component loosening is generally more of a problem than femoral stem loosening beyond 10 years. Charnley recognized the potential problem with the cemented acetabular interface, which usually was composed of fibrous tissue after six months. Over the long term, polyethylene wear particles will degrade this interface, and enhance the aseptic loosening problem. In one recent study of patients in whom 62 Charnley total hips were still in place more than 25 years postoperatively, the prevalence of acetabular revision was 15% compared with 7% for femoral stems [4]. There is generally a higher rate of loosening reported for metal-backed cups compared to analogous reports of cemented all-polyethylene components. Huiskes, and others have been able to demonstrate a poor stress transfer to the underlying bone interface with the interposition of a metal surface.

Cementless Acetabular Components

The clinical results of the use of porous-coated cementless acetabular components in a 5- to 10-year time frame has been reported from a number of centers. Reliable fixation is generally obtained in 95% to 99% of cases [6]. Those results however have focused on the fixation of the titanium mesh metal shell employed which has been most extensively studied with the Harris-Galante I (Zimmer, Inc., Warsaw, IN). Originally, the technique was to use a line to line reaming preparation with insertion of screws for additional fixation. More recently, authors recommend a press-fit of the acetabular prosthetic component with a 1 to 2 mm under-reaming of the acetabulum, depending on the rigidity of the porous surface utilized, using screws only in marginal situations such as the revision or compromised bone stock. As follow-up has progressed, an alarming incidence of osteolytic lesions have been identified with certain modular metal shell acetabular components. Poor locking mechanisms, screw holes in the cups, incongruent backside geometries of the metal polyethylene interface, and exaggerated micromotion against rougher metal surfaces have been factors contributing to this problem. In addition, particle debris from fragmented beads, hydroxyapatite particles, or bone fragments have added to this problem. Recent innovations such as improved locking mechanisms, polished metal back-sided surfaces, or even non-modular implants such as the Trabecular Metal Cup (Zimmer, Inc., Warsaw, IN) with heat pressed polyethylene have been measures to deal with this problem. Though many European centers continue to use threaded screw in cups, the early American experience was dismal, and most centers have abandoned this device.

Acetabular Components
With Alternative Bearing Surfaces

The clinical performance of cementless porous-coated acetabular components over 10 years indicates that problems with component fixation are rare. However, the resulting osteolysis associated with polyethylene wear and modular components has continued to be a concern and has led to heightened interest in alternative bearing surfaces to substitute for polyethylene as the articulation with the femoral head. These alternatives include metal-on-metal and ceramic bearing surfaces, and cross-linked polyethylene.

Chrome cobalt metal-on-metal bearing surfaces have had over 20 years of European clinical experience with favorable results and lack of osteolysis. In one American study of metal-on-metal hip replacements, 70 hips were evaluated at an average of 5.2 years [12]. There was one revision for acetabular loosening, two acetabular component revisions for dislocation, and no femoral component loosening. There was no measurable wear on radiographs and there was no evidence of acetabular osteolysis. It should be noted that these were cemented acetabular components. An underlying concern that yet remains unknown is the long-term problem posed by increase levels of metallic ions in the tissues from these devices. A recent retrieval analysis demonstrated disturbing histological findings in a few cases where there had been impingement or mechanical failure of the metal-on-metal devices creating a concern if wear formation becomes exaggerated. A final area of interest is the cup arthroplasty model such as the McMinn prosthesis which is a metal-on-metal resurfacing device. This device has the advantage of preserving the proximal femur but the disadvantage of proximal fracture that may occur in a few cases as the femur is weakened with insertion.

The other potential hard-on-hard bearing surface is ceramic. The two primary materials are aluminum oxide and zirconium oxide. Both materials have been used as femoral head bearing surfaces against polyethylene but alumina has also been used in a ceramic-on-ceramic configuration. Polyethylene wear against ceramic heads has been reported to be 5 to 10 times lower than that against metal heads in wear simulator studies; however, in clinical radiographic wear measurements the results have been extremely variable. There is conflicting data re-garding ceramic bearing surfaces. Some studies have shown significantly lower radiographic wear rates of the ceramic head against the polyethylene, while an equal number of studies have not shown any significant difference in wear rate. Two major issues associated with the use of ceramic heads are cost and breakage. There have been a number of case reports of fracture of ceramic heads; however, with current specifications fractures should be a rare occurrence. Ceramic-on-ceramic wear rates have been reported to be 10 times less than the lowest polyethylene wear rates. However, a high incidence of lysis and wear has been documented for at least one alumina-on-alumina hip of early design.

The most popular recent approach to enhance the wear characteristics of standard ultra-high molecular weight polyethylene has been to use various methods of cross-linking of polyethylene. A number of highly cross-linked polyethylenes have recently been approved by the U.S. Food and Drug Administration and are currently available on the American market. Laboratory testing would suggest that these materials may reduce clinical wear rates by a factor of ten but these results are unknown in clinical experience. Numerous studies are expected in the coming years that will better delineate the expected rate of wear and osteolysis using the alternative bearing surfaces of metal-on-metal, ceramic-on-ceramic, ceramic-on-polyethylene, metal-on-cross-linked polyethylene, and ceramic-on-cross-linked polyethylene.

Femoral Components

Cemented Stems

The cement technique is recognized as an important factor in increasing the longevity of cemented stem fixation. In the late 1970s, the so-called »second-generation« cement technique was introduced and included the use of an intra-medullary plug, pulsatile lavage of the medullary canal, the use of a cement gun, retrograde filling of the femoral canal with doughy cement, pressurization of the cement, and use of a forged cobalt-chrome stem with rounded corners. Long-term studies at 10 to 15 years and beyond document excellent results with cemented stems implanted with this technique [2]. Despite the excellent long-term results of second-generation cementing, a number of changes in stem design and cement technique occurred in an attempt to further improve fixation of cemented stems. Laboratory evidence indicated that debonding of cement from the stem was potentially the initiating factor in failure of many cemented stems. This provided the rationale for increasing the strength of the bond between stem and cement, which was achieved in some stem designs by increasing the surface roughness of the stem, usually over the proximal portion, and/or the addition of a thin layer of polymethylmethacrylate (pre-coating). Porosity reduction also was introduced in an attempt to increase the fatigue strength of the cement. The major methods of achieving this were with either centrifugation or vacuum mixing. An enhanced stem surface and porosity reduction were components of what was termed »third-generation« cement technique. Recent studies have reported a higher rate of loosening of osteolysis with pre-coated stems attributed to thin cement mantles leading to cement fracture, fragmentation, and subsequent osteolysis or progressive circumferential bone interface osteolysis with relative preservation of the cement-metal interface. As a result, awareness of the importance of stem surface finish as a potential factor in the success or failure of cemented stems has increased.

Surface Finish

A number of clinical series have indicated that at least some stem designs are associated with a higher failure rate with a roughened surface compared with a smooth surface. The Exeter, Iowa, and T-28 stems have had a higher incidence of loosening and osteolysis reported with a rough stem surface finish than with a smooth stem. However, some stems with roughened surfaces have performed well in the 5- to 10-year time frame. Apparently there is an interaction of surface finish with other factors such as stem geometry and length that is important in achieving long-term stability of cemented stems. If a roughened or grit blast surface is applied to a cemented stem it is apparently important that the stem be rotationally stable so that debonding does not occur. Once debonding does occur, a rough stem is more likely to generate wear debris leading to aggressive osteolysis [7].

Charnley Cemented Stem

The most extensively documented results in the literature are with the use of the Charnley cemented stem. In one study of polished flatback Charnley cemented stems, 69 patients (93 hips) younger than 50 years old were followed for 20 to 25 years. Only 5% of stems had been revised whereas an additional 8% were radiographically loose. In another recent study, the results of the Charnley cemented stem were dramatically different than previous reports, with a known rate of aseptic loosening of 2.3% at 5 years, infection rate of 1.4%, dislocation rate of 5%, revision rate of 3.2%, and a radiographic gross failure rate of 5.2% [3]. These results represented an overall failure rate of approximately 10% within 5 years, which may be more representative of the norm rather than the typical reports in the literature that originate from dedicated total joint centers.

Cementless Stems

The use of cementless fixation for primary THA continues to be a popular approach and these stems have been quite successful in achieving fixation consistently. The major problems observed with cementless stems are thigh pain and stress shielding. A number of different uncemented stem designs have been in widespread clinical use for which midterm clinical results of 5 to 10 years have recently become available. Fully porous coated devices such as the AML stem have been noted to have 98% survivorship at 10 years, but substantial changes in the surrounding bone stock have been realized. Proximally coated devices with either porous surfaces or hydroxyapatite coatings have shown survivorship of at least 95% at 10 years, but may have higher rates of thigh pain. Bone preservation however has been shown to be greater when comparing bone densitometry and this may be a valuable trade off in younger patients where long term revision may be inevitable and ease of revision is desirable.

Extensively Coated Stems

Uncemented stems that have a porous coating extending over most or all of the surface previously have been fabricated of cobalt-chrome because of the difficulty in obtaining adequate stem strength with an extensively coated titanium stem [10]. Long-term results beyond 10 years with a fully coated cobalt-chrome stem are documented in the literature. In one recent study that specifically examined the issue of thigh pain in extensively coated stems, a proximally coated stem was found to have twice the incidence of thigh pain as a fully coated stem [1]. The incidence of thigh pain with a fully coated stem was equivalent to that of a cemented stem. A number of studies have suggested that cylindrical cobalt-chrome stems seem to have the best clinical results in terms of thigh pain when they are fully coated rather than proximally coated.

Proximally Coated Stems

Certain proximally coated stems have been associated with a higher incidence of osteolysis, loosening, and revision. One design feature that has been associated with a higher incidence of distal osteolysis is the presence of non-circumferential proximal porous coating. Better results have been documented for proximally coated titanium hips with a circumferential coating. In one series of 100 anatomic proximally coated titanium hips in 88 patients followed for an average of 7.1 years, there was only one revision for loosening, a 5% incidence of thigh pain, and no incidence of femoral osteolysis. Another proximally coated implant system with recently documented long-term results is the Omnifit cementless total hip (Osteonics Corporation, Allendale, NJ). In one series of 76 hips in 67 patients with an average age of 45 years at surgery who were followed for an average of 10 years, two stems and one cup were revised for aseptic loosening for an incidence of 2.6% on the femoral side and 1.3% on the acetabular side. Thigh pain was present in only three patients [5]. Because of the increased incidence of thigh pain and loosening with certain devices, there have been a number of concepts to improve design. There has been a focus on matching the variability of the proximal/distal geometry mismatch often encountered with the normal human femur. Secondly, designs have focused on achieving proximal fit and fixation by abuting the heavy anterior and posterior structures of the femoral neck. Finally, most recent designs have a fully circumferential proximal coating.

Tapered Stems

Another approach to cementless stem fixation has been the use of a stem with a tapered geometry to achieve mechanical stability in the proximal portion of the femur by wedging the component into place rather than using a cylindrical reamer. This design has been a popular concept in Europe for many years. Tapered stems have been used with traditional porous-coated surfaces and roughened titanium surfaces, with or without hydroxyapatite coating. Intermediate-term results are now available for a number of tapered stems with proximal porous coating. Both titanium and cobalt-chrome tapered proximally porous-coated stems have been used with a high degree of success.

In one series of 100 hips (average age of patient, 37 years) followed for a mean of 10.2 years, results showed no femoral loosening. Femoral cortical lysis occurred in seven patients but was considered to be a major event in one. The component used in this study was a plasma spray proximally coated titanium hip (Taperloc, Biomet, Warsaw, IN). Similar results have been reported with a proximally coated tapered cobalt-chrome hip (Trilock, DePuy, Inc, Warsaw, IN). Results of a review of 66 hips followed for an average of 10 years (range, 8.3 to 11.6; average patient age 62 years) showed only one stem revised for loosening and no cases of distal lysis [10].

Hydroxyapatite

The use of hydroxyapatite to help achieve fixation of uncemented femoral stems is a subject of interest. The possibility that hydroxyapatite could increase polyethylene wear and increase the incidence of osteolysis is cause for concern, as well as the possibility that the hydroxyapatite coating may resorb over time and thus fail to maintain long-term fixation. A multicenter study of 316 hips in 282 patients in which a hydroxyapatite coated stem was used assessed patients for an average 8.1 years, only one stem (0.3%) was revised for aseptic loosening and there were no instances of intra-medullary femoral osteolysis [8]. The results of the use of hydroxyapatite with this particular stem did not support concerns over increased wear or osteolysis with a hydroxyapatite stem. In addition, the ability of hydroxyapatite to produce a significant barrier to intrusion of wear debris has been shown in animal studies. This may be an optimum application for the hydroxyapatite technology as the surface not only enhances bone ongrowth to the device but creates a stable implant surface environment for long term stability and bone stock preservation. The acetabulum on the other hand has been a poor application for hydroxyapatite, and retrieval studies have implicated the exaggerated micromotion expected about these devices to cause early particulate debris to form which may exaggerate wear of the polyethylene bearing surface.

Surgical Technique: Options

The primary goal of total hip arthroplasty is the anatomic reconstruction of the hip joint. Mechanically, the goal is to create a stable hip joint throughout the range of motion, while restoring offset and limb lengths. Adequate exposure is required to achieve proper placement of the prosthetic components and should not be compromised simply to minimize the length of the incision. The hip surgeon should be familiar with the anterolateral as well as the posterolateral approaches to the hip since both are useful in particular patients. Preoperative planning is important to achieving success at surgery [11].

Preoperative Planning

A thorough radiographic evaluation of the hip in anteroposterior (a.-p.) and lateral projections should be performed preoperatively. For the a.-p. projection, place both ankles in 15 degrees of internal rotation to position the head and neck parallel to the coronal plane. Center the beam on the symphysis pubis and ensure the proximal femoral shaft is included in the radiograph. The radiographs should include both the acetabulum and the proximal femur. When the affected hip is fixed in external rotation, template the normal hip. Using the a.-p. radiograph, position the template 35–45 degrees to the teardrop so that the medial aspect of the cup abuts the teardrop and the superior-lateral cup is not uncovered.

Anterolateral Approach

The anterolateral (Watson-Jones) approach has been popular for total joint arthroplasty. This approach, combined with release of the abductor mechanism either by trochanteric osteotomy or by release of the anterior portion of the gluteus medius and minimus from the trochanter, offers excellent exposure of the acetabulum and the femoral shaft. The interval between the tensor fascia lata and the gluteus medius is innervated by the superior gluteal nerve, and care must be taken not to dissect more than four centimeters proximal to the tip of the greater trochanter, as a portion of the medius and tensor fascia lata can be denervated. With this precaution, the approach can be safely used for total hip arthroplasty.

The patient is placed supine on the operating table, and a »bump« (rolled sheet) is placed underneath the ischial tuberosity to bring the hemipelvis forward and to allow the buttock to hang freely down from the area of dissection. The area is prepared with povidone-iodine and the lower extremity draped free.

A straight incision is made centered over the greater trochanter but crossing the posterior aspect of the trochanter. A common error when using this approach is to not make the incision posterior enough, thereby allowing the soft tissues to impinge during adduction and external rotation. An anteriorly placed incision makes exposure more difficult, risking injury to the neurovascular bundles during flexion, adduction, and external rotation as the capsule is approached. The incision is taken down through subcutaneous tissue to the tensor fascia lata. The fascia at the distal aspect of the wound is incised and a tonsil clamp inserted to elevate the fascia from the underlying vastus lateralis. The fascia is split proximally, once again taking care to stay toward the posterior aspect of the greater trochanter. Proximal to the trochanter the incision is carried at the interval between the tensor fascia lata and gluteus medius. The fascia is retracted anteriorly and posteriorly. The vessels encountered between the tensor fascia lata and gluteus medius are cauterized with the Bovie cautery, after which the curved end of a Hohmann retractor is used to retract the gluteus muscle proximally and laterally away from the anterior joint capsule.

The hip is then externally rotated, and the origin of the vastus lateralis on the vastus ridge is released, once again with the Bovie cautery. The anterior capsule is dissected free using the periosteal elevator. At this point, the anterior portion of the gluteus medius insertion into the greater trochanter is released with the Bovie cautery and the tendon tagged with a non-absorbable suture; alternatively, a comparatively small anterior trochanteric osteotomy is performed. The tendon is released until adequate exposure can be obtained to allow placement of a retractor over the superior aspect of the acetabulum. The rectus tendon is elevated from the capsule and a sharp Hohmann retractor placed on the anterior rim of the acetabulum (◘ Fig. 6-1). Care must be taken during placement of this retractor, as the neurovascular bundle lies in close proximity medially. Palpating the medial anterosuperior aspect of the acetabulum is an important safety precaution at this stage before placing the sharp Hohmann retractor. After adequate retraction has been

achieved, the capsule may be incised using a T-shaped incision based once again at the acetabular rim. The hip may then be dislocated by further external rotation and abduction. The exposure may be extended down the thigh by extending the incision in the fascia lata distally and splitting the vastus lateralis fascia, then splitting the vastus fibers with a periosteal elevator and elevating the vastus from the surface of the femur with a Bennett retractor.

Hardinge Approach

A modification of the anterolateral approach has been described by Hardinge that attempts to preserve the functional continuity of the gluteus medius and vastus lateralis muscles. With this approach, the fascia lata is divided throughout the length of the incision and reflected anteriorly and posteriorly. The trochanteric bursa is excised, after which the anterior insertion of the gluteus medius and minimus are mobilized using the Bovie cautery to incise in line with the fibers from the posterior one-third of the tendinous portion of the gluteus medius, across the insertion of the anterior two-thirds of the gluteus medius, and into the fascia of the vastus lateralis. This maneuver forms a continuous fascial layer and leaves a stump of tendon attached to the bone as well as a portion attached to the muscle. The anterior fibers of the medius tendon are then split bluntly for 5 to 6 cm in the direction of their fibers, as are the fibers of the vastus lateralis (◘ Fig. 6-2). The gluteus minimus is progressively released from the anterior trochanter using the Bovie cautery. The anterior capsule may be exposed using the periosteal elevator, after which capsulotomy may be performed with external rotation of the femur, allowing dislocation of the femoral head. The bulk of the gluteus medius is retracted superiorly with a sharp Hohmann retractor. Dislocation of the femoral head requires flexion. adduction, and external rotation. after which femoral neck osteotomy is performed. Exposure of the acetabulum is obtained by placing anterior and posterior retractors at the margins of the acetabulum. The danger of a gluteus medius splitting approach is that if the dissection is carried too far proximally the superior gluteal nerve may be injured as it traverses the medius muscle, denervating its anterior portion.

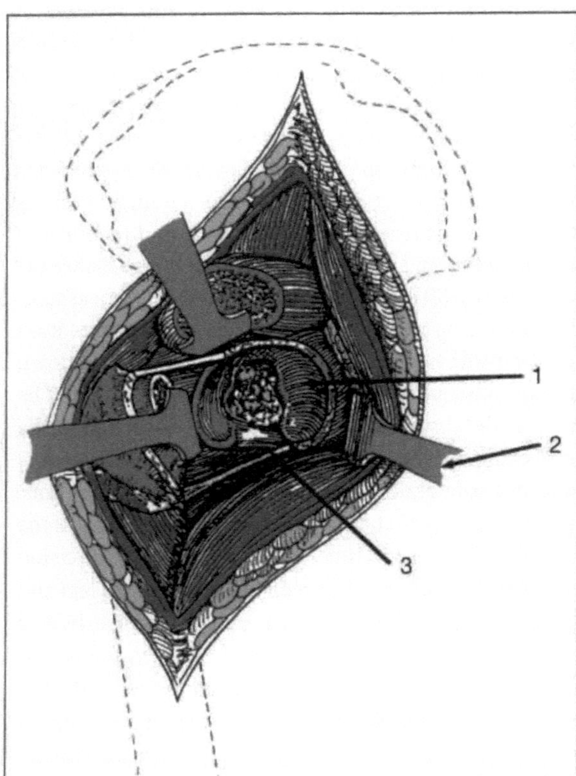

◘ **Fig. 6-1.** Anterolateral approach to the hip. *1* Anterior acetabulum; *2* Retractor placed under the rectus muscle over the anterior lip of the acetabulum; *3* Transverse cotyloid ligament.

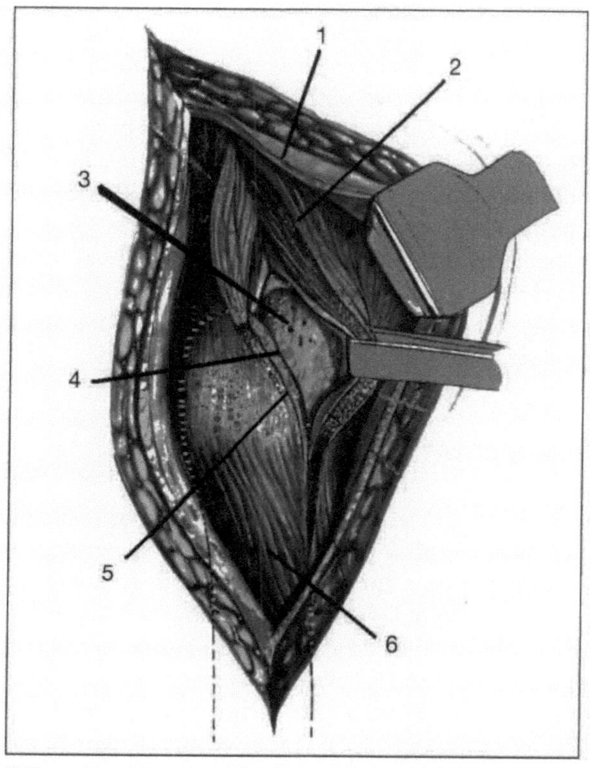

Fig. 6-2. Posterolateral approach to the hip. *1* The femur is internally rotated to stress the posterior external rotators; *2* pyriformis tendon; *3* superior and inferior gemellus, and obturator internus muscles; *4* quadratus femoris muscle; *5* retracted posterior gluteus medius muscle.

Posterolateral Approach

For the posterolateral approach, place the patient in the lateral decubitus position. Ensure that the operating table is parallel to the floor and that the patient is adequately secured to the table to improve accuracy of the external alignment guides. The patient is positioned in the lateral decubitus position and firmly held with padded kidney rests and back support. The skin is prepared with povidone-iodine and the affected limb prepared and draped free. The incision is centered over the greater trochanter and curves posteriorly in its proximal line while following the femoral shaft distally. The fascia lata is split in line with the incision, and the gluteus maximus fibers are spread by blunt dissection at the proximal aspect of the wound. The wound is covered with moist lap sponges, and a Chamley retractor is placed. The leg is maximally internally rotated and the piriformis tendon exposed with

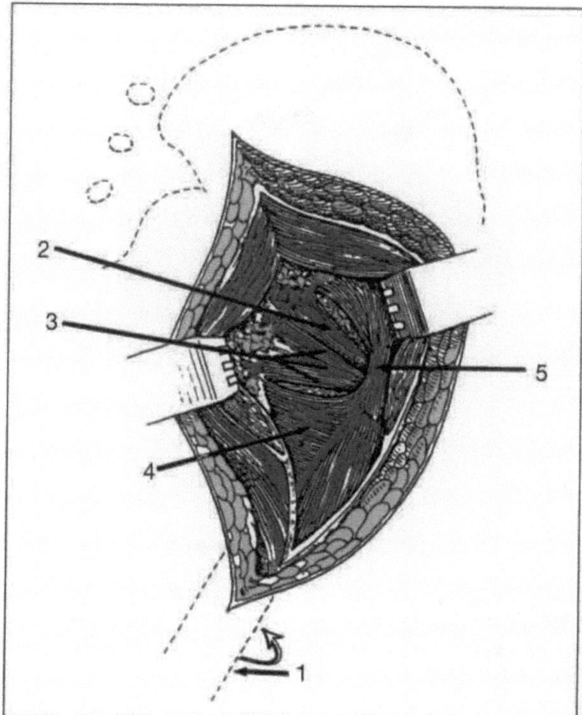

Fig. 6-3. Posterolateral approach

blunt dissection (**Fig. 6-3**). The tendon is found by retracting the posterior border of the gluteus medius, and palpating the tendon as it inserts on the posterosuperior aspect of the greater trochanter. A narrow, bent Hohmann retractor may be placed extracapsularly but deep to the gluteus medius and minimus to facilitate the exposure. The insertions of the piriformis, gemelli, and obturator internus are then released as close to their insertion as possible using electrocautery (**Fig. 6-4**). The proximal portion of the quadratus femoris is also released with electrocautery, and branches of the medial femoral circumflex vessels are cauterized. The obturator externus is identified deep to the quadratus femoris and is divided as well. The tendon of the gluteus maximus is identified as it inserts on the proximal femur and is released with electrocautery after passing a Kelly clamp deep to the tendon to protect the sciatic nerve. The vessels at the distal portion of the gluteus insertion are then cauterized. The piriformis and conjoined tendons are tagged with non-absorbable sutures for reattachment at the end of the case. The capsular incision is begun superiorly and

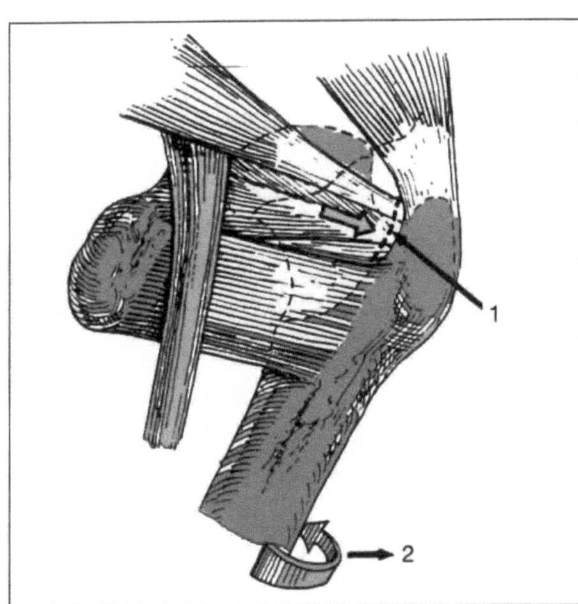

Fig. 6-4. Posterolateral approach to the hip. *1* undertension, the externally rotators are incised at the bony insertion; *2* note internal rotation of the hip joint.

carried parallel to the acetabular rim as far distally as possible. The incision is converted to a T incision cutting from the posterior acetabular rim anteriorly to meet the longitudinal incision. Dislocation of the femoral head is achieved by adduction, flexion, and internal rotation of the leg. A bone hook may facilitate the dislocation. The remaining soft tissue is removed from the posterior femoral neck back to the intertrochanteric crest. The hip is held in internal rotation, with the tibia vertical and the foot toward the ceiling. The neck is exposed with a bent Hohmann retractor superiorly and an Aufranc retractor inferiorly. The neck osteotomy guide is then positioned over the femur, taking care to avoid varus or valgus positioning. Electrocautery is used to mark the femoral neck at the proposed site of the osteotomy, which is then carried out using the reciprocating saw. A curved Aufranc retractor is placed underneath the proximal femur and the tip passed up over the anterior margin of the acetabulum. The tip of the retractor now lies inside the pelvis and allows anterior retraction of the femur to expose the acetabulum. Retraction is completed by placement of an Aufranc retractor inferiorly, a wide, bent Hohmann retractor posteriorly, and a stout Steinmann pin superiorly into the ilium.

The inferior Aufranc retractor is placed first outside the inferior acetabular ligament while soft tissue debridement is carried out and then just superior to the ligament, levered over the inferior bony lip of the acetabulum. The wide, bent Hohmann is gently tapped into the bone of the ischium after being advanced between the posterior capsule and the acetabular labrum. Finally, a Steinmann pin is placed about 2 cm proximal to the superior acetabular rim to retract the abductors. All soft tissue is removed from the rim and base of the acetabulum so the acetabular fossa is well visualized.

Component Placement

One key to proper acetabular component positioning is adequate surgical exposure. Following femoral neck resection, pass a curved retractor, which straddles the pubis, or a blunt cobra over the anterior column to displace the femur anteriorly. Position a second retractor at the acetabular notch, inferior to the transverse acetabular ligament. An additional retractor may be positioned posteriorly to retract the capsule or short external rotators. Care should be taken to position retractors to avoid injury to the sciatic nerve. Obtain an unobstructed view of the acetabulum. Excise the entire labrum and remove osteophytes to identify the true anterior and posterior acetabular margins. Release or resect the transverse ligament, together with any accompanying osteophytes. A branch of the obturator artery is often encountered. Clear all soft tissue from the fovea to define the true medial wall.

The goal of acetabular reaming is to restore the center of the original acetabulum. Initially employ a grater 6–8 mm smaller than the anticipated acetabular component size to deepen the acetabulum to the level determined by preoperative templating. Subsequent reaming should proceed in 1–2 mm increments. Center the reamers in the acetabulum until the deepened socket becomes a true hemisphere. Use a curette to free all cysts of fibrous tissue. Pack any defects densely with cancellous bone. Under-reaming of the acetabulum is dependent on bone quality and the size of the acetabular component. A 1–2 mm under-ream is used since soft bone will more readily accommodate a greater press-fit of the acetabular component than sclerotic bone.

The preoperative a.-p. X-ray can help determine the ideal abduction angle. The lateral ilium is a useful landmark as an intraoperative guide to a proper abduction angle. In a normal acetabulum with good lateral coverage, if the implanted socket lies flush with a normal lateral pillar, the abduction angle is usually correct. However, degenerative sockets often have deficient lateral covering. The preoperative NP X-ray can be helpful in determining how much of the acetabular component should be left uncovered to provide the proper implant abduction angle.

The most reliable method for determining proper anteversion is the use of the bony landmark. Other methods are subject to error through a change in patient position during the procedure. Defining the bony landmarks of the ischium and pubis during exposure greatly facilitates proper acetabular component position. The plane created by the pubis and the ischium can serve as a guide for proper acetabular shell orientation. The cup should be slightly more anteverted than the pubislischial plane. This relationship should remain constant regardless of the depth of reaming.

Depending on the quality of the prepared bone, select the acetabular trial equal to or 1 mm larger in diameter than the final acetabular reamer size. Using shell and liner trials in conjunction with the femoral component trials aids in ensuring optimum position of the components. Place the shell trial in an anatomic orientation with an abduction 35–50 degrees to the transverse plane and 15–30 degrees anteversion. Following positioning and seating of the acetabular shell trial, place a liner trial into the trial shell. With the femoral component trials in position, assess stability and range of motion. Couple the liner trial with the shell trial in the desired position.

Before implanting the real prosthesis, take the hip through a full range of motion and stability assessment with all trial components in position. Anteversion is typically set at 15–30 degrees. Establish this orientation through visual confirmation. After confirming alignment, impact the prosthesis into position. Given the under-reaming of the acetabulum, rim contact will occur before dome seating occurs.

To assess the combined anteversion of the femoral stem and acetabular component, place the patient in the lateral decubitus position with the operative hip gently flexed and internally rotated until the circumference of the femoral head becomes coplanar with the opening of the acetabular liner, placing the axis of the femoral neck perpendicular to the liner face. The angle between horizontal and the internally rotated operative leg provides an estimate of combined anteversion of the acetabular component and the femoral stem. Combined anteversion of 30–40 degrees is recommended.

References

1. Barrack RL, Paprosky W, Butler RA, Palafox A, Szuszczewicz E, Myers L (2000) Patients perception of pain after total hip arthroplasty. J Arthroplasty 15:590–596
2. Bourne RB, Rorabeck CH, Skutek M, Mikkelsen S, Winemaker M, Robertson D (1998) The Harris design-2 total hip replacement fixed with so-called second-generation cementing techniques: A ten to fifteen-year follow-up. J Bone Joint Surg Am 80:1775–1780
3. Callaghan JJ, Forest EE, Olejniczak JP, Goetz DD, Johnston RC (1998) Charnley total hip arthroplasty in patients less than fifty years old: A twenty to twenty-five-year follow-up note. J Bone Joint Surg Am 82: 704–714
4. Callaghan JJ, Albright JC, Goetz DD, Olejniczak JP, Johnston RC (2000) Charnley total hip arthroplasty with cement: Minimum twenty-five-year follow-up. J Bone Joint Surg Am 82:487–497
5. Capello WN, D'Antonio JA, Feinberg JR, Manley MT (1997) Hydroxyapatite-coated total hip femoral components in patients less than fifty years old. Clinical and radiographic results after five to eight years of follow-up. J Bone Joint Surg Am 79:1023–1029
6. Clohisy JC, Harris WH (1999) The Harris-Galante porous-coated acetabular component with screw fixation: An average ten-year follow-up study. J Bone Joint Surg Am 81:66–73
7. Crowninshield RD, Jennings JD, Laurent ML, Maloney WJ (1998) Cemented femoral component surface finish mechanics. Clin Orthop 355:90–102
8. D'Antonio JA, Capello WN, Manley MT, Geesink R (2001) Hydroxyapatite femoral stems for total hip arthroplasty: 10- to 13-year follow-up. Clin Orthop Rel Res 393:101–111
9. McAuley JP, Moore KD, Culpepper WJ II, Engh CA (1998) Total hip arthroplasty with porous-coated prostheses fixed without cement in patients who are sixty-five years of age or older. J Bone Joint Surg Am 80:1648–1655
10. Purtill JJ, Rothman RH, Hozack WJ, Sharkey PF (2001) Total hip arthroplasty using two different cementless tapered stems. Clin Orthop Rel Res 393:121–127.
11. Thomas BJ, Amstutz HC, Yao J (1991) Surgical approaches to the hip joint. In: Amstutz HC (ed) Hip arthroplasty. Churchill Livingstone, New York
12. Udomkiat P, Dorr LD, Wan Z. (2002) Cementless hemispheric porous-coated sockets implanted with press-fit technique without screws average ten-year follow-up. J BoneJoint Surg Am 84-A(7):1195-2000

II A Navigation: Total Hip Arthroplasty

7 Mini-Incision Techniques and Navigation for Total Hip

A. M. DiGioia III, A. Y. Plakseychuk, B. Jaramaz

Introduction

Before the era of navigation surgery, total hip arthroplasty has evolved to the degree that, we thought, it is one of the most predictable and efficacious procedures that ortho-pedic surgery has to offer. Clinical experience with computer-assisted hip systems demonstrated in recent years that synergistic combinations of surgeons and computerized machines may produce results that are better than would be possible otherwise.

Our clinical experience in navigation for total hip arthroplasty is based on the HipNav system [2, 3]. The HipNav system was developed to permit not only accurate placement of implants, but also to couple and tightly integrate preoperative planning with intra-operative execution. The system also can be used as a measurement device that provides timely and accurate intra-operative information to surgeons like the position of the bone, tools, cutting guide orientation or location of the im-plants.

The navigation system includes two components: a preoperative planner with the range of motion simula-tor and an intra-operative image guided navigation. In the planning phase, patient's CT scan is electronically transferred to the planning site and processed to extract bone contours. Wide variety of the implants are available in the planning station database. Implant design, size, orientation, leg length and offset are interactively dis-played. The full 3D virtual anatomic model of the pelvis and femur with artificial joint implanted is taken through the test of range of motion and stability (◘ Fig. 7-1). Joint kinematics are simulated to test and maximize the safe range of motion by minimizing both prosthetic and bone impingement. Once the surgeon has optimized the plan and placement of implant components, all relevant para-meters are stored for the image guided surgical proce-dure. The HipNav intra-operative guidance system navi-gation system consists of software that registers and matches a preoperative CT scan to the position of the patient on the operating table and an infrared optical localization system (Optotrak, Northern Digital Inc, Waterloo, Ontario, Canada) equipped with light emitting diodes (LED) for tracking the position of the pelvis and surgical tools. Prior validation tests have shown high accuracy of the navigation system that matches the pelvic geometry within one millimeter and one degree [7, 13, 14]. The HipNav system developed in such a way that only additional five to ten minutes of OR time required to use the system.

Our clinical experience with computer-assisted navi-gation in THA consists of more than 250 cases at present time. All patients are included in the Total Joint Registry for follow-up and data collection. In this chapter we would like to discuss accuracy of acetabular component placement with mechanical guides and with navigation system, as well as functional results following computer-assisted THA with mini-incision technique.

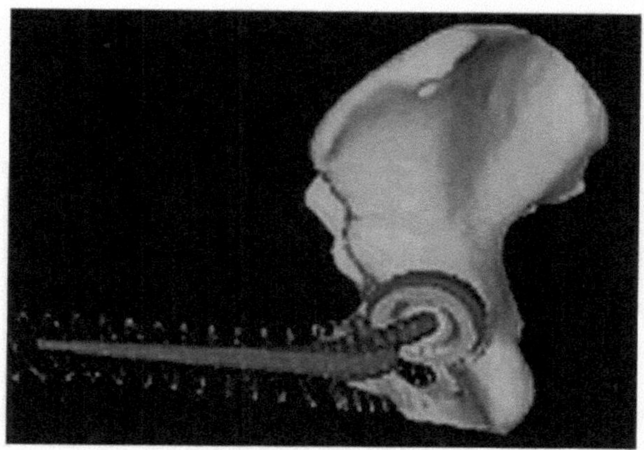

◘ **Fig. 7-1.** The pre-operative planner and range of motion simulator

Accuracy of the Mechanical Acetabular Alignment Guides in THA

Acetabular component orientation has been shown to be one significant factor affecting the risk of dislocation, impingement, pelvic osteolysis, acetabular migration and wear between components in patients undergoing hip arthroplasty. There have been numerous reports on the optimal orientation of the acetabular component in total hip arthroplasty with wide variety of »best parameters« [15]. Harris [5] suggested an abduction angle of 30° and anteversion angle of 20°; Harkess [4] recommended an abduction angle of 45° and anteversion angle of 15±5°; and Lewinnek et al. [9] considered an abduction angle of 40±10°, and an anteversion angle of 15±10°. Although improvements continue to be made in the design of implants and methods of fixation and the development of materials that better resist wear, little effort has been made to provide surgeons with more accurate tool guides or strategies to improve the reproducibility of implant alignment.

The position of the acetabular component is dependent on the orientation of the bony acetabulum and on the position of the patient's pelvis on the operating table. Despite many techniques of stabilizing and positioning the patient's pelvis, most surgeons will admit that it is very difficult to precisely know how the patient's pelvis is oriented during surgery. McCollum and Gray [11] reported that the pelvis may not be reproducibly or correctly aligned with the patient in the lateral decubitus position and that pelvic malalignment could lead to improper cup alignment. Numerous terms are used to describe acetabular orientation including inclination, anteversion, cover, abduction, tilt, opening and flexion [1, 6]. Murray [12] proposed radiographic, operative and anatomical definitions of the acetabular component position, depending on the method of assessment.

The difference in the three definitions of cup orientation results from rotation around different axes after initial abduction of the cup, starting from the face down position (◪ Fig. 7-2a). The operative orientation is associated with the mechanical guides used to align the cup during surgery. During surgical placement, if the pelvis is oriented in the correct position, the cup is initially abducted around the sagittal axis (◪ Fig. 7-2b) and then is flexed around the transverse axis (◪ Fig. 7-2d). The anatomic orientation can be recovered from CT or MRI and consisted of abduction around the sagittal axis and rotation (anteversion) around long body axis (◪ Fig. 7-2c).

Abduction and anteversion are the most commonly used terms to describe true »anatomic« alignment, but is not really what surgeons achieve during surgery. It is important to understand that operative orientation of 45° of abduction and 20° of flexion will be different compared to anatomic orientation with the same set of numbers. Nomograms to convert operative cup orientation to anatomical orientation are available in the literature [12]. All measurements in this particular study were based on abduction and flexion, as our goal was to determine the reliability and reproducibility of the operative definition for acetabular component placement with the mechanical alignment guide.

The purpose of this investigation was to determine the variation of the angular orientation of the acetabular implant placed using the mechanical guide as the sole source of alignment compared to the desired angles, and whether the orientation of the pelvis on the operating room table changes significantly throughout the operation.

The clinical trial was initiated in 1996 using the hip navigation system strictly as an intra-operative measurement tool in seventy-eight patients with 82 hips (4 patients had bilateral hip replacements). No guidance in placement of the cup was provided to the surgeon by the navigation system. studied. The average patient age was 63 years old, (range 37–81), with 40 women and 38 men. The affected hip was right in 50 and left in 32. The Zimmer cup was positioned using the Zimmer Acetabular Cup Impactor-Positioner mechanical guide with an »A-Frame« (Zimmer Inc, Warsaw, IN) in all 82 hips. In 74 of 82 hips the cup position was quantified during surgery by the computer-assisted navigation tool. Eight measurements were not available because of difficulties related to software problems (6 hips) and optical targets visibility during the operation (2 hips).

All patients were positioned and stabilized on the operating table in the lateral decubitus position by orienting the patient's trunk along the longitudinal axis of the operating table. The goal was to align the anterior pelvic plane parallel to the longitudinal axis and perpendicular to the surface of the operating table. The

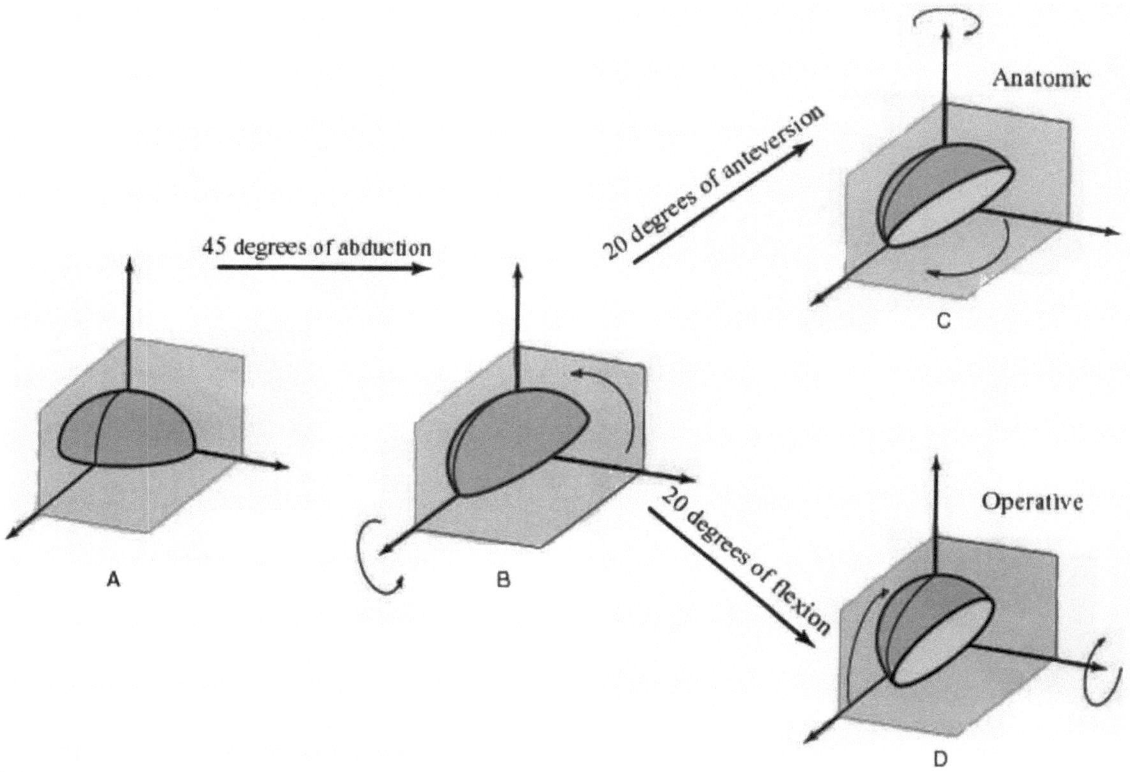

Fig. 7-2a-d. Difference in anatomical and operative cup orientation

pelvis was stabilized with anterior and posterior blocks, supplemented with a suction beanbag. Blocks were placed outside of the beanbag with an anterior block at the level of the pubis and posterior block over the mid sacrum. The beanbag was positioned around the chest prior to inflation in an attempt to prevent anterior or posterior displacement of the torso. A posterolateral approach to the hip was performed in all cases by one experienced surgeon (AMD), who also performed acetabular preparation and implantation in each of the cases. The Zimmer Trilogy press-fit acetabular component with cluster holes (Zimmer Inc, Warsaw, IN) was used in all 82 hips.

The cup was first positioned using the Zimmer Acetabular Cup Impactor-Positioner (Zimmer Inc, Warsaw, IN) with the goal being to orient the cup in 45 degrees abduction and 20 degrees of forward flexion (**Fig 7-3**). Theoretically, when the pelvis is properly oriented, 45° of abduction is achieved by positioning the »A-Frame« parallel with the operating table, and 20° of forward flexion is achieved by positioning the appropriate shoulder of the »A-Frame« parallel with patient's longitudinal axis. When the surgeon was satisfied with the alignment, using only the mechanical guide, the actual orientation of the cup was measured by the navigation tool and documented. During this initial phase of cup positioning with the mechanical guide, the surgeon was blinded to the information provided by the navigation system. Subsequently, after recording mechanical guide alignment measurements, the surgeon was informed of the precise computer anatomic orientation of the acetabular component and could perform necessary corrections to the alignment. For all measurements of cup alignment and pelvic orientation, the pelvic coordinate system or frame of reference (abduction 0, flexion 0, version 0) was set relative to the anterior plane of the pelvis. Most mechanical guides are designed to use this anterior pelvic plane as a baseline for orientation. The anterior

7

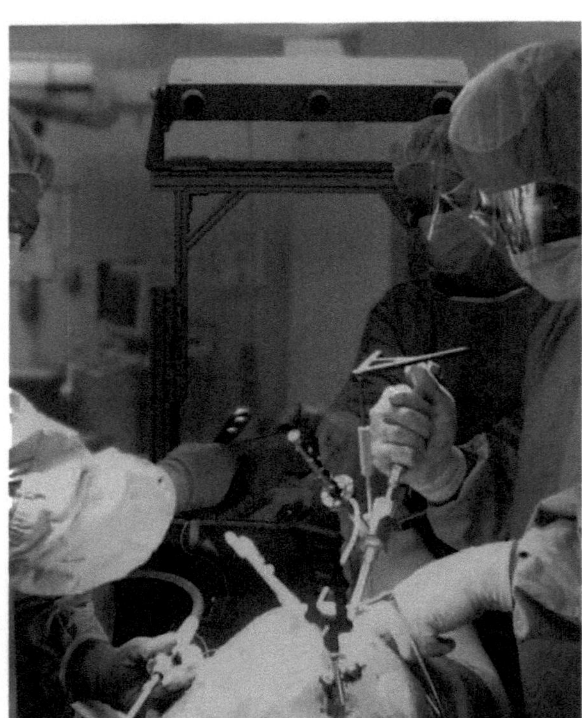

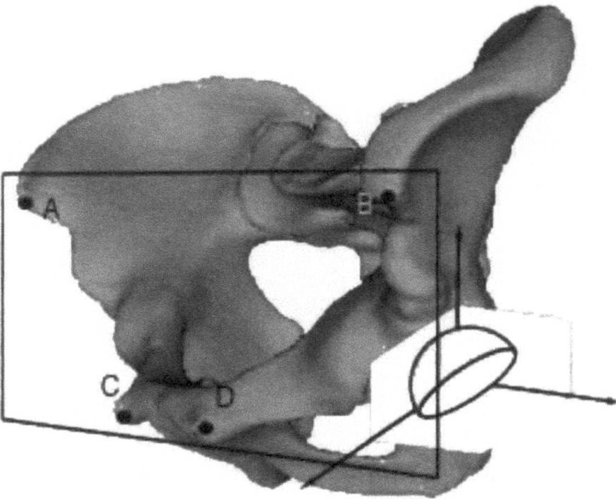

Fig. 7-4. Anterior pelvic plane

Fig. 7-3. Zimmer Acetabular Cup Impactor-Positioner with A-frame and computer-assisted tracking device

pelvic plane was defined on CT-scan by the maximally anterior points on the bilateral anterior superior iliac spines (A and B) and the maximally anterior midpoint of bilateral pubic tubercles (C and D; **Fig. 7-4). The same plane was used to set the longitudinal and transverse axes of the pelvis. The absolute orientation of the pelvis on the operating table was also measured first prior to dislocation (baseline) and then during acetabular alignment. The first measurement reflects how the pelvis was actually positioned on the table, because it was recorded before any manipulations to the lower extremity were performed. The second measurement records any change in the pelvic orientation after hip dislocation and during cup alignment. Pelvic motion was expressed in terms of abduction and adduction, flexion and extension, and anteversion and retroversion. If the patient's pelvis was aligned during surgery in the expected neutral baseline position and there were no changes in pelvic orientation during surgery, all measurements would be zero. A paired t-test (SAS Version 6.12 statistical software, Cary,

NC) was used to assess the statistical significance. A p value of less than 0.05 was considered to be statistically significant.

The orientation of the acetabular component using the mechanical guide measured by the navigation tool was available for 74 hips. Measured cup alignment using the mechanical guide as the sole source of alignment ranged from 35° to 59° in abduction (mean 44° with standard deviation 4°) and from 33° of forward flexion to 26° of extension (mean one degree with standard deviation 10°). The actual angles obtained for abduction and flexion were subtracted from ideal values (45° of abduction and 20° of flexion) and statistical significance of these differences was assessed. The variation of cup orientation from the desired acetabular implant alignment was in the range of –10° to +14° in abduction (mean, minus one degree) (p=0.13) and –46° to +13° in flexion (mean, minus 19°; p<0.001). None of the 74 cups were positioned with 45° of abduction and 20° of flexion. Nine cups were positioned exactly with 45° of abduction. None of the cups were positioned close to 20° of flexion. In 62 of the 74 cases (84%), acetabular implant alignment would have been outside the »safe zone« as defined by Lewinnek et al. [9] of 40±10° of abduction and 15±10° of anteversion. One cup was positioned outside the »safe zone« in abduction and 63 cups in flexion.

The mean difference of the pelvic orientation on the operating room table from desired position (anterior pelvic plane parallel to longitudinal body axis and also parallel to longitudinal axis of the table) was 6° in flexion (range from –7° to 23°) and 3° in abduction (range from –9° to 19°) prior to dislocation ($p<0.05$). During the acetabular alignment, mean anteversion of the pelvis on the table was 18° from the desired orientation (range from 4° to 28°; $p<0.05$) and mean abduction was 3° from the desired orientation (range from –11° to 11°; $p<0.05$). The mean difference of pelvic flexion and extension from desired was 1° and was not significantly different.

The results of this study show that the mechanical guide for acetabular alignment used in this study was inadequate in achieving the desired goal. There was variation in the range of the cup alignment in abduction (range, –10° to +14°) and especially in version (range, –46° to +13°). Sixty three of 74 cups were placed outside of desired anteversion of 20° ± 10°. Only 1 cup was placed outside of desired abduction of 45±10°. With the support system we used, the pelvis was not reliably oriented in the assumed neutral position on the operating room table initially or, more importantly, during acetabular alignment. Position change from optimal was exaggerated following dislocation of the hip. For all patients, the pelvis was rarely aligned in the desired neutral position during any phase of surgery. There was a general trend toward increased flexion and anterior tilting of the pelvis during acetabular alignment. However, the actual variation from patient to patient, and the magnitude of these differences, was variable, which contributed to the inaccurate and unreliable acetabular implant alignment using the Zimmer mechanical guide. Our results are also in agreement with McCollum and Gray [11] who suggested that an unknown and variable orientation of the pelvis is one reason for unacceptable cup alignment contributing to the continued problem of dislocation following total hip replacement. The limitations of this clinical trial are that it represents the experience of a single surgeon and is limited to one surgical approach.

Mini-Incision Technique In THA

All surgeons are taught early in training that wide »surgical exposure« is one of the most important factors in performing successful THA. Traditionally, it was impossible to achieve accurate fixation and orientation of the implant without complete visualization of the bony landmarks. These large exposures permit implant alignment, but at the same time makes total hip arthroplasty a more invasive procedure. Therefore, our goals should be to minimize the amount of soft tissue trauma while still being able to achieve the surgical goal of reconstructing the hip. By definition, performing any procedure less invasively results in less soft tissue disruption which should reduce pain, speed healing, decrease recovery, and potentially reduces complications. Access to surgical navigation technologies and computer-assisted tools has created opportunities to develop less invasive surgical techniques for THA. Surgical navigation permits accurate orientation and fixation of the implant without complete visualization of the bony landmarks [2,3]. The authors have developed a mini-incision technique for total hip replacement based on a modified posterior (Moore) approach that is enabled by surgical navigation tools.

The mini-incision surgical technique was first utilized for primary total hip arthroplasty in October of 1998. One hundred twenty-one patients with 137 hips were operated using this technique. Thirty-three patients (35 hips; Group I) were selected out of 121 patients that had undergone a mini-incision THA matched by diagnosis, sex, average age and preoperative Harris Hip Score (HHS) to thirty-three patients (35 hips; Group II) of 120 patients that had undergone THA using the traditional posterior approach. The same surgeon (AMD) operated all patients and all surgeries were performed with the navigation system. Patients were prospectively evaluated in a Total Joint Registry by an independent observer. Evaluations were performed preoperatively, and at 3 months, 6 months, and 12 months postoperatively. The number of blood transfusions, postoperative complications, and hospital stay were also recorded and statistically compared.

Both groups consisted of patients with osteoarthritis (19 females, 14 males) (◨ Table 7-1). In group I (mini-incision) the average age was 65 years (range, 49–80 years old), in group II (traditional approach) the average age was 65 years old (range, 49–76 years old; $p = 0.86$). The average preoperative HHS was 52.29 (range, 24–74) in group I and in group II was 53.44 (range, 22–76; $p = 0.88$). The affected hip was right in 15 cases and was left in 20 cases in group I. In group II the affected hip was right in 18 cases and was left in 17 cases. In both groups, two patients had bilateral surgery. Average weight in mini-

◻ Table 7-1. Comparison of two groups

	Group I Mini-incision 33 pts., 35 hips	Group II Traditional incision 33 pts., 35 hips	T test [p]
Female	19	19	
Male	14	14	
Bilateral	2	2	
Age (average)	65 (range, 49–80)	65 (range, 49–76)	0.86
Pre-op. HHS	54 (range, 24–74)	53 (range, 22–76)	0.881
3 months HHS	85 (range, 63–96)	81 (range, 63–95)	0.045
6 months HHS	92 (range, 84–100)	87 (range, 71–100)	0.017
1 year HHS	93 (range, 86–100)	94 (range, 79–100)	0.081

incision group was 79.8 kg and average height was 170.6 cm. Average weight in traditional incision group was 79.5 kg and average height was 167.8 cm. Body mass index (BMI) was 27 for mini-incision group and 28 for traditional incision group. It was no significant statistical difference in BMI between groups ($p>0.5$). The Zimmer Trilogy press-fit acetabular component with cluster holes (Zimmer Inc, Warsaw, IN) was used in all hips. In group I, 27 patients received cemented femoral implant Versys Plus (Zimmer Inc, Warsaw, IN) and 6 received non-cemented femoral implant Meridian (Howmedica, Allendale, NJ). In group II, 27 patients received similar femoral cemented implant and 6 patients received non-cemented implant.

Statistical analysis was performed with a student's t-test to compare the differences between these two groups (SAS, version 6.12). Statistical significance was set at a confidence level of $p<0.05$.

The mini-incision surgical approach used in our study is a modification of the traditional posterior approach (Moore). In the proposed technique the skin incision is used as a mobile window in order to permit the visualization of the deeper tissues. The landmarks for initial skin incision are varies significantly from traditional approach. Moore's incision starts approximately 10 cm distal to the posterior superior iliac spine and extended distally and laterally parallel with the fibers of the gluteus maximus to the posterior margin of the greater trochanter. The traditional incision is then directed distally 10 to 13 cm parallel with the femoral shaft and can result in incisions 25–35 cm in length. More recently, mini-incision techniques and modification of the Moore approach have been described in the literature. According the description by A.H. Crenshaw (modification by Sequeira and Khanuja [12]) a straight incision about 13 cm long is made slightly posterior to the trochanter with hip adducted and flexed at 90 degrees. The trochanter is at the midpoint of the incision. In contrast, to this description, we found that for optimal use of the »mobile skin window«, the hip should be flexed about 70–80 degrees (◻ Fig. 7-5). The leg will be in this position following dislocation and during acetabular and femoral preparation and implantation. The greater trochanter is palpated and an eight to ten centimeter straight incision is then made in line with femoral shaft with two thirds of the incision carried proximal and one third distal to the tip of the greater trochanter (◻ Fig. 7-6).

The tensor fascia lata is incised along the incision. The gluteus maximus muscle is split in line with its fibers.

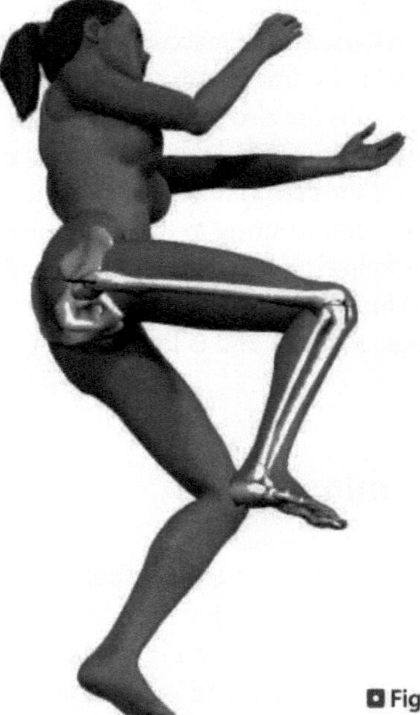

◻ Fig. 7-5. Mini-incision with hip flexed 70–80 degrees

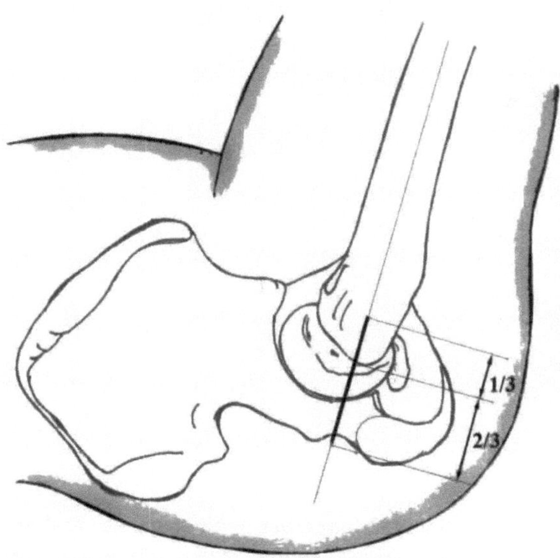

◻ Fig. 7-6. Mini-incision

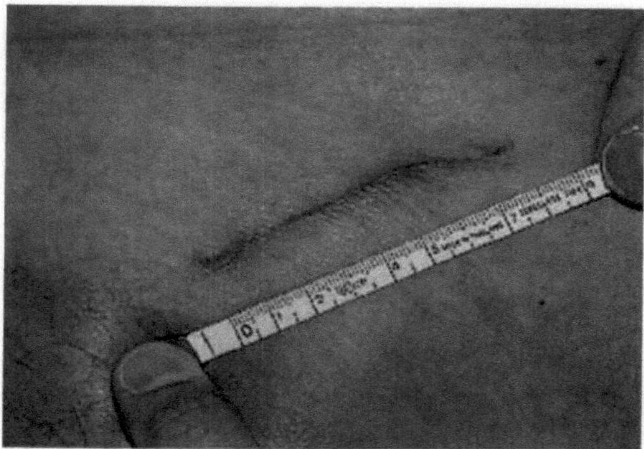

◻ Fig. 7-7. Patient with mini-incision after THA

The leg is then held in maximum internal rotation and neutral or slight extention. The interval between the pyriformis and gluteus medius muscle is identified and the abductors are carefully retracted superiorly. The approach is then performed in a routine manner. Only standard retractors were used during the surgery. Prior to dislocation of the hip, a one centimeter incision is made over the wing of the ilium allowing application of the pelvic tracking clamp. This clamp has optical tracking targets that enable the navigation system to visualize pelvic position and intra-operative motion. After dislocation and the neck resection reaming is performed in a sequential manner. Medialization of the acetabulum is confirmed with the navigation system, which allows direct interactive visualization of the medial wall of the acetabulum to determine the amount of bone resected. During acetabular cup impaction, the navigation system continually measures implant orientation, as the cup is press-fit. Supplemental screw fixation is used as necessary. In this particular series, the femoral component was positioned without navigation, but the updated navigation system measures orientation of the femoral component and real time leg lengths. All patients had similar rehabilitation protocol. Patients had 2 session of physical therapy per day with weight bearing as tolerated on first postoperative day.

The average length of the skin incisions for group II (traditional posterior approach) measured 20.2 cm (range, 14.8–26.0). The length of the skin incisions for group I (mini-incision) averaged 11.7 cm (range, 7.3–13.0; $p<0.001$; ◻ Fig. 7-7). Average surgical time was 2 hours for mini-incision group and 1 h 40 min for traditional approach. Preoperative plan for each cup position was 45° of abduction and 20° of flexion. Acetabular cup alignment for both groups was within five degrees of the preoperatively planned position using the navigation system. After final cup placement average abduction was 46° (range, 42–48°), average flexion was 22° (range, 18–25°). At 3 months, the HHS increased by an average of 34 points (range, 63–96) in the mini-incision group, and by 27 points (range, 63–95) in group II, and this difference was statistically significant ($p=0.045$; ◻ Table 7-2). At 6 months, in the mini-incision group the HHS increased an average of 41 points (range, 84–100) in group I, and by 34 points (range, 71–100) in group II, and was again statistically significant ($p=0.017$). At the one year follow-up, the average HHS was 96 points (range, 86–100) for group I and 94 points (range, 79–100) for group II, and there was no significant difference in the HHS between groups ($p=0.08$).

A more detailed evaluation of the pain, limp, distance walk, need of support, ability to walk stairs, and range of motion was then performed to examine these significant differences at the 3 and 6 month follow-up. At the 3 month visit, patients in the mini-incision group had significant improvement in limp ($p=0.04$) and stair climbing ($p=0.009$) compared to group II (see Table 7-2). The

□ Table 7-2. Functional results of THA

	Preoperative			3 months			6 months			1 year		
	TI	MI	T test [p]	TI	MI	T test [p]	TI	MI	T test [p]	TI	MI	T test [p]
Pain	18	19.7	0.25	38	40	0.1	40.7	41.8	0.28	43	43	0.59
Limp	4.6	3.91	0.31	7[a]	8.3[a]	0.04	7.9[a]	9.36[a]	0.01	10	10	0.8
Support	8.4	8.8	0.6	8.8	9.7	0.1	9.8	10.2	0.48	11	11	0.3
Distance	6.2	5.2	0.1	7.9	8.6	0.2	8.4[a]	10.1[a]	0.001	9.2	10	0.1
Stairs	1.5	1.4	0.6	2.1[a]	2.8[a]	0.009	2.2[a]	3.2[a]	<0.001	3.1	3.5	0.1
Socks	1.8	1.7	0.6	2.5	2.4	0.6	2.8	2.9	0.7	3.3	3.5	0.4
Sitting	4.3	4.2	p = 0.7	4.7	4.9	0.2	4.8	4.9	0.3	4.9	5	1
Transport	0.8	0.9	p = 0.5	0.9	1	0.08	1	1	0.9	1	1	1
Range of motion	86.4	83.8	p = 0.6	95	94.3	0.6	94.94	96.78	0.16	96.7	97.9	0.15

[a]Statistically significant; *TI* traditional incision (n=34); *MI* mini-incision (n=34).

remainder of the parameters of HHS evaluation had no statistical difference. At the 6 month follow-up, the mini-incision group was significantly better in terms of limp (*p*=0.01), distance walked (*p*=0.001), and stair climbing (*p*<0.001). There was no difference between groups in pain, limp, need of support, stair climbing or range of motion at one year follow-up (*p*>0.05).

Patients in the mini-incision group received an average 0.7 units of blood in the postoperative period (range, 0–2 units), while the patients in traditional group averaged 1.1 units of blood transfused (range, 0–2 units; *p*<0.05). The difference in hospital stay was not statistically significant between group I and II and averaged 3.8 and 3.9 days respectively (*p*=0.6). There were no dislocations or nerve injuries in either group within the 1 year follow-up period.

Little clinical research has been undertaken to relate the extent of the surgical approach to postoperative complications or patient function. The Norwegian Arthroplasty Register reported a 0.8% mortality rate (standardized mortality ratio = 1.39) in 39,543 patients during the first 60 postoperative days after total hip replacement [10]. Also, despite the good overall results of THA, the recovery time to improved function can be lengthy. Knutsson and Engberg [8] reported significant improvement in patients' total physical and psychosocial quality of life 6 months postoperatively compared to prior to the operation, but at 6 weeks after the THA the level of pain and discomfort was higher than prior to the surgery. Our study demonstrated, that less invasive surgery will improve clinical outcomes by speeding patients' recovery to a more functional status earlier. Achieving these goals will result in quality driven health care that will reduce costs. Access to surgical navigation technologies and computer-assisted tools also create many opportunities for clinician-scientists and research. With the ability to precisely measure intraoperative implant alignment, these navigational devices will now permit less invasive and more accurate surgical technique for THA.

References

1. Ackland M, Bourne W, Uhthoff H (1986) Anteversion of the acetabular cup: Measurement of angle after total hip replacement. J Bone Joint Surg 68B: 409–413
2. DiGioia AM, Jaramaz B, Colgan B (1998a) Computer assisted orthopaedic surgery: image guided and robotic assistive technologies. Clin Orthop Rel Res 354: 8–16
3. DiGioia AM, Jaramaz B, Blackwell M et al. (1998b) Image guided navigation system to measure intraoperatively acetabular implant alignment. Clin Orthop Rel Res 355: 8–22
4. Harkess WJ (1992) Arthroplasty of the hip: dislocation and subluxation. In: Crenshaw AH (ed) Campbell's Orthopaedics, 8th edn. Mosby, St. Louis, pp 541–547
5. Harris WH (1980) Advances in surgical technique for total hip replacement: Without and with osteotomy of the greater trochanter. Clin Orthop Rel Res 146: 188–204
6. Herrlin K, Pettersson H, Selvik G (1988) Comparision of two- and three-dimensional methods for assessment of orientation of the total hip prothesis. Acta Radiologica 29: 357–361
7. Khadem R, Yeh CC, Sadeghi-Tehrani M et al. (2000) Comparative tracking error analysis of five different optical tracking systems. Computer Aided Surgery 5: 98 – 107

8. Knutsson S, Engberg S (1999) An evaluation of patients' quality of life before, 6 weeks and 6 months after total hip replacement surgery. J Adv Nurs 30: 1349

9. Lewinnek GE, Lewis JL, Tarr R, Compere CL, Zimmerman JR (1978) Dislocations after total hip replacement arthroplasties. J Bone Joint Surg 60A: 217–220

10. Lie S, Engesaeter L, Havelin L, Gjessing H, Vollset S (2000) Mortality after total hip replacement: 0–10-year follow-up of 39.543 patients in the Norwegian Arthroplasty Regisrter. Acta Orthop Scand 71: 19

11. McCollum DE, Gray WJ (1990) Dislocation after total hip arthroplasty: Causes and prevention. Clin Orthop Rel Res 261: 159–170

12. Murray DW (1993) The definition and measurement of acetabular orientation. J Bone Joint Surg Br 75: 228-232

13. Rohling R, Munger P, Hollerbach JM et al. (1995) Comparison of relative accuracy between a mechanical and an optical position tracker for image-guided neurosurgery. J Image Guided Surg 1: 30–34

14. Simon D, Hebert M, Kanade T (1995) Techniques for fast and accurate intrasurgical registration. J Image Guided Surg 1: 17–29

15. Visser J, Konings J (1981) A new method for measuring angles after total hip arthroplasty. J Bone Joint Surg 63B: 556–559

8 Acetabular Cup Navigation with the *OrthoPilot* System

H. Kiefer

Introduction

Optimal positioning of both cup and shaft is essential for both reduction of the risk of dislocation and for the improvement of longevity [1]. During the last five decades significant progress in hip arthroplasty was achieved due to improvement of materials, fixation techniques, reduction of wear and longevity [1, 20]. Still it is not always possible to achieve perfect individual cup position. The final result usually depends on experience and subjective intuition of the surgeon. Improper cup positioning may lead to reduced range of motion, impingement [8], increased wear [3, 11] and to a higher risk of dislocation. It is reported to occur between 1 and 9% [1, 6]. The »safe zone« [16], with $45\pm10°$ for inclination and $15\pm10°$ for anteversion, cannot be reached when using conventional technique even by experienced surgeons in up to 42% [9]. The range varies from 14 to 65° for cup inclination and from 27° of retroversion up to 47° of anteversion [15]. The main cause for these facts is the lack of information about the three-dimensional position of the pelvis due to unknown amounts of lordosis or kyphosis [5]. Assuming a patient's straight position, the surgeon uses the position of the operating table as his only eye-controlled orientation on which his manual instruments are based on. Even when using fluoroscopy, the angle of lordosis, and therefore inclination and anteversion angles, cannot be defined exactly.

Modern navigation technologies might offer the possibility to achieve better control over the three-dimensional position of the pelvis and the implants. CT-based techniques compete with kinematic procedures. In theory, the CT-based techniques might provide higher precision [4, 10], but they are time consuming, expensive, require high technical efforts and inflict radiation. Kinematic procedures provide less information about the individual skeletal anatomy, but are easier and faster to use [2].

The kinematic navigation system OrthoPilot [2] was proven to be efficient in knee arthroplasty for four years and more than 5000 applications [12, 14, 17]. This technique now was adapted for hip surgery. As the cup position is more crucial than the shaft orientation [9, 15], the navigation device for the cup was developed first. Since the first application of the system 18 months ago the surgeons grew more experienced [13].

Material and methods

Principle

In human upright standing position the plane defined by both anterior iliac spines and the symphysis runs more or less vertical and parallel to the coronal plane. In a normally configured pelvis there is a highly significant anatomical relationship of the acetabular position to this plane. Intraoperatively this plane is defined via surface matching by palpation of these bony landmarks with a pointer. The kinematic navigation system works by showing the surgeon via computer screen how to guide the acetabular reaming and cup positioning instruments. The cup can be firmly implanted in the desired position with respect to the pelvis, independent on the patient's position on the table.

OrthoPilot

The OrthoPilot system consists of optoelectronic Polaris stereo cameras that detect the infrared signals of the so-called »rigid bodies«. These carry infrared transmitters and are firmly attached to the supra-acetabular bone and the surgical instruments in use (i.e. pointer, acetabular reamer, cup placement jig). A computer program calculates the hip center from the data obtained by surface matching and kinematic acquisition. Acetabular position, direction and depth of reaming, and the orientation of trial and final cup are calculated by a sophisticated algorithm [2]. The results are displayed and shown to the surgeon step by step on the monitor, as surgery is going on. Easily understood graphical and numerical elements as well as virtual instruments on the screen help the surgeon during the entire procedure. In case of a technical malfunction manual surgical procedure is always possible.

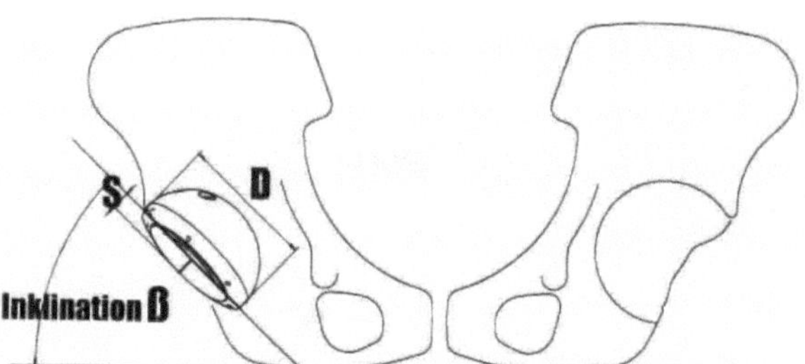

Fig. 8-1. Pelvis scheme with lines to measure the (projected) inclination angle and to calculate the anteversion angle. The angle of cup inclination can be obtained from the tangent to the sciatic bones and the axis through the acetabular poles (osteophyts excluded) in preoperative X-ray and the cup poles in the post-operative X-ray, respectively. The calculation formula for the cup anteversion angle α is [19]:

$$\alpha = \arcsin \frac{S}{D/2}$$

Surgical Technique

The OrthoPilot device along with the stereo cameras is positioned on the opposite side of the surgeon two meters away from the rigid bodies. The patient is in a supine position and a standard lateral surgical approach is used. Next, a trocar shaped Steinman pin is inserted firmly into the cancellous bone cranial to the acetabular roof. The pin works as a soft tissue retractor and follows, together with the firmly attached rigid body, every movement of the pelvis. By rotation of the best fitting trial cup with an insertion instrument, which carries another rigid body, the rotational center of the acetabulum is defined. An additional surface matching with a pointer to determine the maximum depth of the acetabular fossa is performed. While a rigid body is attached to the reamer, depth and direction of reaming are displayed and can therefore be controlled on the screen. After defining the desired inclination and anteversion angles within the »safe zone« using the trial cup, the final implant is inserted in this very position. Again, the positioning can be checked on the computer screen.

Clinical Application

From April 2001 to January 2002 147 patients underwent cementless total hip arthroplasty for primary coxarthrosis using the kinematic navigation technique. In all cases a porous coated Plasmacup and a Bicontact stem were press-fit implanted. Patients were mobilized from the first postoperative day, and increasing weight bearing was allowed with respect to pain, wound healing, muscle function and joint motion. The average age of the 62 men and 86 women during surgery was 68±8 (48–88) years; the body mass index was 26,3±3,7 (21,5–39,1) kg/cm².

In nine cases, at the beginning of the learning curve, the navigation procedure had to be interrupted because of software and hardware problems. The surgical procedure was then finished using conventional technique. In the meantime improving both camera software and instruments has solved these problems.

The cup inclination angle can be measured directly on the pre- and postoperative pelvioradiographies between the cup axis and the tangent at both ischia. For the evaluation of the anteversion angles a mathematical calculation formula according to Pradhan [19] was used (Fig. 8-1).

Results

The data of the 138 remaining patients was evaluated. Nine patients had to be excluded because of poor referencing due to obesity, early loosening of the Steinman reference pins in osteoporotic bone and rigid body cable defects. No specific intraoperative complications were seen. The average blood loss as measured with the cell caver system was 1350 ml. The surgical time was 90±19

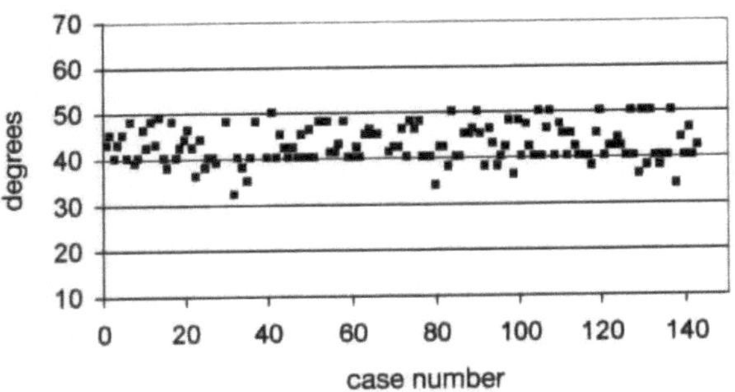

Table 8-1. Cup inclination angle

Inclination (degrees)	Mean	Standard deviation	Range
Preoperative	50	7	30–70
Planning	42	5	38–55
Trial cup	40	4	26–50
Cup intraoperative	41	5	29–48
Cup postoperative	42	5	34–50

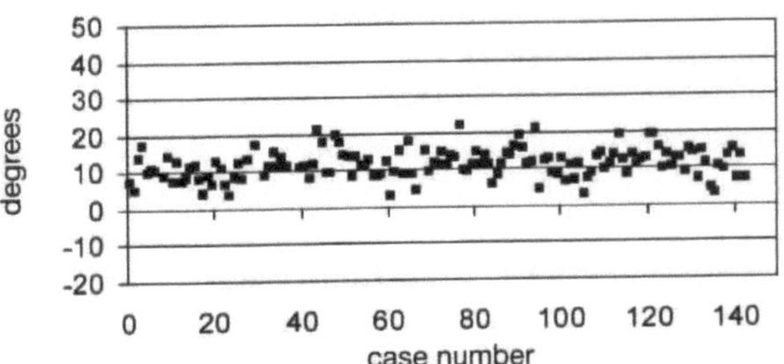

Fig. 8-3. Range of the postoperative anteversion angles in 138 patients from 3–22°, mean 11°, derived from Pradhan [19]

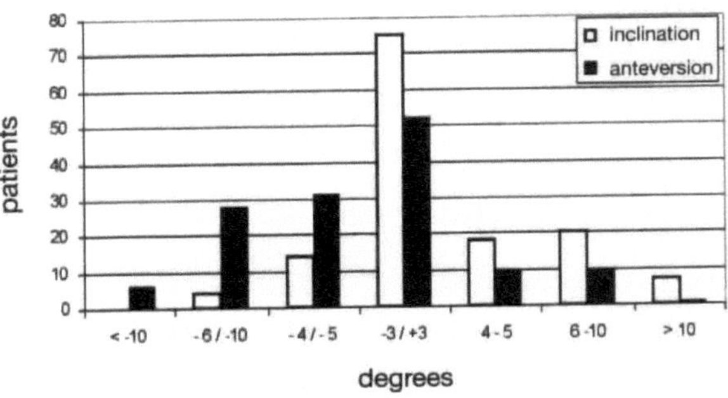

Fig. 8-4. Deviation of intraoperatively measured angle data from postoperative measured and calculated data from X-ray projection. Depiction of the case numbers in groups. The precision of concordance was somewhat higher for inclination compared to the anteversion data

(55–130) min including standard fluoroscopic controls. It was prolonged for 9 min with respect to a conventionally treated collective. The mean pre-operative inclination angle was 50±7°. Intraoperatively, the mean inclination angles were determined with the OrthoPilot system as 40±4° for the trial cup and 41±5° for the definite implant, and thus were close to the postoperatively measured data of 42±5° (■ Table 8-1).

The single data varied from 29° to 54° intraoperatively, and from 32° to 55° postoperatively (■ Fig. 8-2). The results for the mean intraoperative and postoperative anteversion angles were found as 15° and 11° (■ Table

8-2), while the single data varied relatively higher between 3° and 22° (■ Fig. 8-3).

The variation between the intraoperative and postoperative evaluated cup angles is displayed in ■ Fig. 8-4.

Two postoperative hip dislocations occurred during the rehabilitation period due to poor compliance of the patients. One patient slipped in the shower room and fell while externally rotating her leg. The second patient was an alcoholic and was found sleeping in the clinic garden with a dislocated hip. The postoperative cup angles with 42° of inclination and 16° of anteversion were found within the »safe zone«.

All patients demonstrated a normal postoperative recovery with respect of wound healing, range of motion, and time conform mobilization. A typical radiological example demonstrates pre- and postoperative findings including the planned and evaluated inclination and anteversion angles (■ Fig. 8-5).

Fig. 8-2. Range of the postoperative inclination angles in 138 patients from 34–50°, mean 42°, directly measured prom the pelvis a.-p. projection

Table 8-2. Cup anteversion angle

Anteversion (degrees)	Mean	Standard deviation	Range
Trial cup	15,4	4,8	0–30
Cup intraoperative	15,9	4,5	3–29
Cup postoperative	10,9	4,8	3–22

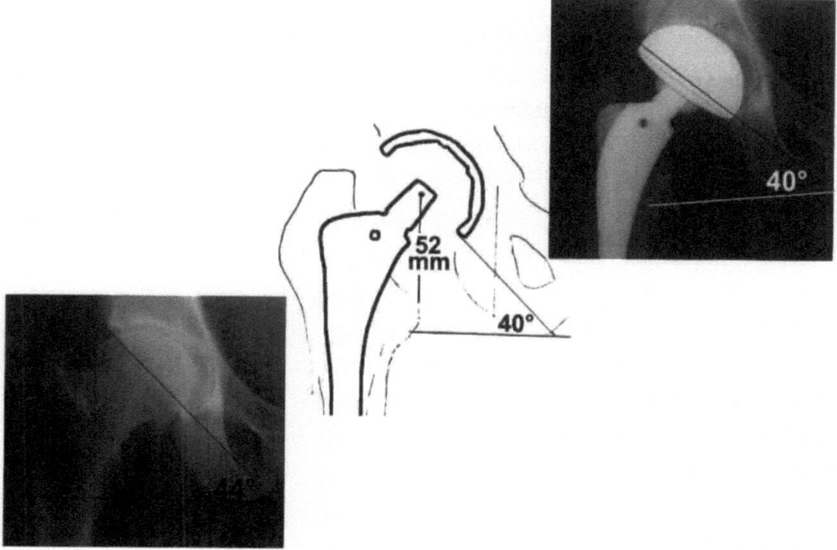

◘ Fig. 8-5. 61-year-old patient with coxarthrosis on the right hip, pre-operative inclination angle 44°. The preoperatively planned angle of 40° was matched exactly by intra-operative navigation, as it is proved by the postoperative radiologic results. The intraoperatively naviga-ted anteversion was 13°, the post-operative calculation showed 11°

Discussion

The experience of three years of OrthoPilot navigation technique [14] in more than 400 of our own navigated knee arthroplasties was a helpful basis for the application of the technology to the cup navigation. After some minor technical difficulties had been solved, the application of the OrthoPilot system for the cup navigation has been proved as a simple and safe procedure. The learning curve is short with this approach. After a few cases, the additional time consumption is only 7 to 10 min. Expensive CT scans [10] and other additional costs are not necessary. There is no need for any other specific pre-operative planning besides the standard drawing with templates and goniometer. Initial technical problems, as there were loosening of connecting screws between Steinman reference pin and rigid body caused by vibrations of hammer impacts, have been solved. Initial insufficiencies of the software also have been excluded by some updates.

The preliminary results confirm the prediction that the desired cup position within the »safe zone« [7, 16] can be reached precisely. The cup position can always be oriented with respect to the pelvis, not worrying about the pelvis position itself. So the mean deviation of the radiological postoperative to the intraoperatively displayed data was only 1±4,8° for inclination and 4±6,1° for anteversion. The range of inclination between 34° and 55° and

of 3–22° for the anteversion led to a significant improvement of the cup position [9, 15]. Malpositions outside the »safe zone« could be avoided.

The cup inclination angle on the postoperative pelvioradiographies, as projected to the coronal plane, seems to be increased by few degrees as compared to the intraoperatively measured data. The cup anteversion angle, as it is calculated with the formula of Pradhan [19], is few degrees lower than it is displayed during navigation.

Specific complications were not found. The Steinman reference pin must not be inserted deeper than into the intern lamina of the pelvis. This can be done easily by listening to the sound during hammering. Thus, an injury of the iliac vessels can be avoided. In case of loosening of this reference pin, the registration and navigation procedure has to be repeated or the surgery can be finished manually.

Both dislocations occurred from poorly compliant patients. In both cases there were no malpositions of the cups, the navigation procedure worked without any difficulties and the radiological result was perfect as well as the soft tissue tension around the joint.

The limits of kinematic navigation are related to the lack of information about the specific individual bony anatomy as there is no CT data needed. While a »normally« shaped pelvis has an acetabulum position within the range of the »safe zone« with 45±10° of inclination and 15±10° of anteversion, the cup position in a dysplastic pelvis and acetabular shape cannot be defined clearly from standard X-ray projections [5]. The optimal individual acetabular position for a single person without CT scans can be estimated only approximately and thus not determined exactly by the surgeon [10]. Here further research is necessary.

When using the OrthoPilot navigation technique the desired cup position can by achieved precisely in standard cases with a normal anatomical configuration. Severe cup malpositions, as they happen even to experienced surgeons, can be avoided with high reliability [9, 15]. The variation of the single data for the cup angles is also reduced markedly.

Preview

In the near future, additional updates for the kinematic hip navigation will be developed. There will be a module for navigation of leg length, antetorsion, and axial direction of the shaft. An intraoperative simulation of hip motion and stability prior to implantation of the final implants would offer a chance of an individual optimal position of the cup and stem with respect to each other. Consequently, impingement phenomena and dislocations might be avoided in most cases. If CT or MR data is available, it also might be included in further kinematic navigation technique development as well as the images of the new intraoperative three-dimensional fluoroscopy, which offers almost CT quality.

Summary

The kinematic cup navigation procedure is a surgically simple technique for improving the precision of cup placement. With a navigated CT-free system, acetabular cup positioning can be optimized. The rate of desired cup inclination and anteversion angles is markedly increased as shown by the first results of 147 navigated cups. While the inclination is reached precisely with a tendency to a slightly larger angle than desired, the postoperative anteversion angle shows a somewhat larger variation than the intraoperatively navigated angle with a tendency to less

anteversion. This might be due to a lack of information about the actual pelvic position depending on spinal lordosis.

Clinical relevance: Dislocations of the prostheses might be reduced significantly. The kinematic cup navigation with the use of the OrthoPilot is an additional and useful tool for the surgeon. The procedure is simple, quick, and cost effective, does not cause specific complications and does not require additional CT or MRI scans. It may lead to a reduced dislocation rate, improved joint mobility and reduced impingement syndrome and therefore theoretically to reduced wear.

Further improvement can be expected by additional shaft navigation techniques in the near future.

References

1. Berry DJ (1999) Dislocation. In: Steinberg ME, Garino JP (eds) Revision total hip arthroplasty. Lippincott, Williams & Wilkins, Philadelphia, pp 463–481
2. Blömer W (2000) Knieendoprothetik – Herstellerische Probleme und technologische Entwicklungen. Orthopäde 29: 688–696
3. Del Schutte H Jr, Lipman AJ, Bannar SM, Livermore JT, Ilstrup D, Morrey BF (1998) Effects of acetabular abduction on cup wear rates in total hip arthroplasty. J Arthroplasty 13: 621–626
4. DiGioia AM, Jaramaz B, Blackwell M et al. (1998) The Otto Aufranc Award. Image guided navigation system to measure intraoperatively acetabular implant alignment. Clin Orthop 355: 8–22
5. Eddine TA, Migaud H, Chantelot C, Cotten A, Fontaine C, Duquennoy A (2001) Variations of pelvic anteversion in the lying and standing positions: analysis of 24 control subjects and implications for CT measurement of position of a prosthetic cup. Surg Radiol Anat 23: 105–110
6. Ekelund A, Rydell N, Nilsson OS (1992) Total hip arthroplasty in patients 80 years of age and older. Clin Orthop 281: 101–106
7. Hirakawa K, Mitsugi N, Koshino T, Saito T, Hirasawa Y, Kubo T (2001) Effect of acetabular cup position and orientation in cemented total hip arthroplasty. Clin Orthop 388: 135–42
8. Gondi G, Roberson JR, Ganey TM, Shahriari A, Hutton WC (1997) Impingement after total hip arthroplasty related to prosthetic component selection and range of motion. J South Orthop Assoc 6: 266–272
9. Hassan DM, Johnston GH, Dust WN, Watson G, Dolovich AT (1998): Accuracy of intraoperative assessment of acetabular prosthesis placement. J Arthroplasty 13: 80–84
10. Jaramaz B, DiGioia AM 3rd, Blackwell M, Nikou C (1998) Computer assisted measurement of cup placement in total hip replacement. Clin Orthop 354: 70–81
11. Kennedy JG, Rogers WB, Soffe KE, Sullivan RJ, Griffen DG, Sheehan LJ (1998) Effect of acetabular component orientation on recurrent dislocation, pelvic osteolysis, polyethylene wear, and component migration. J Arthroplasty 13: 530–534
12. Kiefer H (2000) Navigation gibt Sicherheit. Gibt die Navigation einen wirklichen Vorteil im Implantate-Einbau? Implant 1: 5–6

13. Kiefer H (2001) Navigationssystem Orthopilot: Erste Ergebnisse und Erfahrungen in der Hüftnavigation. Implant 2: 5–7

14. Kiefer H, Langemeyer D, Schmerwitz U (2001) Computergestützte Navigation in der Knieendoprothetik. Eur J Trauma [E-Suppl] 1: 128–132

15. Lahmer A, Wiesel U, Börner M (2000) Besteht eine Notwendigkeit der rechnerunterstützten Implantation der Pfanne bei der Hüfttotalendoprothese? Deutscher Orthopädenkongress, Wiesbaden, 11.–15. Oktober 2000

16. Lewinnek GE, Lewis JL, Tarr R, Compere CL, Zimmerman JR (1978) Dislocations after total hip-replacement arthroplasties. J Bone Joint Surg 60A: 217–220

17. Miehlke RK, Clemens U, Jens JH, Kershally S (2001) Navigation in der Knieendoprothetik – vorläufige klinische Erfahrungen und prospektiv vergleichende Studie gegenüber konventioneller Implantationstechnik. Z Orthop 139: 109–16

18. Paterno SA, Lachiewicz PF, Kelley SS (1997) The influence of patient-related factors and the position of the acetabular component on the rate of dislocation after total hip replacement. J Bone Joint Surg 79A: 1202–1210

19. Pradhan R (1999) Planar anteversion of the acetabular cup as determined from plain anteroposterior radiographs. J Bone Joint Surg 81B: 431–435

20. Soderman P, Malchau H, Herberts P (2001) Outcome of total hip replacement: a comparison of different measurement methods. Clin Orthop 390: 163–172

9 Acetabular Cup Navigation with the *VectorVision* System

W. H. Kluge, J. Babisch, R. A. Venbrocks

Introduction

Despite technical improvements misplacement of implants leading to complications like dislocation or loosening [2, 3] are still observed in total hip arthroplasty (THA). Especially correct anteversion of the cup can prove difficult if the operating table is used as the only reference level regarding pelvic tilt. Computed tomography (CT) allows for three-dimensional reconstruction of individual pelvic and femoral anatomy providing basic information for modern navigation systems. The navigation system VectorVision has been employed in our hospital since the year 2000. Soft- and hardware are currently the phase VectorVision hip 2.0.

Planning the Operation

Individual patient data are acquired according to the CT protocol developed by BrainLAB. Pelvis, proximal and distal femur have to be included in the CT. Data sets are converted from scanner format to BrainLAB data format at the planning station before being saved on a ZIP-disc ready to be read by the navigation system.

The planning program allows for fine tuning of gray scales which is important to minimize artifacts on the reconstructed 3D-image of the pelvis. A frontal plane is placed automatically on the pelvis and must be adjusted manually to be situated exactly on the anterior iliac spines and the most anterior part of the pubic bones adjacent to the symphysis (■ Fig. 9-1).

Segmentation of femur and pelvis is being performed automatically after precise manual separation of the femoral head from the acetabulum (■ Fig. 9-2). Thereby pelvic and femoral osteophytes can be clearly identified in the final images.

The navigation system will suggest a starting position for the cup which will need adjustment according to biomechanical aspects and to the surgeons preference. Cup fine tuning is first performed on 2D-images demonstrated in 3 planes simultaneously to define depth, craniocaudal, and anterior-posterior positioning (■ Fig. 9-3).

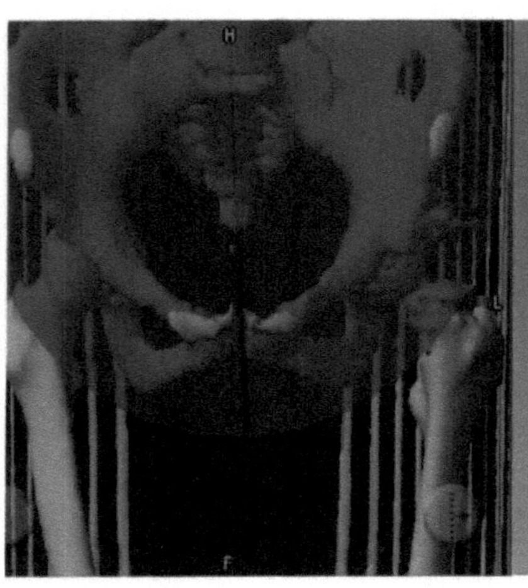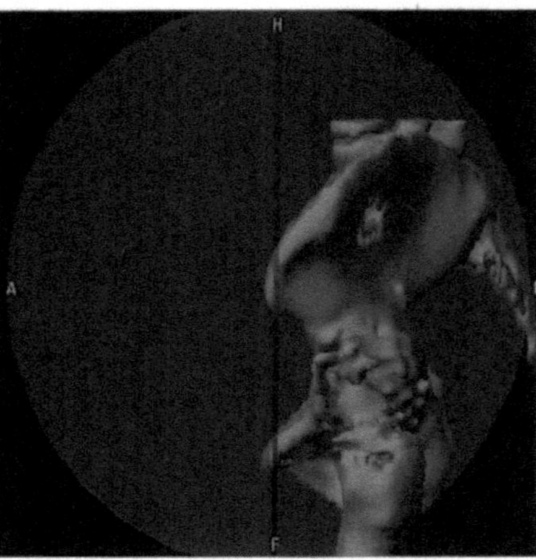

■ **Fig. 9-1.** Determination of frontal and sagittal pelvic plane

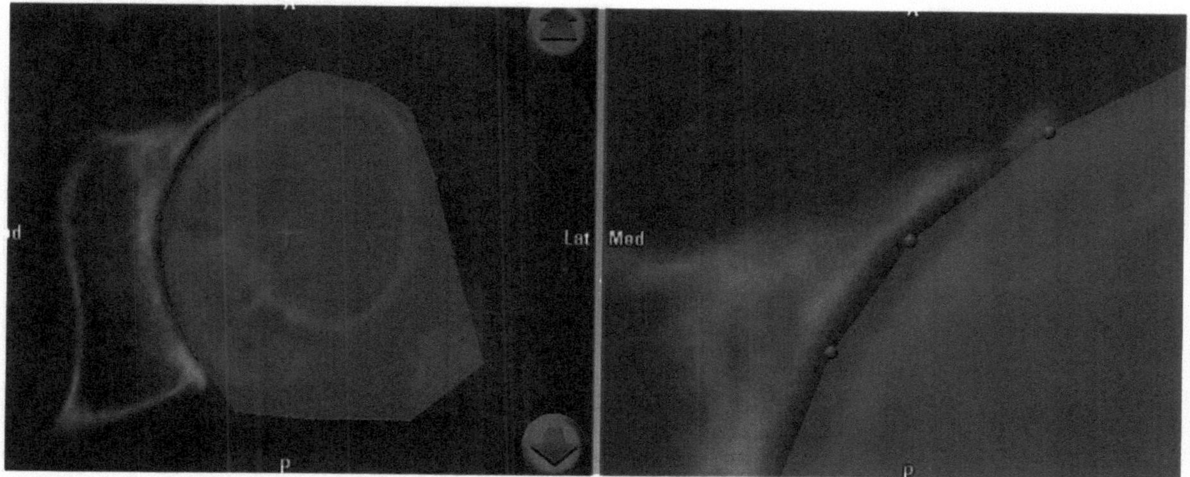

Fig. 9-2. Manual adjustment of segmentation between femur and pelvis allows for precise identification of osteophytes

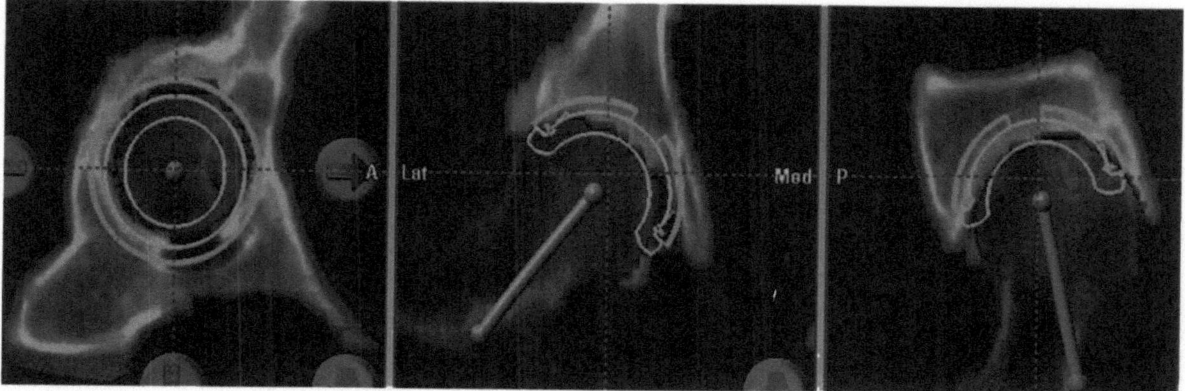

Fig. 9-3. Planning – cup: definition of depth, craniocaudal and anterior-posterior position

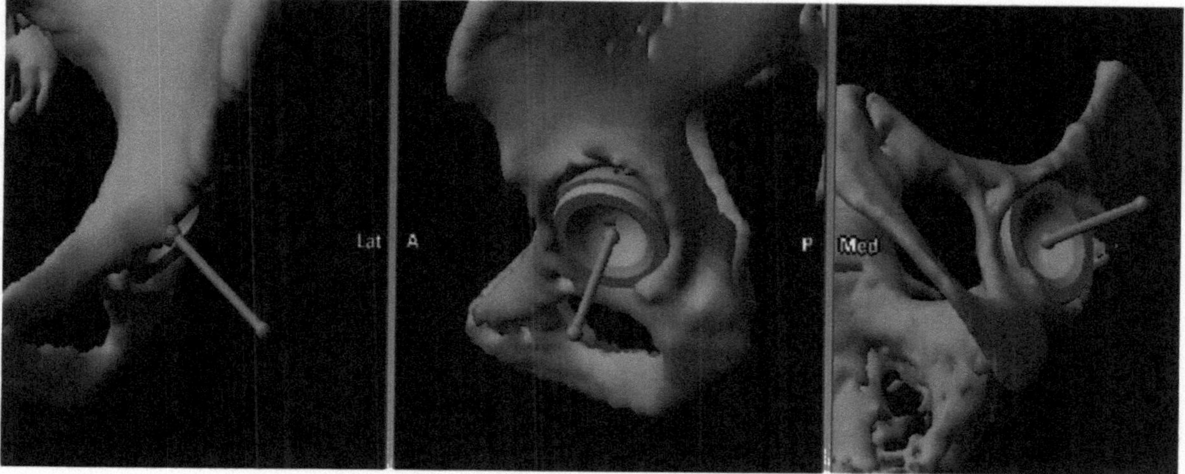

Fig. 9-4. Planning – cup: anteversion and inclination are related to pelvic planes and can be adjusted using a 3D image

Anteversion and inclination of the implant are being related to the frontal and to the sagittal pelvic plane and can be adjusted using the 3D-image (■ Fig. 9-4).

Remarks: We still prefer to place the cup in the »safe zone« defined by Lewinneck [4]. Femoral stem planning should supplement the acetabular planning procedure in order to use the module for preoperative determination of leg length differences and range of joint motion.

The planning procedure for the acetabulum is complete after definition of the registration areas for the surface- and paired-point matching on the iliac crests, and surrounding the acetabulum. Data can be saved on disc and recalled at surgery.

Navigated Surgery

The infrared camera of the navigation platform Vector Vision should be placed about 2 m from the patient's pelvis. We prefer to perform primary hip surgery with the patient in supine position using a transgluteal anterolateral approach. The touchscreen – covered with a sterile transparent drape – should be placed within easy reach of the surgeon or his/her assistant. If the surgeon only intends to navigate the cup the femoral head can be resected before the acetabulum is exposed. Iliac bone is exposed just 3 cm cranial to the acetabulum for placement of the dynamic reference base (DRB). Bony fixation of the DRB is achieved by means of a Schanz-srew penetrating the outer as well as the inner iliac cortical layer being fastened by a special fixation sleeve. Registration of the pelvis (matching of the actual anatomy with the computer image) is now performed within the registration areas (anatomical landmarks) which had been defined during the planning procedure. The navigation system calculates and displays the exactness achieved during the registration process. Vector-Vision hip requires an accuracy of less than 3 mm before navigation can be started. The result of the registration procedure should always be double-checked by placing the pointer on an anatomical landmark visible to the surgeon.

Calibration of the first cup reamer applied must be performed utilizing the calibration device in case ordinary surgical tools are used. Pre-calibrated reamers are also available. In any case the size of the cup reamer has to be adjusted touching the appropriate button on the screen. While reaming the acetabulum the surgeon can exactly follow up the position of the reamer within the pelvic bone. The screen continuously displays the actual anteversion and inclination of the reamer in relation to pelvic planes (■ Fig. 9-5 and 9-6).

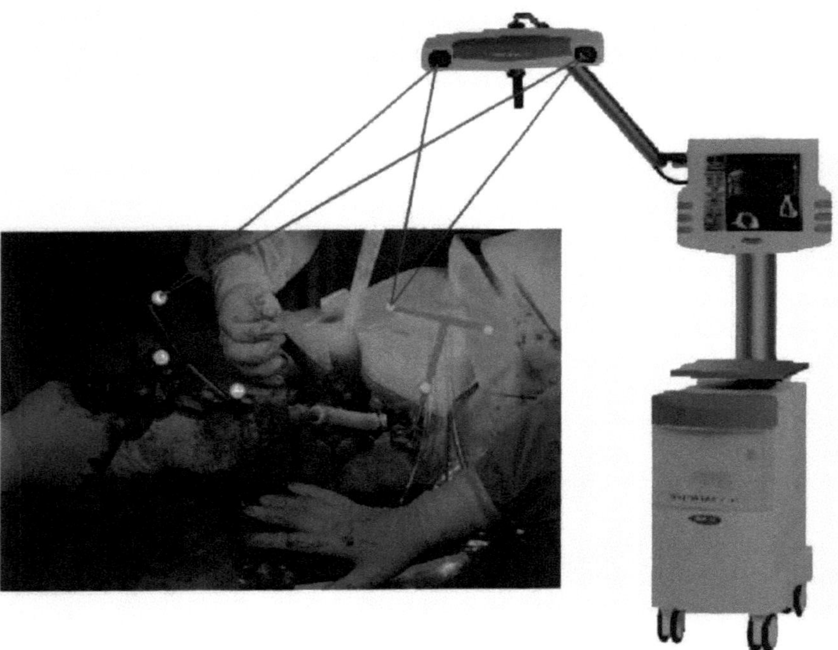

■ **Fig. 9-5.** Reflective spheres of registration arrays fixed to the pelvis and to instruments are recognized by the infrared camera

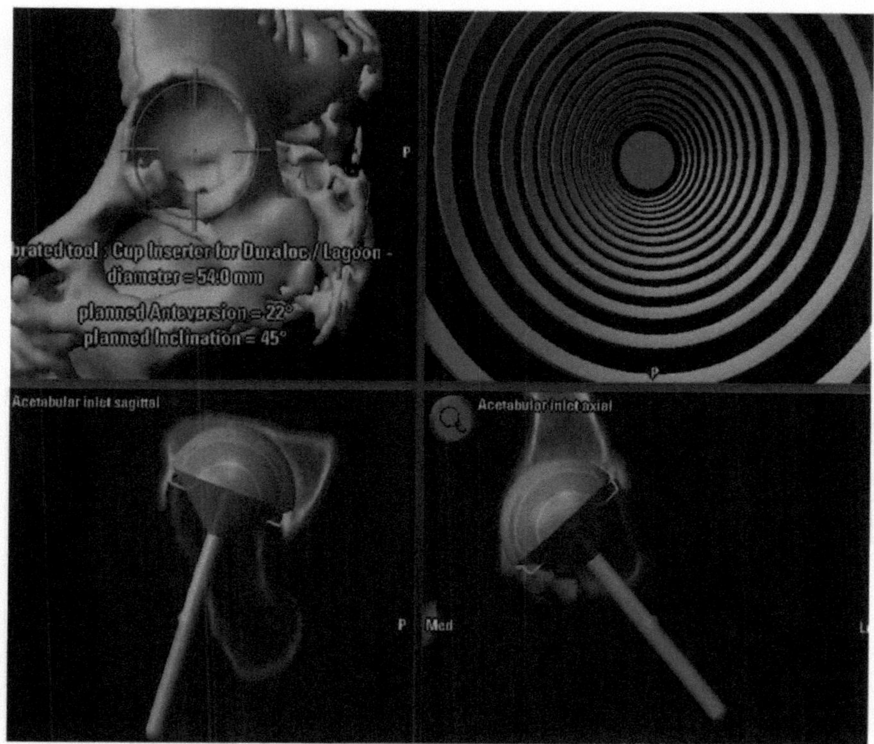

◨ **Fig. 9-6.** Navigation – cup: During navigated surgery 2D or 3D images can be chosen to track the actual position of the instrument (cup reamer or cup inserter) within the pelvic bone. Anteversion and inclination are being displayed online

Remember: The navigation system does not relieve the surgeon of his duty to keep direct visual control of the operating procedure.

After reaming of the implant bed within the acetabulum the cup inserter has to be calibrated once for the trial- and the definitive implant. The position during impaction of the cup can be followed up on the screen in real time (see Fig. 9-6). Again anteversion and inclination are being displayed.

Using the button »cup verification« the final position of the cup can now be compared to the plan regarding anteversion, inclination, depth, craniocaudal- and anterior-posterior shift. This result as well as every step of planning and navigated operative procedure is automatically saved in the operation protocol which can be recalled for quality control.

Clinical Experience, Recommendations

A reliable cup navigation system has been developed within a relatively short period of time by close teamwork between producers of implants, navigation system and clinical applicants. The surgeon does not have to rely on the support of a technician to handle the system during planning and surgery. Optional manual adjustment of basically automatic segmentation between pelvis and femur improves the planning procedure in case of complicated anatomy. Implant positioning can be planned either on 2D or 3D images allowing for a deeper insight it to the pelvic anatomy. Pelvic planes being **the** important reference system for cup placement are independent of the pelvic tilt on the operating table. In the long term it can be anticipated that detailed recommendations regarding precise cup positioning will be available as numbers of navigated surgical procedures are growing. Current clinical experience and radiological studies [4] could be compared to exact 3D data. Producers of implants would thus be able to precisely suggest the most reliable position of a special cup to the surgeon. So far manuals have been rather vague for understandable reasons.

Planning an operation on a 3D image for the first time can be difficult even for the most experienced surgeon. An optional »X-ray view« provided by VectorVision ought to ensure the clinician of the satisfactory result of the planning procedure.

Correct placement of the infrared camera can be confirmed by looking at a special 3D image available showing registration arrays on bony structures and surgical instruments only. Passive optical markers are registered by the camera and displayed on the screen in real time. Thereby any movement of the pelvis or surgical instruments can be watched simultaneously on screen.

Using a registration landmark far from the operative area, i.e. on the contralateral anterior-superior iliac spine has proved helpful to improve the accuracy of registration. In our experience also an increased number of registration points per surface area have improved registration exactness. In principle the navigation system accepts an endless number of registration points – this of course will lead to time-consuming calculations which might lengthen the operating time. According to our experience »pivoting« as recommended by the system does not increase registration accuracy and is only required if the femoral stem is to be navigated (the femoral neck cut being navigated at the same time). Currently femoral stem navigation is not as much advanced as cup navigation and further improvements are to be expected.

Intraoperative calibration of non-flexible surgical instruments (i.e. cup inserter) is reliable and done within seconds. Conventional flexible instruments (cup reamer) allow a certain angular give between the reaming device and the power tool. If the DRB is fixed to the powertool unreliable images can be caused by these unwanted angular movements. We therefore recommend the use of a special pre-calibrated instrument with the registration array fixed to a sleeve on the rotating reamer (■ Fig. 9-7).

One of the most important goals regarding the use of a navigation system in hip replacement surgery is quality control. As mentioned before a protocol of the navigated surgical procedure is provided automatically by the system. The surgeon should also consider to take screenshots of important operative stages to for instance recall why and how he had decided to adapt the intra-

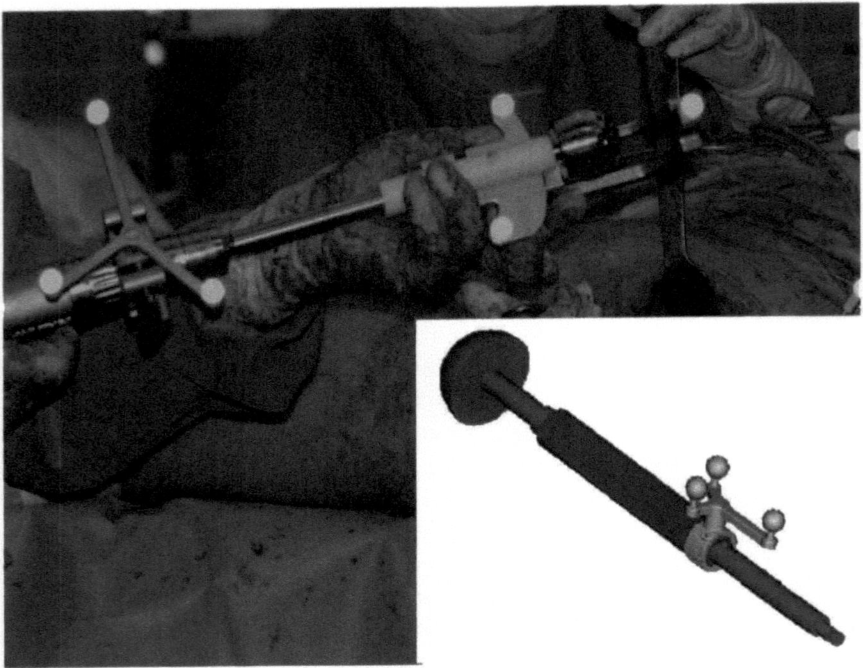

■ **Fig. 9-7.** Calibration of conventional cup reamer. Insert: Pre-calibrated cup reamer, the registration array being fixed to a sleeve on the rotating instrument

operative procedure in comparison to the preoperative plan.

Twenty-four cup- (Duraloc DePuy, Johnson & Johnson) and ten femoral stem navigations (Vision 2000 DePuy, Johnson & Johnson) have so far been performed at our hospital applying various developmental stages of VectorVision hip. Taking clinical applicability into account planning and navigation of the acetabular component can be considered reliable and precise. While preoperative planning of the femoral stem placement proved to be useful the actual stem navigation is still at the stage of further development.

Preoperative planning including the stem currently does not take longer than 45 min even in complicated cases. Registration procedures can be time-consuming if accuracy achieved is not satisfactory after the primary attempt.

Surgeons at our hospital are convinced that cup navigation using VectorVision hip in cases presenting with complicated anatomy offers considerable advantages compared to conventional methods of planning and monitoring THA. Surgery performed exactly according to the plan providing a biomechanically well-positioned cup will permit improved joint movement. Short term clinical studies including advanced gait analyses [1] show that navigation in THA is justified despite the substantial technical effort and time consuming procedures. Comparable long term results will not be available for the next two decades. If navigation will become accessible as a standard method for complicated cases it seems justified to predict a smaller number of complications in THA.

References

1. Babisch J, Seidel EJ, Conradi S (2001) 3D-Ultraschall-Ganganalyse ZEBRIS bei Dysplasiekoxarthrose vor und nach der Hüft-TEP-Inplantation. Phys Med Rehab Kuror 11: 139
2. Grossmann P, Braun M, Becker W (1994) Dislocation following total hip endoprosthesis. Association with surgical approach and other factors. Z Orthop Ihre Grenzgeb 132: 521–526
3. Hassan DM Johnston GH, Dust WN, Watson G, Dolovich AT (1998) Accuracy of intraoperative assessment of acetabular prosthesis placement. J Arthroplasty 13: 80–84
4. Lewinnek GE, Lewis JL, Tarr R, Compere CL, Zimmermann JR (1978) Dislocations after total hip-replacement arthroplasties. J Bone Joint Surg Am 60: 217–220

10 Computer-Assisted Planning and Navigation of Total Hip Arthroplasty Using the *Navitrack* and *mediCAD* System

J. Babisch, F. Layher, R. A. Venbrocks

Introduction

Evolving orthopaedic diagnostics and surgery requires increasing precision. With the help of modern medical imaging technologies such as CT and MRI allowing for 2D and 3D anatomical reconstructions, accurate anatomical diagnostic and therapy becomes available. CT scan reconstruction of bone morphology is common practice and a useful tool in planning and performing individual prosthetic surgery [1]. 3D imaging provides a number of advantages compared with conventional radiographs including metric accuracy, magnification factors, and bone morphology. Preoperative planning on 3D models is more accurate and gives hints for possible intraoperative problems. These are important factors for computer-assisted surgery (CAS), a technology that has recently been established as a tool for the orthopaedic-surgical therapy [7, 12, 13]. The most important innovations being the development of surgical robots and advanced navigation systems [5, 17].

Current Concepts in Navigation

The principle of intraoperative CT-guided navigation includes virtual imaging of anatomical key structures and surgical tools allowing the surgeon to compare the real surgery online with a planned operation calculated via CT data preoperatively. With the help of visual control, navigated surgery can be executed on the monitor comparing implant and positioning permanently with the real situation. Continuous updating of calculated versus actual instrumentation are the primary goals. In passive computer navigation surgical tools are virtually imaged in 3D views, but manually guided by the surgeon, whereas a robot takes over surgical actions such as bone resections or reaming in active navigation systems.

Navigation of Total Hip Arthroplasty

Why Navigation?

Despite increasing advantages in biomaterials, prosthetic design, and implant fixation clinical outcome of total hip arthroplasty (THA) has a 10% failure rate after 10 years. Aseptic loosening is the by far most common reason for revision surgery followed by septic loosening counting for 7%. Fractures and prosthetic dislocation have a likelihood of 5%, and failures of surgical technique (implant position) add up to 3% of all complications requiring revision surgery [8, 9, 15, 16]. Improved implant alignment (with use of navigation) is an important factor contributing to fewer complications following THA. The number of misalignment in THA can be reduced and the longevity increased with the use of preoperative planning of implant size and position together with navigation during surgery.

The safe zone of acetabular component implantation is defined with 40 degrees (±10) of inclination and 15 degrees anteversion (±10) as described by Lewinneck et al.

[15]. Implantation of the acetabular component should be independent of the patients position on the operating table, because this factor represents a common potential error, that is difficult to influence by the surgeon [7, 9]. The rotational hip centre is another factor contributing to optimal results. The goal is optimal reconstruction of the primary hip rotation centre particularly in secondary hip arthritis, which has the best potential for excellent long-term results [19].

At the beginning, navigation in THA was focused on acetabular component positioning [7, 14], however, stem positioning has recently been added. This technology will enhance accuracy of both antetorsion angle of the femur and proper leg length. Particularly improved management of anatomically challenging surgeries and less invasive technique would be advantageous for the surgeon.

Navigation with the Navitrack System

Navigation in THA traditionally required digital CT scan data, an expensive, time-consuming technique with additional radiation risk. This led to development of CT-free navigation systems; however, CT navigation is to date still advantageous in cases with severe pathological morphology such as dysplastic hips or posttraumatic. The hip module Navitrack is a CT-based optoelectronic system, which was first used for cup implantation in 1999. Stem navigation and CT-free navigation is currently investigated. Planning and navigation is performed with the same hardware. During the intervention an infrared camera using passive markers attached to the instruments, which are then represented on a monitor, tracks the surgical instruments. Each surgical step will be described and illustrated (◘ Fig. 10-1).

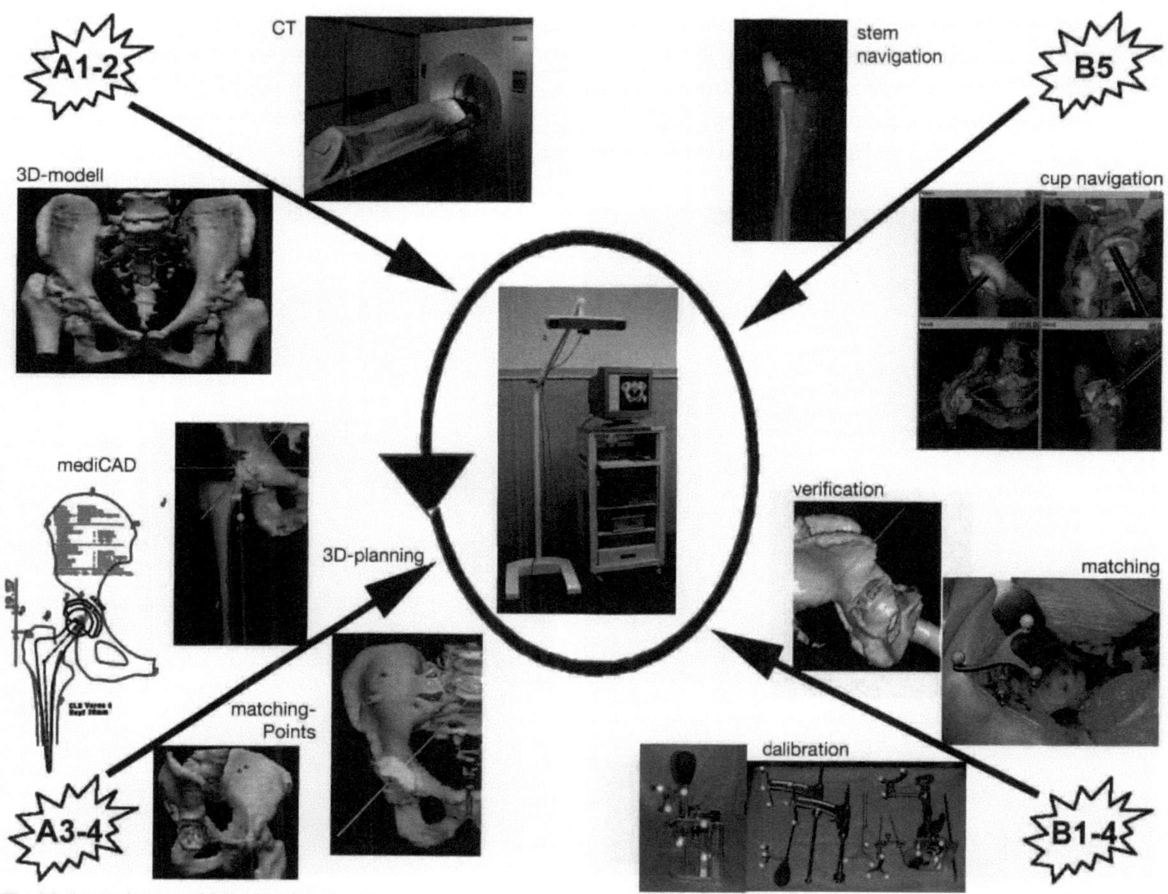

◘ **Fig. 10-1.** Worksteps with Navitrack navigation

Preoperative Planning

1. **CT-investigation:** CT scan data are transferred either via intranet or transportable storage media followed by picture editing with regards to threshold and gray-scale clipping.
2. **Segmentation and creating of a 3D pelvis model** (and femur) from CT data with isolated picture of either pelvis or femur. Following recent suggestions the frontal pelvic plane is defined via both anterior superior iliac spines and both pubis tubercle.
3. **Planning:** A virtual operation is performed with selection of component size and position on 3D and optional 2D image [see p. 85]. Here the operation is performed on a 3D image. The surgeon can choose the preferred implant from a databank. Optimal acetabular component position can be checked on a free rotational translucent pelvic model. The system allows metric measurements as well as cup antetorsion and cup inclination. In cases of stem navigation, femoral data are available with calculation of leg length.
4. **Matching:** Marking of anatomical landmarks on the 3D image as matching points for later registration using the acetabulum and ipsilateral and contralateral iliac spines (◼ Fig. 10-2). Landmarks for stem navigation are both femoral condyles and the trochanter. In the newest software version additional bone surfaces for free point collection for the use in later surface matching can be determined and marked.

Intraoperative Navigation

1. Preoperative **calibration of surgical tools** such as pointer, rasp, acetabular reamer and impactor. All tool tips are positioning into a defined contact area of a calibration block and recognized via a three-pointed LED reference star.
2. **Fixation of DRB:** The dynamic reference base (DRB) is firmly attached to the pelvis using a Schanz screw, which allows recognition of relative pelvic motion on the operating table. In femoral navigation the Schanz screw is attached to the middle third of the femur.
3. **Registration:** Matching of the 3D pelvic image and the patient pelvic bone by pair point matching of anatomical landmarks with additional surface matching using the calibrated pointer.
4. **Verification** of plausible intraoperative anatomical landmarks using the pointer. If landmarks are not compatible with either the patient's anatomy or 3D

◼ **Fig. 10-2.** Registration points on a 3D pelvis model

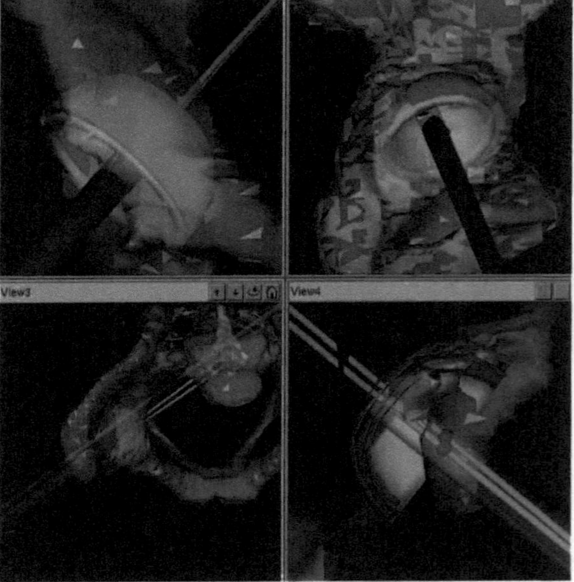

◼ **Fig. 10-3.** Cup navigation; planning = green, execution = yellow

image, point matching has to be confirmed as described above.

5. **Navigation:** Reaming of the acetabulum and impacting the cup under continuous observation of the 3D model with the aim to match the planned acetabular component position (Fig. 10-3). The introduction of the rasp into the intramedullar canal is navigated in case of the femoral navigation in similar manner.

Indication of THA Navigation

There is no contraindication for THA navigation, however, consideration of costs, radiation, and additional operating time involved with this technology may rightfully limit its use. Therefore, CT- based hip navigation is not routinely used at our institution, but is the preferred method in complicated cases, particularly secondary hip arthritis, which this usually represents a difficult operation without navigation. Optimal component position as well as proper leg length is difficult in these cases, especially orientation on altered anatomical landmarks can be problematic. The ideal position of the prosthesis is often clearly different from old joint geometry. We therefore consider navigation a very useful tool for the experienced surgeon in difficult THA.

Exact Positioning of Hip Components with the mediCAD System

Investigations performed at our center demonstrated a considerably increased variability of implant positions after intuitively positioned components on two- or three-dimensional images, especially with difficult secondary arthrosis on both sides, by different surgeons. Reconstructions of a new optimal joint geometry done with subjective experiences of surgeons are difficult to check for optimal anatomical fit, cup-to-stem relation, range of motion and impingement. Potential changes of hip joint forces which may result from the new prosthesis position and a possible change of hip center, offset, and trochanter position cannot be calculated without additional devices. In combination with an attempt of correction of leg length differences they require a preoperative

planning, which should be done for conventional surgical techniques as well as for CT-free navigation.

Computer-assisted calculation of hip biomechanics have been time-consuming and, therefore, not practical for routine use [6, 10, 11]. Musculoskeletal models of hip joint biomechanics are seldom used in THA, but have been practiced in our clinic for planning hip arthroplasty using the 2D mediCAD software on 1:1 scaled radiographs. This method allows a biomechanical analysis of virtually implanted prosthetic components with regards to geometry, joint forces, and hip center in the frontal plane. [2] After simulation of stem implantation ten reference points are marked at the pelvic and femoral bone surface indicating traction of the abductors and the spinocrural muscles in the frontal plane. Additional patient data such as height and weight are registered. The software analyses the newly defined joint geometry for determination of optimal cup position. This position is marked in green on the monitor radiograph and has to overlap with both cup and head center (Fig. 10-4a). Results of positioning are judged automatically using a 12 point score (BLB-Score) [2]. Stem position should be altered in cases of scores lower then 10 points or a surgical unrealistic cup position.

The 2D mediCAD software allows optimal cup and stem positioning and includes a vast majority of currently used prosthetic data. There is FDA approval of this software (ENDOMAP). Initial 2D raw data are transferred into a 3D visualization with the 3D Navitrack system on a frontal plane on which distances of landmarks can be measured and compared with the radiograph (Fig. 10-4b). Alternatively, the resulting postoperative radiographs can be transferred and checked for optimal positioning and joint biomechanics using the mediCAD software (Fig. 10-4c).

Materials and Preliminary Results

Our center has experiences with THA navigation using the Navitrack system since 1999. 43 patients with a mean age of 53 years (31 to 75) underwent this procedure. Indication for THA was primary osteoarthritis in 10 cases, idiopathic femoral head necrosis in 2 cases, and dysplastic hips in 31 cases. Femoral head bone grafting for reconstruction of the acetabular wall in dysplastic hips was

10

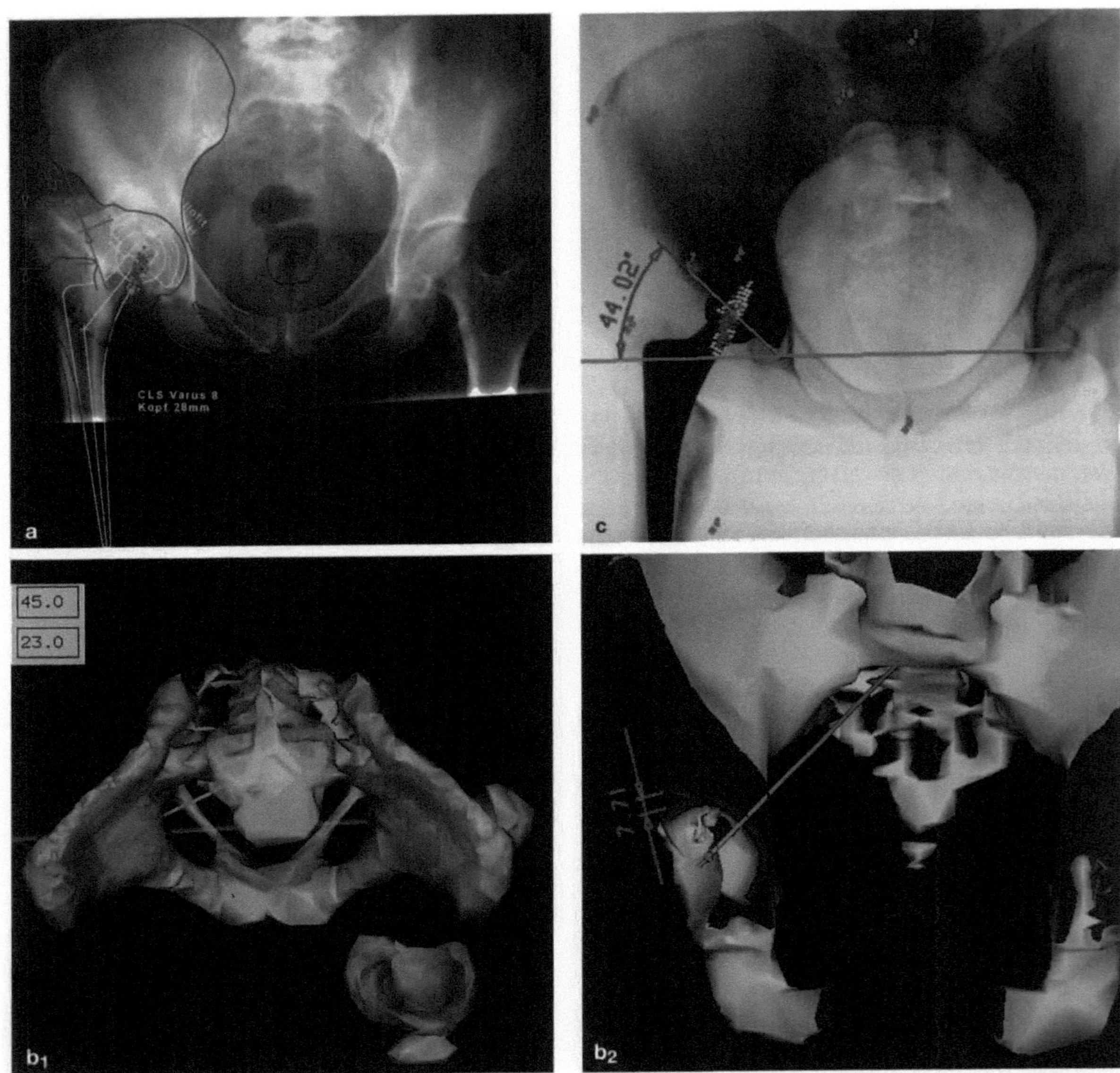

◘ Fig. 10-4a-c. a 2D mediCAD planning in dysplastic hip arthritis right side. **b$_{1/2}$** 3D Navitrack planning in a cross section plane (yellow) with 45 degrees inclination and 23 degrees anteversion. **c** Postoperative 2D mediCAD control, ideally reconstructed joint geometry, BLB score = 12

performed in 12 cases. Thirty-three patients were operated in the supine and ten in lateral decubitus position. Components used were Allofit (Centerpulse, Winterthur, Switzerland) press-fit cups. In the results all cup angles were in the safe zone between 35 and 55 degrees of inclination and 5 to 25 degrees of anteversion. Three cases demonstrated 2 mm medial wall migration according to the navigation; however, radiographs could not confirm this problem. Alteration of cup position were encountered due to improper impaction of the cup or deliberate acceptance of different angles by the surgeon, often in combination with bone grafting.

Registration and calibration errors during navigation were analyzed retrospectively in postoperative CT scans. In 11 selected cases there was a maximum of 5 degrees difference for inclination and 10 degrees difference for anteversion when comparing both preoperative planning and postoperative CT scans of navigated hips. These observations led to implementation of the contralateral superior anterior iliac spine as an additional matching point. Following this technique accuracy of anteversion improved. Preoperative cup size planning was identical in 29 cases and altered in 14 with only 2 mm difference.

There is a learning curve when employing navigation in THA, which leads to a considerable decrease in time consumption and application errors. Additional preoperative time for CT segmentation and planning averages 40 to 50 min and intraoperative surgery time is about 15 min longer. Due to the fact that the majority of cases belonged to a subgroup of complicated secondary OA patients, planning and navigation often required changes in biomechanical aspects such as the hip center and leg length.

There were 43 THA cases that underwent mediCAD software analysis pre- and postoperatively. 27 had excellent results (BLB-Score 11 to 12), 14 had satisfactory results (BLB-Score 8 to 10) and in two cases cup position was not ideally reconstructed. Gait analyses 6 months postoperatively using 3D ultrasound technique revealed a positive association with regained muscle function and reconstructed hip biomechanics as seen in BLB-Score [3]. Stem navigation commenced in August 2001 showing advantages with regards to stem and cup positioning; however, stem navigation is still improving.

To date, a CT-free navigation system for cup and stem navigation is currently being tested. Preliminary results seem promising as the preoperative phase is reduced to standard 2D planning, thus eliminating time intensive reconstructions. During navigation the cup placement relative to the original center of the hip and the angular orientation of the cup are being monitored. This allows for an easy intraoperative comparison to the 2D planning. On the femoral component the preparation of the canal with the rasp is tracked where the orientation of the intra-medullar canal is digitized and used to prevent varus/valgus misalignment. As a result of the rasp and cup tracking the leg-length changes can be monitored in real time while the canal is prepared. Postoperative X-ray analysis shows similar results in component placement as with CT-based applications.

Summary and Perspectives

The Navitrack hip navigation system allows accurate 3D planning and implantation of both cup and stem. Additional information such as 3D orientation and feedback are helpful tools for the operating surgeon, which allows proper execution of THA with little alterations from preoperative planning. Navigation complements the experience of the surgeon, who is still the basis for a good surgical result. An intraoperative plausibility check of the preoperative planning and prosthetic selection is always required, where bony fixation and soft-tissue management should be evaluated. Ideally, one should aim for a combination of secure and precise bony fixation, reattachment of muscle insertions and correction of the leg length, in anatomic difficult cases this might result in a compromise. THA navigation appears to improve component position and increased clinical results. However, long-term data are still required for further proof. There is remaining future potential with navigation in THA including improved planning and execution of the procedure.

Whereas implant position is more or less defined in total knee arthroplasty, ideal component alignment in THA is still discussed. Our experience with difficult secondary osteoarthritic hip cases using CT-based navigation has demonstrated the individually different anatomy of the pelvis, which can be observed by the definition of the frontal plane. Anatomic pelvic variances and pelvic tilt variances should be considered for implant positioning, but rules are not yet clearly established (❑ Fig. 10-5a,b). Because of this, additional biomechanical planning tools for the range of motion, hip joint forces and impingement analysis should be incorporated, as they provide supplementary information for an ideal component placement to the surgeons intuitive, experience-based choice of component placement [2, 4, 18]. Our experience with the 2D planning system mediCAD show first results for those requirements.

Additional time and costs associated with navigation as well as the limited number of compatible implants do not allow general use of this technology, however, CT-free

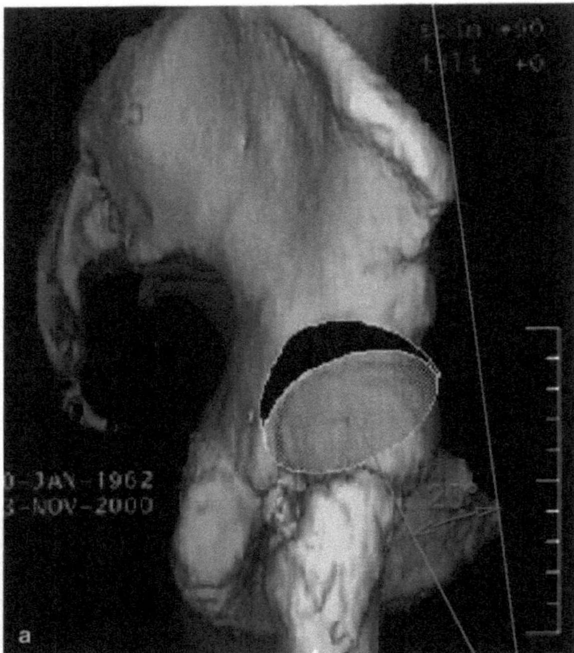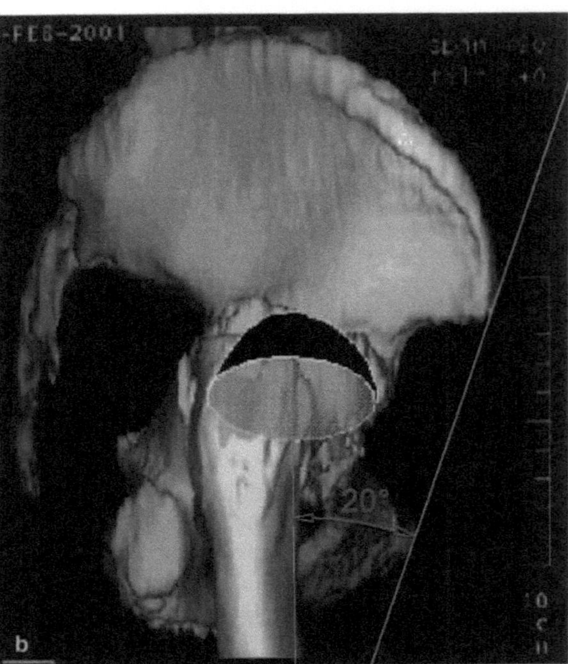

■ Fig. 10-5a, b. Variations of the frontal plane lead to significantly different cup position when 20 degrees anteversion is chosen (*blue line*)

navigation of primary straightforward THA cases is becoming available to overcome some of those limitations. Nevertheless, CT navigation is recommended in difficult hips and revision cases. Finally, the relation of expenses and benefit for this new technology still has to be confirmed in further long-term studies.

References

1. Aldinger G, Fischer A, Kurtz B (1983) Computer assisted manufacturing of individual endoprostheses (preliminary report). Arch Orthop Traumatol Surg 102: 31

2. Babisch J, Layher F, Ritter B, Venbrocks R (2001) Computergestützte biomechanisch fundierte zweidimensionale Operationsplanung hüftchirurgischer Eingriffe. Orthop Praxis 37: 29—38

3. Babisch J, Seidel EJ, Conradi S (2001) 3D-Ultraschall-Ganganalyse ZEBRIS bei Dysplasiecoxarthrose vor und nach der Hüft-TEP-Inplantation. Phys Med Rehab Kuror 11: 139

4. Bader B, Willmann G (1999) Keramische Pfannen für Hüftendoprothesen. Teil 6: Pfannendesign, Inklinations- und Antetorsionswinkel beeinflussen Bewegungsumfang und Impingement. Biomed Technik 44: 212–219

5. Börner M, Wiesel U (1999) Einsatz computerunterstützter Verfahren in der Unfallchirurgie. Trauma Berufskrankh 1: 85–90

6. Steffan H, Breitenhuber W, Sodia F, Reimann R, Moser A (1997) Angewandte Biomechanik — Dreidimensionale Kräfteanalyse und interaktive Operationsplanung. In: Tschauner C (ed) Die Hüfte. Enke, Stuttgart, S 13–18

7. DiGioia AM, Simon D, Jaramaz B et al.)1998) Intraoperative measurement of pelvic and acetabular component alignment using an image guided navigational tool. Trans Orthop Res Soc 23: 198

8. Dorr LD, Wan Z (1998) Causes of and treatment protocol for instability of total hip replacement. Clin Orthop 355: 144–151

9. Hassan DM, Johnston GH, Dust WN, Watson G, Dolovich AT (1998) Accuracy of intraoperative assessment of acetabular prosthesis placement. J Arthroplasty 13: 80–84

10. Johnston RC, Brand RA, Crowninshield RD (1979) Reconstruction of the hip. A mathematical approach to determine optimum geometric relationships. J Bone Joint Surg 61-A: 639–652

11. Kummer B (1991) Die klinische Relevanz biomechanischer Analysen der Hüftregion. Z Orthop 129: 285–294

12. Kurth A, Wassum P, Dietz U, Scale D (1997) Dreidimensionale Darstellung der Becken- und Hüftregion am Computer zur präoperativen Planung von orthopädischen Eingriffen und Operationssimulation. Z Orthop 135: 120–123

13. Lahmer A, Börner M, Kappus M, Skibbe H (1999) ORTHODOC- ein Planungssystem für das rechnergestützte Operieren und zur Visualisierung von Befunden am Skelettsystem. Trauma Berufskrankh 1: 96–103

14. Langlotz U, Lawrence J, Hu Q, Langlotz F, Nolte LP (1999) Image Guided Cup Placement. CARS 99: 717–721

15. Lewinnek GE, Lewis JL, Tarr R et al. (1978) Dislocations after total hip replacement arthroplasties. J Bone Joint Surg 60A: 217–220

16. Malchau H et al.(2000) Prognose der totalen Hüftarthroplastik.67rd Annual Meeting AAOS

17. Nolte LP (1995) Computer-aided fixation of spinal implants.J Imag Guid Surg 1:88–93

18. Robinson RP,Simonian PT,Gradisar IM et al.(1997) Joint motion and surface contact area related to component position in total hip arthroplasty.J Bone Joint Surg 79B:140—146

19. Yoder SA, Brand RA, Pederson DR, Gormann TW (1988) Total hip acetabular component position affects component loosening rates.Clin Orthop 228:79–87

11 Hip Cup Implantation Using the *SurgiGATE* System

M. Stockheim, J. Krämer

Experiences gained with systems developed for placement of pedicle screws led to the transmission of this new knowledge to the field of hip cup placement. DiGioia et al. [4] presented a system in 1998 which enabled CT-based planning of the position of the hip cup, simulated the range of motion especially with regard to impingement and made it possible to achieve the exact planned position by the means of an intraoperative navigation system [5].

Furthermore, this system was used in a number of studies on the precision of hip cup placement. This work pointed out, that conventional planning tools such as templates and scales could not in the least meet the requirements for precision [5]. The knowledge about the optimal hip cup geometry was well-known in literature [1, 6, 9, 12, 13, 15], only the transferral of this knowledge to the insitus was not possible with the conventional, so far developed positioning devices. A similar system was developed by Langlotz et al. at the Maurice E. Mueller Institute in Bern, Switzerland, in 1999 [10]. This newly developed software was integrated as the Hip-Module to the Surgi-GATE-System manufactured by Medivision, Switzerland, and thus introduced to the market.

First clinical experience with the CT-based Surgi-GATE Hip Module was reported by Bernsmann et al. in 2000 [2]. In this work, 70 computer-assisted hip cup placements were examined. It could be shown, that the procedure was approximately only 15 to 20 min prolonged compared to the conventional surgical procedure, that blood loss did not exceed the values given in the literature, but, quite the opposite was rather less (630 ml) and that no complications due to the computer assistance had occurred. In a further analysis Bernsmann et al. differentiated between press-fit and screw cups both placed with image guidance and again reported an overall good precision of the procedure [3].

The further progress in the development of the software, made it possible to orientate the implant position with direct regard to the patients anatomy. Until then, the the OR table had been the reference. This development was achieved by calculating the implant position with respect of the anatomic pelvis plane as determined by the anterior superior iliac spines and the pubic tubercles. This plane represents 90° of cup anteversion. The implant position is determined with reference to this plane and therefore with regard to the patient's anatomy.

The SurgiGATE system consists of a northern digital infrared camera, a Unix workstation running the Sun operating system Solaris. The software developed by Medivision runs on this platform. The software has a modular structure, which gives the user the opportunity to customize the system precisely to his needs. One hardware platform may run different applications, from which the hip module is only one of many (Fig. 11-1).

The instruments for the computer-aided implantation of hip endoprostheses are quite similar to the conventional instruments. One major difference are the infrared transducers, with which the instruments are equipped. These transducers make the instruments visible to the infrared camera. The instruments are equipped with a cable connection to a special connecting box, the Strober box, from where the connection leads to the computer system. The computer system can identify each instrument individually and determines the position of the instruments in space.

Three special instruments are needed in addition to the instruments used in the conventional operating method. There is a foot switch, so that the surgeon can operate the computer system. The pointer is an instrument to point out anatomical structures intraoperatively to the computer system on the skeleton of the patient. The virtual keyboard is an aluminium plate on which special

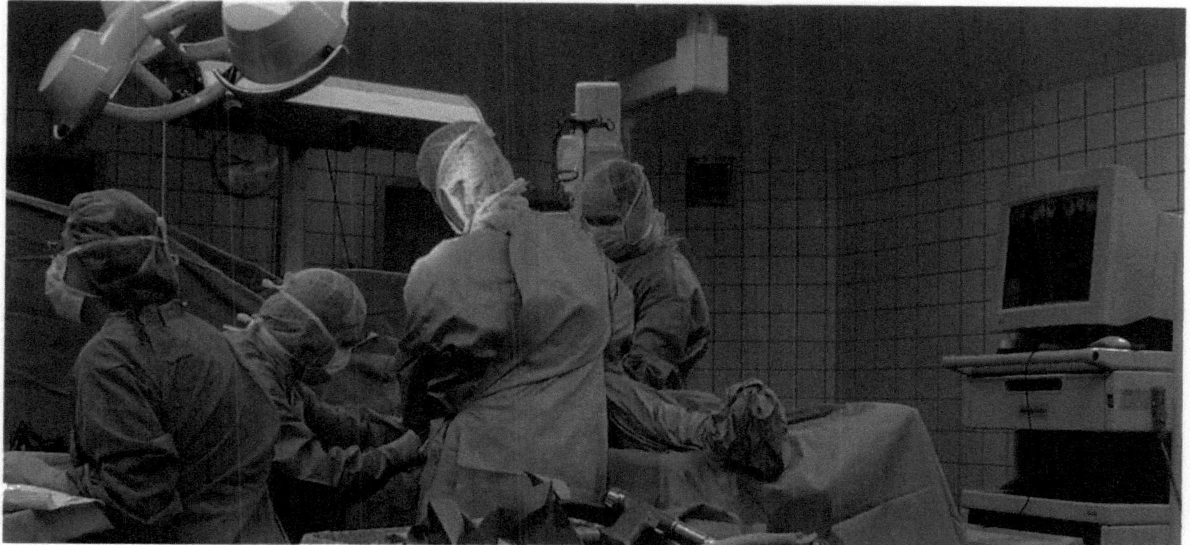

□ Fig. 11-1. The SurgiGATE system

function keys are marked. The virtual keyboard identifies itself through infrared transducers, just as the other instruments. By the means of the infrared transducers the virtual keyboard can be tracked in space. The virtual keyboard is an aluminium plate on which special areas are marked. These areas do not represent keys in a conventional manner, but are only areas in space, which, if touched by the pointer give to certain commands to the computer system. The virtual keyboard, in conjunction with the foot switch, gives the surgeon full control over the SurgiGATE system without depending on other people or impairing the sterile conditions of the operative field.

Just as tracking the instruments in space, the SurgiGATE system needs to track the position of the patient's pelvis as well. For this purpose a dynamic reference base, the DRB, an instrument also equipped with infrared transducers, needs to be securely fastened to the pelvic skeleton of the patient. This is usually done by using a Steinman's pin, which is applied approximately 2 cm cranial of the acetabular roof, using the surgical access according to Bauer. Varying from this procedure, the DRB can alternatively be fixed on the anterior superior iliac spine. The fixation of the DRB is in general variable, taking into account the preferred positioning of the patient on the OR table and the preferred surgical access. It is important

that the DRB is tightened securely to the pelvis and is protected from manipulation (□ Fig. 11-2).

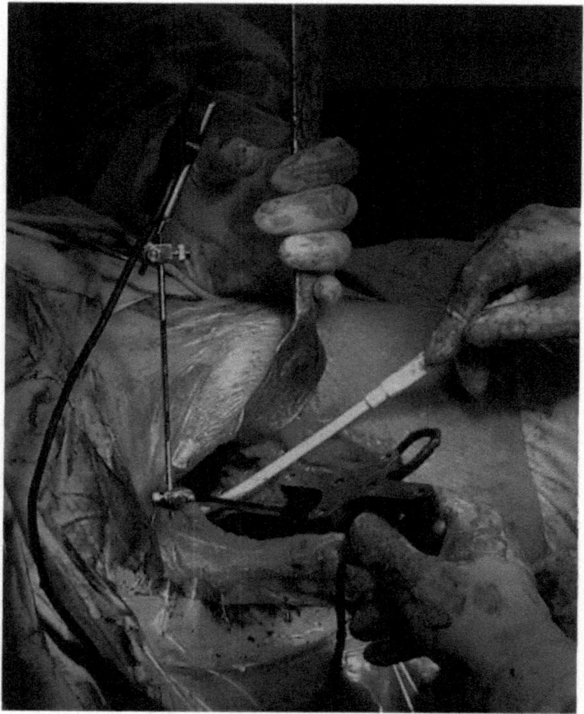

□ Fig. 11-2. Situs. *On the left* DRB fastened to the pelvis. Pointer in use

The computer navigation is separated into preoperative planning and intraoperative navigation. At first, the preoperative planning will be described.

Initially, a CT-scan of the patient's pelvis, done with 3 mm slices and a 1 mm gap, is fed into the computer system. The CT data is either transferred to the Surgi-GATE station by magnetooptical disc or via the hospital network. The SurgiGATE system than reconstructs a three-dimensional model of the pelvis. The femoral head is manually separated from the 3D model. This makes it necessary to remove the femoral head from approximately 20 CT-slices. The femoral head has to be circled in each image using the mouse and the marked area will then be removed. Separation algorithms would be desirable but wouldn't make the manual work on the single CT slices obsolete. Advanced coxarthrosis always melts the bone structure of the acetabulum and the femoral head in X-ray and CT scans. The up to now developed separation algorithms usually follow contrast differences and can therefore be only of little help in arthritic joints.

Next, two sets of landmarks have to be chosen on the 3D model. The landmarks of the first set are called the reference landmarks, they determine the pelvis entry plane, which is defined through both iliac spines and both pubic tubercles. The computer than calculates a plane which touches all four points. Anteversion and inclination are determined with reference to this plane. Only when this pelvic plane has been defined, will the cup position be calculated with respect to the patients anatomy. If this step in the preoperative planning is skipped, the system will position the cup referring to the CT reference of the OR table.

Secondly, another set of landmarks has to be chosen: the landmarks for the pair-point matching. Commonly both iliac spines are used, however at least one of them should be marked. Furthermore, one selects 3 to 4 convinient anatomic structures of which 2 or 3 should be placed in the acetabular floor. Usually one point is placed on the ventral edge of the acetabular notch, the second on the dorsal edge of the acetabular notch and the third in the depth of the second acetabular floor. These points have to be marked during surgery to align the created 3D model and the real patient's pelvis.

From the 3 D model virtual X-ray projections are generated: an a.-p. and an axial view. During surgery the planned axis of the implant and the actual axis of the tool in use will be projected into these virtual X-rays. These projections will give the surgeon a quick overview over the difference between actual tool position and the planned cup position.

In a further planning step the centre of the femoral head is marked. This step has been introduced to the planning software in anticipation of the stem navigation and is not necessary for cup positioning only. Stem navigation with the SurgiGATE. System is covered in detail in chapter 13 of this book by F. Langlotz et al.

Next, the sagittal view on the 3D model is adjusted, matching a plane over the acetabular inlet. The Surgi-GATE system automatically maintains a 90° orientation between the sagittal, frontal and axial plane. This step will give the surgeon a view to the plan corresponding to the operative field.

After these steps the virtual cup may be positioned. The initial course position of the implant is set by two mouse clicks in the a.-p. view. Then the desired implant can be chosen from the SurgiGATE database and can be inserted in the computer images. The virtual cup can be positioned freely and the size can be adjusted to the patient's individual needs. The operation plan is now ready to use and can be saved to the computer hard drive (◘ Fig. 11-3).

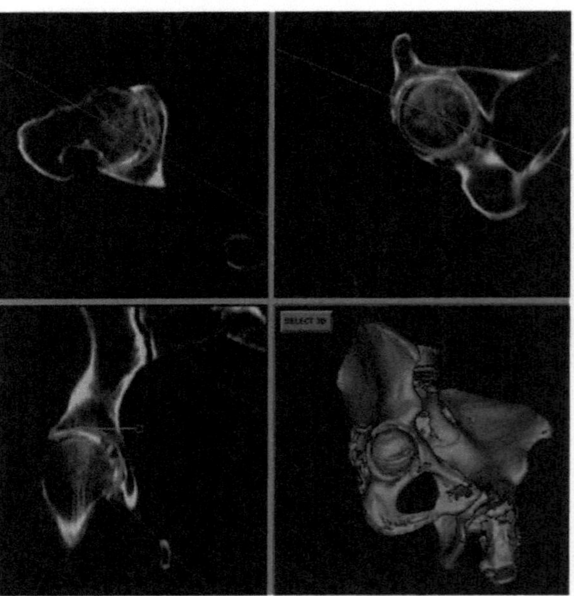

◘ **Fig. 11-3.** Screenshot of a complete hip plan

The choice of available implants implemented in the SurgiGATE software is growing continuously. The SurgiGATE system is an open system and not bound to certain implants. On request, individually preferred implants can be introduced to the software by Medivision. We have regularly achieved good results using the Stratec PPF screw cup, (Boesch cup) and the screw cup according to Hofer-Imhoff, produced by Pentamedical. As press-fit cups we frequently use the PTP-monoblock press-fit cup and the ECM-modular press-fit cup, both manufactured by Stratec-Medical. Stratec has recently sold the endoprothesis section to Biomed Merck. Furthermore, we use the DePuy Duraloc cup. In case of a cemented THR, we consequently use the Stratec Mueller PE cup.

Talking about anteversion and inclination this text always refers to the operative angles. The reader should bear in mind, that there is a difference between the radiologic, anatomic and intraoperative view. Because the three views are based upon different three-dimensional contexts, the numeric values for the angles differ in the three different views. For a detailed overview over this problem the works of Murray [14] and Jaramaz et al. [8] may be recommended.

The intraoperative navigation can be divided in two major steps. First, the instruments and the reference base need to be checked. Then the infrared camera has to be positioned with good view to the operative field and the dynamic reference base (DRB) is fastened to the patient's pelvis. Following these steps, the so-called pair-point matching is done. Pair-point matching means to show the system the pair-point landmarks as determined during preoperative planning. Afterwards, the surface matching has to be done, in which a cloud of points, consisting of at least 12 separate points, is placed on the patient's pelvis. The surface matching shows the computer system parts of the pelvic surface. Preferred areas are the anterior superior iliac spines, the area cranial to the acetabular roof and the parts of the pelvis dorsal to the acetabulum. A few points should be placed inside the hip socket as well. These points taken from the actual patient's pelvis are fed into the SurgiGATE system. For these steps the pointer has to be used.

The SurgiGATE system then tries to find a good alignment between the demonstrated points and the virtual 3D model as generated in the preoperative planning. The precision with which the computer system can align the actual and the virtual pelvis, is expressed in dimensionless figure, the quality index. The manufacturer of the system gives limiting values for these steps. According to the limit given by the manufacturer, the quality index of the pair-point matching should be less than 10.

We regularly choose 5 pair points in preoperative planning, because, after initial processing of the pair-point matching, the SurgiGATE system offers the surgeon the possibility to delete the pair point with the poorest correspondence between preoperative plan and intraoperative mark, as the pair-point matching requires at least four pair points. Choosing five points, one can delete the poorest point with a simple »click« to the virtual keyboard and improve the pair-point matching without additional expenditure.

After pair-point matching, the surface matching has to be done. For surface matching at least 12 points have to be marked on the surface of the patient's pelvis. These points show the SurgiGATE system parts of the pelvic surface. The areas of the pelvic surface to be marked can be chosen quite freely, however, the manufacturer gives a recommendation to the areas that will quickly deliver most reliable results.

The recommended areas are the corpus ossis ilii in the fossa supra acetabularis, the corpus ossis pubis next to the acetabulum, the area of both spinae iliaca anteriores superiores as well as inside the acetabulum. It is recommended to choose more than the required minimum of surface marks, because, same as with the pair point marks, the surface point with the poorest alignment – in this case meaning the point that is placed at the fare most distance from the surface of the 3D model of the pelvis – can be erased and a new calculation can be conducted. When the computer processes the surface points it »pulls« the marked points onto the surface of the 3D model of the pelvis that has been reconstructed from the CT scans. After this calculation the real pelvis and the virtual pelvis are aligned. The achieved precision in this calculation is also expressed as a quality index. After surface matching the value should be less than two.

Following the matching, verification is necessary. The matching is a purely mathematical procedure, during which the system searches for the best suitable solution for the task »align virtual and actual pelvis!«. It is therefore possible that in very few cases the system finds a quality index within the manufacturers limitations, but the actual alignment is only poor. To get a vivid picture of this problem, one may think of the glove example: A right hand glove turned inside out, can be worn on the left hand. This will result in a flawless fit of the glove, but is not the intended solution.

During verification the surgeon points out different prominent anatomic structures in the area surrounding the hip socket and the pelvic skeleton available through the surgical access. The pointer position is displayed on the monitor of the SurgiGATE system. If the SurgiGATE system always reproduces the pointer at the precise place, where the surgeon has put it, the matching has been mathematically precise and has reached good alignment with reality. To strain the above given example again, the right hand glove is actually worn on the right hand.

Since the dynamic reference base (DRB) is placed inside the surgical access it is within reach of the instruments used during surgery. This can lead to dislocation of the DRB. If the DRB is dislocated the referencing will be lost. Minor manipulations of the DRB may happen undetectedly. It is therefore useful to mark a so-called confidence point. To collect a confidence point, the pointer has to be placed onto a structure, that can be identified easily and reliably. This position is saved. In case of an obvious manipulation of the DRB, or if the surgeon is under the impression that the DRB has been moved, the surgeon can place the pointer upon the structure initially marked and have the computer system compare both points. This is called the accuracy check. If the initially marked position and the repeatedly marked position differ more than 3 mm, the movement of the DRB has exceeded the accepted range and the referencing is lost. The matching has either to be repeated or the navigation has to be cancelled. Experience has shown, that it is often difficult to re-identify the initially marked confidence point. It may therefore be advisable to mark the confidence point with a small screw.

After matching and verification, the actual navigation starts. The operation is performed in the conventional technique, only direction and depth of the tools are additionally displayed on the computer screen.

The visualization of the tool direction is done in different ways. The greater part of the computer screen is taken by three reticules, each for one dimension in space. If all three reticules are brought to alignment, the tool runs on the path determined in the preoperative plan.

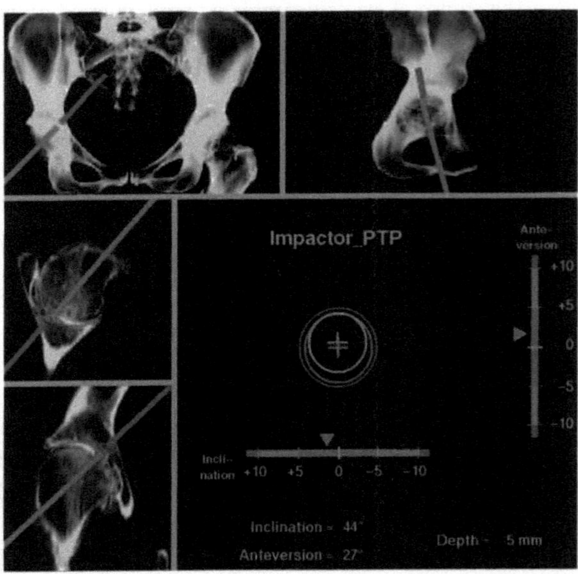

◨ Fig. 11-4. Screenshot of the navigator. *Red* the planned implant axis, *green* the actual tool axis. In the big window the 3-way redicule

Besides there are two scales, one for anteversion and one for inclination, which show the deviation of the actual position from the planned position on a scale and also give the deviation in degrees. Third, there are trajectories of the actual and the planned implant position projected into the virtual X-rays reconstructed from the CT scans (◨ Fig. 11-4).

After the cup implantation an accuracy check is carried out to see if the system has worked inside the given tolerance. If this is the case, the computer-assisted cup placement has been successful.

The Medivision has introduced the CT-free cup navigation in 2001 [11]. The CT-free cup navigation acquires the necessary image data from a fluoroscope. The C-arm has to be equipped with a calibration grille which is necessary for size and distorsion correction. To perform the surgery one image in a.-p. view and one image in lateral view are acquired. The surgery is than guided with virtual fluoroscopic images. The principles of fluoroscopy-based image guided surgery have been published by Hofstetter et al. [7] in 1999.

In CT-free cup navigation preoperative planning and intraoperative matching is not necessary. To determine the pelvic entry plane the spina iliaca anteriores superiores are marked with the pointer, the tubercula pubicae are

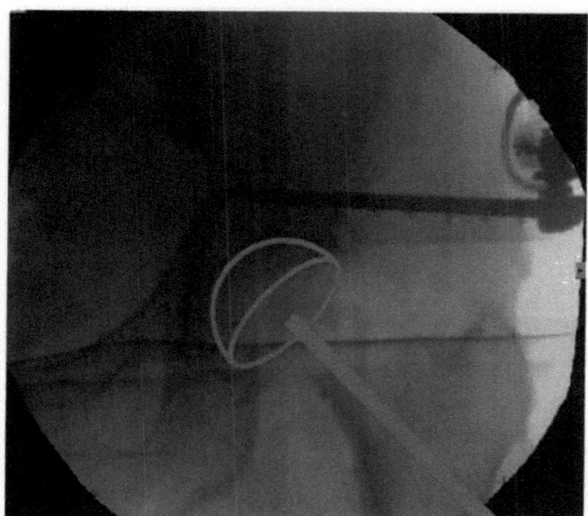

◼ Fig. 11-5. Screenshot from the SurgiGATE C-arm. The virtual cup projected into the fluoroscopic image

marked virtually with two stereoscopic fluoroscopic shots. The determined plane is equivalent to 90° anteversion and is identical to the pelvic entry plane which has been described above with the CT-based cup navigation. To keep track of the patient's movement, a dynamic reference base (DRB) has to be fastened to the patient's pelvis just as in the CT-based navigation.

The benefits of fluoroscopic navigation are obvious. First, there is the significantly reduced radiation exposure of the patient. Hospital logistics are relieved from acquiring preoperative CT scans and transferring the image data to the department that will perform the surgery, besides reducing logistic problems, this leads to a cost reduction as well (◼ Fig. 11-5).

Apart from the considerable advantages of fluoroscopy-based navigation, the renunciation of preoperative planning can be a disadvantage in special indications. Marked dysplastic hips are an important indication for preoperative planning, as described in chapter 12 of this book by R. Haaker and J. Krämer. Only the CT-based preoperative planning gives the surgeon the chance to precisely chose a suitable implant, reinforcement rings and the extent of necessary acetabuloplasty prior to surgery.

When this book is in print the stem navigation will be available in the CT-free as well as in the CT-based

SurgiGATE hip module as described in chapter 13 of this book by F. Langlotz et al.

References

1. Bader R, Willmann G (1999) Ceramic acetabular cups for hip endoprosthesis: 7: How do position of the center of rotation and CCD angle of the shaft modify range of motion and impingement? Biomed Tech (Berl) 44: 345–351

2. Bernsmann K, Langlotz U, Ansari B, Wiese M (2000) Computer-assisted navigated acetabulum placement in hip prosthesis implantation – application study in routine clinical care: Z Orthop Ihre Grenzgeb 138: 515–521

3. Bernsmann K, Langlotz U, Ansari B, Wiese M (2001) Computer-assisted navigated cup placement of different cup types in hip arthroplasty – a randomised controlled trial: Z Orthop Ihre Grenzgeb 139: 512–517

4. DiGioia AM, Jaramaz B, Blackwell M et al. (1998) Image guided navigation system to measure intraoperatively acetabular implant alignment. Clin Orthop 355: 8–22

5. DiGioia AM, Jaramaz B, Nikou C, LaBarca RS, Moody JE, Colgan BD (2000) Surgical navigation for total hip replacement with the use of HipNav. Operative Techniques in Orthopaedics 10: 3–8

6. Fontes D, Benoit J, Lortat-Jacob A, Didry R (1991) Luxation of total hip endoprothesis. Statistical validation of a modelization, apropos of 52 cases. Rev Chir Orthop Reparatrice Appar Mot 77: 163–170

7. Hofstetter R, Slomczykowski M, Sati M, Nolte L-P (1999) Fluoroscopy as an imaging means for computer-assisted surgical navigation. Comput Aided Surg 4: 65–76

8. Jaramaz B, DiGioia A, Blackwell M, Constantinos N (1998) Computer assisted measurement of hip cup placement in THR. Clin Orthop 354: 70–81

9. Jerosch J, Steinbeck J, Stechmann J, Güth V (1997) Influence of a high hip center on abductor muscle function. Arch Orthop Trauma Surg 116: 385–389

10. Langlotz U, Lawrence J, Hu Q, Langlotz F, Nolte LP (1999) Image guided cup placement. In: Lemke HU, Vannier MW, Inamura K, Farman AG (eds) Computer assisted radiology and surgery. Elsevier Science B.V., Amsterdam, pp 717–721

11. Langlotz U, Grützner PA, Bernsmann K et al. (2003) A hybrid CT-free navigation system for acetabular cup placement. J Arthroplasty (submitted for publication)

12. Lengsfeld M, Bassaly A, Boudriot U, Pressel T, Griss P (2000) Size and direction of hip joint forces associated with various positions of the acetabulum. J Arthroplasty 15: 314–320

13. Lewinnek GE, Lewis JL, Tarr T, Compere CL, Zimmermann JR (1978) Dislocations after total hip-replacement arthroplasties. J Bone Joint Surg Am 60: 217–220

14. Murray DW (1993) The definition and measurement of acetabular orientation. J Bone Joint Surg Br 75: 228–232

15. Seki M, Yuasa N, Ohkuni K (1998) Analysis of optimal range of socket orientation in total hip arthroplasty with use of computer-aided design simulation J Orthop Res 16: 513–517

12 Hip Navigation Using the *SurgiGATE* System in Dysplastic and Revision Cases

R. G. Haaker

Introduction

Opponents to CT-guided navigation of acetabulum components in total hip arthroplasty (THA) argue that this technique is not problem oriented, time consuming with additional radiation, and too inconvenient for practical routine use. Therefore, two- and three-dimensional fluoroscopic systems have been developed as well as on purely kinematics based systems, such as the OrthoPilot (Aesculap, Tuttlingen, Germany).

Having gained considerable experience in the field of CT guided hip acetabulum navigation in two controlled comparative trials with 150 CT cases, we now extended the indication to perform SurgiGATE CT navigation on dysplastic and revision THA as well. There were 20 dysplastic hips that entered the second study, in which the alignment of the acetabular cup was confirmed by CT scan. Revision cases had preoperative CT scans. Due to considerable artifacts caused by the metal cups, we recommend CT scans in loosened cemented polyethylene cups only, however, even metal head makes interpretation and planning difficult (see Fig. 12-2).

Cup Navigation in Dysplastic Hip Joints

CT-based planning of cup alignment in dysplastic hips offers the advantage of exact calculation and prediction of component positioning with regards to the hip center. Both 2D fluoroscopy and fully kinematics based system software are not able to accomplish these goals. Dysplastic hips are usually combined with pathologic femoral shaft versions, which require implant adaptation in terms of a deviation from the norm. This technique has been established using the conventional technique and individually increases range of motion. A variety of implant products is needed (screwed cups, press-fit cups, etc.), therefore, open navigation systems become a necessity with a »library« that allow for different manufactures implants.

Case Report 1

This case demonstrates a secondary dysplastic hip OA 20 years after Chiari osteotomy. The opposite side was treated conventionally 4 years ago using a Burch-Schneider cage and autologous bulk bone grafting with 5 cm leg lengthening (■ Fig. 12-1). A screw in cup plus autologous bone grafting was planned for navigation of the remaining dysplastic hip. Preoperative radiographs included artifacts from the metal implants, which led to software and cup positioning problems in comparison to the mediCAD system (■ Fig. 12-2). However, cup size and cranial acetabular reconstruction could be planned (■ Fig. 12-3).

Since the acetabular congruency was pathological, the anterversion angle was changed from an ideal 25 degrees to 15 degrees with 45 degrees inclination. The hip center was calculated from the opposite side radiographs, because of the missing tear drop structure (■ Fig. 12-4). Required anatomical landmarks were non-existing in this case, therefore, intraoperative pair-point matching as described in chapter 11 is impossible. Preoperative planning and surgical execution should be performed by the same person (■ Fig. 12-5). Intraoperative navigation necessitates both two-plane orientation and perfect acetabular positioning. Preoperative planning and postoperative results show excellent correlation (■ Fig. 12-6).

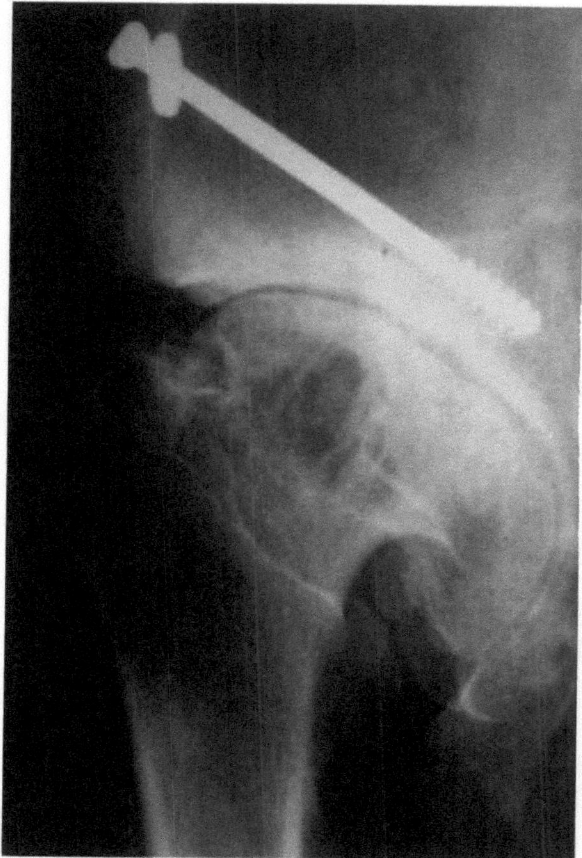

Fig. 12-1. Preoperative a.-p. radiograph 20 years post Chiari osteotomy

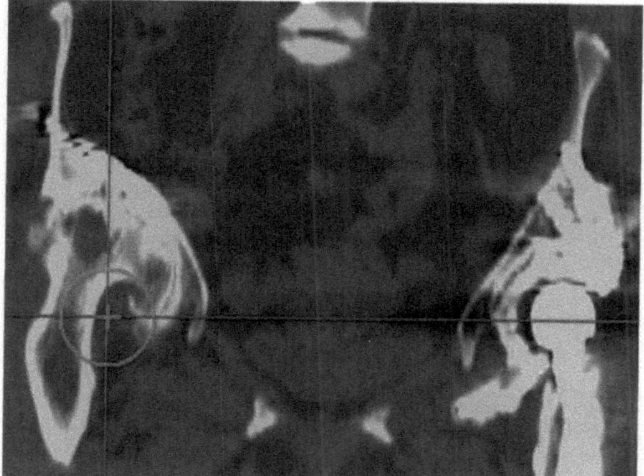

Fig. 12-2. Preoperative planning of the hip center using the Surgi-GATE module. Artifacts caused by metal components

The surgeon can check upon the accuracy of the navigation system throughout the operation. The implantation of an acetabular 2.7 mm temporary reference screw, which carries a reproducible pointer housing has proven to be useful.

Case Report 2

The challenge in this case was complicated by high hip dislocation with 5 cm limb shortening of the right side with a normal opposite hip joint (■ Fig. 12-7). Soft tissue attachment would not allow full leg length restoration, but preoperative expander treatment was refused. According to the literature medium term Harris Hip Score results were comparable with the hip center located either in the primary, secondary or tear-drop position.

The goal was to use a press-fit implant (ECM-Cup, Stratec), which allows fixation of bulk autograft via component implemented screw holes. In order to accomplish vertical screw positioning the cup had to be put into 45 to 50 degrees of inclination and 15 degrees of anteversion. Preoperative planning led to a less than ideal hip center and decreased anteversion compared with the opposite side because of pathological shaft position (■ Fig. 12-8).

Although resorption of autologous bulk bone grafts remains an issue of concern, some authors accept cup inclinations of up to 50 degrees in order to improve host bone contact with the cup [5, 8]. Considerable autograft resorption in seven (9%) of 77 cases was reported in one series [6]. Whether or not bulk graft requires screw fixation is controversial.

Although CT data indicated dysplastic anterior and posterior columns, a satisfactory positioning of the cup could be achieved intraoperatively, a difficult maneuver when performed by conventional methods (■ Fig. 12-9 a,b). One of the main advantages of 3D preoperative planning is the possibility of predictive cup positioning despite massive bone defects and acceptable compromises (■ Figs. 12-10 and 12-11).

In the remaining 18 cases the final cup positioning was within 2 mm of tolerance compared with preoperative planning, a figure that is likely to improve with a more precise preoperative planning. In some cases a perforation of the caudal acetabular floor with a cage was

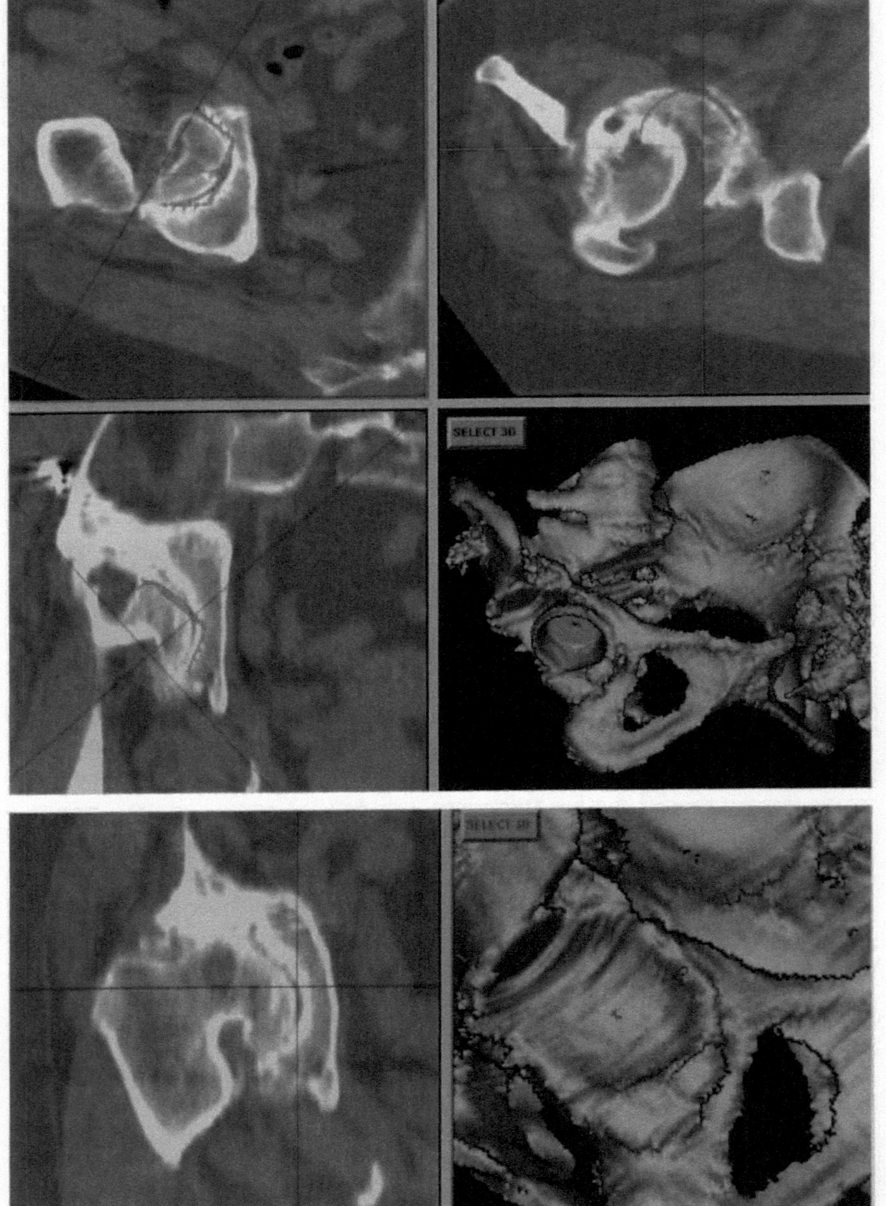

Fig. 12-3. 3D preoperative planning using a virtual screwed cup implant (Stratec, PPF) in a 3D pelvis module

Fig. 12-4. Definition of the hip center, cup positioning and probing of landmarks

attempted, but abandoned during surgery. A precision of two to three degrees cup version could be achieved with most procedures. Figures of cup and stem versions were higher than the normal group depending on the severity of preoperative hip pathology.

Cup Navigation in Revision Cases

In revision cases, intraoperative matching is complicated by metal artifacts including markers in cemented polyethylene (PE) cups. In addition, a loosened PE cup does

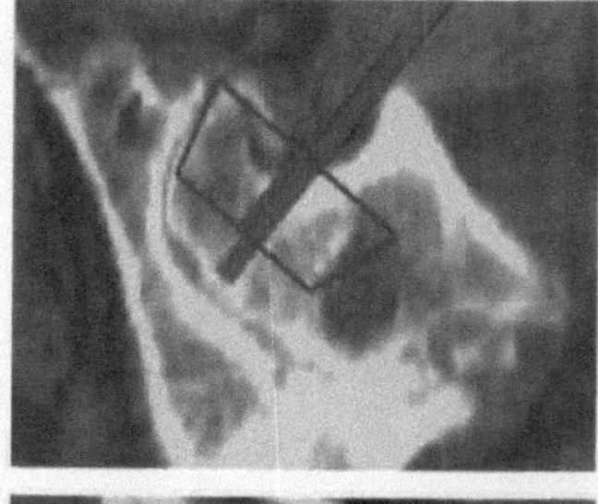
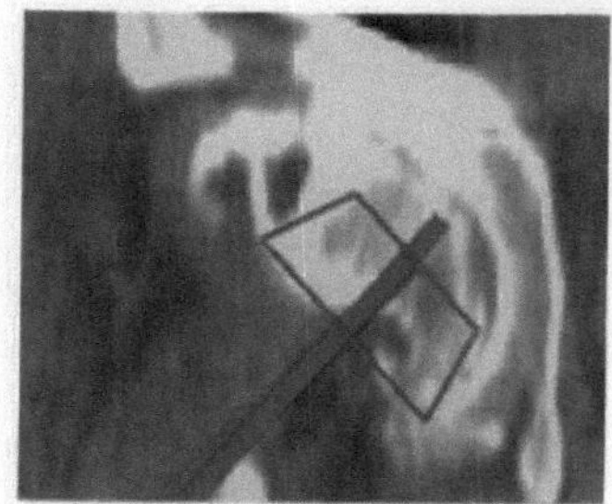
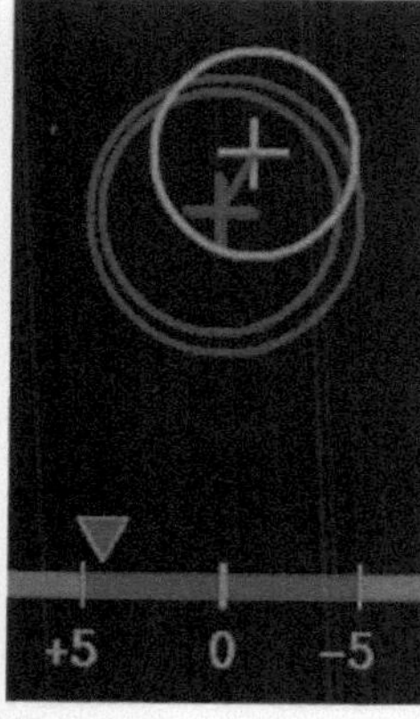

Fig. 12-5. Intraoperative navigation of the cup in two planes of autograft (anteversion of 26 degrees is accomplished)

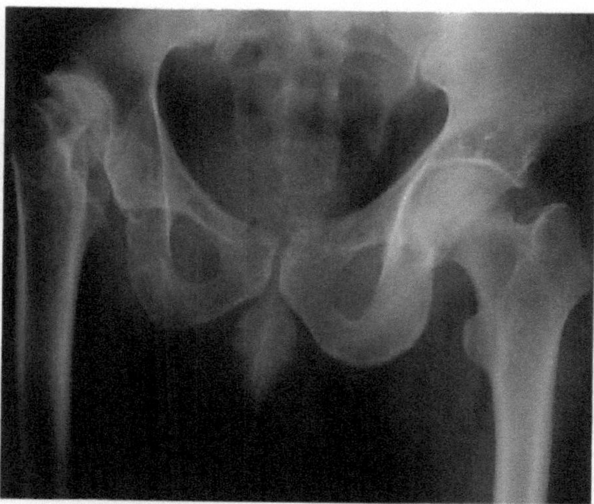

Fig. 12-7. Preoperative status with 5 cm leg length deficit left in a dysplastic hip joint

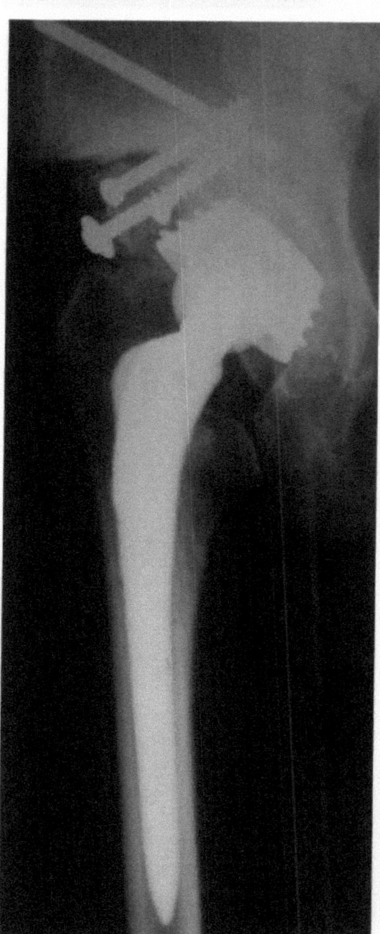

Fig. 12-6. Post-operative radiograph showing perfect alignment of both autograft and cup

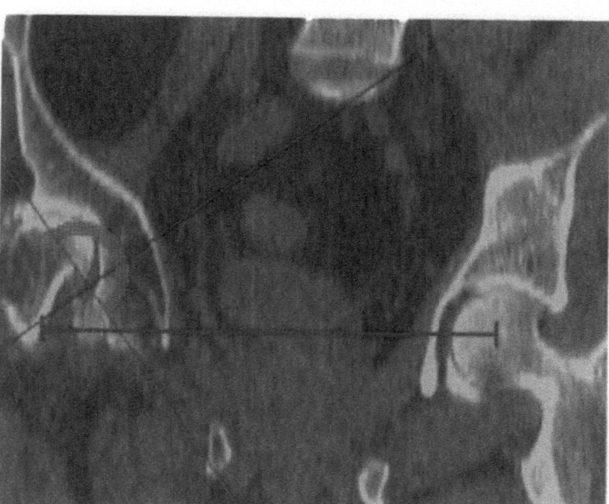

Fig. 12-8. Preoperative planning with the SurgiGATE module. Calculation of the rotational hip center

not represent a fixed landmark for matching purposes. Therefore, severely loosened or subluxed cups can make navigation impossible. In those cases a laser surface mapping and matching as used by neurosurgeons can be helpful. Another advantage is the 3D fluoroscopic C-arm.

As demonstrated both implantation and correct version of a cemented cup or cage version is possible with this navigation system. Satisfactory solutions are not available with current software module.

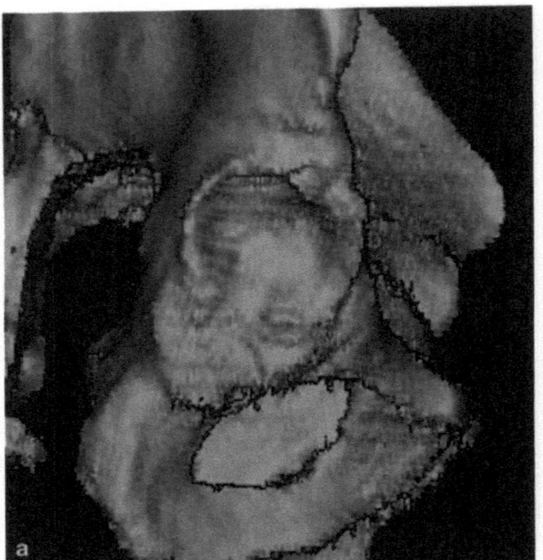
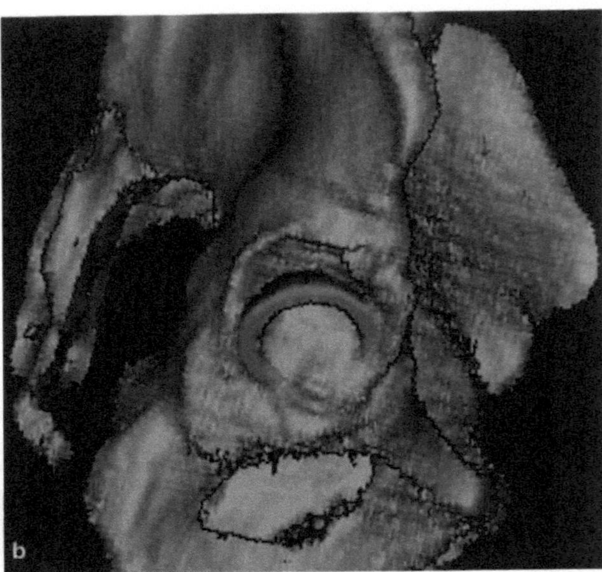

Fig. 12-9a, b. a 3D model of the acetabulum; **b** planning of the virtual press-fit cup (Stratec, ECM). Space left cranially for planning of the bone graft

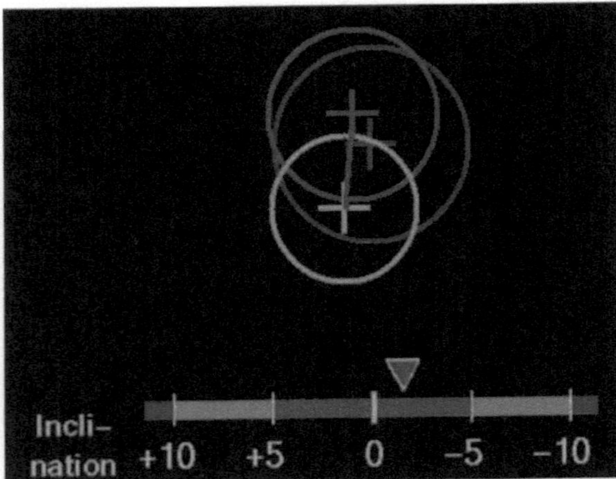

Fig. 12-10. Intraoperative navigation with depth data (lower left = 1 mm)

In summary, CT-based navigation of cups using the SurgiGATE system in dysplastic hip cases showed promising applications. Additional 3D geometric preoperative planning as is available with the mediCAD system (see chapter 10) would enhance the accuracy and reproducibility of the right hip center. Virtual implantation and reconstruction of the acetabular bone defect with the

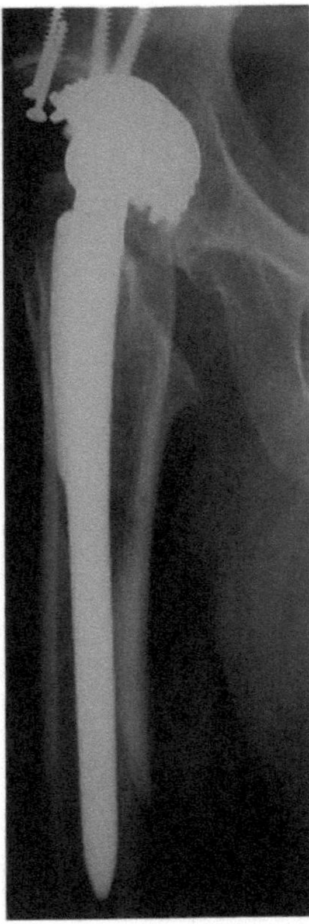

Fig. 12-11. Postoperative radiograph showing considerable external rotation of the stem because of strong muscle tension after 3.5 cm leg lengthening

patient's own femoral head would be desired. The current SurgiGATE system is not recommended for revision cases yet.

Future Perspectives

For perfect soft tissue balancing of total hip arthroplasties a combination of both cup and stem navigation is required. Data for best cup positioning with a low risk for dislocation in the so-called „save zone" were first advocated by Lewinnek in 1978 and were recently confirmed in 2001 by Widmer et al. and Bader et al. with 40 degrees inclination and 26 degrees anteversion plus a stem anteversion of 15 degrees. Dysplastic hip joints are frequently associated with an increased shaft anteversion raising the question whether anatomical reduction of this anteversion is desired or whether balancing of the shortened soft tissues have priority. We believe that these key questions may be answered with new evolving computer navigation of total hip arthroplasty, which includes correct anatomical positioning of the hip center, alignment of the cup, stem anteversion, off-set and soft-tissue balancing.

References

1. Bader R, Willmann G (1999) Ceramic acetabular cups for hip endoprothesis: How do position of the center of rotation and CCD angle of the shaft modify range of motion and impingement? Biomed Tech (Berl) 44: 345–351
2. Bader R, Willmann G (2000) Einfluß von Implantatdesign und -lage auf Range of Motion und Impingement bei künstlichem Hüftgelenkersatz. Z Orthop 138: 19–20
3. Bernsmann K, Langlotz U, Ansari B, Wiese M (2000) Computerassistierte navigierte Pfannenplatzierung in der Hüftendoprothetik – Anwendungsstudie im klinischen Routinealltag. Z Orthop 138: 515–521
4. Bernsmann K, Langlotz U, Ansari B, Wiese M (2001) Computerassistierte navigierte Platzierung von verschiedenen Pfannentypen in der Hüftendoprothetik – eine randomisierte kontrollierte Studie. Z Orthop 139: 512–516
5. Büttner-Janz K, Jessen N (1998) Dysplasie-Coxarthrose mit Sekundärpfanne – Endoprothesen-Impalntation in die Primär- oder Sekundärpfanne? Z Orthop 136: A47
6. Gleißner F, Wessinghage D, Fitzek JG (1991) Der Pfannenerkeraufbau – eine spezifische Ergänzung des totalendoprothetischen Hüftgelenkersatzes. Z Orthop 129: 188–193
7. Haaker R, Tietjen K, Rubenthaler F, Stockheim M (2003) Computer-Assisted Navigated Cup Placement in Primary and Secondary Dysplastic Hips. Z Orthop 141: 105–111
8. Hauser R (1991) Die Balgrist-Pfanne in der zementfreien Endoprothtik von Dysplasiecoxarthrosen und von anderen Acetabulumdefekten. Z Orthop 129: 183–187
9. Jerosch J, Hasselbach C, Filler T, Peuker E, Rahgozar M, Lahmer A, Witzel U (1999) Roboterassistierte Implantation der femoralen Komponente einer Hüftendoprothese – eine experimentelle Untersuchung. Orthop Praxis 35: 632–641
10. Jerosch J, Steinbeck J, Stechmann J, Güth V (1997) Influence of a high hip center on abductor muscle function. Arch Orthop Trauma Surg 116: 385–389
11. Widmer KH, Ackermann JP, Bereiter H (2001) Ergebnisse der manuellen und computernavigierten Implantation einer Monoblock-press-Fit-Pfanne mit Tantalumoberfläche. Z Orthop 139: S 59

13 Femoral Stem Navigation with the *SurgiGATE* System

F. Langlotz, A. Marx, M. Kubiak-Langer, G. Zheng, U. Langlotz

Introduction

While robotics in total hip replacement (THR) is applied during the preparation of the femoral cavity, surgical navigation for THR has its roots in the placement of acetabular cups. Based on anatomical bony landmarks, a pelvic coordinate system was defined allowing for precise computer-assisted alignment of the implant. Different approaches have been realized to optimize cup placement. Navigation systems based on preoperative CT scans compete with those using direct digitalzation or kinematic analysis for landmark acquisition. Recent developments led to a CT-free navigation system based on registered fluoroscopy and direct landmark digitization. Neither time-consuming preoperative planning nor error-prone intraoperative registration is required with this approach. The existing systems have a patient-specific pelvic reference coordinate system in common, enabling exact realization of the correct anteversion and inclination of the cup independently from the intraoperative position of the patient.

A number of studies could demonstrate the direct relation between the malpositioning of hip prostheses and an increased risk of postoperative complications such as luxation, excessive wear, or early loosening [6]. Computer integrated techniques enabled the development of surgical navigation systems for THR yielding first positive results with CT based approaches [6,7].

The development of the two SurgiGATE navigation systems for femoral stem placement was largely based on experiences gained in the area of computer-assisted cup placement. Two alternative approaches were followed in order to complement the cup navigation systems presented in chapter 11 and 12 with navigation support for the femoral side. The following paragraphs cover the developmental basics of both systems for computer-assisted stem placement.

What is Required of a Prosthetic Stem Navigation System?

None of the systems should have a decisive influence on current surgical techniques. Thus, the surgeon should remain free to choose both the position on the operating table and the surgical approach to the hip joint. Navigation should not influence or prohibit specific surgical techniques. Supine and varied lateral positioning on the operation table must be possible. The type of surgical approach must conform to the anatomical situation and/or the surgeon's preferences. This also includes the surgeon being free to choose the osteotomy of the femoral neck. In both the system variants presented here, a navigation aid for the incision is omitted. As an advantage compared to robotics, introducing navigation should reduce the approach and so be able to reduce invasiveness and trauma from the operation. Moreover, the surgeon – as the operator – shall actively use the computer as an orientation aid, and the success of the operation must not be compromised by a system failure.

When navigating only the cup, it is sufficient to align the implant in the frontal and transverse plane. The main focus is to exactly determine the angle of inclination and anteversion. By registering the final femoral and pelvic position of the prosthesis, the displacement of the hip's center of rotation along the longitudinal axis may be calculated. The size of the implant introduced in each case and/or the size of the inlay and the head can be taken into account here. A preoperative difference in the length of the leg can be exactly corrected for by selecting the appropriate implant and/or inserting the prosthesis, with the aid of navigation, to an appropriate depth. Similarly, the displacement of the center of rotation in the transverse plane can be registered and the altered offset thus determined, which also allows its possible influence on the function of the gluteal muscles to be assessed. Graphically visualizing a possible postoperative result intraoperatively enables the given situation to be adapted at any time. Extreme changes in the length of the leg can be taken into account as the prosthesis is permanently implanted, and possible insufficiency in the muscles encompassing the hip can be compensated for.

One purely stem-specific parameter is the exact alignment of the prosthesis in the frontal plane of the femur. Varus and valgus malpositioning is to be avoided. Varus mispositioning is significantly more common and thus clinically more relevant. Inserting the stem prosthesis insufficiently laterally in the region of the ridge of the trochanter causes a danger of a biomechanically unfavorable, varus mispositioning of the stem prosthesis. Navigation is intended to help achieve an exact alignment in the frontal plane and precise rotational alignment in the transverse plane. Femoral anteversion, in combination with the inclination of the cup, has a decisive influence on the range of motion of the prosthesis. This information forms the basis for developing the necessary simulation software intended to minimize postoperative impingement; the development of this software is planned for both systems. Thus, a pre- and/or intraoperative diagnostic tool will be provided, using which restrictions of motion for the prosthesis may be registered.

System Description

Hardware

The standard SurgiGATE (Medivision, Oberdorf, Switzerland) components make up the computer hardware of the two modules that were developed by the Maurice E. Müller Institute for Surgical Technology and Biomechanics in collaboration with Medivision. An optoelectronic camera (Optotrak 3020, Northern Digital Inc., Waterloo, Ontario, Canada), mounted onto a mobile cart, measures the position of objects with attached infrared light emitting diodes (LED). This setup enables the precise three-dimensional (3D) tracking of surgical instruments, the operated anatomy, and – in the case of fluoroscopy-based navigation – the C-arm (see below). The navigation software runs on an Ultra-10 Workstation (Sun Microsy-

stems, Volketswil, Switzerland). This computer is responsible for all graphical output of navigational information, the control of user interaction, and the communication with the tracking camera. All hardware components are assembled in a mobile cart that facilitates flexible usage of the system in different operating theaters of a hospital.

Instruments

For the described applications, the standard SurgiGATE tool set, consisting of pointer, dynamic reference base (DRB) [11], and virtual keyboard [12], was extended by navigated broaches (◘ Fig. 13-1). The current software version supports the PPF prosthetic stem system (Biomet-Merck, Darmstadt, Germany; formerly Stratec Medical, Oberdorf, Switzerland). Due to design of this stem, a direct navigation of the implant insertion process is not possible. A navigation adapter attached directly to the stem could damage the implant's surface, which cannot be accepted. Instead, the rasps are navigated during the preparation of the femoral canal, and an appropriate LED shield was developed. Since various rasp sizes are required for the preparation of the cavity intraoperatively,

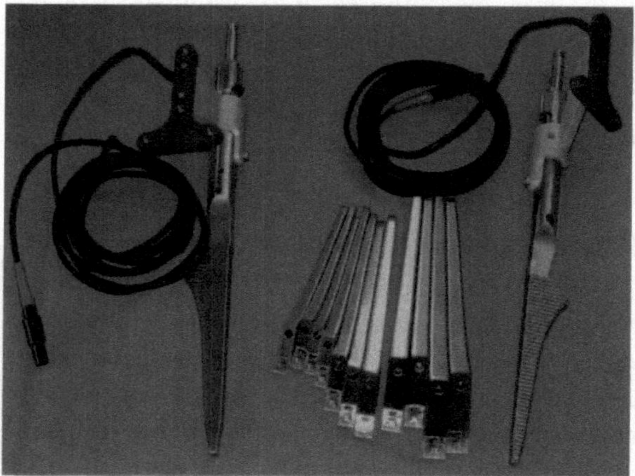

◘ **Fig. 13-1.** Newly developed modular rasps of the PPF system are used during the navigated preparation of the femoral cavity. A quick-link attaches the different sizes of the instrument to a navigation shield holder that connects to the standard manual or pneumatic hammer. Additionally, this holder houses the infrared LEDs enabling tracking of the rasp's position. Depending on the operated side, the navigation shield may be mounted to the holder in two alternative orientations

a special modular rasp handle had to be developed, which carries one LED shield for each of the broaches. Its coupling mechanism has been optimized, allowing any of the available rasps to be attached rigidly and without play. Intraoperatively, the handle may be impacted with a manual sliding or air-driven automatic hammer. The rasp, once placed within the femoral canal, acts as a trial implant as well, i.e., any head and neck of the implant system may be attached for trial repositioning.

New methods had to be developed for the fixation of the DRBs to the bones. Two separate LED shields are required for the two bony structures involved in a THA procedure: pelvis and femur. Tests have proven an anchoring with two self-drilling screws or K-wires to be extremely stable. Since bone quality in the area of the greater trochanter is often poor in patients scheduled for THA surgery, a secure DRB fixation cannot always be achieved. Therefore, in CT-free THA navigation, the DRB is attached to the distal part of the femur. The exact location and orientation of the navigation reference may be adapted to case-specific needs. In CT-based navigation the femoral DRB is attached after femoral head resection and repositioning of the leg. Especially in the lateral decubitus position, this enables the surgeon to place the DRB close to the lesser trochanter. An additional trauma of the distal femur can therefore be prevented. Depending on the image modality used for navigation, as well as the surgical approach and technique, the camera position within the OR may have to be changed during the procedure to achieve optimal intraoperative visibility of the navigated instruments.

gistration in the two implemented systems, two strategies were realized, both of which require the acquisition of image data, either pre- or intraoperatively. Precise digitization with direct physical contact, as used for navigated acetabular cup placement, is obviously impractical for the femur. Both presented system variants differ completely in the way they implement solutions for this problem (see below).

In both modules, the individuality of the employed reference coordinate system is an essential feature for the anatomically correct placement of an endoprosthesis. Only with the help of navigation, stem-specific complications such as cortex perforations can be avoided.

The two alternative modules that have been mentioned several times already shall be presented in detail now. Chapters 11 and 12 is suggested as supplementary reading. It describes the associated SurgiGATE modules for computer-assisted acetabular cup placement.

CT-Based Femoral Stem Navigation

Based on experiences with the existing CT-based acetabular cup navigation system, an associated module for the navigated implantation of femoral prosthesis components was developed. Preoperatively, a CT scan is required of the hip to be operated. The scanned volume has to cover the acetabulum and the proximal femur as well as approximately 3–4 cm of the distal femur. This latter area is required to define the patient-individual coordinate system.

Patient-Specific Coordinate System

Noble et al. demonstrated the nonexistence of one universal femoral canal, but rather individual femoral anatomy is considerably variable [10]. Consequently, it is necessary to define a patient-specific frame of reference, in which planning of the femoral canal preparation can be performed. Such a coordinate system must be based on anatomical landmarks to make it patient-specific. The authors are not aware of any published work on femoral coordinate systems that defines methods for the individual determination of the proximal femoral shaft axis. Depending on the preferred method of landmark re-

Patient-Individual Coordinate System

For the CT-based module, a femoral coordinate system is established by the preoperative digitization of five anatomical locations within the CT scan. The axis of the femoral shaft is defined by two points in the proximal area. To minimize rotational errors, both points shall be selected as far away from each other as possible. The calculation of femoral antetorsion is based the transcondylar axis, which is derived from Dunlap's definition of a femoral reference plane [4]. This plane is constructed through the posterior aspects of the femoral condyles and the posterior aspect of the lesser trochanter.

Preoperative Planning

The possibility to precisely plan the intended intervention preoperatively is a major advantage of CT-based navigation. The existing cup-planning module [7] was extended to facilitate determination of correct implant size, position, and orientation, as well as all navigation relevant parameters. The planning of all data for the acetabular component is completed first. The surgeon performs the following steps in order to establish the required information for the femoral shaft.

Definition of Anatomical Landmarks

Two sets of landmarks need to be selected. Five points serve as reference locations according to the aforementioned definition. They establish the patient-individual coordinate system that is used to calculate femoral antetorsion and potential varus/valgus orientation of the implant. Additionally, characteristic anatomical landmarks are chosen on the intraoperatively accessible bone surface. They are required for the intraoperative registration [9] of the CT data with the operated femur and function as input to a »paired-points matching« algorithm that is used in combination with a »restricted surface-matching« procedure [1].

Planning of Size, Position, and Orientation of Prostheses

In analogy to the acetabular implant planning, a three-dimensional model of the femoral prosthesis stem is loaded into the software. Manipulation with a computer mouse allows the interactive moving of a contour of the implant over the CT images – similarly to conventional planning using implant templates. In this way, the surgeon is able to select the optimal component size and to determine the ideal spatial position and orientation of the stem. The planning of the femoral implant is carried out after planning of the acetabular component. Therefore, the software can predict the postoperative position of the rotational center of the hip. Important measures such as antetorsion, varus/valgus orientation, leg length, and lateralization of the joint can be derived from this information and are displayed continuously representing valuable planning aids. Finally, all planning data is stored for the intraoperative navigation.

Intraoperative Application

Following conventional surgical approach and resection of the femoral head, the acetabular cup is replaced as described in chapter 8. Next follows the fixation of the DRB (◘ Fig. 13-2). Screws or pins are used as anchors and are placed into the proximal region of the femur, avoiding the increased invasiveness that would come along with a distal transmuscular fixation. This placement was suggested by F. Kerschbaumer (Frankfurt/M., GER), who supported the clinical evaluation of the CT-based module. Using a tracked pointer, those landmarks are digitized that were selected for »paired-points matching« during the planning phase. The accessible femoral anatomy is usually lacking a sufficient number of precisely identifiable landmarks disallowing accurate navigation based on »paired-points matching« alone. Consequently, a subsequent surface registration is carried out, requiring 12–20 additional points to be captured on the accessible femoral anatomy. The acquisition of data from the distal area of the scanned data volume is advised for both registration steps. Initial studies could demonstrate that the precision improvement resulting from the larger distance of these points to the operation field overrule the inac-

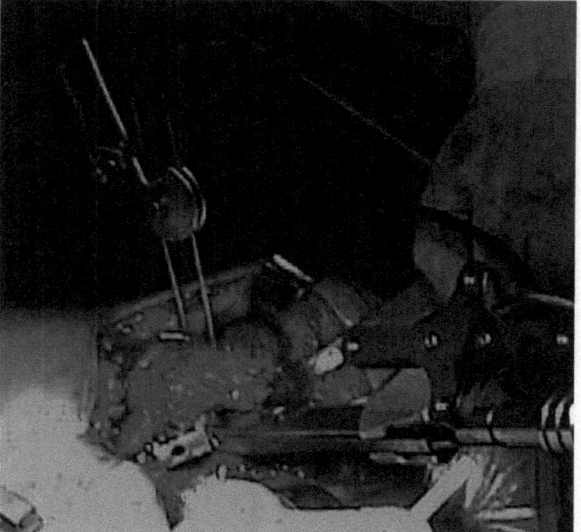

◘ **Fig. 13-2.** During the intraoperative usage of the CT-based femoral stem navigation system (here: lateral positioning), the DRB may be attached near the lesser trochanter, avoiding transmuscular fixation at the distal femur (permission granted by F. Kerschbaumer, Frankfurt/M., GER)

curacies that result from a cutaneous digitization of the points.

Following successful registration and subsequent verification, the system presents the postoperative implant position as given by the current broach position. This information is displayed graphically within different sections through the CT volume as presented in ◘ Fig. 13-3. The current broach size is selected with the help of a foot switch. To complement this very intuitive representation, deviations between current instrument and planned implant position are visualized numerically as well as with the help of graphical aiming tools.

Fluoroscopy-Based Femoral Stem Navigation

A CT-free navigation system was recently introduced which offers a reliable solution for placing the cup, by combining intraoperative fluoroscopy with modern surgical free-hand navigation [8]. In this system, the hybrid strategy for registering landmarks described below was successfully used for the first time, and was combined with transcutaneous, pointer-based point digitalzation. This enabled landmarks to be spatially reconstructed non-invasively, using registered fluoroscopic images. Using the application presented here, these concepts were extended to the prosthetic stem. Combining the two systems enables both implant components to be inserted with the aid of CT-free navigation. An associated clinical pilot study was carried out in collaboration with K.-H. Widmer (Bruderholz, CH).

Hardware

The hardware used in this system only slightly differs from the setup described above.

Instrumentation of the fluoroscope using infrared LEDs is required for C-arm based navigation as well as

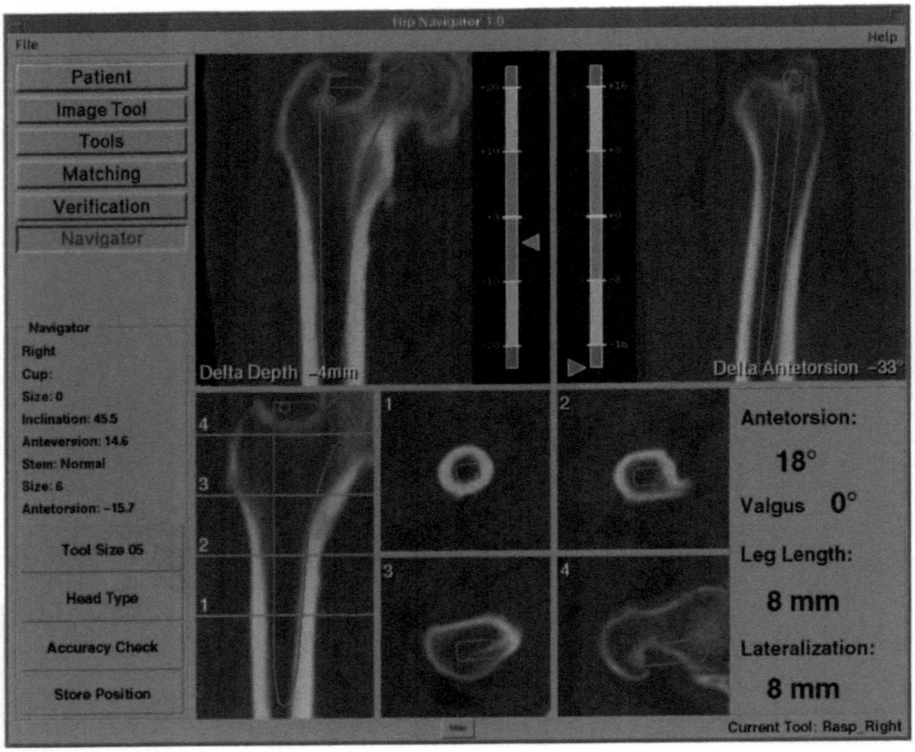

◘ **Fig. 13-3.** On the left side of the screen the planned prosthesis parameters as well as the currently selected rasp size are displayed numerically. The CT window in the *lower left corner* shows the planned position of the femoral implant as well as the location of the horizontal sections 1 to 4. The upper half of the screen presents the current rasp position (visualized as the contour of the matching implant) and the deviation from the planned location. A numerical summary as well as the predicted postoperative joint parameters are provided by the data in the *lower right corner* of the screen

subsequent calibration of the device [5]. Image information is transferred through the video-out line of the C-arm and into an Osprey-150 frame grabber board (Osprey Systems, Cary, NC, USA) installed in the workstation.

Hybrid Landmark Acquisition Concept

Although stereotactic basics were established as early as at the beginning of the 20th century [3], they can be transferred easily to modern computer-assisted surgery systems [2]. Basically, a representation of the surgical object in the form of a virtual object is required. Not only can this representation be based on preoperative 3D information, such as e.g. a CT scan, but intraoperatively acquired fluoroscopic images are suitable as well. The inherent registration of a navigated fluoroscope provides a mathematical link between the therapeutic and virtual object [2], which enables the digitization of landmarks in either of the two objects. For the therapeutic object, i.e., the patient anatomy, landmarks are usually acquired using a special pointing device.

Fluoroscopy-based landmark acquisition requires two independent images of the anatomic landmark. In both images the point of interest is identified on the computer monitor. Two lines of interest can be calculated by back-projecting the two points to the corresponding positions where the X-ray source used to be at the time of image acquisition. These lines intersect at the 3D coordinate of the landmark. This technique allows determination of the position of bony landmarks non-invasively, even if they are seated deeply within the body, as no direct access to the landmark in required.

The intraoperative control of the software within the sterile OR environment is facilitated with the so-called »virtual keyboard« [12]. Precise definition of specific points in fluoroscopic images, as required for C-arm-based reconstruction, requires direct interactive control of the computer cursor by the surgeon. For this purpose a so-called »virtual joystick« extends the functionality of the virtual keyboard. Once the pointer is placed into a dedicated indent on the keyboard plate, pivoting motion of the tool is translated into synchronous cursor movements. Capturing desired point locations is then carried out with the help of a foot switch.

Patient-Specific Coordinate System

While the CT-based variant of this system relies upon intraoperatively accessible landmarks, CT-free navigation technology completely abandons manual digitization and reconstruction of points. The patient-specific coordinate system is solely built on structures digitized with the technique described above.

Five points define the patient's coordinate system. The posterior condyles c_1 and c_2, the medullary canal axis of the proximal femur (defined by a_1 und a_2) as well as the center of rotation of the hip joint (h). The transcondylar plane is defined as the plane that includes c_1 and c_2 and is parallel to the medullary canal axis. Measurements of leg length are carried out along the axis linking the middle of the condylar axis (c_1, c_2) with the hip center (h).

Intraoperative Usage

Once the dynamic reference base has been transmuscularly fixed in the distal femur using two Schantz screws, three pairs of registered fluoroscopic images are taken in

Table 13-1. To determine the patient's individual coordinate system during fluoroscopy-based navigation, three image pairs are acquired. Five points are digitized interactively in these images. The points allow calculation of various parameters that are presented in real-time as navigational aids

Visualized anatomy	Digitized points	Derived parameters
Femoral head	Center of the femoral head	Lateralization of the hip joint, change of leg length
Proximal femur	Proximal and distal point in the center of the femoral canal	Frontal plane, varus/valgus orientation
Distal femur	Lateral and medial aspect of the posterior condyles	Antetorsion

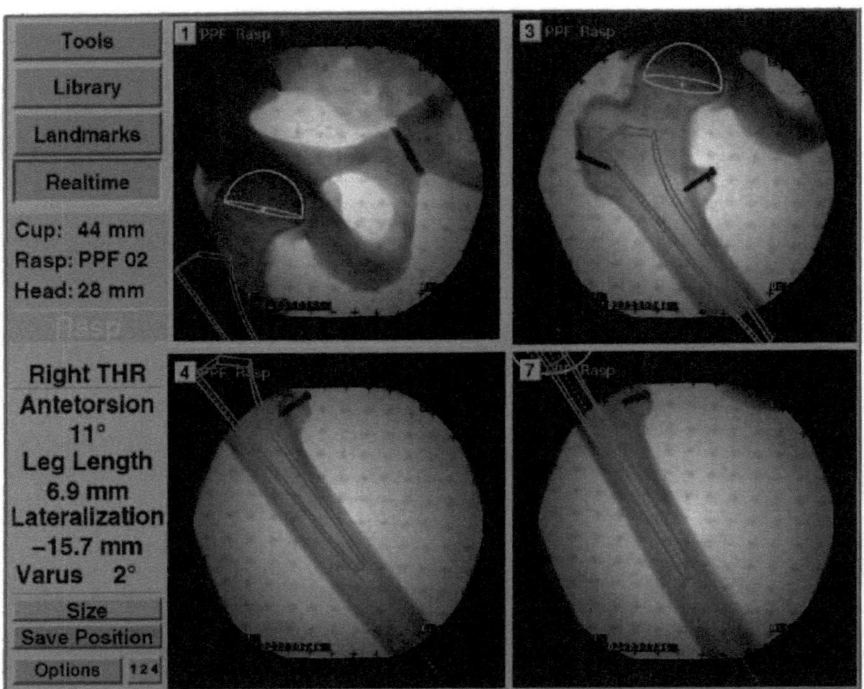

Fig. 13-4. During the preparation of the femoral cavity, the final position of the implanted acetabular component is visualized in its correct size. Femoral antetorsion, postoperative change in leg length, lateralization of the femoral head, and the current varus/valgus orientation are presented numerically on the *left* of the screen. The screws that are visible near the trochanters of the plastic model were used during an accuracy analysis

each of the anterior-posterior direction and the lateral-medial direction, with the aid of which the five landmarks mentioned above are ascertained, thus enabling the individual patient coordinate system to be determined (**Table 13-1**).

While the femoral canal is surgically prepared, a wireframe display of the rasp geometry is projected simultaneously onto four different fluoroscopic images of the pelvic and proximal femur region (**Fig. 13-4**). In addition, the femoral antetorsion of the prosthesis, the lateralization of the femoral center of rotation, the varus/valgus angle of the rasp with respect to the axis of the femur, and the change in the length of the leg are continuously calculated and displayed as numerical navigation aids.

Outlook

The presented systems for femoral stem navigation, in combination with their cup navigation counterparts, enable complete computer-assisted support during total hip arthroplasty for the first time. The CT-based modules in addition allow the preoperative planning of the final implant position. Using this technology, the individual postoperative situation can be influenced with respect to both implant components and the optimal functioning of the endoprosthesis, can be granted. Nevertheless, further improvements can be foreseen already at this point in time. The simulation of impingement will help to achieve maximal range of motion of the artificial joint. On the hardware side, additional prosthesis models should be integrated. According to current knowledge, a modular rasp design is required to enable navigation of the rasping process. Prior to a potential extension of the presented technology to cemented total hip replacement, the instrumentation not only of the rasps but also of the prosthesis must be realized. Navigation of the implant would then guarantee the central insertion of the stem into the femoral cavity, ensuring a homogenous cement mantle.

References

1. Bächler R, Bunke H, Nolte LP (2001) Restricted surface matching – numerical optimization and technical evaluation. Comput Aided Surg 6: 143–152

2. Bowersox JC, Bucholz RD, Delp SL et al. (1997) Excerpts from the final report for the second international workshop on robotics and computer assisted medical interventions. Comput Aided Surg 2: 69–101

3. Clarke RH, Horsley V (1906) On a method of investigating the deep ganglia and tracts of the central nervous system (cerebellum). Br Med J 2: 1799–1800

4. Dunlap K, Shands AR, Hollister LC, Gaul JS, Streit HA (1953) A new method for determination of torsion of the femur. J Bone Joint Surg 35A: 289–311

5. Hofstetter R, Slomczykowski M, Sati M, Nolte L-P (1999) Fluoroscopy as an imaging means for computer-assisted surgical navigation. Comput Aided Surg 4: 65–76

6. Jaramaz B, DiGioia AM, Blackwell M, Nikou C (1998) Computer assisted measurement of cup placement in total hip replacement. Clin Orthop 354: 70–81

7. Langlotz U, Lawrence J, Hu Q, Langlotz F, Nolte L-P (1999) Image guided cup placement. In: Lemke HU, Vannier MW, Inamura K, Farman AG (eds) Computer-assisted radiology and surgery. Elsevier Science B.V., Amsterdam, pp 717–721

8. Langlotz U, Grützner PA, Bernsmann K, Wälti H, Rose E, Bächler R, Korber J, Tannast M, Nolte L-P (2002) A hybrid CT-free navigation system for acetabular cup placement. J Arthroplasty (submitted)

9. Lavallée S (1996) Registration for computer-integrated surgery: methodology, state of the art. In: Taylor RH, Lavallée S, Burdea GC, Mösges R (eds) Computer-integrated surgery. MIT Press, Cambridge, pp 77–97

10. Noble PC, Alexander JW, Lindahl LJ, Yew DT, Granberry WM, Tullos HS (1988) The anatomic basis of femoral component design. Clin Orthop 235: 148–165

11. Nolte L-P, Zamorano L, Visarius H, Berlemann U, Langlotz F, Arm E, Schwarzenbach O (1995) Clinical evaluation of a system for precision enhancement in spine surgery. Clin Biomech 10: 293–303

12. Visarius H, Nolte L-P, Berlemann U, Ozdoba C, Schwarzenbach O, Arm E, Jost B (1995) Computer-assisted orthopaedic surgery – an application in spine surgery. In: Lemke HU, Inamura K, Jaffe CC, Vannier MW (eds) Computer-assisted radiology. Springer, Berlin Heidelberg New York Tokyo, pp 838–843

14 Minimally Invasive Hip Surgery with Imageless Navigation

M. Nogler, M. Krismer, F. Rachbauer, J. Sledge

Introduction

The concepts of minimally invasive surgery and computer-assisted surgery have recently come to the forefront of total hip arthroplasty (THA). These techniques have been borrowed from other surgical disciplines and have been introduced to Orthopedics independently. Minimally invasive techniques and surgical navigation have both been used, to some degree, in THA for several years, but only recently have the techniques been merged. With the introduction of specialty instruments and imageless navigation the combined technique has matured to a point were we can demonstrate a measurable early postoperative benefit and hopefully a long term benefit as measured by clinical outcome. Total hip arthroplasty is one of the most successful surgical procedures performed today. The history of THA is littered with attempts to improve outcome that have, with time, shown disappointing results. Few, however, would disagree with the goals of creating less soft tissue damage at the time of the procedure and being able to more accurately and reproducibly position the components; it being understood that long term hip function and implant survivorship are not decreased.

Over the years the field of total hip arthroplasty has seen new materials and new prosthesis designs, but for a procedure that has consistently displayed excellent clinical result real innovation has been difficult to achieve and even more difficult to prove scientifically. Huge numbers of patients and a long-term follow-up are needed to measure outcome parameters such as long term clinical outcome and implant survival. All lines of development in computer-assisted orthopedic surgery (CAOS) can be seen as an attempt through innovation to advance the field. Present systems are mainly designed to address the need for perfect implant placement and joint alignment as these parameters can be assessed early. These parameters will decrease the complications seen by mal-position of the components such as dislocation and leg length discrepancy, but they are only surrogate parameters, which may – or may not – give us some estimation, for long term clinical outcome and implant survival.

Another field of new developments is the surgical technique of THA. Minimized approaches to the hip – no matter if they are called »minimally invasive«, »less invasive« or »mini incision« techniques – are an important and new development in hip arthroplasty. New techniques have been developed for both the posterior approach with the patients lying on their side and for the anterolateral or lateral approaches with the patient in supine position. Different approaches have been described and early clinical results have been reported [1, 4, 6–8]. These techniques allow for a reduction of in the incision length and a reduction in soft tissue damage which results in a faster postoperative rehabilitation [9].

Minimally invasive approaches offer decreased exposure and a more limited view of the boney anatomical landmarks when compared to traditional approaches. It has been noted by surgeons performing THA utilizing minimally invasive approaches that this decreased visualization makes anatomical orientation more difficult and can result in greater variation in the placement of the implants. As surgical navigation in THA is aimed to decrease the variations in the placement of the components, independent of the surgeon or the technique, this should be particularly beneficial in minimally invasive techniques. Since imageless surgical navigation has been shown to improve the accuracy of components placement during standard THA, it would follow that it would show the same or greater benefit for minimally invasive techniques. Minimally invasive techniques with and without surgical navigation have been compared and an increase in the accuracy of components placement during the navigated procedures has been shown by DiGioia et al. [2] for their mini-incision dorsal approach.

The Need for an Imageless Navigation System

There is a need for a navigation system thats design and implementation is optimized for minimally invasive techniques regardless of surgical approach. The ideal system would require as little extra preoperative setup as possible, require the least amount of operative time, be as accurate as possible and incur the least amount of additional soft tissue damage. For the development of such a system the authors propose the following criteria:

- No additional pre- and intraoperative radiation for planning purpose or the addition of as few additional steps as necessary. This goal requires an intraoperative, imageless system which allows acquiring all reference frames intraoperatively.
- Trackers should be attached rigidly through small incisions. For future development non-invasive or through existing incision fixation of trackers is desired.
- Acetabular component orientation should be navigated based on a pelvic reference frame.
- Femoral component orientation should be navigated in reference to a femoral reference frame.
- The acetabular reference frame and the femoral reference frame should be referencable to each other through a fixed point common to them both.
- Such as system should allow determination of leg length and offset during placement of the broaches and the implant.
- The range of motion during the trial reduction and the final reduction should be calculated.

Approaches

For the adaptation of the Stryker navigation system three distinct approaches have been chosen:

1. A direct anterior single-incision approach based on the Smith Petersen approach.
2. A double incision approach with an anterolateral incision for cup preparation and a lateral incision for stem placement.
3. A posterior mini-incision approach based upon the Kocher-Langenbach approach.

Patients are positioned in the supine position for the first approach and lying on their side for the other two approaches.

Cup Navigation with the Stryker Hip Navigation System

The Stryker (Stryker-Navigation, Freiburg, Germany) hip navigation system is a completely intraoperative, imageless navigation system. The system is equipped with boom-mounted infrared cameras, which are able to track and

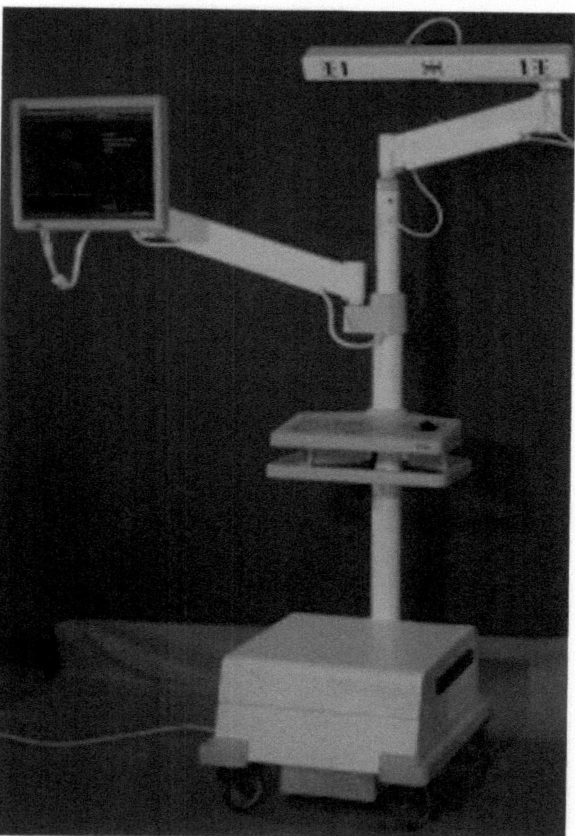

◻ **Fig. 14-1.** The Stryker navigation system unit

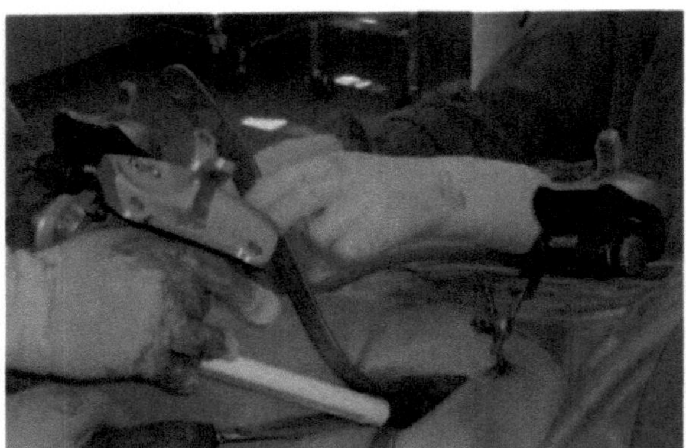

Fig. 14-2. A minimally invasive direct anterior approach with both Trackers in place. The angulated reamer is inserted

communicate with active battery powered instruments with LEDs. The system's software runs on a standard laptop and comes as a single easily mobile unit (**Fig. 14-1**).

The system requires the placement of a pelvic tracker that gets screwed into bone in the area of the anterior superior iliac spine (ASIS) on the operated side through a very small incision. An active pistol grip pointer is used to operate the software and to digitize anatomic landmarks percutaneously (**Fig. 14-2**). The pelvic reference frame is constructed by registering the ASISs on both sides as well as both pubic tubercles (PT). These points are digitized by the surgeon percutaneously with the pointer. Coordinates of these points are recorded relative to the pelvic tracker. The distance between the two PTs is

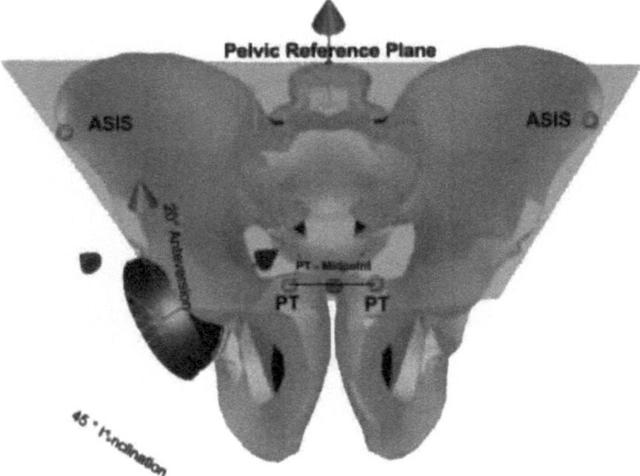

Fig. 14-3. The definition of the pelvic reference frame with a cup in correct orientation

calculated and the midpoint between them is taken together with the two ASIS in order to calculate a pelvic reference plane (PRP; **Fig. 14-3**) [5].

Additionally, a series of points is digitized in the acetabulum after dislocation of the femoral head to create a graphic representation of the acetabular rim, articular surface and the acetabular fossa in the navigation software. Navigation of the acetabular cup reamer and the cup inserter can be achieved using specialized minimally invasive instruments that have a post for mounting the instrument tracker (see Fig. 14-2). The specific geometric data of the instruments and implants is known to the software thereby eliminating the step calibrating each instrument for all degrees of freedom during each case. Each instrument tracker is checked once during each case to insure that it has not been damaged or bent. The reaming of the acetabulum and the cup impacting are navigated in real time showing the instrument's position and orientation on screen as well as numerical values of cup inclination and version (Fig. **14-4**) The system calculates the cup position relative to the PRP [3].

Stem Navigation with the Stryker Hip Navigation System

The system allows navigation of the femoral component so it can be placed more accurately, but more importantly it allows for calculations to be performed between the two reference planes so that leg length and offset can be determined. In order to define a femoral reference frame, a femoral tracker is placed in the distal femur. Before dislocation of the femur the rotational centre is detected kinematically through movements of the leg about the centre of rotation. In addition the anatomical landmarks at the piriformis fossa, the popliteal fossa and the achilles tendon are digitized. From these landmarks the mechanical axis, anatomical shaft axes and a femoral reference plane are calculated.

As neither the mechanical axes nor the anatomical shaft axes provides a valid orientation for varus/valgus alignment of the femoral component, the proximal shaft axes is measured intra-medullarily. This proximal shaft axes defines the references axes to which broaches and implant are aligned. As in the case of cup positioning on the pelvic side the system supports navigation of ream-

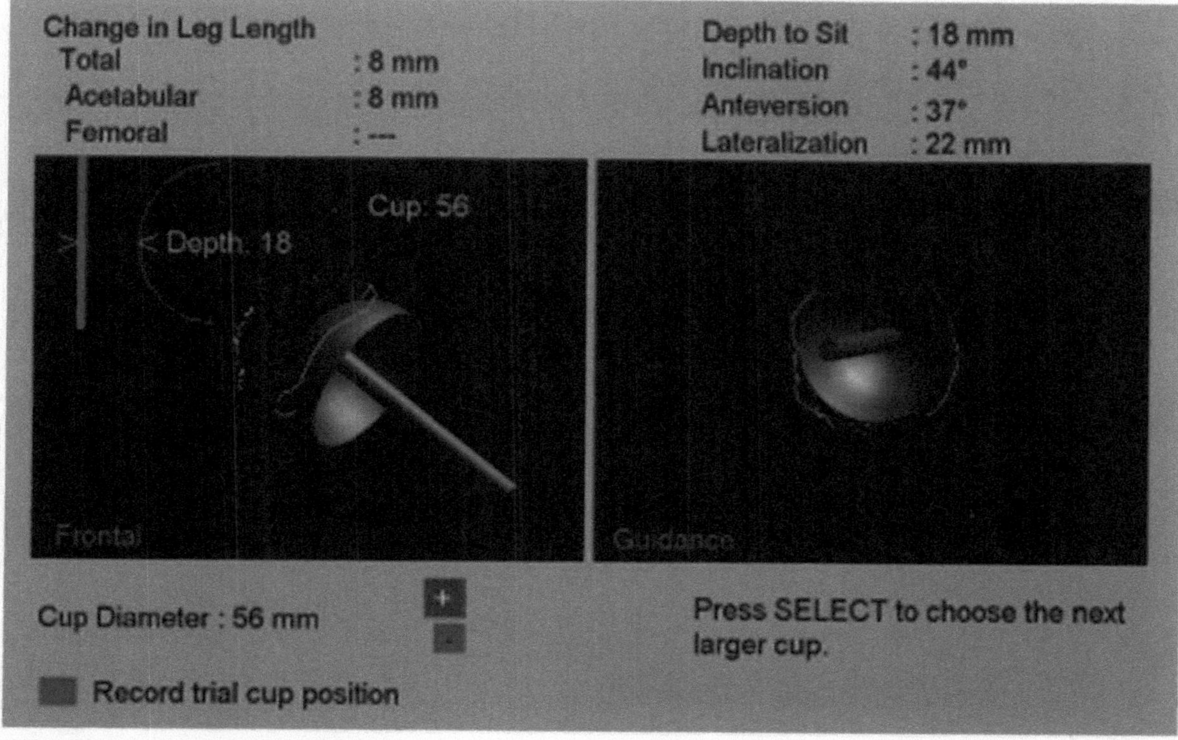

Fig. 14-4. Visualization of cup navigation

ing, broaching and placement of trial and final implant on the femoral side. While these steps are being performed, the varus/valgus angle, the rotation, the change in leg length and change in offset due to the femoral component are visualized on screen. These can all be calculated based upon the position information from the trackable instruments all relative to the femur reference frame.

Leg Length, Offset and ROM Navigation with the Stryker Hip Navigation System

During the process of acetabular and femoral preparation the instruments current position and the calculated implant position are determined and relative changes of leg length and offset are calculated and displayed. The implants current position is calculated using a data base of the geometrical data of the instruments and of the implants. After the placement of trials the system allows for a trial reduction. Real leg length change and resulting offset, as compared to the calculated ones during the surgery, can be displayed at this stage. Through changes in implant position, or implant size, the surgeon has the chance to intraoperative accurately assess all parameters. The final selection can then have the resulting range of motion determined as well as the point the joint starts to sublux prior to dislocation determined during a kinematics motion test (**Fig. 14-5**).

This gives the surgeon a valuable tool at hand to exactly control these crucial parameters even with a limited view to the surgical field.

A Need for Specialized Instruments

With the advent of the mini-approaches, manufacturers have had to rethink their concepts for implants and instruments. So far we have seen the development of new instruments for standard implants but as these instruments open up new avenues for minimally invasive techniques

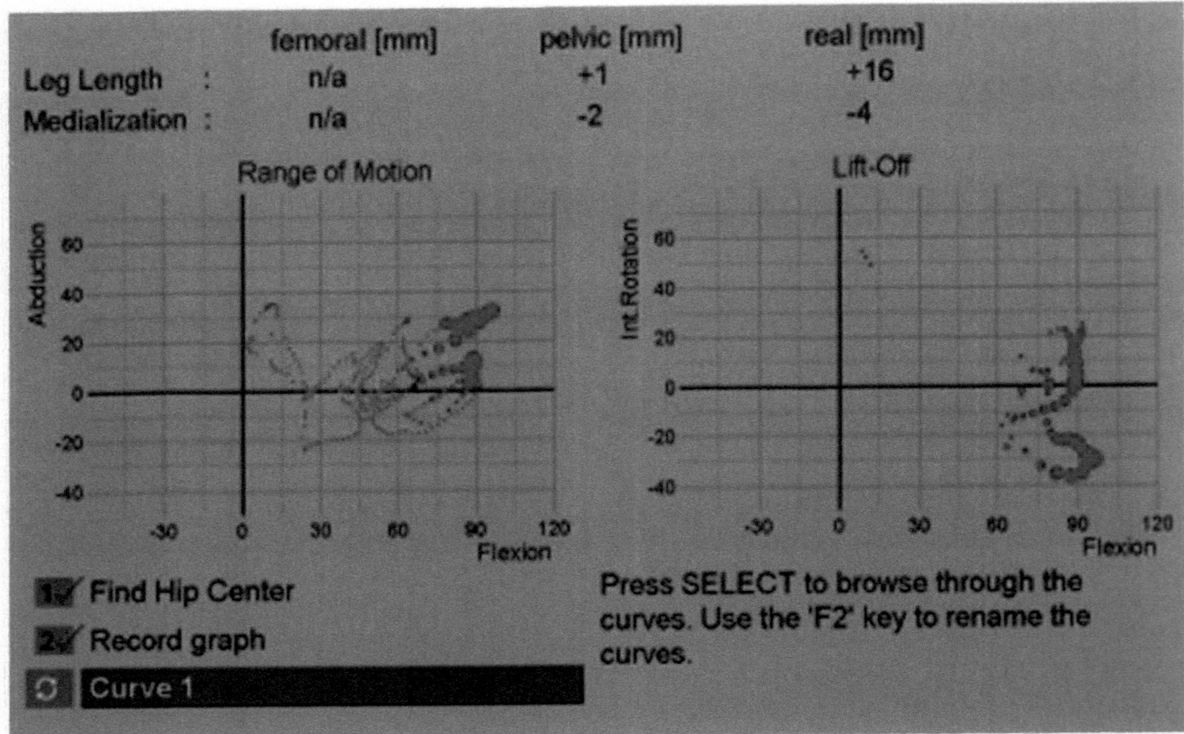

Fig. 14-5. Visualization of range of motion and impingement in the reduced joint

we are starting to see the development of a new generation of implants to better address the problems presently being encountered. Such new instruments have to be smaller and allow for insertion through small wounds and in unfavorable directions. In certain circumstances new instruments and implants are being introduced for newly created problems such as the attachment of the head in a very narrow space (**Fig. 14-6).

One of the main problems created by the minimally invasive techniques is the anatomic visualization previously required to allow accurate placement of the implants. The maturation of minimally invasive techniques has reached a point that visualization for orientation is now limiting the advancement of the technique. While the surgeon traditionally is used to orienting components in relation to anatomic landmark, such as the tip of the greater trochanter or the depth of the fossa, a navigation system allows for precise implant positioning without a constant view of these landmarks. Now that only limited or percutaneous access to anatomical reference points are required visualization of the anatomy is no longer a limiting factor so the size and type of approach are now independent to the accuracy and reproducibility of implant positioning.

And all these instrument should be equipped with interfaces for the mounting of tracking devices.

Conclusion

Minimally invasive techniques make total joint arthroplasty technically more demanding. Yet, first reports lead us to expect major benefits such as shorter hospital stays, earlier rehabilitation and consecutively decreased cost of joint replacements for our patients. As we have seen for other fields of surgery, minimally invasive techniques offer potential value for both surgeons and patients. Even though it will be awhile before we can clinically prove for the superiority of small incisions in THA, we should be able to expect improved patient outcomes due to less soft

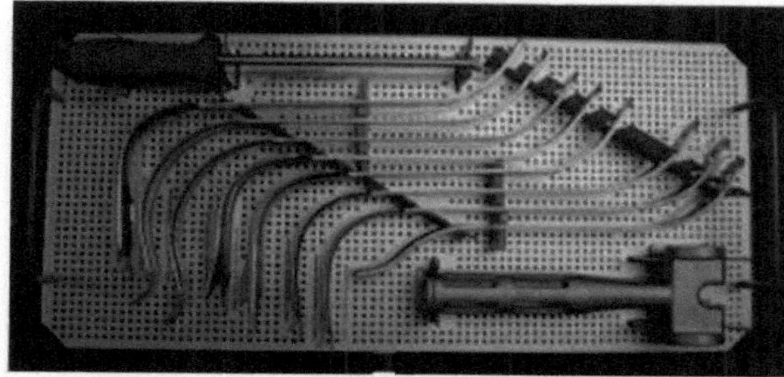

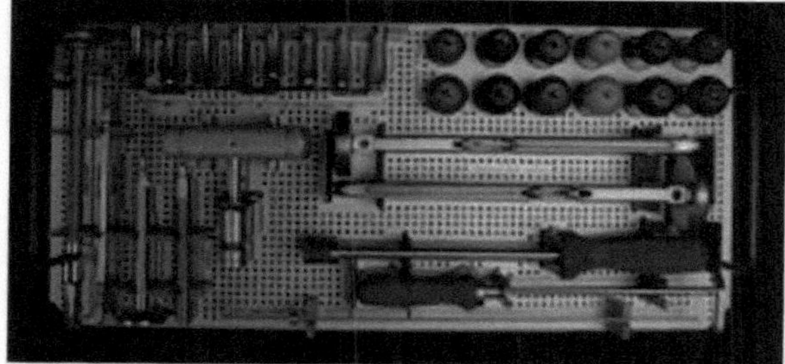

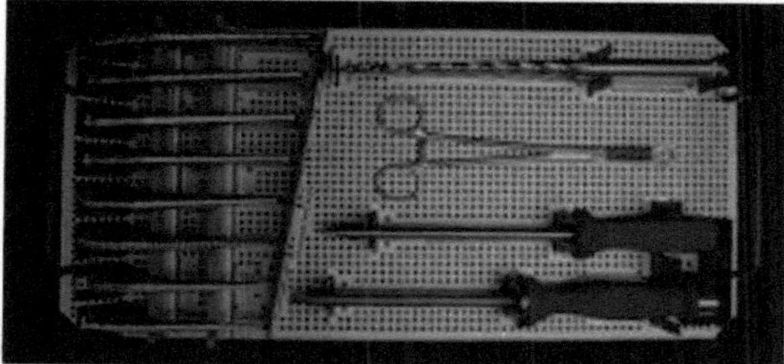

■ **Fig. 14-6.** A set of specialized instruments for minimal invasive THA

progressed rapidly over the past few years. The first step was the development of minimally invasive surgical techniques, this required the creation of the specialty instruments to solve exposure issues created by these new techniques and now it is the introduction of imageless navigation to solve the problem of implant positioning. The design of new implants to solve the limited space issues seen with minimally invasive techniques is already underway and the design of new implants to solve the position and range of motion issues seen with navigation is just starting. For minimally invasive techniques to continue to develop they must be merged with surgical navigation techniques; only in this way can we hope to maximize the potential benefits offered by minimally invasive techniques without jeopardizing our current excellent clinical results.

tissue damage as seen in other surgical fields. The goal is to obtain the short term advantages offered by minimally invasive techniques without adversely affecting the excellent long term outcome that we presently enjoy with THA. The way to do this is to develop innovative solutions to the difficulties created by minimally invasive techniques.

The concepts of minimally invasive surgery and computer-assisted surgery in total hip arthroplasty have

References

1. Berger RA (2002) Mini-incisions: two for the price of one! Orthopedics 25:472–498
2. DiGioia AM 3rd, Plakseychuk AY, Levison TJ, Jaramaz B (2003) Mini-incision technique for total hip arthroplasty with navigation. J Arthroplasty 18:123–128
3. DiGioia AM, Jaramaz B, Blackwell M et al. (1998) The Otto Aufranc Award. Image guided navigation system to measure intraoperatively acetabular implant alignment. Clin Orthop 355:8–22
4. Mathias JM (2001) MIS total hip implant speeds recovery. OR Manager 17:5–7
5. McKibbin B (1970) Anatomical factors in the stability of the hip joint in the newborn. J Bone Joint Surg Br 52:148–159
6. Rodrigo JJ (2002) Juan J. Rorigo, MD on minimally invasive hip surgery. Orthopedics 25:1016, 1028
7. Sherry E, Egan M, Warnke PH, Henderson A, Eslick GD (2003) Minimal invasive surgery for hip replacement: a new technique using the NILNAV hip system. ANZ J Surg 73:157–161
8. Waldman BJ (2002) Minimally invasive total hip replacement and perioperative management: early experience. J South Orthop Assoc 11:213–217
9. Wenz JF, Gurkan I, Jibodh SR (2002) Mini-incision total hip arthroplasty: a comparative assessment of perioperative outcomes. Orthopedics 25:1031–1043

II B Robotics: Total Hip Arthroplasty

15 Robotic Hip Surgery and Current Development with the *ROBODOC* System

W. Bargar

Introduction

Why use a robot in joint replacement surgery? The answer is, it allows the surgeon to execute the preoperative plan, and to machine the bone interface to maximize contact.

ROBODOC was the first »active« surgical robot. Although the ROBODOC system actually began the era of computer-aided surgery, it is probably the most intrusive of the entire new computer aids used in surgery. So why should surgeons put up with this intrusion? Most surgeons do not precisely plan their operations. They may have a general idea of what they want to accomplish, but mostly, they rely on their skills in the operating room, »eyeballing,« to accomplish their goals. They have good reason not to trust planning that is based on traditional radiographs. Because of rotational effects and variation in magnification of standard radiographs, the size and positioning of the implants are difficult to predict. Relying on surgical skills, however, can result in unintended errors. Not only do surgical skills vary, but also the information available to surgeons during an operation is limited. The reasons are that the operative field is relatively small, and there is unrecognized movement of the pelvis or femur.

In cementless hip replacement surgery the goals are clear and universal:

1. In the femur, the implant must fit the endosteal canal as closely as possible in order to achieve a stable implant for fixation and to distribute load as uniformly as possible. By doing so, they avoid stress shielding and thigh pain due to stress concentrations. The new prosthetic head center should reproduce, as closely as possible, the horizontal offset, anteversion and leg length of the normal femur.
2. In the acetabulum, the center of the new hip should be located as close as possible to the original anatomic hip center, and the size should be chosen to maximize host bone contact with healthy bleeding bone, while preserving bone stock. The orientation of the component should complement the femoral neck orientation so as to maximize the range of motion without impingement or dislocation.

Although most surgeons accept these goals, the methods used to accomplish them vary widely. Most surgeons agree, however, that proper preoperative planning is the best way to insure that these goals are accomplished, but planning using inaccurate images can be worse than having no plan at all.

The key, then, is to have accurate three-dimensional images on which to plan. Further, it is important to have a method that will accurately and reproducibly execute that plan. This can only be accomplished using an active surgical robot and a preoperative planning computer workstation based on CT images. These goals are accomplished with ROBODOC.

Development

ROBODOC took advantage of tremendous advances in the fields of medical imaging and robotics. The speed and accuracy of CT images has undergone astounding quantum leaps over the past 20 years. Care must be taken however not to confuse pictorial accuracy with dimensional accuracy. When the ROBODOC system was in early development, it was discovered that most commercially available three-dimensional models created from raw CT data contained dimensional inaccuracies up to 3 mm. This inaccuracy is acceptable for diagnostic purposes, but for positioning of implants in hip replacement surgery it is unacceptable. We performed a study to show that the raw CT data is accurate to approximately the size of one pixel. We then had to develop our own proprietary software that would yield a three-dimensional image upon which the surgeon could plan, but still retained the inherent dimensional accuracy of the raw CT data.

The field of robotics has undergone a similar development and refinement. Industrial robots were developed 30 years ago. Their speed and accuracy, as well as safety, have improved dramatically. What was lacking when ROBODOC was being developed in the late 1980s, was an ability to program robots quickly and efficiently. IBM, Inc., had developed an experimental language at that time to allow robots to be programmed similar to computers. That language allowed us to program ROBODOC for the complex individualized tasks required for surgery.

The chronology of the early development of the ROBODOC system has been published elsewhere [6] and the reader is referred to that reference for a more detailed account. Dr. Howard A. Paul, DVM (deceased) and I conceived the idea in 1986. A feasibility study was undertaken in 1987 at the IBM Thomas Watson Research Center, Yorktown Heights, NY. This was followed by two consecutive 2-year grants from IBM made to The University of California Davis Orthopaedic Research Laboratories. A canine study preceded the first hip replacement performed on a human done on November 12, 1992. In 1991, Integrated Surgical Systems, Inc., was formed to commercialize the project. A 10-patient feasibility study was performed in 1992. This was followed by an FDA multicenter trial carried out from 1994 to 1996. This study required 2-year minimum follow-up. The results of that study have also been published [1].

In 1994 ROBODOC was approved for sale in the European Union, and that year Prof. Boerner at the Unfallklinik in Frankfurt, Germany, performed the first case. That center now has three robots and serves as a major training and development site for ISS. There are now over 40 installations in Europe and 7 in Japan and there have been over 9000 robot-assisted joint replacements performed.

As a result of experience gained in Germany and in the US FDA trial, ROBODOC has evolved into a more efficient and user-friendly device. Our original version required that a separate operative procedure be performed before the CT scan was made. In this preliminary operation, fiduciary markers were implanted in the distal and proximal femur under local anesthetic in an outpatient setting. At the hip replacement operation, these pins were exposed and used to register the robot. Developing the new Digimatch software has now obviated the need for this additional surgery, and the time and morbidity in exposing the implanted pins at the hip replacement surgery. With this software, the unique anatomy of the bone can be used for registration, thereby avoiding the need for fiduciary markers.

»Pinless« ROBODOC

The Digimatch software developed by ISS utilizes the unique shape of the femur to register the robot at the time of surgery. From the CT scan a surface model of certain key areas of the femur is created. During the operative procedure, the proximal part of the femur is easily visualized through the standard incision (either anterior, direct lateral or posterior), and can be reached using a digitizing probe. Distally at the mid-shaft of the femur, three small 1 cm incisions are made to allow access for the digitizing probe. Points are collected both proximally and distally and a proprietary pattern recognition program is run to match these points to the surface model from the CT scan. Additional points are then obtained in these same areas to verify the accuracy of the registration. Two temporary »recovery markers« are placed in the femur, one proximal in the greater trochanter and the other distally through one of the 1 cm incisions used for point collection. These markers are also digitized to allow quick recovery if unintended bone motion is detected. The markers are removed at the end of robot milling.

Over 2000 cases have been successfully performed in Europe using this new technology. A new randomized FDA clinical trial is underway in the U.S. to establish the equivalence of this methodology to the previous study. Other modifications include faster cutting times and a more robust error recovery system. Our experience indicates that on average the total surgery time for ROBODOC primary total hip replacement cases is approximately 20 min longer than conventional methods, and the blood loss is substantially equivalent.

Additional Applications

Two other applications for ROBODOC have been developed in Europe. The first relates to revision surgery. The task of removing the cement from the femur while simultaneously preparing the bone for the implant makes the ROBODOC method for revision surgery not only safer but also faster than non-robotic methods. The literature [2–5, 7] shows that complications such as shaft perforation and fracture were frequently encountered in revision surgery performed without robot-assistance. The gentle and accurate removal of old cement, using robotically controlled high-speed milling, minimized these risks. Upon completion of robotic milling the implant can be inserted, since the cavity prepared for the implant includes the cavity resulting from cement removal. Significant time can be saved as compared to conventional methods while decreasing the complications.

The other application relates to total knee replacement. Most surgeons agree that among the keys to a successful total knee replacement are accurate alignment and appropriate implant sizing. Preoperative planning using CT scan data, and execution of that plan by ROBODOC virtually assures that these goals are met. In addition, the accuracy of the milling process achieves an accuracy of surface preparation greater than can be achieved with hand held tools. This helps to ensure excellent stability and bony ingrowth in those cases where the cementless method is chosen.

Both the applications have achieved clinical success in Europe and will be discussed by Professor Boerner in his contribution to this book (see chapter 17). US FDA clinical trials are planned for both applications following completion of the current trial of the Digimatch system.

Minimally Invasive Surgery

Minimally invasive surgery (MIS) in both hip and knee replacement holds the promise of faster, less painful recovery from operation. To accomplish these goals, the techniques must be truly **minimally invasive** rather than merely using a minimal incision. In addition, there can be no compromise of accuracy of the operation. We have already shown the superiority of the ROBODOC technique in achieving fit and alignment, as compared to conven-

tional techniques. Since the surgeon has greatly limited exposure of the operative field in MIS, there is little question that techniques using ROBODOC would be superior to those performed by hand. Currently some MIS techniques use fluoroscopy to guide the surgeon. This exposes the surgeon and the patient to significant levels of radiation, and requires the surgeon to be exceptionally skilled at mentally converting two-dimensional data into three-dimensional reality. Even though computer-assisted navigation potentially offers to improve the accuracy of MIS techniques, it still requires the surgeon to move the surgical tools along a very specific path to avoid errors and inaccuracies. Only a surgical robot offers the ability to accurately and reproducibly execute the preoperative plan despite the limited visual exposure of the operative field in MIS. Applications of ROBODOC to MIS techniques in the hip and knee are under development.

The Future

At the present time the field of surgical robotics is exploding. Many centers around the world are developing new applications and devices. There are »active systems« (such as ROBODOC and CASPAR), »passive systems« (navigation and CAS) and »semi-active systems« (such as robotic tool guides). New societies are being formed. There are now acronyms galore: CAOS, MRCAS, MICCAI, CARS and many more. Areas of concentration in orthopaedic surgery are not confined to joint replacement surgery. Osteotomies of the hip and knee, ACL reconstruction, arthroscopy, pelvic and long bone fractures and, of course, spine surgery is all candidates for robot-assistance.

I believe there will be two categories of future developments: those that offer to improve existing surgical procedures, and those where procedures would only be possible using robots. There are limitations, however, on these possibilities. The first is the natural resistance of surgeons to adapt to a new technology. This reluctance is certainly justified considering the number of highly touted technologies that have not fulfilled their promise, or worse, have resulted in inferior results or higher complications. Another limitation is that resulting from the reluctance of insurance companies and other third party payers to compensate surgeons for new technologies. A third area of limitation is that resulting from governmental regulation. It has been ten years since the first ROBODOC surgery, and U.S. FDA approval is still a year away. These regulatory delays are extremely costly and many small companies cannot financially sustain such delays. Ultimately, political and economic forces will dictate progress throughout the entire field of medicine.

The true key to success in the future will be proving »clinical utility.« This term was introduced in the U.S. by the Clinton administration, and is now part of the FDA mandate for new devices. It is not a defined term, but it is required. My interpretation is that it involves cost-effectiveness. In essence, clinical utility is »true marketability.« To have true marketability a new device must answer four questions:

- Does it solve a real problem in clinical medicine?
- Does it improve the clinical outcome?
- Does it result in monetary savings without lowering quality?
- Is it worth the investment?

If just one of these questions can be answered in the affirmative, the new devices will have clinical utility. To paraphrase a famous quote: »If you prove it, they will come!«

References

1. Bargar WL, Bauer A, Borner M (1998) Primary and revision total hip replacement using the Robodoc system. Clin Orthop 354: 82–91
2. Engh CA Jr, McAuley JP, Engh C Sr (1999) Surgical approaches for revision total hip replacement surgery: the anterior trochanteric slide and the extended conventional osteotomy. Instr Course Lect 48: 3–8
3. Gardiner R, Hozack WJ, Nelson C, Keating EM (1993) Revision total hip arthroplasty using ultrasonically driven tools. A clinical evaluation. J Arthroplasty 8: 517–521
4. Hubble MJ, Smith EJ (1996) Revision of failed total hip replacement. Br J Hosp Med 55: 432–436
5. Lombardi AV Jr (1992) Cement removal in revision total hip arthroplasty. Semin Arthroplasty 3: 264–272
6. Paul HA, Bargar WL, Mittlestadt B et al. (1992) Development of a surgical robot for cementless total hip arthroplasty. Clin Orthop 285: 57–66
7. Pierson JL, Jasty M, Harris WH (1993) Techniques of extraction of well-fixed cemented and cementless implants in revision total hip arthroplasty. Orthop Rev 22: 904–916

16 Robotically Milled Bone Cavities in Comparison with Hand-Broaching in Total Hip Replacement

M. Thomsen

Introduction

Long-term results and clinical success of a cementless hip stem decisive depend on the primary stability at the time of operation and is the most important factor for osseo-integration [1, 6, 13, 15]. Noble et al. [14] have emphasized the difficulties of achieving press-fit and demonstrated the influence of stem design and anatomical variations of the proximal femur. Gaps between implant and bone may particularly occur when contemporary broaching techniques are used which are susceptible to surgical error [18]. As a consequence, more sophisticated methods of bone cavity preparation have emerged. Experimental work has led to the development and clinical introduction of robotic systems for orthopaedic surgical application [17].

Two mainly preferred systems: ROBODOC of Integrated Surgical Systems (ISS) and CASPAR by URS/Ortomaquet, are implemented in Europe with the majority in Germany. Both systems cost about $ 400,000–500,000.–. Moreover, for each case an additional $ 700–1000.– for drills, pins and preparation kit have to be encountered.

Preoperative planning and exact subsequent intra-operative execution by the robot are considered the most striking advantages [5].

Improved stem fit and enhanced primary stability have been proposed by the distributing companies and supporting surgeons. In a cadaver study [2] superior bone-implant-contact has been demonstrated.

With our investigations [21, 22] we wanted to discuss the effectiveness of computer assisted bone preparation with regard to primary rotational stability of different cementless stems in comparison to hand broaching.

Investigations

For the investigation a standardized protocol for cementless hip stems is performed using a special device [9, 20]. Eight different types of cementless femoral components: ABG I and II, Antega, G_2, Osteolock, S-ROM, VerSys ET, Vision 2000 were tested. ABG I, II and Antega were anatomic designs. All other stems were straight and tapered (◻ Fig. 16-1).

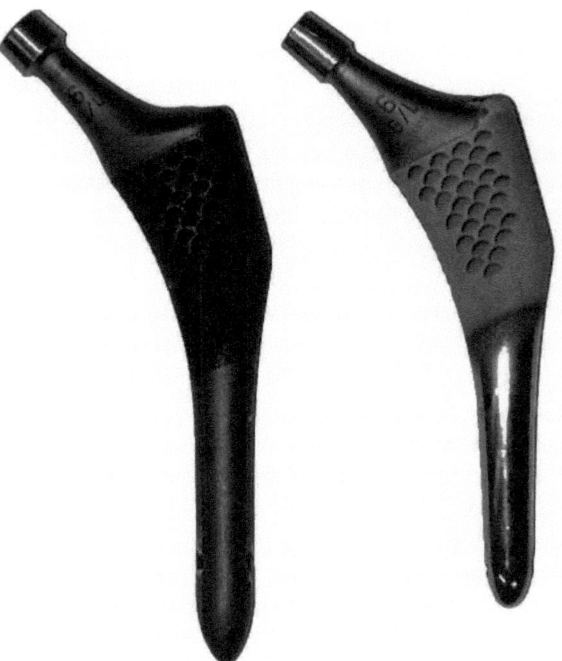

◻ **Fig. 16-1.** Design differences of the ABG I (*left*) and the shorter ABG II (*right*). The proximal part in both stems is comparable. The cone in the ABG II was changed to the 12/14 Euro cone

To ensure standardized experimental conditions synthetic femora (composite bone) from Pacific Research Lab (Vashon Island, WA, USA) with mechanical properties and dimensions closely resembling the human femur and with proven low inter-femur variability [8] were used.

Cortical structures were mimicked by longitudinally laminated fibers bound by epoxy wax, and the spongiosa was simulated by polyurethane foam. Its mechanical properties had the following characteristics: bending strength = 276 N/mm^2; tensile strength = 172 N/mm^2; Young's modulus = 14.200 N/mm^2; and geometry: length = 46.0 cm (0.2 cm), femoral neck-shaft angle = 136.3° (1.2°); anteversion = 8.2° (0.9°); and shaft diameter = 3.1 cm (0.3 cm).

A femoral neck osteotomy was performed at identical levels on all synthetic femora one centimeter above the lesser trochanter. The femora (three per stem design) were prepared by hand broaching by an orthopaedic surgeon familiar with the system and in attendance of a company representative. All systems provide undersized broaches/reamers to ensure press-fit fixation.

The femora for the robotic implantation had been CT-scanned prior to planning.

The virtual planning and robotic milling for G_2, VerSys ET and Vision 2000 stems was done by the author clinically using the CASPAR (Computer-assisted Surgical Planning and Robotics) system (URS/orto, Rastatt, Germany). ABG I and II, Antega and S-ROM were planned and milled by surgeons using the ROBODOC system [Integrated Surgical Systems Inc. (ISS), Davis, CA, USA]. Milling for Osteolock stems was done with both robotic systems.

After canal preparation all specimens were embedded in Plaster of Paris at the level of the femoral condyles to produce a rigid attachment of the femur to a support. The stems were then pressed into the femora in a stepwise manner by 25 cycles of 2000 N followed by 25 cycles of 4000 N using a universal test machine (Frank-Universal-Testing machine 81816/B, Karl Frank GmbH, Weinheim, Germany). We chose this force according the maximal force acting upon the hip joint during walking and jogging as reported by Bergmann et al. [4]. Anterior-posterior and straight lateral radiographs were taken to ensure comparable stem alignment in both groups.

Testing Mode

The femora with implanted stems were mounted into a specially designed device for torsion measurements [9, 20]. In principle, relative motion (i.e. stem displacement, defined as »slip«) and deformation of stem and bone (i.e. torsion, defined as »twist«) were measured in millidegrees/Nm (mdeg/Nm). As neither the femur nor the stem can be considered rigid bodies, measurements at several levels (both on femur and implant) were necessary. In discrepancy to other devices, the apparatus used here allows the measurement of movements of a volume element (i.e. spatial dimensions of measurement points) of stem or cortex in six degrees of freedom (three for translation and three for rotation) using 6 linearly variable differential transducers (LVDT) with a resolution of 0.1 micrometers (μm).

The volume elements measured were taken at five different levels, two at the implanted stem (#1: shoulder, #2: tip) and three at the synthetic cortex (#3: 8 cm below lesser trochanter, #4: at the same level as #2, #5: 20 cm below lesser trochanter). The external loading system was applied to the neck taper. To maintain the press-fit situation achieved during implantation a continuous coaxial force (F=70 N) acting along the longitudinal axis of the femur was applied during all measurements.

To produce the variable axially acting torque two weights (30 Newton each) were shifted by distance d in an anti-parallel fashion so that the varying axial torque T was given by the equation: $T = 2d \times F_R$. The torque was applied in six cycles. Each cycle swept along the interval ±6 Nm and was carried out by 150 increments. After each increment the position of the respective volume element was determined in relation to that of the volume element of the lesser trochanter, which was chosen as the reference coordinate system. [N.B.: The S-ROM stems consist of two parts: an inner stem core and an outer sleeve. Therefore, an additional measurement had to be taken from the outer sleeve (# 1b).]

In the following, we refer to the axial rotation angles of the volume elements as α_1–α_5 corresponding to the measurement levels #1–#5:

- α_1: proximal axial slip between stem and cortex at the »shoulder« (# 1) of the stem.
- α_{1b} (S-ROM only): proximal axial slip between outer sleeve and the cortex.

- α_5: axial twist of the cortex between reference and volume element #5. The level #5 is far below the apex of the stem, where the torque T is fully transferred from the stem to the cortex. a5 exclusively depends on the location of the center of torque transfer from the stem to the cortex, and is therefore a measure for the distance from the level #5 to that point on the cortex, where the torque transfer is completed. This point is more proximal, the greater α_5 is.

To enable calculation of both slip and twist (see above) the following parameters were calculated:

- α_{2+4}: axial rotation between the volume elements #2 and #4 thus representing the distal axial slip between stem tip and cortex.
- α_{1-2}: axial rotation between the volume elements #1 and #2 thus representing the axial twist of the stem (Note: smaller α_{1-2} indicate more proximal location of torque transfer from stem to femur).

Data Evaluation Protocol

From the six loading cycles, measured in 150 increments each, only small hystereses curves were determined. The rotational angle α of each volume element and the applied axial torque T were almost proportional to each other. Hence, the axial rotations could be standardized by the average inclination of α/T. As a consequence, the values we refer to as α_1–α_5 (in the results section) represent these standardized axial rotations which were calculated with a resolution of 0.2 mdeg/Nm.

To visualize the contact areas the stems in a second step the stems were painted and reimplanted. After explantation the contact areas were photographed.

Results

Evaluation of the measurement data showed that – except for rotational stem displacement – all other components of stem movement were negligibly small. Hence, only rotational data is presented.

Rotational Stability

All stems evaluated showed minor rotational displacement and no increasing slip throughout the testing process (i.e. 6 cycles with 150 increments each). The sets of all three measurements per stem type resulted in reproducible data with a maximum standard deviation of 0.1–1.2 mdeg/Nm.

For S-ROM stems hand-broaching resulted in smaller rotational slip (decrease of 18 percent) between stem and femur, proximally more pronounced than distally (α_1 and α_{2+4}). Additionally, robotic milling resulted in a significant distal shift of the center of torque transfer. All S-ROM inner stem cores showed slips relative to the synthetic femur as well as to the outer sleeve. The S-ROM patterns became comparable when we performed distal over-reaming in the hand preparation group (■ Fig. 16-2).

Independent of the way of preparation of the femurs, ABG I and II (see Fig. 16-3), Antega, Osteolock and Vision 2000 (see Fig. 16-4) showed comparable proximal fittings.

Stems with Increased Stability by Hand-Broaching

Both anatomic stems (ABG I and Antega) yielded significantly less proximal slip (α_1) in hand-broached specimens.

Stems with Increased Stability by Robotic Milling

G_2 and the VerSys ET stems yielded smaller proximal slips in the robotically milled specimens, with a pattern of more proximal fixation compared to hand-broaching.

The Osteolock data showed only small differences between hand-broaching and the two robotically prepared implants. Solely, the three specimens milled by the ROBODOC showed a significantly higher value for the proximal slip.

In contrast to the ABG I, the ABG II had higher stability in the robotic group (■ Fig. 16-3) whereas there was no difference for the hand preparation of the two ABG designs.

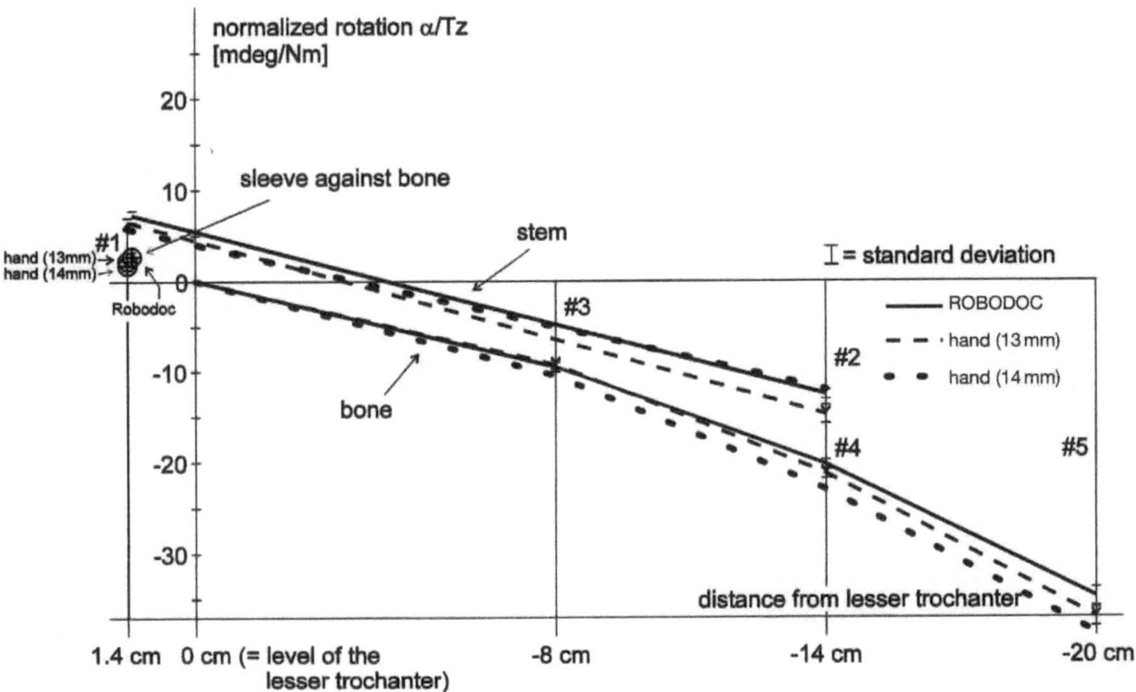

Fig. 16-2. Rotational angle curves of the S-ROM prostheses, size 18F. The *dotted line* indicates the results of the 3 hand-reamed specimens with a 13 mm reamer. The *fat dotted line* represents the 14 mm reamer. The *straight line* shows the results of the ROBODOC milling. The standard deviations (I) were minimal indicating high reproducibility. 0 cm indicates the level of the lesser trochanter, #1–#5 the levels at which measurements were taken. The curve of bone twist is marked in the lower section starting with 0 degree of rotation. The circles show the results of the sleeves, which had highest contact to the bone

Vision 2000 stems yielded significantly reduced proximal and distal stem slip in robotically milled specimens (**▪** Fig. 16-4). In the stems with more lateral stem positioning increased distal torque transfer/distal fixation pattern (indicated by significantly increased stem twist = α_{1-2}) and increased overall fixation were found. The explanation for this phenomenon is a distal-lateral fixation as seen in **▪** Fig. 16-5.

Macroscopic Findings (Contact Areas)

In all samples we found differences between robotic milled and hand-broached femora regarding the surface roughness and/or contact areas of the implant »bed«.

For the S-ROM the contact areas of the hand-reaming is more smooth than the robot preparation, were you can see the prints of the 9 mm drill head.

In the ABG I the robot-reaming especially respects the proximal anatomic design with a very smooth, homogeneous proximal contact zone (**▪** Fig. 16-6, right picture), which could not be reproduced with the hand-broaching (**▪** Fig. 16-6, left picture). But a little bit more distally the robot milling looses contact.

For the ABG II group the hand-broaching contact patterns were comparable with those of the ABG I. The contact area of the robot preparation differs with those of ABG I. We now have also a better distally contact area (Fig. 16-6, right).

The Antega, Versys, Vision 2000 and Osteolock stems just differed regarding the surface roughness. The G_2 stem performed especially in the lateral shoulder a better contact area with the CASPAR milling (**▪** Fig. 16-7, right). Again the prints of the 9 mm drilling head are seen. For this stem the lateral contact of fit was pointed out for the robot preparation.

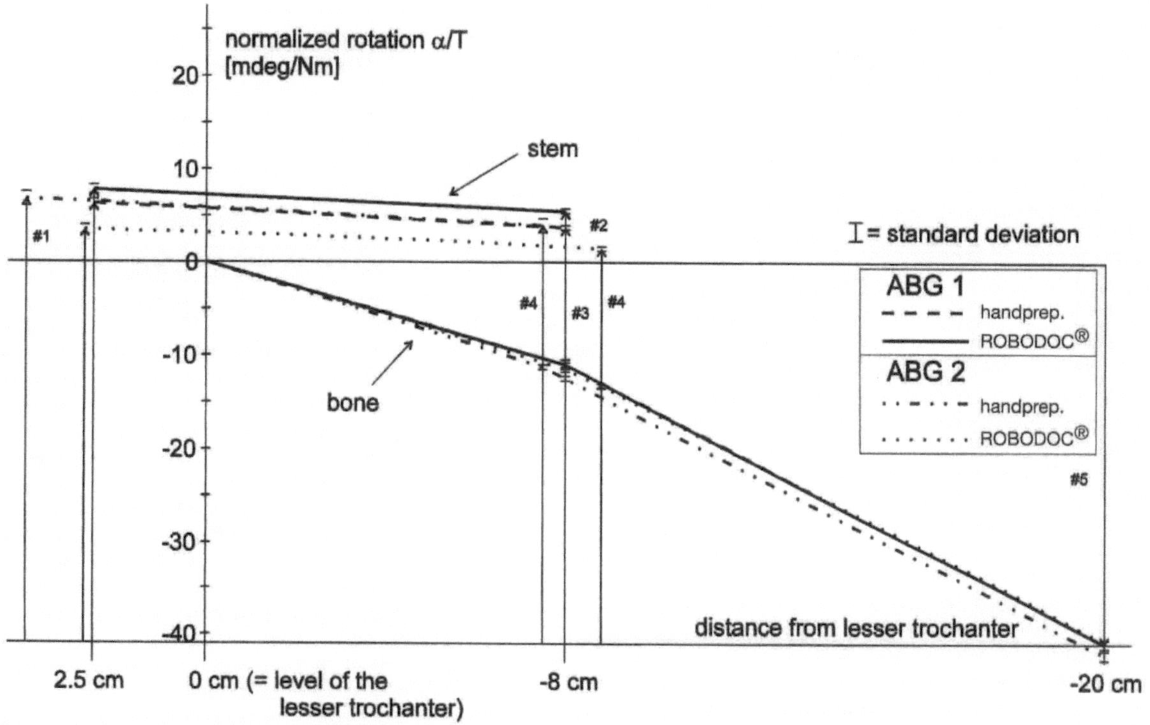

■ **Fig. 16-3.** Rotational angle curves of the ABG I and II stems, size 6. The *dotted line* indicates the results of the 3 ROBODOC preparation for the ABG II, showing the better stability. The *straight line* shows the results of the 3 ROBODOC milling for the ABG I and the other two lines the comparable pattern of the 6 hand-broached femora. The standard deviations (I) were minimal indicating high reproducibility. 0 cm indicates the level of the lesser trochanter, #1–#5 the levels at which measurements were taken. The curve of bone twist is marked in the lower section starting with 0 degree of rotation

Discussion

Computer navigation and robotic machining systems have been suggested to provide both improved femoral component alignment and improved initial press-fit fixation and stability of the femoral stem [3, 5, 16]. Although we did not evaluate all benefits of computer-guided stem insertion, there is some evidence in the literature that reduced rates of stem malpositioning occur with the use of robotic systems [10, 11].

Interestingly, our results failed to demonstrate the total benefit of robotic canal preparation (with regard to enhanced stability), as currently advocated [3, 5], in four of the eight implants investigated (■ Table 16-1). Two of these implants were anatomic. We believe that the robot needs additional space for maneuvering the drill head around the curved shoulder thus resulting in gaps between stem and bone bed. Gaps between the implant and bone created by inaccurate bone preparation may lead to implant instability and decreased bone ingrowth [14]. Paravic et al. [16] compared the accuracy of manual broaching and robotic reaming and observed significantly more gaps in the mid-shaft and distal regions between stem (Osteolock) and bone in the hand-broached group.

Similar to our findings, Alexander et al. [2] found no enhanced rotational stability of Osteolock stems in robotic-machined human femora compared to conventional hand-broaching. The authors suggested, that both compaction of the bone bed and critical contact areas in the hand-broached specimens may be responsible for their findings. Interestingly, they described a large variability in

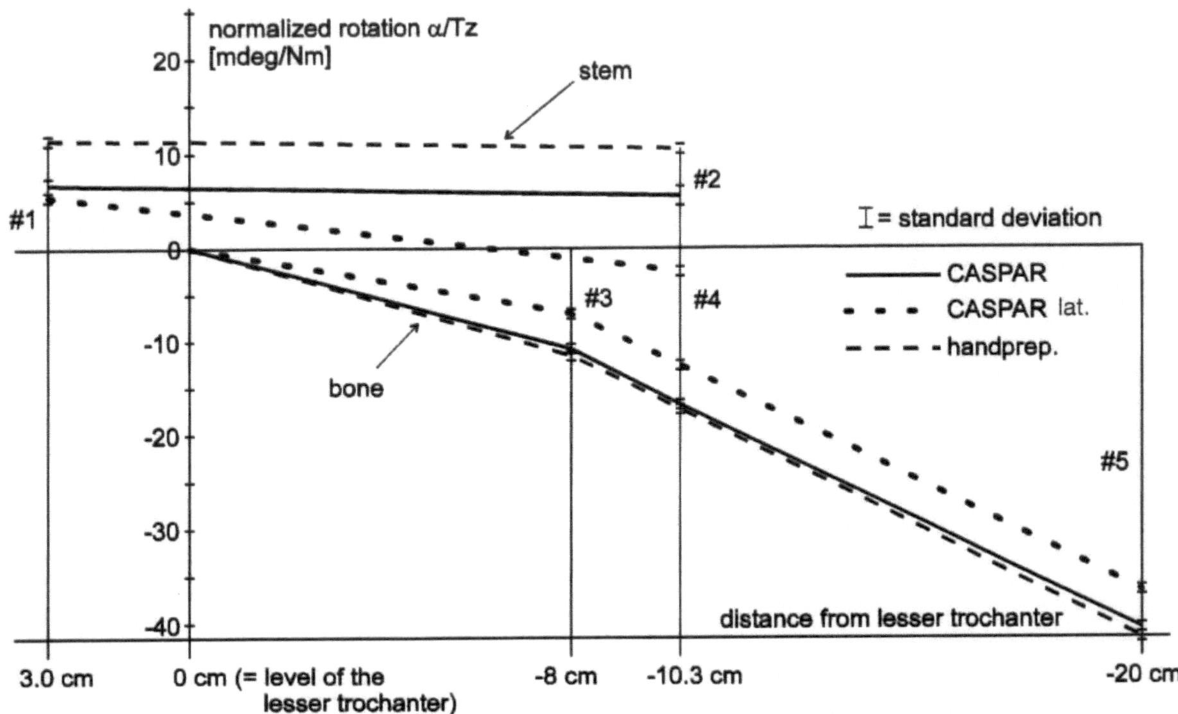

◘ Fig. 16-4. Rotational angle curves of the Vision 2000. The dotted line indicates the results of the 3 hand-broached specimens. The *interrupted line* shows the results of the CASPAR milling and the straight line the results achieved with lateral stem positioning. The standard deviations (I) were minimal indicating high reproducibility. 0 cm indicates the level of the lesser trochanter, #1–#5 the levels at which measurements were taken. The curve of bone twist is marked in the lower section starting with 0 degree of rotation

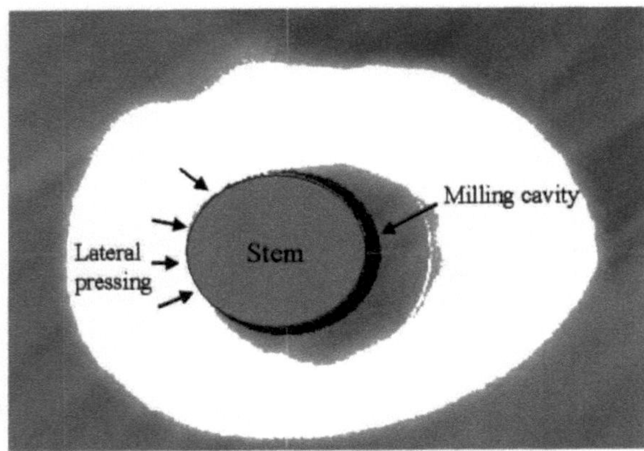

◘ Fig. 16-5. Distal transversal CT scan of the planning station for the Vision 2000 stem. The *black area* is the milling cavity of the robot. The *gray area* represents the prostheses at this level. Laterally is a close cortical contact (*arrows*) which produces some kind of press fit, whereas medially there is much space

the hand-broached group. This is in contrast with our results which have featured small standard deviations. Differences between robotic and manual canal preparation may have been more or less pronounced if paired human femora with genuine cancellous bone had been used.

ABG, Antega, Osteolock, VerSys ET and the Vision 2000 stems showed a pattern of proximal fixation with little proximal slip. In the Swedish hip registry [12] promising short-term results for the ABG Ha stem implanted with hand-broaching have been reported. Interestingly, by positioning the Vision 2000 stem more laterally the fixation pattern was altered from a proximal to a more distal fixation and torque transfer. However, this did not result in increased proximal slip but in an increased overall stability and increased stem twist as a consequence. Similarly, robotic milling changed the pattern of fixation to an even more proximal one in G_2 and

▣ Table 16-1. Showing the different types of prostheses, manufacturer, the robotic system used, were we saw proximalisation of the fitting, increasing of the primary stability

Prostheses (manufacturer)	Size	CASPAR	ROBODOC	Proximalisation	Increase of primary stability	Additional findings
ABG 1	6		×		×	Changed contact areas
ABG 2 (Styker/Howmedica)	6		×			
Antega (Aesculap)			×			
G2 (DePuy/J&J)	7	×		×	×	
Osteolock (Styker/Howmedica)	3×	×	×		(×)	
S-ROM (DePuy/J&J)	18 F		×			Distal over-reaming
Versys ET (Zimmer)	13	×		×	×	
Vision 2000 (DePuy/J&J)	13	×			×	Cave lateral positioning

VerSys ET stems. In hand-broached specimens due to the altered (more distal) torque transfer G_2 stems seem subjected to significantly higher levels of implant twist.

The S-ROM stem showed a mixed pattern of proximal, mid-shaft and distal fixation with a high stem twist and reduced stem stiffness thus resembling a deformation pattern closer to (synthetic) femora. Reduced stem stiffness had lead to reduced proximal bone loss and distal cortical hypertrophy at short-term in a dog model [19]. However, from our data material no valid conclusions can be drawn to the clinical phenomenon of pro-ximal (radiographically evident) stress shielding, as this represents a bone remodeling response over time.

Early clinical results have been favorable with the S-ROM stem even in dysplastic hips [7]. However, we are concerned about the micromotion we measured between the sleeve and inner core of the S-ROM system. It is difficult to believe that fretting and metal wear should not occur.

These findings highlight that the mode of preparation, the definition of implant bed dimensions and the implant position significantly influence the pattern of

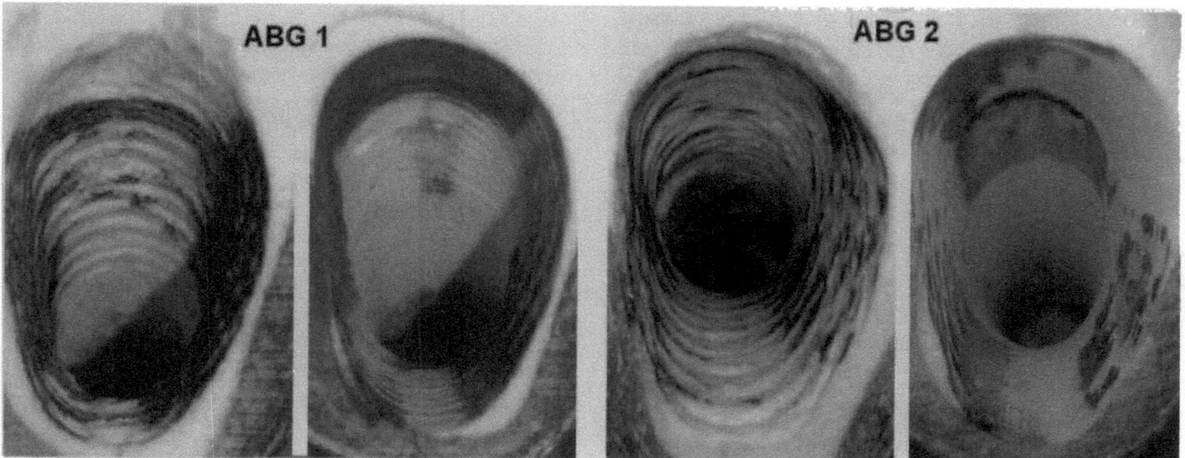

▣ Fig. 16-6. Pictures of the contact areas of the ABG 1 (left pair) and the ABG 2 (right pair), showing the difference between the hand-broached (left) and robotically milled (right) stems of each pair. The rough contact areas in both hand-broached stems are but comparable. The robotic preparation in the ABG 1 respects the anatomical design of the lateral shoulder (white area). The area in the ABG 2 robotic preparation, shows good contact also distally

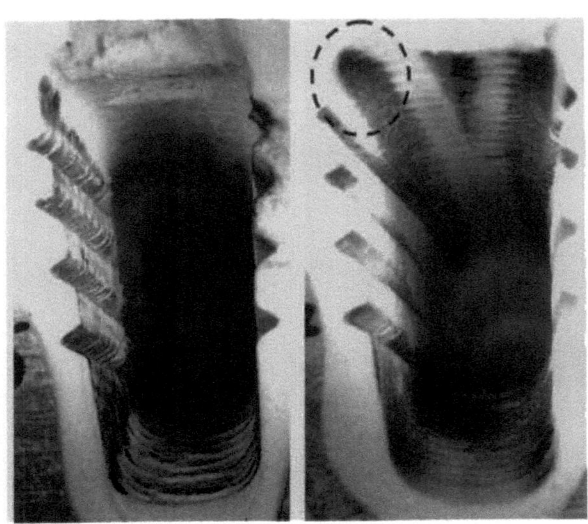

Fig. 16-7. Rough structure medial and only rare contact area laterally in the hand broached G2 (left). In contrast in the CASPAR-preparation high press-fit in the lateral areas. This is a result of the round drilling head, which keeps the lateral rim untouched.

fixation, even for the same implant type. Furthermore, more distal fixation of a stem may not necessarily lead to reduced proximal stability. Increased implant deformation occurred in this instance. This observation was surprising to us, as it not only confirmed that femoral implants do not represent rigid bodies which primarily deform bone, but they also undergo deformation themselves, which seems to depend on the pattern of fixation.

Some of our findings highlight the difficulty in creating the perfect robotically milled cavity as compromises regarding size and maneuvering of the drill head have to be made by the manufactures.

With the ABG I and ABG II the influence of the different definitions of the cavity is demonstrated. The ABG II has a much better fit in the robot group than the ABG I.

Prior to robotic implantation of a cementless stem in vitro studies are essential to understand individual patterns of fixation and to assure reproducibility and adequate primary stability. We consider these experimental studies of great value to the designing companies and are concerned about clinical introduction (of robotic milling) without preceding in vitro studies. Considering the significant additional cost, we find the widespread use of robotic milling devices currently difficult to justify as no proof exists that better primary stability and ultimately improved outcome will result. However, at centers where prospective, comparative studies can be performed the clinical implication of robotic systems should be further evaluated.

References

1. Albrektsson T, Bränemark PI, Hansson HA, Lindström J (1981) Osseointegrated titanium implants. Requirements for ensuring a long-lasting, direct bone-to-implant anchorage in man. Acta Orthop Scand 52: 155–170
2. Alexander JW, Kamaric E, Noble PC, McCathy JC (1999) The effect of robotic machining on the micromotion of cementless femoral stems. 45th Annual Meeting, Orthopaedic Research Society, Anaheim
3. Bargar WL, Bauer A, Boerner M (1998) Primary and revision total hip replacement using the Robodoc system. Clin Orthop 354: 82–91
4. Bergmann G, Graichen F, Rohlmann A (1993) Hip loading during walking and running measured in two patients. J Biomech 26: 969–990
5. Boerner M, Bauer A, Lahmer A (1997) Computerunterstützter Robotereinsatz in der Hüftendoprothetik. Unfallchirurg 100: 640–645
6. Callaghan JJ, Fulghum CS, Glisson RR, Stranne SK (1992) The effect of femoral stem geometry on interface motion in uncemented porous-coated total hip prostheses. J Bone Joint Surg (Am) 74: 839–848
7. Cameron HU, Botsford DJ, Park YS (1996) Influence of the Crowe rating on the outcome of total hip arthroplasty in congenital hip dysplasia. J Arthroplasty 11: 582–587
8. Cristofolini L, Viceconti M, Cappello A, Toni A (1996) Mechanical validation of whole bone composite femur models. J Biomech 29: 525–535
9. Görzt W, Nägerl UV, Nägerl H, Thomsen M (2002) Spartial micromovements of uncemented femoral components after torsional loads. J Biomech Eng (ASME) 124 : 1–8
10. Hasselbach C, Lahmer A, Witzel U, Rahgozar M (1999) Operationsroboter beim Hüftendoprotheseneinbau. 116. Meeting of the German Society of Surgery, München
11. Jerosch J, Hasselbach C, Filler T, Peuker E, Rahgozar M, Lahmer A (1998) Qualitätssteigerung in der präoperativen Planung und intraoperativen Umsetzung durch die Verwendung von computerassistierten Systemen und Operationsrobotern – eine experimentelle Untersuchung. Chirurg 69: 973–996
12. Malchau H, Herberts P, Söderman P, Odén A (2000) Prognostics of total hip replacement. 67th Annual Meeting of the AAOS, Orlando
13. Morscher E (1995) Der zementfreie Femurschaft. In: Morscher E (Hrsg) Endoprothetik. Springer, Berlin Heidelberg New York Tokyo, S 255–267
14. Noble PC, Alexander JW, Lindahl LJ, Yew DT, Granberry WM, Tullos HS (1988) The anatomic basis of femoral component design. Clin Orthop 235: 148–165
15. Nourbash PS, Paprosky WG (1998) Cementless femoral design concerns. Rationale for extensive porous coating. Clin Orthop 355: 189–199
16. Paravic V, Noble PC, McCarthy JC (1999) The impact of robotic surgery on the fit of cementless femoral prostheses. 45th Annual Meeting, Orthopaedic Research Society, Anaheim

17. Paul HA, Bagar WL, Mittelstadt B et al. (1992) Development of a surgical robot for cementless total hip arthroplasty. Clin Orthop 285: 57–66

18. Sugiyama H, Whiteside LA, Engh CA (1992) Torsional fixation of the femoral component in total hip arthroplasty. The effect of surgical press-fit technique. Clin Orthop 275: 187–193

19. Sumner DR, Galante JO (1992) Determinants of stress shielding: design versus materials versus interface. Clin Orthop 274: 202–212

20. Thomsen M, Görtz W, Nägerl H (1999) Characterization of modern hip endoprostheses. Z Orthop Ihre Grenzgeb 137: A32

21. Thomsen M, Breusch SJ, Aldinger P et al. (2002) Robotically milled bone cavities. A comparison with hand broaching in different types of cementless hip stems. Acta Orth Scand 73: 379–385

22. Thomsen M, Aldinger P, Görtz W et al. (2001) The importance to generate robotically milled cavities for total hip implantation. Unfallchirurg 104: 692–699

17 An Anatomically Shaped Prosthesis Stem –

In Vitro Comparison Between Robot-Assisted and Manual Implantation

K. Knabe, C. Hurschler, C. Stukenborg-Colsman, F. Gossé

Introduction

»We had these beautiful implants that were made to fit the individual extremely accurately. We had also broaches that were the same sizes as the implant ... but then we had to take a 2 1/2 lb mallet and ram it down the bone in order to cut inside of the bone out. The bone sometimes were cracking and the implants were sitting up too high or down too low ... We found that other surgeons around the country were having the same problems.«

HOWARD A. PAUL

»... Luckily robots can do all this better.«

RUSSEL H. TAYLOR

These quotes from two of the greatest pioneers in robotic surgery were, among other things, motivation for carrying out the following comparative study.

The introduction of the computer-controlled surgical robot into the areas of general surgery and orthopaedic surgery has simultaneously opened a new chapter in the history of the operational theater, while also creating demand for a new research specialization. Since its introduction, many studies comparing the advantages and disadvantages of robot-assisted surgery over the best available conventional methods have been published.

The main motivation for the implementation of robots in the operational theater are derived from increased precision and an associated improvement in quality, as well as improved preoperative planning and better reproducibility.

Different terms of reference that must be differentiated in the context of robot-assisted surgery are »display systems«, »tracking« or »passive navigations systems«, »semiactive navigations systems« and finally »active navigation systems«, which is the relevant term to be applied in the study presented herein. An active navigation system, in addition to positioning alone, utilizes certain instruments attached to the robot arm in the field of operation.

The goal of the presented study was to determine the relationships between preoperative planning and the actual result obtained postoperatively.

The question to be answered was whether or not preoperative planning was more effectively realized with a robot-assisted technique than with a conventional manual one.

In order to permit such a comparison, it was first necessary to establish the following measurement parameters for manually implanted as well as robot-assisted hip prostheses: antetorsion angle, CCD angle, medial-lateral offset and femur length (with respect to leg length).

Materials and Methods

Two matched groups of ten femurs each (n=10) were formed from 10 human cadaver femur pairs. The first femur of each pair was randomly assigned either to the manually or robot-assisted implantation group.

Reference pins were implanted and computer tomographic (CT) images were taken of all femurs to permit preoperative planning. All stem implantations were planned on an Orthodoc station from these CT images. After manual or robotic implantation respectively, all femurs were again CT scanned and analyzed on the Orthodoc station.

The Antega Prosthesis Shaft

The philosophy of the Aesculap Antega prosthesis shaft (◘ Fig. 17-1) is based on the concept of a proximal anchoring. The proximal stem has an anteversion of 10° and is surface-treated with a rough Plasmapore surface, which in combination with the compressed cancellous bone of the proximal femur improves the primary stability of the prosthesis. The antetorsion of 14° integrated into the prosthesis neck contributes to an anatomic reconstruction of the joint. The cylindrically shaped distal stem guarantees a reliable implant insertion without a cortical press-fit.

Secondary stability of the prosthesis should be achieved by ingrowth into the microscopically porous surface of the proximal stem.

Furthermore, the proximal-ventral fin is intended to establish an increased rotational stability.

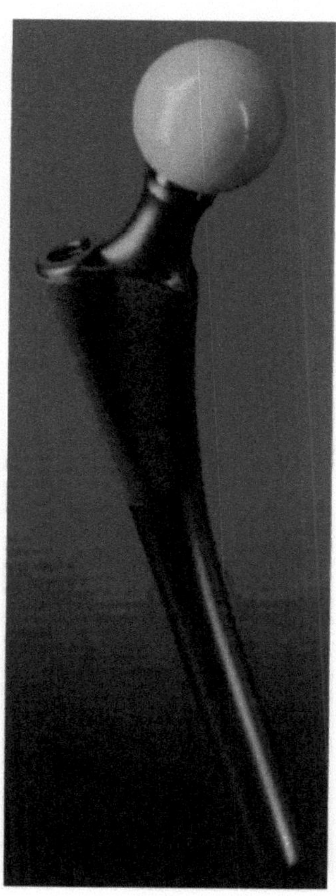

◘ **Fig. 17-1.** The Antega prosthesis stem

Orthodoc Planning

The data, which are stored on optical disc, are transferred onto the planning-station and loaded into the program after CT scanning of the specimens. Image data are displayed only after the data are successfully checked for adherence to the scanning protocol, control of patient motion, and localization of the registration pins.

The size of the prosthesis can be altered at any time without changing its actual position. The position of the prosthesis is verified multiple times in all three planes of view, during which particular attention is paid to the ventral localization of the prosthesis in the proximal surface coated region of the femoral-stem.

Implantation of the Prosthesis

After all 20 femora had been prepared and optimally planned in the Orthodoc station, they were randomly assigned to one of the two experimental groups. Thus, one specimen from each of the femoral pairs was assigned to either the manual or robot-assisted groups. The manual implantation of the Antega prosthesis stem was performed by an experienced attending physician of orthopaedic surgery. The femur shaft was prepared in four steps according to the manufacturers guidelines.

Before the robot-assisted implantation can proceed, the data from the planning workstation are entered into the robot, and the robot is calibrated. This calibration step is performed before every cutting procedure performed by the robot [2]. If the calibration protocol fails, it must be repeated before cutting can begin.

After successful completion of the calibration protocol, the robot is ready to begin cutting the femur according to the preoperatively executed planning. After completion of the cutting procedure, the prosthesis can be tapped into a firmly seated position in the femur.

Analysis and Statistics

Both groups of femurs were analyzed with respect to leg length, medial-lateral offset, CCD angle (neck shaft angle), as well as the antetorsion angle. On the one hand, the physiological values of the unprepared femurs were compared to the parameters achieved in the planning phase, while on the other, the planned parameters were compared to the actually achieved postoperative results. The Students' t test was used to compare means at a significance level of α=0.05.

Results

Physiologic versus Planned Parameters

The results of this analysis (Fig. 17-2) represent the difference between the values of the physiological bones and the values chosen during planning of the prosthesis position.

During planning, the primary goal was to maintain the original leg length, although this was not always possible while maintaining the optimal positioning of the prosthesis. The average leg-length increase in the manual group compared to physiologic was +1.1 mm (SD 1.2), which means that an average increase of leg length of 1.1 mm had resulted already during the planning phase. In the ROBODOC group, leg length increased by an average of +1.7 mm (SD 2.0) compared to the physiological geometry. No significant differences in leg length (p=0.45) were observed between the manual and the ROBODOC groups.

The **medial-lateral offset** was reduced by an average of −7.4 mm (SD 5.4) in the manual group, and by an average of −5.7 mm (SD 7.6) in the ROBODOC group. The difference in offset between the manual and robot-assisted groups was not significant (p=0.56). The **CCD angle** was increased in planning in both groups compared to the physiological situation. The manual group was thus increased by an average of +17.3° (SD 2.5), and the ROBODOC group by an average of +17.1° SD 2.0), which means that a valgus orientation of the prosthesis was planned in all cases.

The antetorsion angle was also increased in the manual as well as the robot-assisted groups. This increase averaged +11.3° (SD 3.7) in the manual, and +8,7° (SD 4.6) in the robot-assisted groups, although the difference was not significant (*p*=0.18).

Planned Versus Postoperative Parameters

This part of the analysis (Fig. 17-3) describes the translation of the planned implantation into a postoperative result. It illuminates whether or not the intended planned implantation was actually realized.

The difference in **leg length** in the manual group was always positive (>0) which means that the leg was always lengthened in the manual group; this was not the case in the ROBODOC group. The average amount of lengthening thus amounted to +6.8 mm (SD 3, p=0.0004) in the manual group, whereas lengthening in the robot-assisted group was limited to an average of +0.3 mm (SD 2.8). The **medial-lateral offset** was reduced in the ROBODOC group by an average of −0.2 mm (SD 2.1), while it was increased an average of +0.6 mm (SD 3.8) in the manual group compared to the planned implantation.

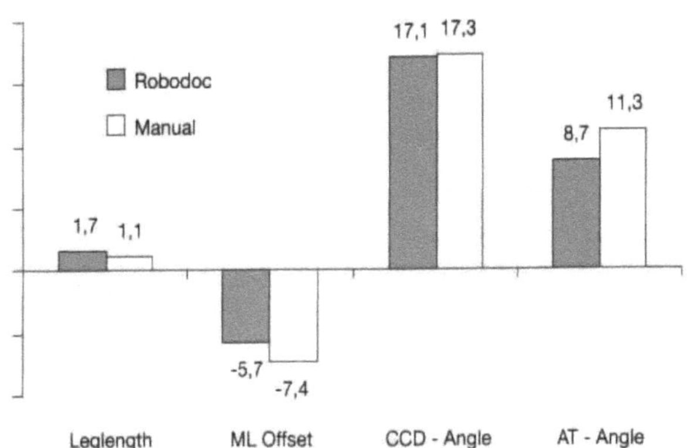

Fig. 17-2. Results physiologic versus planned

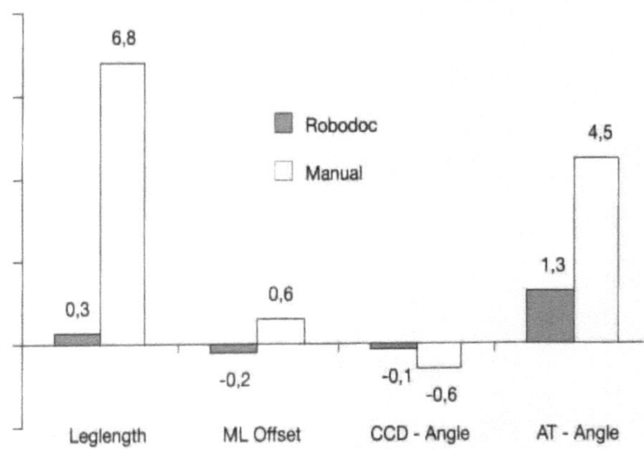

Fig. 17-3. Results planned versus postoperative

The difference in the CCD angle relative to the planned implantation amounted to –0.6° (SD 1.5) in the manual group, and –0,1° (SD 0.5) in the ROBODOC group while no significant difference was observed between the groups ($p=0.23$). The translation of the **antetorsion angle** from planning to the postoperative result tended to be more precise in the ROBODOC group than during manual implantation. Thus, the analysis of the manually implanted group resulted in several outliers. The average antetorsion values for the manual and ROBODOC groups was +4,5° (SD 12.3), and +1,3° (SD 2.1), respectively.

Physiologic Versus Postoperative Data

A comparison between physiologic parameter and postoperatively achieved parameters can be made with the data values from the section above (physiologic versus planned and planned versus postoperative). A comparison between physiologic parameters and postoperative results was thus made (◨ Fig. 17-4).

Leg length was increased an average of +7.9 mm (SD 3.9, p=0.001) in the manually implanted group, and an average of +2.0 mm (SD 2.8) in the ROBODOC group compared to the preoperative (physiologic).

The **medial-lateral offset** was reduced by implanting a prosthesis in 90% of all cases. The average reduction in offset was –6.8 mm (SD 3.9) in the manually implanted group, and –5.9 mm (SD 7.9) in the ROBODOC group, although this result was not statistically significant ($p=0.75$).

The **CCD angle** in all specimens was greater postoperatively than preoperatively, which means the prosthesis stem was implanted in a valgus orientation in both groups. The CCD angle was increased by +16.7° (SD 2.2) after manual implantation, and +17.1° (SD 2.2) in the ROBODOC group, although, again the result was not statistically significant ($p=0.68$).

The average increase in **antetorsion** was 15,9° (SD 15.0) in the manual group and +10,0° (SD 5.9) in the ROBODOC group, the difference is not significant ($p=0.27$).

Rate of Fracture

Two macroscopically visible fractures were observed during manual implantation of the prostheses (◨ Fig. 17-5). These arose in each case upon tapping in of the prosthesis stem. In contrast, no visible fractures were observed in the robot-assisted group.

Discussion

Total hip arthroplasty has presented a thoroughly successful operative procedure over the last 40 years. It has become the most commonly performed procedure, and is most widely accepted among patients [3]. Nonetheless, a series of problems exist, the most important of which is aseptic loosening, which in the long term determines the fate of the implanted prosthesis [4].

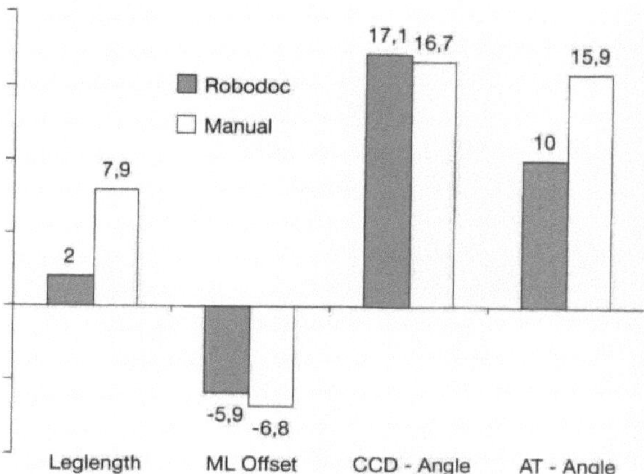

◨ **Fig. 17-4.** Results physiologic versus postoperative

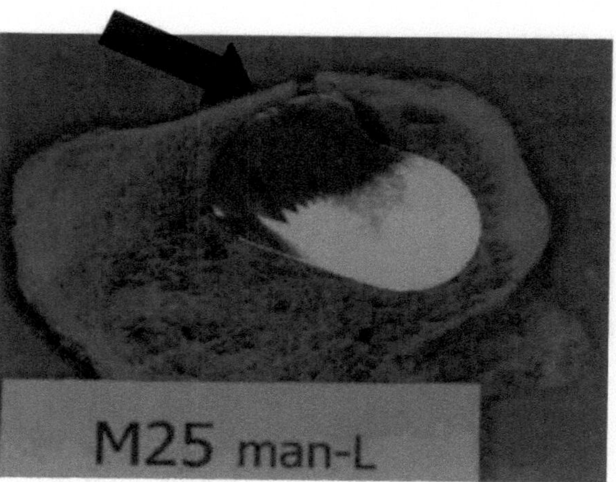

◨ **Fig. 17-5.** Proximal cross-section, manual group

17

Aseptic loosening can be caused by, among other things, primary instability which could for example be the result of poor operative technique. Thus, primary stability must be achieved intraoperatively, under which the following secondary definitive biological stability can result. This secondary biological stability is played out predominately at the cellular level of the implant-bone interface [4]. One expects a better mechanical stability based on close bone-implant contact, through which relative motion is minimized or eliminated.

Additional factors discussed as possible causes for aseptic loosening are biomechanical factors (varus-positioning) for example, or also a suboptimal design of the prosthesis stem.

Prosthesis Design

Posterior Over-Cutting

Since the Antega stem is an anatomically formed prosthesis with a proximally curved neck (anteversion angle of 10°), it is necessary to proximally over-cut a limited area to permit full cutting of the insertion volume. Only after this over cutting is it possible to cut the distal section of the implantation cavity for the Antega stem. The area of this over-cutting is located in the lower third of contact of the Plasmapore surface coating. The size of the over-machined area is dependent on the selected prosthesis size. The volume of the proximally cut cavity is not sufficient to allow the straight cutter to reach distally with the smaller prosthesis sizes.

The over-cutting results in a not insignificant loss of contact surface area in the important proximal area of the surface coating (◘ Fig. 17-6). A portion of the theoretically larger contact surface area is thus lost through use of the surgical robot.

Over-Cutting of the Greater Trochanter

A further problem with the robot-assisted implantation is the partially massive over-cutting of the greater trochanter (◘ Fig. 17-7). This thinning of the trochanter area is similarly necessary to provide the rigid robot-guided cutting head a sufficiently large access tunnel into the femur cavity. The actual advantage of the minimization of bone loss in the region of the trochanter through the use of a anatomic prosthesis design are thus not realized. This can lead to bone loss in the area of the gluteus musculature insertion and thus to concomitant gluteus insufficiency as well as to trochanter fractures.

Okoniewski [6] observed three trochanter fractures in a group of 44 robot-assisted hip stem implantations, although this was with the Osteolock straight shaft prosthesis (not an anatomic prosthesis).

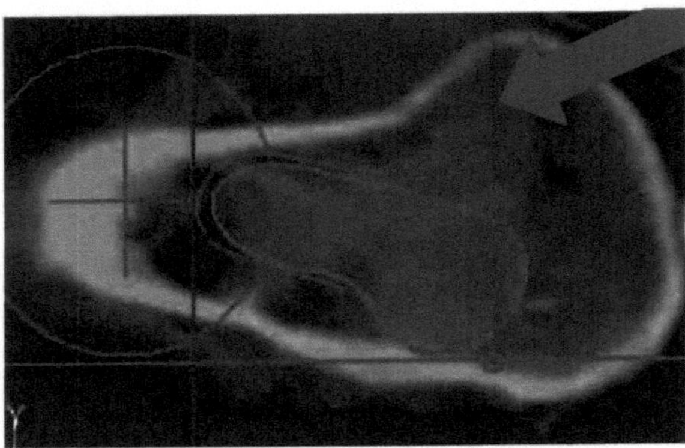

◘ Fig. 17-6. Posterior over-cutting

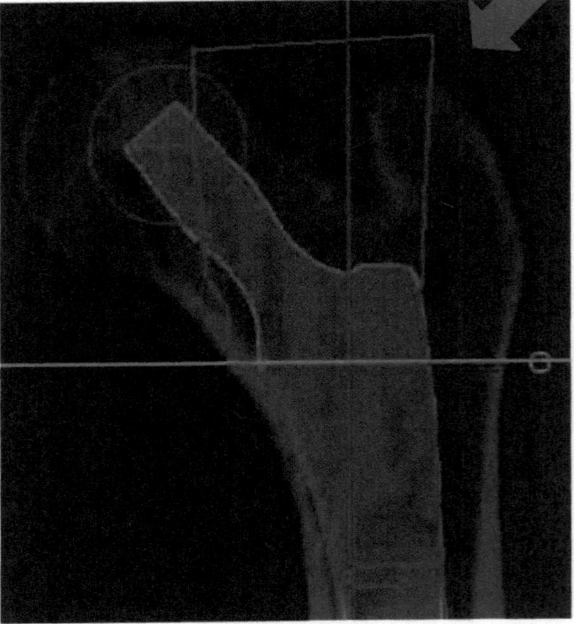

◘ Fig. 17-7. Cut tunnel greater trochanter

Leg Length

The problems of exactly translating a preoperative plan into a postoperative result were particularly well illustrated by the problems observed during the manual total hip prosthesis implantation, which resulted in a large variation in postoperative leg length [2, 8].

In our study, preoperative planning was translated very well into postoperative results by robot-assisted surgery. Thus, in addition to the leg length increase due to planning of the implantation of 1.7 mm, leg length was lengthened by only another +0.3 mm postoperatively, resulting in a total increase of +2.0 mm.

During manual implantation, leg length was increased by +6.8 mm compared to the planned length. Thus, with a planned leg lengthening of +1.1 mm, postoperatively, a leg lengthening of +7.9 mm was observed.

These leg length increases agree with those experienced clinically. Here, too, one observes large variability in leg length, and a clearly more often occurring leg lengthening than shortening [3].

Medial-Lateral Offset

It is noteworthy that in order to obtain optimal positioning, in 19 of 20 cases medial-lateral offset was decreased already during planning of the implantation on the Orthodoc planning station. On average this decrease amounted to −5.7 mm in the robot-assisted group, and −7.4 mm in the manual group. This planning was translated into a postoperative result as well in both the manual (+0.6 mm) and robot-assisted (−0.2 mm) groups.

As a result, a reduced offset was attained postoperatively in both groups (robot-assisted −5.9 mm, manual −6.8 mm).

This is nonetheless justified by the planning guidelines of the prosthesis manufacturer. The goal of the planning was to achieve good alignment of the prosthesis with the femoral shaft. During this optimization, a reduced medial contact of the prosthesis was accepted in compromise. The result was a valgus implantation, which is manifested in the results for the CCD angle (see page 138).

The medial-lateral offset is reduced through a valgus implantation of the prosthesis stem. This can result in muscle imbalances, primarily of the gluteus muscles, and

thus lead to an alteration of the biomechanics of the joint postoperatively [9].

One must view the design of the prosthesis itself as a second reason for the consistent reduction of the medial-lateral offset. The Antega prosthesis itself displays a smaller medial-lateral offset than other anatomically designed stems.

Antetorsion Angle

In 1998 Jerosch [5] emphasized the importance of the postoperative antetorsion angle, the biomechanics of the joint are altered, even in the absence of joint instability (i.e. caused by a large antetorsion angle). This is caused in particular by the small hip rotators, but also by the more horizontally oriented aspects of the gluteus musculature [5].

In this study, the antetorsion angle was increased in the manual group by an average of +15.9°, and in the robot-assisted group by and average of +10.0°. Hereby, one must take into consideration that a greater antetorsion angle results in the preoperative planning alone due to reasons associated with planning objectives and demands. The antetorsion angle was planned to be +11,3° greater during manual, and +8.7° greater during robot-assisted implantation.

The antetorsion angle was additionally slightly increased in the intraoperative implementation of the planning (manually by +4.5°, robot-assisted by +1.3°), so that a distinctly increased antetorsion angle was observed postoperatively (SD 0.42).

One reason for the consistent increase in the angle is most probably the design of the prosthesis.

Good anterior contact is necessary in order to obtain adequate primary stability of the prosthesis. This required contact can be adequately achieved in the area of the anterior fin, which contributes to rotational stability (◘ Fig. 17-8). On the other hand, in order for the prosthesis to be in contact along it's whole width anteriorly, a rotation of the prosthesis in the anterior direction – and hereby an increase in the antetorsion angle – would be necessary. A compromise between anterior fixation and antetorsion angle must be met here, independent of whether the prosthesis in implanted manually, or robot-assisted.

17

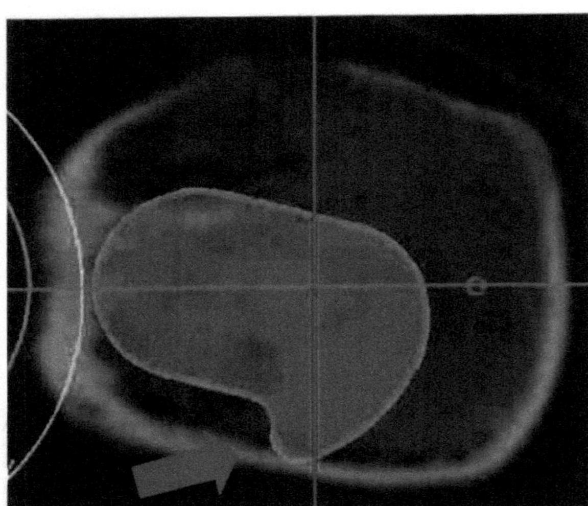

◘ **Fig. 17-8.** Anterior contact of the fin

Furthermore, it is difficult to avoid increased antetorsion while maintaining the principle of an anterior fixation whilst simultaneously being constrained by the anteversion angle of 10°, and the antetorsion angle of 14° dictated by the design of the prosthesis.

CCD Angle

In the analysis of the planned CCD angle one notices that all 20 femurs were planned with a valgus orientation, i.e. that the CCD angle was greater in all cases: in the robot-assisted femurs by +17.1°, and in the manually implanted femurs by +17.3°.

The reasons for this increase are similar as those responsible for the increased medial-lateral offset, i.e. that alignment was assigned a higher priority than medial contact. According to contemporary clinical experience with the Antega prosthesis, changes have been implemented to improve medial contact and afford a more varus planning of the implantation.

The stipulated CCD angle of 145° of the design of the Antega prosthesis corresponds more with the upper end of the physiologic range which is one of the reasons for the valgus planning.

The planning could be implemented well in both groups. Thus, the difference between the planned and postoperative CCD angle was small, averaging 0.1° for the robot-assisted, and –0.6° for the manually implanted groups.

A further problem of the valgus implantation is the over-cutting of the major trochanter (discussed on page 136). A more varus implantation would be desirable here in order to minimize bone loss in this area.

In the typical manual prosthesis implantation, up to 20% of cases are reported with a postoperative varus position, only 1 to 2% with a valgus position.

Precision of Fit

Already in 1992, Paul [7] judged the most important result of his study to be that the direct connection between preoperative planning and surgical implementation is the greatest advantage of a robot-assisted system in comparison to a manual implantation.

Boerner [2] assumes that better ingrowth of the bone will be given based on the significantly improved bone contact and increased primary stability made possible by the exact cutting of the femur. Only thus can micromotion be prevented and rotational instabilities be avoided which furthermore lead to bone resorption and the formation of a fibrous membrane around the prosthesis [2].

It seems logical that although bone is a relatively adaptable tissue which can forgive a certain degree of inprecision of the surgeon, that higher precision in the preparation of the femur cavity would lead to the expected better middle- and long-term results.

Despite the discussions about a better precision of the femoral cavity afforded through the robot, the positioning and fixation of the acetabulum still remain the key problems in the total joint replacement of the hip.

References

1. Aesculap Antega (1998) Hip System
2. Boerner M, Bauer A, Lahmer A (1997) Computerunterstützter Robotereinsatz in der Hüftendoprothetik. Unfallchirurg 100: 640–645
3. Debrunner AM (1994) Das Hüftgelenk. Orthopädie Orthopädische Chirurgie – Die Störungen des Bewegungsapparates in Klinik und Praxis. 3. Auflage, Verlag Hans Huber, Bern, Stuttgart, Toronto
4. Debrunner AM (1994) Degenerative Krankheiten (Arthrosen). Orthopädie, Orthopädische Chirurgie – Die Störungen des Bewegungsapparates in Klinik und Praxis. 3. Auflage, Verlag Hans Huber, Bern, Stuttgart, Toronto

5. Jerosch J, v Hasselbach C, Filler T, Peuker E, Rahgozar M, Lahmer A (1998) Qualitätssteigerung in der präoperativen Planung und intraoperativen Umsetzung durch die Verwendung von computerassistierten Systemen und Operationsrobotern – eine experimentelle Untersuchung. Chirurg 69: 973–976

6. Okoniewski M, Birke A, Schietsch U, Thoma M, Hein W (2000) Frühergebnisse einer prospektiven Studie bei Patienten mit computerunterstützter Femurschaftpräparation bei Hüft-TEP-Implantationen (System Robodoc) –Indikationen, Ergebnisse, Komplikationen. Z Orthop 138: 510–514

7. Paul HA, Bargar WL, Mittlestadt B et al. (1992) Development of a surgical robot for cementless total hip arthroplasty. Clin Orthop 285: 57–66

8. Reichelt A, Botterer H (1993) PM – Prothesen. Z Orthop 131: 532–538

9. Schidlo C, Becker C, Jansson V, Refior J (1999) Änderung des CCD-Winkels sowie des femoralen Antetorsionswinkels durch Hüftprothesenimplantation. Z Orthop 137: 259–264

10. Wixson R, Stuberg D, Mehlhoff M (1991) Total hip replacement with cemented uncemented and hybrid prostheses. J Bone Joint Surgery Am 73: 257–270

18   Clinical Experiences with *ROBODOC* in Total Hip Arthroplasty

M. Boerner, U. Wiesel

The most important precondition for the durability of an implant is its primary stability. The goal of any cementless THA is osteointegration. This means direct contact between the implant and the bone. Besides implant design, implant surface and materials, the surgical technique is a major factor for long-lasting stability. A conical fixation of femoral implants guarantees a high primary stability in cementless THA. The way of fixation of the implant in the femoral cavity and the load transfer play a major role in durability of the implant. To gain an optimal fixation of the implant a robot has been used for cementless THA at BGU Frankfurt since 1994. The 3D preoperative planning data is transferred to the robot that mills out the femoral cavity and guarantees an optimal press-fit of the implant. So far the system has been used on more than 5000 patients. Due to the excellent postoperative results three robots are in daily use at BGU Frankfurt by now.

Many publications show varus and valgus malpositionings in the postoperative radiologic controls. A deviation of the implant position from the proximal femoral axis causes incorrect load transfer to the femur and subsequently early loosening of the implant.

Varus and valgus malpositionings of the femoral implant can easily be detected in the a.-p. X-ray. Besides the correct alignment of the implant in the a.-p. view the positioning in the lateral femoral axis is another important biomechanical factor for correct load transfer. In most studies, however, this is not taken into consideration, mainly, because the lateral view is insufficient in most standard X-rays.

Different attempts to improve primary stability have been made in changing implant and broach design. Implants with sharp edges tend to have a high primary stability (including the rotational stability). In most cases the broaches tend to achieve a higher density of cancellous bone for better primary stability. We do think, however, that it is not considered that that kind of cancellous bone results in a slower osteointegration. A different principle to achieve high primary stability is very close contact between the implant and cortical bone. The anteversion of the femoral implant is an important factor for achieving normal gait.

In conventional THR the anteversion of the femoral component is not taken into consideration. In conventional THR templates are used for preoperative planning. The use of those templates can cause quite a few problems. They can only be used for the given magnification which means that a standardized X-ray technique is absolutely necessary. Even with that it is very hard to achieve exact a.-p. and lateral views. The planning with templates gives only limited information about the implant size and the osteotomy level of the femoral neck. This results in a wide variation of postoperative leg length.

In daily clinical use there is a great discrepancy between preoperative planning and intra-operative execution. In many cases the planned implant size cannot be used which means that frequently no preoperative planning is done at all. As most cementless implant have a press-fit that means that any implant that is too small has an insufficient primary stability. This results in subsidence of the implant. If there is more than 4 mm of subsidence per year this is considered a sign of early loosening due to suboptimal implantation.

Computer-Assisted Robotic THA

To achieve the greatest possible bone-implant contact a new planning and surgical system was developed by Integrated Surgical Systems (ISS) in Sacramento in 1987 (Hap Paul). The goal was to be able to perform exact pre-

operative planning and subsequent intra-operative execution. The system consists of two components:
- Orthodoc: preoperative planning workstation
- ROBODOC: computer-controlled robot

Using CT-slices the proximal femur and the femoral condyles are analyzed. The CT-slices provide information on bone density. The Orthodoc is constructed similarly to CAD systems that are used to plan 3D bodies.

Preoperative Planning

Pin Implantation (1994–1998)

To be able to perform a robot-assisted surgery it was necessary to implant pins in an additional surgery. The pins should be implanted in the greatest possible distance to get exact data on the femur. They were implanted in the greater trochanter, the medial and lateral femoral condyle. After pin-implantation the CT scan was performed.

Pinless Procedure*

The pinless procedure is a major advantage. No additional surgery is needed. During surgery the femoral cavity is prepared before the acetabulum. A digitizer collects 3 points at the distal femur and 14 points at the femoral neck (surface matching). A 3D surface model is created that is matched with the preoperative 3D model (CT scan). If the matching is successful the robot starts milling the femoral cavity. The cutting is shown on a control screen and can be stopped by the surgeon at any time.

CT Scan

The patient is positioned in the CT-scanner. An aluminium rod is attached to the leg to detect bone motion during the CT-Scan.

---

* Since 1998, only ROBODOC, not in the CASPAR system

The scan starts with 3 mm slices at the femoral head until the lesser trochanter (except in the pin areas where there are used 2 mm slices). Below the lesser trochanter 6 mm slices are sufficient. The slices are created in a manner that the whole implant area can be seen. In the area of the femoral condyles 2 mm slices are used again. The data is transferred to the Orthodoc workstation.

Orthodoc Planning

The scan data is checked by Orthodoc. Bone motion during the CT scan is also checked using the aluminium rod. If bone motion is beyond a certain tolerance the scan has to be repeated. If pins were used the Orthodoc also checks the pin position.

Selection and Planning of the Implant

Orthodoc shows a 3D view of the bone in the following aspects: a.-p., lateral and cross-section (similar to CAD technology in engineering). The fourth view is a 3D view. Moving the bone in one view automatically moves the other views as well. Each view can be defined as the active view. The view can be rotated and moved in any direction. The precision is 0.1° and 0.1 mm. Details can be seen in three different views. A magnification of details is possible in all views. Different implant types can be selected from an implant library. Basically any implant can be used. Implants with a good proximal fixation seem to be of advantage. The correct alignment of the femur is important.

Straight-stem type of implants seem to be ideal for robot-assisted THR as the manual implantation is mostly performed with rotating instruments which allows an easy software creation for the robot.

The implant can be moved and rotated in any direction, the precision is 0.1° and 0.1 mm. To get a better view of the femur for planning the bone density is shown in different colors. The implant can also be shown transparent with green lines at the interface.

The implant is planned in a manner that as little as possible cortical bone is sacrificed and that there is the greatest possible contact between the implant and cortical bone.

The center of the femoral head and the implant head should be identical. To adapt the leg length the center can

18

be moved proximally or distally. A great advantage is the possibility to correct pathologic anteversion by comparing it to the opposite joint.

The planning data is stored on a CD-ROM and loaded into the ROBODOC control unit. A special short-stem implant was developed by us for exclusive use with ROBODOC. The rotational and translational stability of that implant was higher than comparable straight stem implants. This was shown doing an FEA and biomechanical testings with Professor Noble in Houston.

Intraoperative Execution by ROBODOC

Before the surgery the robot has to be calibrated. After that it is draped and sterile tools are attached. The surgery is performed in the conventional manner: The patient is positioned on the OR table, a standard antero-lateral approach is used. The cup is implanted manually, the size was planned on the Orthodoc. The patient's leg is positioned on a special leg holder, the robot is moved to the OR table and connected to the patient with a special proximal leg holder. The registration algorithm is started, if pins are used the robot registers the two pins and their angles. When the pinless system is used points are collected. The data is matched with the CT-data. After successful registration the cutter and the irrigation system are installed.

The robot starts milling out the femoral cavity, the progress can be seen on the control screen. The milling process lasts between 12 and 18 min depending on type and size of the implant. After the cutting is finished the robot is moved away from the OR table, the pins (if any) are removed and the planned implant is inserted by the surgeon manually. The implant head with the planned neck length is attached, the implant is reduced and the exposure is closed by the surgeon.

Since 1994 more than 5000 patients have been operated on using the ROBODOC system at BGU Frankfurt. In all cases the planned implant could be used. There was no intra-operative fracture or fissure of the femur. An optimal press-fit could be achieved in all cases. Ever since the first 30 cases we have allowed the patients full weight bearing immediately.

In 20% of our patients ROBODOC THA was performed on both hips. In these cases we were able to measure the position of the already implanted prostheses. There was no deviation from the preoperative planning. We used the greater and lesser trochanters and the femoral condyles as landmarks. This way we were able to measure the implant position in all 3 dimensions.

The radiologic positioning of the femoral implant was the same as in the preoperative planning. The average bone-implant contact was 96%. In 67.5% the primary diagnosis was osteoarthritis, dysplasia in 15.5%. The OR time went down from 210 min to 90–100 min average. Shorter cutting times should be possible in the future.

Our follow-up (3, 6 12 and 24 months postoperative) have shown that there was no case of subsidence in spite of immediate full-weight bearing. Since the introduction of the pinless system there was no more postoperative knee pain (that had been caused by the distal pin(s)).

The results of 4000 ROBODOC THAs are shown in ◘ Table 18-1. A follow-up (2001) of the patients operated on in 1994/1995 (443 patients, 94.4%) showed only one case of septic loosening 2.5 years after primary implantation. No other case of early loosening was seen (◘ Table 18-2).

◘ Table 18-1. Results of 4000 ROBODOC THAs

Complications	%
Infections	0.84
Nerve lesions	1.9
Muscular deficiency	1.7
Fracture/fissure	0.0
DVT	1.6

◘ Table 18-2. ROBODOC surgeries November 1994 until December 1995 (n=433), follow up 2001

Complications	%	n
Periprothetic fracture	0.0	0
intraoperative fracture/fissure	0.0	0
Vessel damage	0.0	0
Aseptic losening	0.0	0
Infections	0.2	1
Postoperative bleeding	0.2	1
Sunsidence 1–3 mm	0.4	2
DVT	1.8	8
Dislocation	2.3	10
Muscular deficiency	2.8	12
Nerve lesions	3.2	14

Conclusion

Robot-assisted THA can be performed without unforeseeable risks for the patient. The use of Orthodoc in preoperative planning is a revolution. The robot guarantees the precise execution of the preoperative planning. Femoral fractures can be avoided. The OR time is longer but acceptable. ROBODOC is a dependable technology that can be used by a trained surgeon without the presence of an engineer.

The introduction of the pinless system in 1998 was an important step as it saves cost and an additional surgery. Since the end of 2001 we have been testing the ROBONAV system. This system combines a robot and a navigation system, and as a synergy the advantages of both systems are combined and at the same time the disadvantages are eliminated.

The use of a specially designed implant – the Life Quality Hip – was started at BGU in May 2002 and presently we perform a clinical study on the new implant. The OR time is greatly reduced while at the same time soft tissue and bone is saved and the implant shows the greatest possible stability.

By January 2002 more than 5000 patients had been operated on using the ROBODOC system. All this shows the great importance of surgical robotics for the future.

Overview of the Advantages of Robot-Assisted Surgery at BGU Frankfurt

- Optimal preoperative planning and execution by the robot (precision: $0.1°, 0.1$ mm)
- Greatly increased bone-Implant contact: 95–98% robot/35% manually
- Pinless procedure: no additional surgery
- High primary stability, immediate full-weight bearing
- Successful osteointegration
- No fractures or fissures intraoperatively
- Modular implant system, individual planning and combination for each patient
- No increased rate of infections, muscular deficiencies, nerve or vessel lesions
- Revision surgeries save healthy bone and soft tissue
- Exposure not greater than in conventional method
- OR time increased by about 20 min compared to conventional method

After 5000 patients operated on with ROBODOC with THA and TKA and constant improvements in surgical technique we can say: There are no robot-specific complications.

References

1. Bargar WL, Bauer A, Boerner M (1998) Primary and revision total hip replacement using the ROBODOC system. Clin Orthop 354:82–91
2. Bargar WL, Bauer A, DiGioia A, Turner R, Taylor JK, McCarthy J, Mears D (1999) ROBODOC clinical trial status. Center for Orthopaedic Research, http://www.cor.ssh.edu/projects/robodoc/status.html.
3. Bauer A, Boerner M, Lahmer A (1997) Tierstudie: Roboterassistierte vs. handgeraspelte Endoprothese. Langenbecks Arch Chir I (Forumband 1997):465–469
4. Boerner M, Wiesel U (1999) Einsatz computerunterstützter Verfahren in der Unfallchirurgie. Trauma Berufskrank 1:85–90
5. Börner M, Bauer A, Lahmer A (1997) Computerunterstützter Robotereinsatz in der Hüftendoprothetik. Unfallchirurg 100:640–645
6. Börner M, Bauer A, Lahmer A (1997) Rechnerunterstützter Robotereinsatz in der Hüftendoprothetik. Orthopäde 26:251–257
7. Boerner M, Wiesel U, Lahmer A (2000) European experience with an operative robot for revision total hip. Proc Hip Society Meeting, Orlando, FL, March 18th, p 44
8. Cain P, Kazanzides P, Zuhars J, Mittelstadt B, Paul H (1993) Safety considerations in a surgical robot. ISA Paper #93–035:291–294
9. DiGioia AM (1998) What is computer-assisted and image guided orthopaedic surgery? Clin Orthop 354:2–4
10. DiGioia AM, Colgan BD (1997) Robotics, image guidance, and computer assisted orthopaedic surgery. Proc Second Annual North American Program on Computer-Assisted Orthopaedic Surgery (CAOS/USA), pp 35–49
11. Jerosch J, v. Hasselbach C, Filler T, Peuker E, Rahgozar M, Lahmer A (1998) Qualitätssteigerung in der präoperativen Planung und intraoperativen Umsetzung durch die Verwendung von computerassistierten Systemen und Operationsrobotern – eine experimentelle Untersuchung. Chirurg 69:973–976
12. Kazanzides P, Mittelstadt B, Musits B et al. (1995) An integrated system for cementless hip replacement: robotics and medical imaging technology enhance precision surgery. IEEE Engineering in Medicine and Biology, May/June:307–313
13. Lahmer A, Boerner M, Bauer A (1997) Experiences with an image directed workstation (Orthodoc) for cementless hip replacement. Proc 11th International Symposium and Exhibition on Computer Assisted Radiology and Surgery (CAR'97), pp 939–943
14. Lahmer A, Bauer A, Hollmann G, Börner M (1998) Is there a difference between the planning and the real position of the shaft 300 days after a robot assisted total hip replacement? Proc 12th International Sym-

posium and Exhibition on Computer Assisted Radiology and Surgery (CAR '98), pp 694–698

15. Mittelstadt BD, Kazanzides P, Zuhars J, Williamson B, Cain P, Smith F, Bargar W (1994) The evolution of a surgical robot from prototype to human clinical use. Proc First International Symposium on Medical Robotics and Computer Assisted Surgery 1, Pittsburgh, pp 36–41

16. Mittelstadt B, Paul H, Kazanzides P et al. (1993) Development of a surgical robot for cementless total hip replacement. Robotica 11: 553–560

17. von Loewenich C, Wiesel U, Stuhler T, Müller A (2001) Perioperative Komplikationen bei Primärimplantationen von Hüftendoprothesen-Vergleich von manuellen mit ROBODOC-assistierten Implantationen. Deutscher Orthopädenkongress Berlin, 2001, Z. Orthop 139 (2001) p 59

18. Wiesel U, Lahmer A, Boerner M, Skibbe H (1999) ROBODOC at Berufsgenossenschaftliche Unfallklinik Frankfurt (BGU) – Experiences with the pinless system. CAS 6: 342

19. Wiesel U, Lahmer A, Börner M, Skibbe H (1999) Robodoc at Berufsgenossenschaftliche Unfallklinik Frankfurt (BGU) – Experiences with the Pinless System.« Third Annual Program on Computer Assisted Orthopaedic Surgery (CAOS/USA '99), Pittsburgh, PA, pp 113–117

20. Wiesel U, Lahmer A, Tenbusch M, Boerner M (2000) Comparison of hand-broached vs. robot-assisted total hip replacement. Proc CAOS/USA, Pittsburgh 2000, pp 171–172

21. Wiesel U, Boerner M (2001) Does medical robotics influence the implant design in THR? CAOS España 2001, Marbella

19 Minimally Invasive Total Hip Replacement – Applicaton of Intra-operative Navigation and Robotics

F. Kerschbaumer, S. Kuenzler, J. Wahrburg

The classical extensive approach to the hip joint used for total hip alloarthroplasty usually gives the surgeon a good view and orientation. On the other hand, patients prefer minimally invasive operations. This applies also to total hip replacement surgery. The advantages of a minimally invasive surgical technique are accompanied with higher demands to the surgeon because the limited field of view makes spatial orientation difficult. To compensate the surgeon's limited three-dimensional coordination and to ensure an optimal spatial orientation of the implants, intraoperative navigation and mechatronic instruments like robots are useful.

Minimally Invasive Approach to the Hip Joint

The patient is to be positioned strictly on the side with supports at the os sacrum and symphysis. The unaffected leg is fixed about 40 degrees bent on the operation table.

The skin incision of about 7,5 cm (just large enough to extract the femoral head and insert the implants) is made behind the trochanter major (Fig. 19-1). The incision of the fascia lata and the m. gluteus maximus is done in the direction of fibres. For better exposure, a spreader that was originally developed for spinal surgery is inserted (Figs. 19-2 and 19-3). After that, a bent Hohmann retractor is inserted underneath the tendon of the m. glutaeus medius. The short external rotating muscles are transsected. The leg is internally rotated and the femoral head dislocated. The next step is the osteotomy of the collum ossis femoris and removal of the femoral head. A bent retractor is inserted at the anterior border of the acetabulum and a second retractor behind the ligamentum

transversum. The caput reflexum of the m. rectus femoris is transsected and the femoral shaft is levered forward

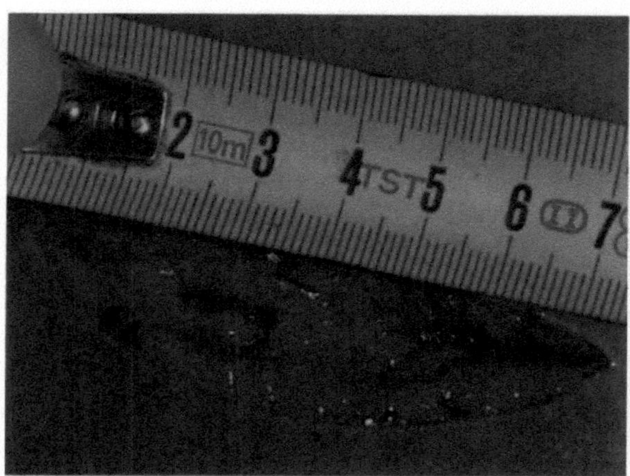

Fig. 19-1. Skin incision for total hip replacement surgery

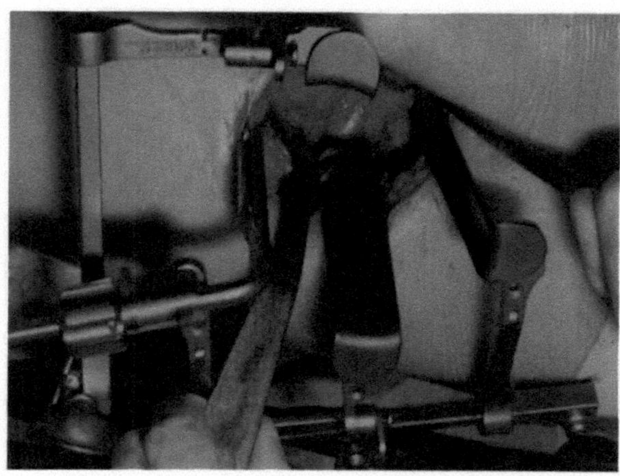

Fig. 19-2. Arrangement of retractors for the minimally invasive approach

19

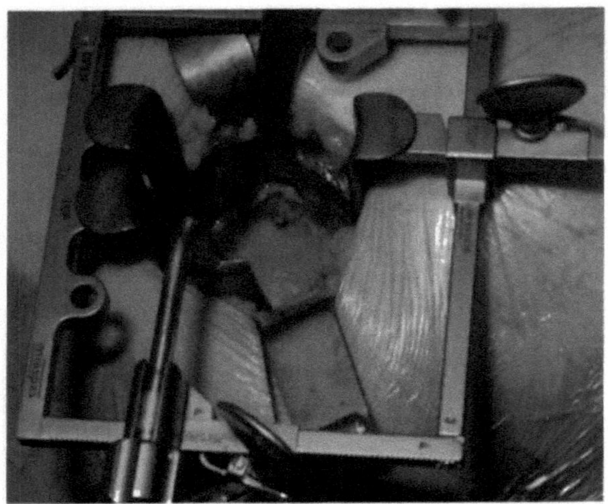

◘ Fig. 19-3. View on the acetabulum after resection of the femoral head

to get a good view of the acetabulum. Now the operating table may be tilted towards the surgeon to provide a better view, but has to be reset into horizontal position during the reaming procedure. After the preparation of the acetabulum and the removal of osteophytes the bed for the acetabular implant may be reamed and the cup component implanted.

For the next step, a bent retractor is positioned underneath the gluteal muscles at the trochanter major and the m. glutaeus medius retracted. Now the tip of the trochanter is fenestrated with a box chisel. After broaching, the

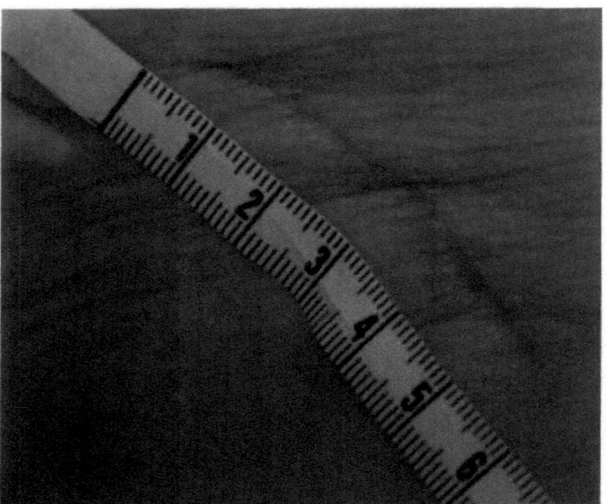

◘ Fig. 19-4. Scar one year after total hip replacement surgery

trial stem with a head of appropriate length attached can be inserted. After reduction, control of implant stability and range of motion the definitive stem can be implanted. The control of leg length is done by palpation of the kneecaps. The capsule is refixed to affect proprioception as little as possible. The detached rotators can be refixed with bone-anchors.

A clinical investigation with patients one year postoperative (◘ Fig. 19-4) was accomplished with two groups of 28 patients each using matched pairs for the variables diagnosis, gender, type of implant, age. Investigative device was the hip score described by Johnston et al. [1].

The descriptive statistics, based on the average values, showed less pain, less consumption of analgetics, less limping and less intraoperative blood loss in the minimally invasive group.

Requirements

We think that congruence between the reamed bed and the acetabular implant is a precondition for a good primary and secondary stability of the acetabular implant. Our own investigations on artificial bones and animal bones show that manual reaming does usually not produce a satisfying congruence. The continuous monitoring und display of the position of manually guided instruments with the aid of intraoperative navigation systems offers a good help to improve the spatial positioning and orientation during the preparation of the bony bed and the positioning of the implant. Nevertheless, it cannot be avoided that during the preparation of the bony bed the instrument starts to vibrate or is deflected by zones of different resistance, which results in a geometric deviation of the reamed bony bed. The use of robotic systems may offer advantages. However, the commercially available systems are not configurable for minimally invasive surgical technique and they do not support the acetabular component in total hip replacement at all.

To use computer- and robotic-assisted surgical techniques with the highest advantage and to achieve a broad acceptance of these methods, some objectives have to be accomplished:

— High precision and reproducibility of the intervention. It has to be ensured that intraoperatively the implant is placed at exactly the desired spatial position and with the spatial orientation that has been planned by the surgeon.

- A simple and quick handling of the system, which does not prolong the procedure.
- A modular concept, which offers different and adaptable solutions both for planning and intraoperative performance.
- No significant disadvantages compared to manual surgery.
- Planning and performance of surgery should be documented.
- New, less invasive surgical techniques should be used.

Concept

The commercially available surgical robots and surgical navigation systems do not conform to the requirements stated above. Since 1996 we have been working on a concept, which tries to avoid the disadvantages and deficiencies of the systems that are currently in use [2, 5, 6].

The basic idea is to combine an optical three-dimensional localizing system that is the core component of commercially available surgical navigation systems and a robot as an integrated system (◘ Fig. 19-5). This combination enables us to utilize the specific advantages of both systems:

The localizing system measures the position of styli, tools and reference bodies, which are equipped with light emitting diodes or reflective balls. It does not have its own drives and therefore it is classified as a passive system. Its advantage is that through the manually guided stylus the surgeon can register points, edges and surfaces of bony structures very quickly. Because it is a passive system, there are no problems with safety and no elaborate precautions have to be taken, in contrast to using a robot for registration.

The advantages of the robot are its ability to move a tool exactly along a given trajectory or to hold the tool at a calculated position. This precision cannot be reached with manual tool handling, even when there is a continuous feedback of spatial position and orientation.

Components

The system idea has led to the design of a modular interactive system. It consists of the following components, which can be added one to the other and thus allow different stages of expansion:

- A newly developed planning system. It allows pre- and intraoperative planning of the intervention using CT- or X-ray data and can be used as a stand-alone system (◘ Fig. 19-6) [7].

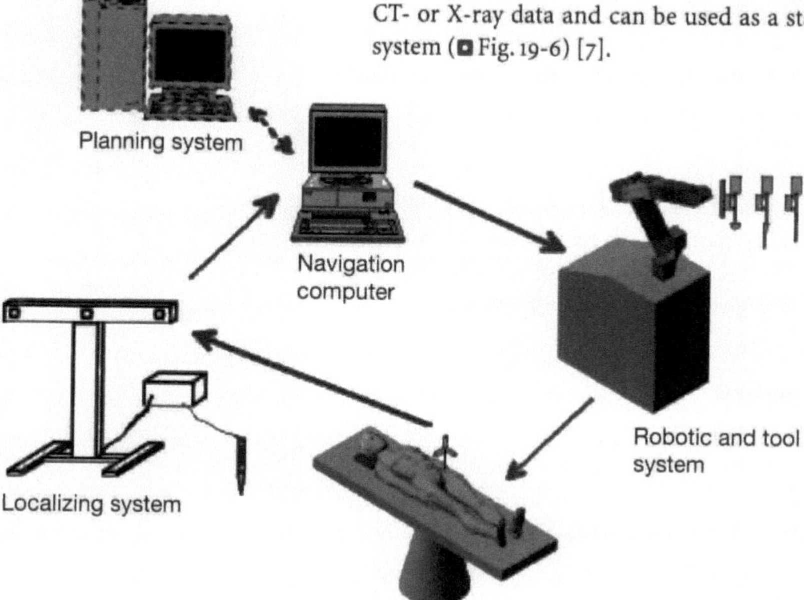

◘ **Fig. 19-5.** Components of the system

19

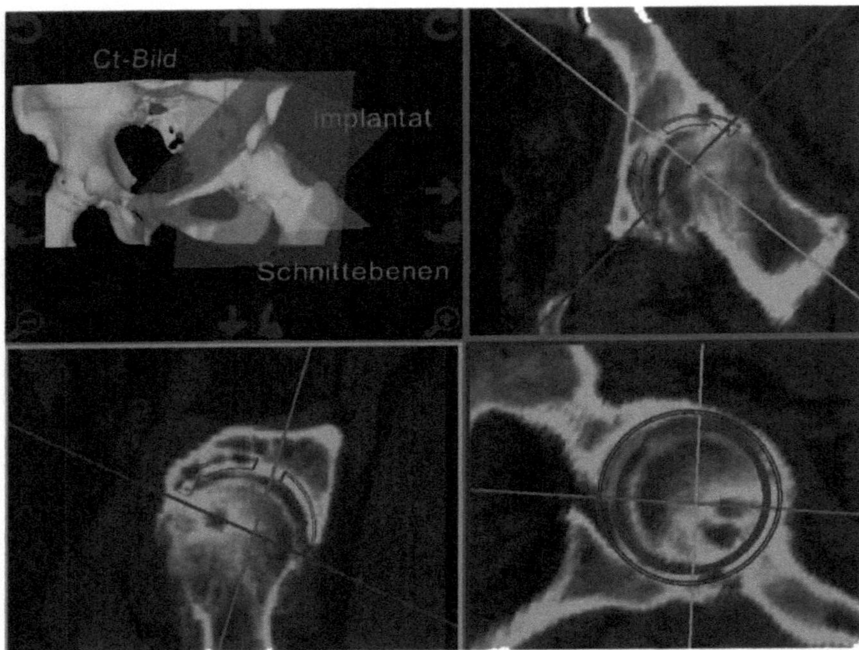

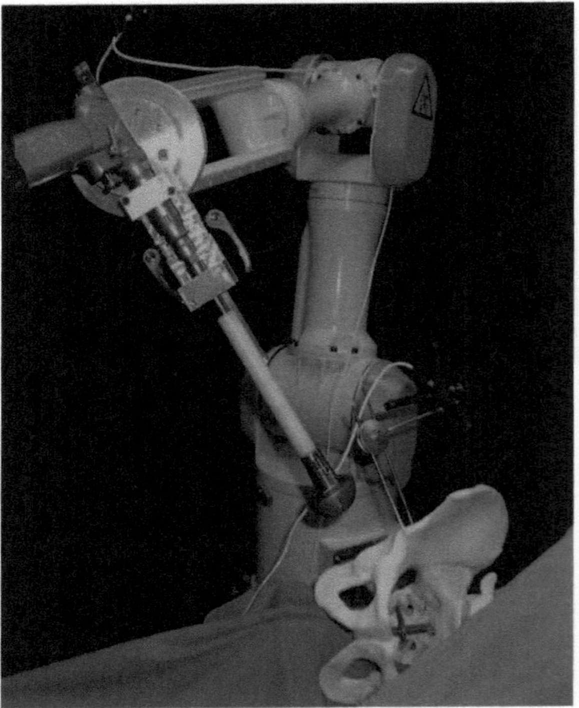

Fig. 19-6. Positioning of the acetabular implant using the planning system

- An optical three-dimensional localizing system with partly passive and partly active position markers. Equipped with software modules for intraoperative registration and matching it can be used as a surgical navigation system.
- A slender robotic arm on a small mobile base frame. This robot may, completely covered with sterile draping, be positioned very close to the operating table and the surgeon (**Fig. 19-7**). Combination with the other two modules creates a navigated intraoperative robotic system [9].
- A modular tool system. The diverse tools will be attached to the flange of the robotic arm. This concept allows the adaptation to other surgical fields by developing specially adapted tools (**Fig. 19-8**) [8].

Functionality

The planning system offers universal planning tools and allows the surgeon the virtual planning and documentation of an intervention. Possible data sources can be X-ray images, CT- or MRI datasets. It is also possible to guide a surgical intervention without any preoperative imaging

Fig. 19-7. Positioning of the acetabular implant using the planning system

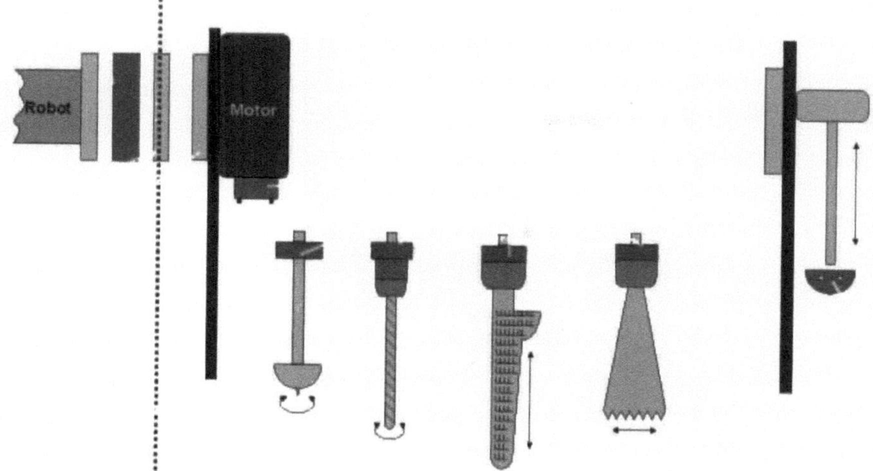

◘ Fig. 19-8. Modular tool system

using only intraoperatively recorded spatial points. The planning system has been developed from scratch because the existing solutions do not offer freely configurable interfaces, which are needed for communication with the navigation system and the robotic arm.

For the registration of bone motion a reference body with infrared light emitting diodes, which is called dynamic reference base (DRB), is firmly attached to the bone during surgery. In the case of hip surgery, this will be the pelvic bone or the femur. The DRB is tracked by the localizing system and the exact position and spatial orientation of the bone relative to the surgical tools can be continuously calculated by the system. The position of the robotic arm will be continuously corrected in adaptation to the dislocation of the bone so that the relative position remains unchanged. This is done in real time and does not prolong surgery. By the use of this technique, it is no longer necessary to create a rigid connection between the base of the robot and the bone of the patient. In this way, minimally invasive surgery is supported and accelerated.

Use of Robotics in Total Hip Replacement

Our concept makes use of conventional or only slightly modified surgical tools. These tools are attached to a linear carriage, which is positioned by the robotic arm in an exactly planned position relative to the bone. This position is controlled and corrected in real time in case the patient moves. The machining of the bone is done by pushing the surgical tool manually forward. The direction of infeed is precisely limited by the linear carriage, which is positioned by the robotic arm. The infeed is done by the surgeon manually under direct visual and haptic control. The manual infeed of the slider is limited by a femoral bedstop, in order to prevent too deep intrusion of the surgical tool.

On the linear carriage, it is also possible to attach components supporting the implantation of the acetabular component and tools supporting the implantation of the femoral component, drills and saws. In this way, the system will be able to support the whole procedure of THA.

Clinical Use

The first clinical use of the system is the implantation of the cementless spherical acetabular components in total hip arthroplasty (◘ Fig. 19-9). Preliminary results of the current clinical trial are encouraging but must be controlled further. The quality of the reamed cavity and the spatial positioning and orientation of the implant are. The prolongation of surgery does not exceed 15 min compared to conventional total hip replacement surgery.

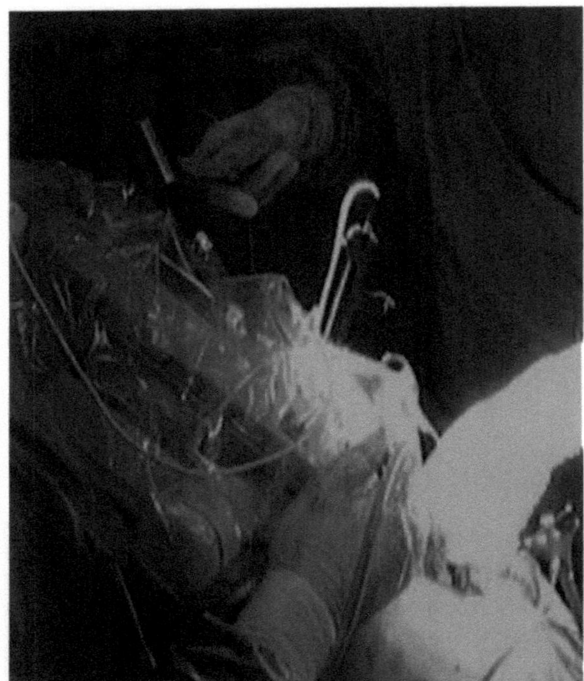

Fig. 19-9. Clinical use

Advantages

The described concept offers, in our opinion, the following advantages:

- The manual infeeding of the tool gives the surgeon a feedback of the applied force the possibility to interfere at anytime.
- The possibility to control the bone machining directly gives the surgeon a better control of position and orientation of the tool and the possibility to change the position, rotation frequency and deepness of the reamer if necessary.
- The system can be used for the acetabular and the femoral component in total hip alloarthroplasty.
- The system is adaptable to different surgical techniques, including minimally invasive approaches.
- Possible patient movements are continuously monitored and corrected in real-time. In this way, a rigid fixation of the patient or the bones is not necessary.

- The duration of robot-assisted THR will, after the necessary learning curve, not be longer than that of conventional THR.

Future Applications

The future fields of application of the described concept will be knee replacement surgery, spinal surgery and corrective osteotomies.

References

1. Johnston RC, Fitzgerald RH, Harris WH, Poss R, Müller ME, Sledge CB (1990) Clinical and radiographic evaluation of THR. J Bone Joint Surg Am 72: 161–168
2. Kerschbaumer F, Wahrburg J, Kuenzler S (2001) A mechatronic system for the implantation of the acetabular component in total hip alloarthroplasty. In: Niessen WJ, Viergever MA (eds) Medical image computing and computer-assisted intervention – MICCAI 2001. Lecture Notes in Computer Science, vol 2208. Springer, Berlin Heidelberg New York Tokyo, pp 1433–1434
3. Knappe P, Gross I, Pieck S, Kuenzler S, Kerschbaumer F, Wahrburg J (2002) Design of an interactive navigated robot for surgical interventions. In: Troccaz J, Merloz P (eds) Surgetica 2002, Computer-aided medical interventions: tools and applications. Sauramps Medical, France, pp 83–89
4. Kuenzler S, Knappe P, Gross I, Pieck S, Wahrburg J, Kerschbaumer F (2002) Evaluation of a new navigated robot system for minimally invasive total hip alloarthroplasty. In: Troccaz J, Merloz P (eds) Surgetica 2002, Computer-aided medical interventions: tools and applications. Sauramps Medical, France, pp 345–348
5. Wahrburg J, Kerschbaumer F (1998) Using robots to increase the accuracy of surgical interventions. Proceeding of the 24th Conference of the IEEE Industrial Electronics Society (IECON '98), Aachen, Germany, 31st Aug – 4th Sept 1998, pp 2512–2516
6. Wahrburg J, Kerschbaumer F (2000) Überlegungen zum Einsatz mechatronischer Implantationshilfen bei Minimalzugängen für Hüftendoprothesen. Orthopäde 29: 650–657
7. Wahrburg J, Gross I (2000) Computer-assisted planning for total hip replacement procedures based on multiple 2D images. Computer Assisted Orthopaedic Surgery Meeting CAOS/USA 2001, Pittsburgh, USA
8. Wahrburg J, Knappe P (2000) A modular mechatronic tool-system for robot assisted surgical interventions. IEEE International Conference on Mechatronics and Machine Vision in Practice M2VIP 2001. Hong Kong, China
9. Wahrburg J, Pieck S, Kerschbaumer F (2002) A navigated robot system to assist in orthopaedic interventions. In: Hoffmann K-H, Keeve E (eds) Computer aided medicine. Proceedings of the Third Caesarium held November 12–13, 2001 in Bonn, Germany. Springer, Berlin Heidelberg New York Tokyo

20 Cement Removal with the *ROBODOC* System in Total Hip Arthroplasty Stem – Revision

M. Nogler, M. Krismer

In the case of aseptic or septic loosening of a cemented femoral component in a total hip arthroplasty (THA), the old stem, including the complete cement has to be removed [5]. After removal of the prosthesis, which usually can be performed without any problems, two distinct portions of cement remain in the cavity (◻ Fig. 20-1). In the area of the prosthesis usually a relatively thin layer of cement can be found. Underneath the tip of the prosthesis a solid cement plug remains. The removal of proximal parts of the cement mantle is easy whereas distal mantle parts and the cement plug often constitute more complex problems.

For cement removal different procedures have been propagated. Mechanical tools such as chisels, drills and hooks are in use in order to remove the cement through the proximal opening of the femur. Such procedures are performed under C-arm control, yet the risk to perforate or fracture the femur remains high. Extended surgical approaches and distal fenestration [2, 7, 9, 14] in the are of the cement plug have been propagated as well as controlled perforation [18] or a transfemoral approach [13]. Beside mechanical solutions ultrasound removal systems [4, 6, 20], laser [16, 21] and extra corporal shock waves (ESWT) have been studied [8, 15, 17].

The ROBODOC system (ISS, Integrated Surgical Systems, Davis, CA) has modules for primary total knee and hip arthroplasties. In addition to that, a module for cement removal in revision THA is available. First clinical experiences with this system have been reported [1, 2, 19]. Like in primary total hip arthroplasties the system is based on computer tomographic scans of the operated hip. For the revision module two fiducial markers, two screws (pins) are required. These pins have to be implanted into the greater trochanter and the medial femoral condyle (anterolateral approach) or the lateral femoral condyle (posterior approach) in a surgery prior to the revision. Data from the CT scan are transferred into the Orthodoc planning station. After assuring that no motion had occurred during the scan, the screws are detected semi-automatically in the CT dataset. Due to artefacts from prosthesis metal, it is usually necessary to separate the smaller proximal screw manually. After pin recognition (◻ Fig. 20–2) the orientation of the femur is calculated from screw positions.

Consequently, the planning of the cutting path is performed on the Orthodoc planning station. First the cutting tool has to be chosen. Currently a 22 cm cylindrical cutter with a diameter of 12,5 mm is available. This tool is visualized in the CT dataset and can be used for the planning. The tool itself confounds the minimal cutting

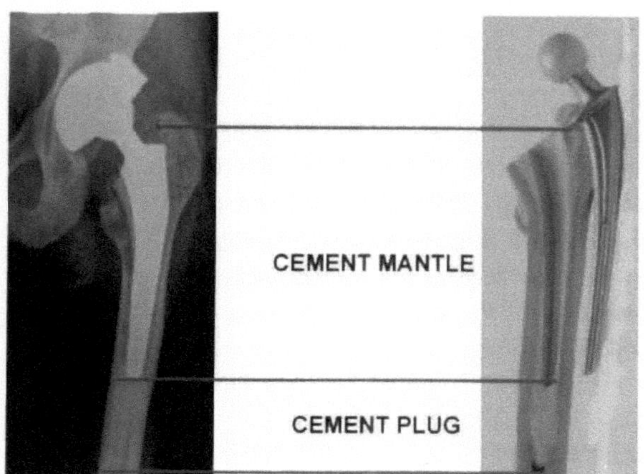

◻ **Fig. 20-1.** In the area of the prosthesis a cement mantle remains after it's removal. Underneath the tip of the prosthesis a solid cement plug can be found

20

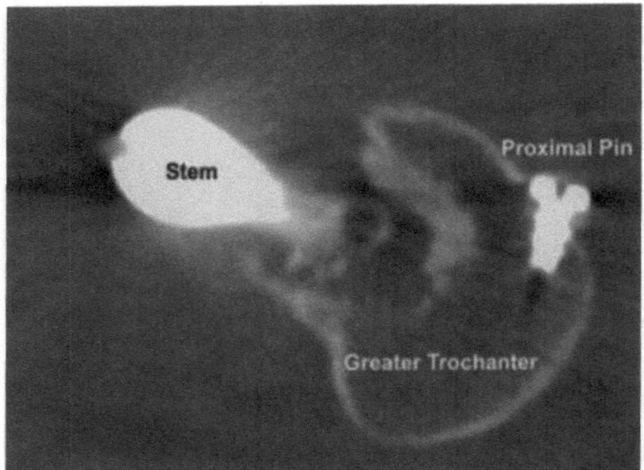

◘ Fig. 20-2. Proximal pin (screw) implanted into the greater trochanter in a prior surgery

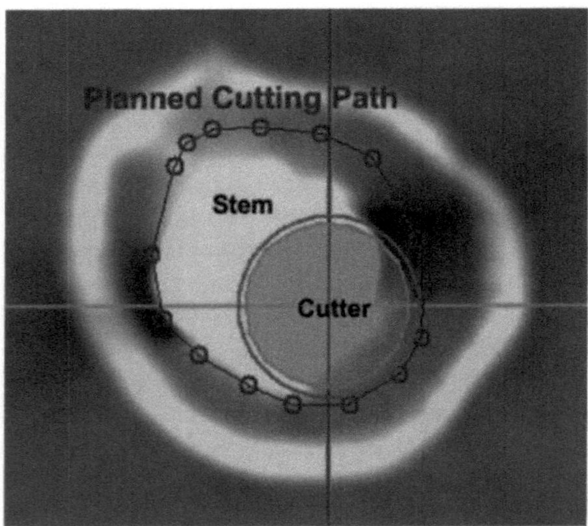

◘ Fig. 20-3. Planning of the cutting path around the cutting tool on a cross section. The pictures shows total extinction in the axis of the prosthesis

path. In different cross-sections the exact cutting path can be defined (◘ Fig. 20-3). The user has to draw lines around the planned cutting area on each section. He has to define the cement-bone interface, which can be invisible in some areas due to total extinction caused by metal artefacts from the prosthesis in place. We always decide in favor of preserving bone stock and accept, that little islands of cement remain.

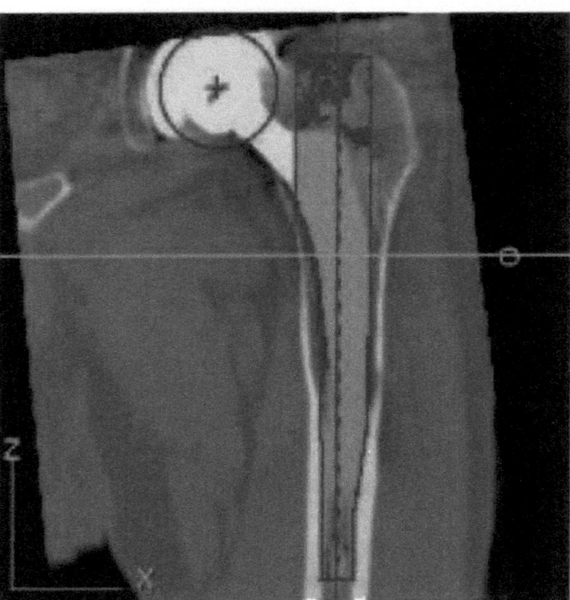

◘ Fig. 20-4. Final cutting path based on the planning

If a sufficient number of planes (a minimum of 8 is necessary) has been sequenced, the computer is able to calculate a cut cavity by interpolating, all remaining areas between the planes. In several steps the cutting path has to be checked and if necessary to be adjusted until the desired shape of the cavity has been reached. After the final cutting path has been calculated (◘ Fig. 20-4) it is stored on a tape which is used to transfer data to the operating room.

A version of the ROBODOC revision module for the anterolateral approach to the hip with the patient in a supine position is available as well as one for the posterior approach with the patient lying on the side. After exposing the femur and extracting the old stem, the leg has to be fixated rigidly to the table. Usually this is easier achieved in the posterior approach with the leg falling onto the table than in the supine position in which an additional fixation platform has to be attached to the table in order to support the patient's leg. After fixation the robot is moved to the table and docked to the femur. The system's bone clamp has to be attached to the proximal femur. If bone stock is poor and the clamp cannot be attached directly to the bone, it has turned out to be useful to support the bone with a metal mesh placed between bone and clamp.

In the next step the orientation of the femur in space is detected based on the position of the two screws. In order to do so first the distal screw is probed (medial in the anterolateral approach, lateral in the posterior approach). After that the robot arm with the ball probe has to be positioned at the proximal screw and automatically probes this screw, too. Due to the usually poor bone stock in the proximal area of the femur the cement mantle should remain during this step in order to support the bone.

After calculating the orientation of the femur the ball probe can be removed and the cutter is installed to the robot arm. The cutting procedure is performed with constant irrigation through an integrated irrigation system. In our own studies we could show that high temperatures are possible during cutting, especially in the distal part [10]. The use of a high-flow irrigation system is recommended. In addition to that, irrigation assures the rinsing off the cavity from cement debris, which could block the cutter. Also with regard to irrigation and cooling the dorsal approach seems to be superior to the anterolateral approach. In the latter the femur is directed upwards. Therefore, irrigation solution has to be pumped upwards, whereas in the posterior approach the femur is directed downwards and the fluid can follow gravity. In this case with sufficient flow only the fluid surplus has to be collected. In any case, aerosol generated during the use of high-speed cutters in wet areas, especially in infected patients has to be minimized [12].

The cutter is equipped with a force sensor, which stops the cutter, if high forces occur. While the cutting procedure in the proximal mantle area usually can easily be performed, such stops commonly occur in the area of the cement plug. Useful methods to avoid such stops are:
- changing the cutter before the cement plug area,
- slowing down cutting speed to 50% (25%),
- sufficient and constant irrigation.

During the cutting progress of the cutter is visualized on screen. Afterward the cutting the robot is removed from the patient and the table. An inspection of the femoral cavity usually reveals some remaining cement islands, areas which were invisible during the planning in the CT-dataset due to metal artefacts. They never extend over the whole circumference of the cavity. Therefore, it is easy to remove them with hooks and chisels. A smooth cement-free femoral cavity remains (■ Fig. 20-5).

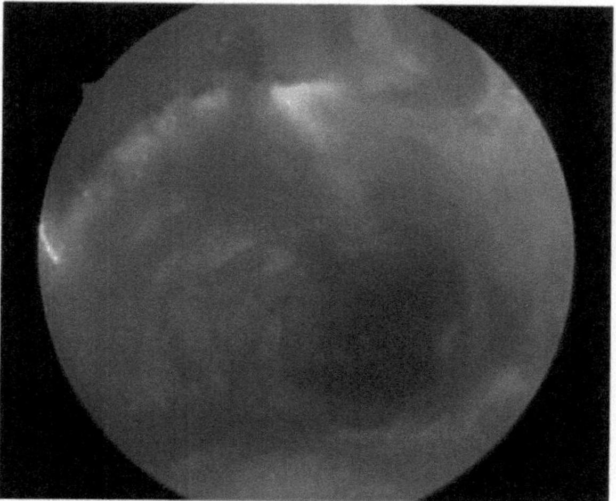

■ **Fig. 20-5.** Smooth cement-free femoral cavity

Areas of Further Development

Tool Length

The length of the cutter is currently restricted to 22 cm. Only cement to that depth can be removed. The cutting path starts at the most proximal point of the greater trochanter. In the case of an only 15 cm long prosthesis usually the tool is just long enough to reach to the bottom of the cement. The polyethylene cement plug often cannot be reached. Yet, in our experience, this plug can easily be removed under arthroscopic view.

Cutting Path

Currently only a straight cutting path is implemented in the system. The cutter remains in the primarily defined angle of entrance. Angulations of the tool are not possible. This results in sometimes severe bone loss at the greater trochanter in order to reach the most distal points in the cutting path. This effect is aggravated by the antecurverture of the femur (see Fig. 20-4). During planning a compromise between an optimal cutting path and preservation of bone stock has to be made.

Pin Implantation

For primary THA a pinless registration module is available. The pinless procedure is based on surface matching at the femoral neck. As the neck is not existing in a revision, the pinless procedure cannot be used. Pin implantation in an additional surgery is an additional morbidity for the patient and causes additional costs. Patients also have reported long lasting, severe pain at the medial femoral condyle [11].

Conclusion

In our experience it is possible to remove cement from the femoral cavity totally and safely with the ROBODOC system. The procedure is demanding. Yet, it is possible to save time, if the cement could otherwise only be removed through extended approaches or complex osteotomies. By the use of the system it is certainly possible to reduce the extension of the surgical approach. Using the system, there is a learning curve for the whole team. Due to our experience, it is possible to reduce the robot utilization time in complex THA revisions to below one hour. The use of the system is limited in cases of extremely poor bone stock, which either make it impossible to place the pins or the fixation clamp cannot be supported.

Overall, cement removal in cemented THA is a rather rare procedure. The use of the ROBODOC revision system seems to be recommended where the robot is already in use for primary arthroplasties or in specialized orthopaedic centers with sufficient numbers of cases.

References

1. Bargar WL, Bauer A, Börner M (1998) Primary and revision total hip replacement using the Robodoc system. Clin Orthop 354: 82–91
2. Boerner M, Bauer A, Lahmer A (1997) Computer-assisted robotics in hip endoprosthesis implantation. Unfallchirurg 100: 640–645
3. Buehler KO, Walker RH (1998) Polymethylmethacrylate removal from the femur using a crescentic window technique. Orthopedics 21: 697–700
4. Caillouette JT, Gorab RS, Klapper RC, Anzel SH (1991) Revision arthroplasty facilitated by ultrasonic tool cement removal. Part I: In vitro evaluation. Orthop Rev 20: 353–357
5. Dennis DA, Dingman CA, Meglan DA, O'Leary JF, Mallory TH, Berme N (1987) Femoral cement removal in revision total hip arthroplasty. A biomechanical analysis. Clin Orthop 142–147
6. Klapper RC, Caillouette JT, Callaghan JJ, Hozack WJ (1992) Ultrasonic technology in revision joint arthroplasty. Clin Orthop 147–154
7. Klein AH, Rubash HE (1993) Femoral windows in revision total hip arthroplasty. Clin Orthop 164–170
8. May TC, Krause WR, Preslar AJ, Smith MJ, Beaudoin AJ, Cardea JA (1990) Use of high-energy shock wave s for bone cement removal. J Arthroplasty 5: 19–27
9. Moreland JR, Marder R, Anspach WE Jr (1986) The window technique for the removal of broken femoral stems in total hip replacement. Clin Orthop 245–249
10. Nogler M, Krismer M, Haid C, Ogon M, Bach C, Wimmer C (2001) Excessive heat generation during cutting of cement in the Robodoc hip-revision procedure. Acta Orthop Scand 72: 595–599
11. Nogler M, Maurer H, Wimmer C, Gegenhuber C, Bach C, Krismer M (2001) Knee pain caused by a fiducial marker in the medial femoral condyle: a clinical and anatomic study of 20 cases. Acta Orthop Scand 72: 477–480
12. Nogler M, Wimmer C, Lass-Florl C, Mayr E, Trobos S, Gegenhuber C (2001) Contamination risk of the surgical team through ROBODOC's high-speed cutter. Clin Orthop 225–231
13. Rinaldi E, Vaienti E (1992) The trans-femoral approach in prosthesis replacements: results after two years. Acta Biomed Ateneo Parmense 63: 79-83
14. Savvidis E, Loer F (1989) Surgical technique in femur shaft fenestration within the scope of revision operations following hip joint total endoprostheses. Z Orthop Ihre Grenzgeb 127: 228–236
15. Schreurs BW, Bierkens AF, Huiskes R, Hendrikx AJ, Slooff TJ (1991) The effect of the extracorporeal shock wave lithotriptor on bone cement. J Biomed Mater Res 25: 157–164
16. Sherk HH, Lane G, Rhodes A, Black J (1995) Carbon dioxide laser removal of polymethylmethacrylate. Clin Orthop z: 67–71
17. Stranne SK, Callaghan JJ, Cocks FH, Weinerth JL, Seaber AV, Myers BS (1993) Would revision arthroplasty be facilitated by extracorporeal shock wave lithotripsy? An evaluation including whole bone strength in dogs. Clin Orthop 252–258
18. Sydney SV, Mallory TH (1990) Controlled perforation. A safe method of cement removal from the femoral canal. Clin Orthop 168–172
19. Taylor RH, Joskowicz L, Williamson B et al. (1999) Computer-integrated revision total hip replacement surgery: concept and preliminary results. Med Image Anal 3: 301–319
20. Yaffey MA (1968) Ultrasonic cement removal. JPO J Pract Orthod 2: 418.
21. Zimmer M, Klobl R, De Toma G et al. (1992) Bone-cement removal with the excimer laser in revision arthroplasty. Arch Orthop Trauma Surg 112: 15–17

21 Advantages of Custom-Made Stems Using Adaptiva Components

G. Gruber

Introduction

The first custom-made stem was implanted by Aldinger in Tuebingen, Germany, in 1987. Based on these experiences the third generation cementless Adaptiva stem design was developed by Prof. Kusswetter in Tuebingen. In contrary to older round stem designs the new custom-made stem has a square cross-section and three metaphyseal fins and consists of Titanium-Aluminum-Vanadium alloy ($TiAl_6V$). With this fit without fill design high primary and rotational stability is warranted within the femoral shaft. When stems are implanted without cement, a funnel shape stem and a rotationally stable design of the stem are required for optimal results. Both factors lead to a primary stable stem implantation, since loosening of the stem appears to occur within that proximal Gruen zone 1.

Martini et al. [20] have shown a 5% decrease in bone density in 27 cases after 21.2 months follow-up. The press-fit principle achieves primary stability as according to Wolff's law. Lewis et al. [18] confirmed the principle of primary stability in an infinite element analysis. Two principle conditions are required: primary stability in the contact zone immediately after implantation and a maximum contact area at the rough bone-prosthesis interface (◘ Fig. 21-1).

A high degree of primary stability and rotational security are necessary demands for stable and long-term secondary osseointegration of the implant. Götze et al. [13] showed in a comparative biomechanical study on 18 cadavers a five fold improved stability (reversible test) of the Adaptiva stem compared with other commonly used stems in Germany. New bone formation is dependent on

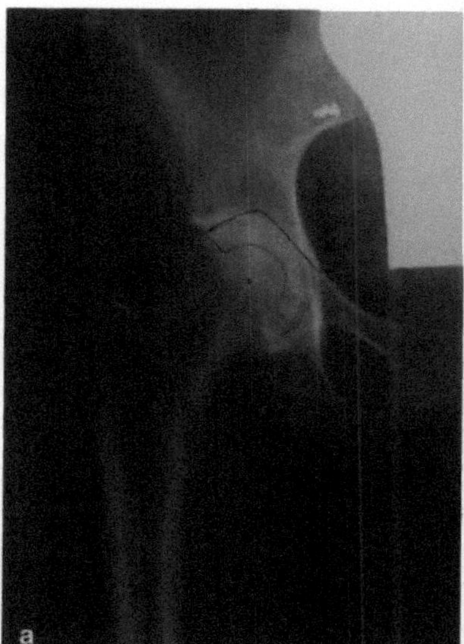
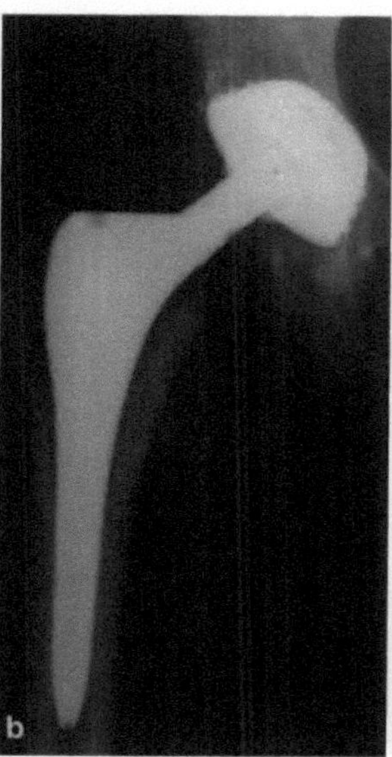
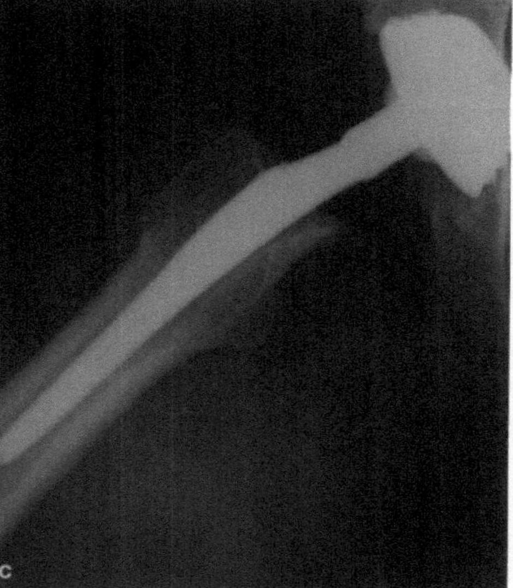

◘ **Fig. 21-1a-c.** 57-year old patient with primary hip OA right side: preoperative radiographs, pelvis a.-p. **(a)**, and post-operative pelvis and hip views **(b,c)**

the porosity, the interface contact, and stem fit with the living host bone. Osseointegration is decreased when the interfacial space is too large and in cases with increased stem motion. The following factors increase the likelihood of osseointegration:

- correct axes of implantation,
- primary and rotational stability,
- large interface contact area,
- Titanium alloys as a biologically inert metal,
- stem surface enlargement with a porosity of 3–5 μ,
- physiologic stress patterns.

Planning and Manufacturing of the Custom-Made Prosthesis, Logistics

Plane radiographs of the pelvis, the hip joint and a 3D-CT scans of the femur are raw data for planning stem size and position on a monitor in cooperation with a surgeon and an engineer. Further helpful parameter for developing the stem are bone size, femoral neck angle and anteversion, offset, rotational hip center, leg length, and position of the acetabular cup. The Adaptiva stem and the accompanying rasp are custom-made and the finally manufactured via CT data stored on a tape. Implant and rasp sizes are principally identical, although the stem has a smooth surface, but the rasp a rough toothed surface for femoral preparation. The Adaptiva stem is manufactured to fitting the femur in comparison to robotics, where the femur is reamed to fit the stem. Hence, the individual femur is the model for the manufactured stem and rasp. Planning and manufacturing of the final stem and rasp take about 3 to 4 weeks. This time window allows perfectly for patients' own blood sampling without wasting time. Therefore, Adaptiva stems are not applicable for femoral neck fracture cases.

Indications, Relative Indications and Contra-Indications

The Adaptiva custom-made stem is not a designed prosthesis for anatomical variances, but an optimal cementless implant for routine and individual total hip replacement of both primary and secondary hip arthritis cases. Therefore, the indication equals all hip patients warranting cementless THA.

Indications for Adaptiva Stem System

- Primary coxarthrosis
- Secondary coxarthrosis
- Posttraumatic coxarthrosis
- Postarthritic/postinfectious coxarthrosis
- Dysplastic coxarthrosis
- OA due to M. Legg-Calvé-Perthes
- OA due to slipped upper epiphyseolysis capitis femoris
- AVN
- Coxarthrosis in rheumatoid arthritis
- Coxarthrosis secondary to hyperuricaemia
- Coxarthrosis secondary to psoriasis

Advantages of the Adaptiva custom-made hip stem include individual and perfect anatomical fit.

Advantages of Adaptiva Stem System

- Perfect fit due to individual anatomical stem
- Stem is formed to anatomy, not vice versa
- High-contact area at the implant-bone interface
- High-primary stability
- High-rotational stability
- Early mobilization
- No additional surgery time

Relative indications include patients with osteoporosis, high intake of alcohol and nicotine, or other drug abuse, since these risk factors are now to decreasing osseointegration of cementless components in THA. There is, however, no scientifically defined age limit for not using cementless stems. As a rule of thumb we consider 70 years of age or older as a relative indication (□ Figs. 21-2 and 21-3).

Surgical Technique and Clinical Experience

Surgery is performed in supine or lateral position with a routine standard approach. After resection of the femoral neck and cup implantation the proximal femur is

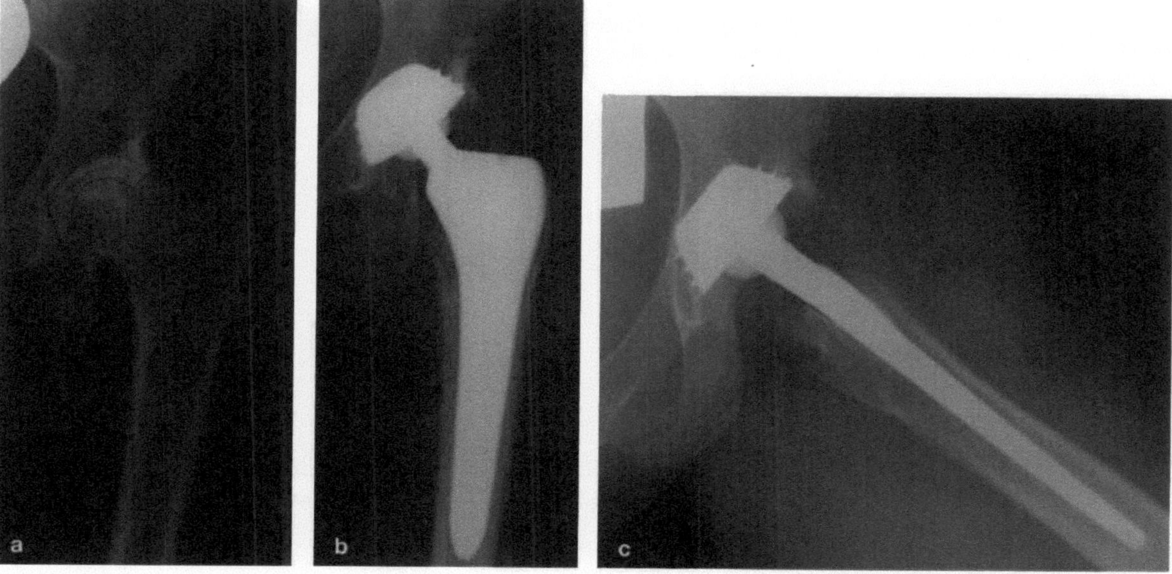

▣ Fig. 21-2a-c. 63-year old patient with primary hip OA left: preoperative radiographs, pelvis a.-p. (**a**), and postoperative pelvis and hip views (**b, c**)

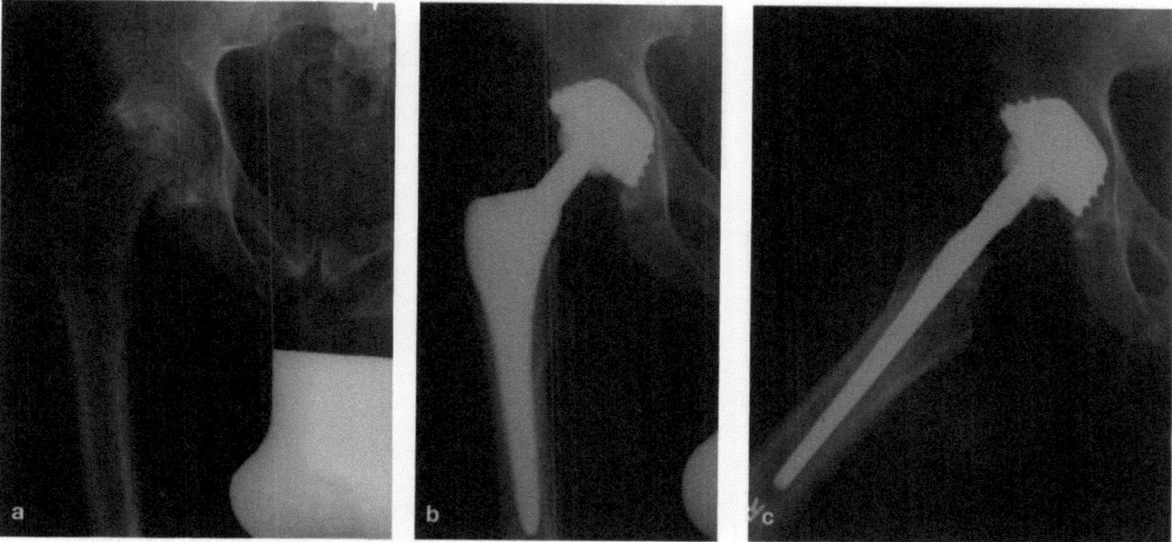

▣ Fig. 21-3a-c. 55 year old man with secondary hip OA right: preoperative radiographs, pelvis a.-p. (**a**), and postoperative pelvis and hip views (**b** and **c**)

reamed with standard-rasps with increasing sizes until the final custom-made rasp can be used. Any cup can be combined, however, we recommend a cementless version. According to CAD planning the surgeon is provided with the following reference parameter:
- height of neck resection,
- angle and anteversion of implantation,
- depth of implantation,
- maximal size of conventional rasp.

Over 1000 Adaptiva stems have been implanted in Germany since 1993. Hartwig and Reize [16] reported a mean follow-up of 6 years in 68 cases. No stem loosening was encountered in that time frame. In another series Reize et

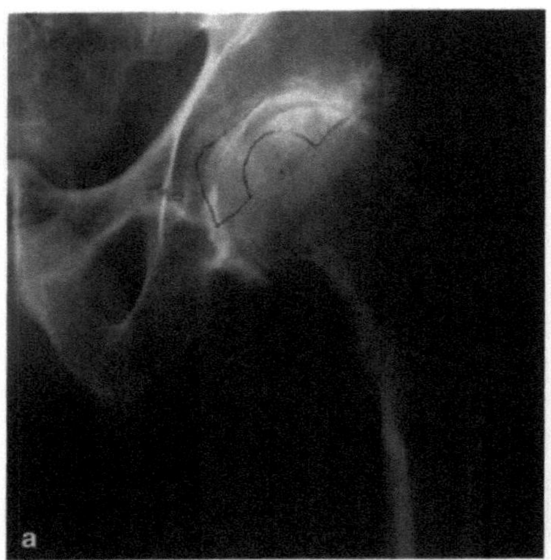
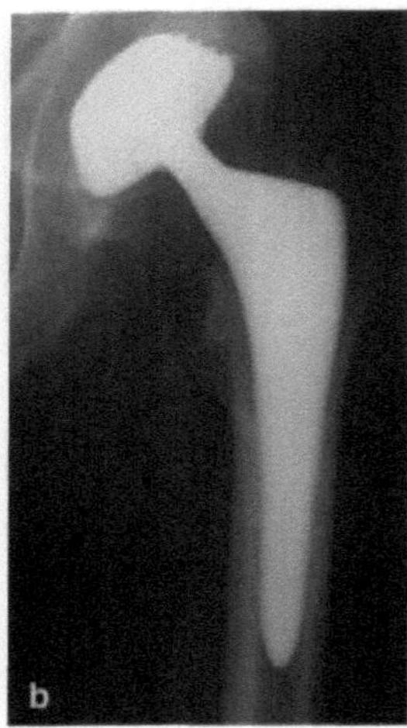
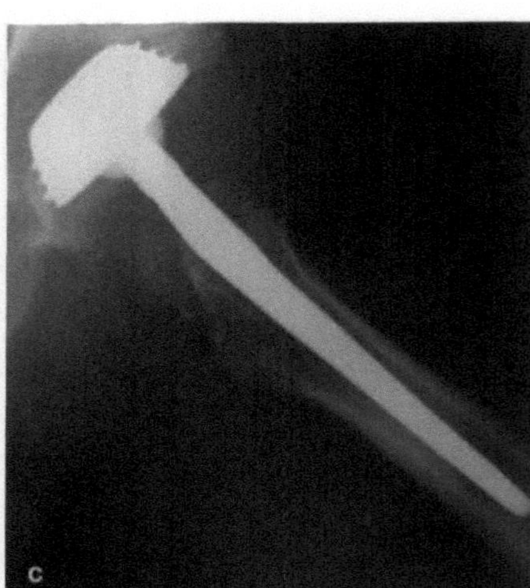

■ **Fig. 21-4a-c.** 63 year old patient with hip OA left: preoperative radiographs, pelvis a.-p. (**a**), and postoperative pelvis and hip views (**b** and **c**)

al. [23] report of 95% excellent results in 177 cases after 65 months without radiographic signs of loosening or radiolucent lines or stem migration around the stem. In an own series of 101 Adaptiva stems with a follow-up of 1.5 years the following complications were observed: One THA dislocation, one neurological complication, and three femoral fissures, but none required revision (■ Fig. 21-4).

The Adaptiva custom-made stem represents a future concept in primary THA of secondary coxarthritis. Both routine and difficult anatomical hips are suitable for this system. During planning of the stem cup parameters such as rotational hip center, offset, and antetorsion angle can be optimized. Navigation of this stem is part of the planning process and is currently tested. Short and long-term data available today are encouraging, however, long-term data over 10 years have yet to prove the success of this new implant.

We believe that the patient has a considerable benefit of a potentially long lasting custom-made stem because of factors including individuality of the component, optimal press-fit and primary stability providing sound biomechanics for secure secondary osseointegration.

References

1. Albrektsson T, Albrektsson B (1987) Osseointegration of bone implants. Acta Orthop Scand 58: 567

2. Albrektsson T, Brånemark P-I, Hansson H-A, Lindstrom J (1981) Osseointegrated titanium implants. Acta Orthop Scand 52: 155

3. Aldinger G, Fischer A, Kurtz B (1983) Computer-assisted manufacturing of individual endoprostheses (Preliminary report). Arch Orthop Traumat Surg 102: 31

4. Aldinger G, Kurtz B (1984) Fortschritte in der Endoprothetik durch die Computertomographie? Fortschr Röntgenstr 141: 509–511

5. Bargar WL (1989) Shape the implant to the patient. Clin Orthop 249: 73–78

6. Brånemark P-I, Breine U, Adell R, hansson BO, Lindstöm J, Ohlsson A (1969) Intra-osseous anchorage of dental prostheses. Scand J Plast Reconstr Surg 3: 81–100

7. Brånemark P-I, Aspegren K, Breine U (1964) Micricirculatory studies in man by high resolution vital microscopy. Angiology 15: 329–332

8. Breine U, Adell R, Hansson BO, Lindstöm J, Ohlsson A (1969) Intra-osseous anchorage of dental prostheses. Scand J Plast Reconstr Surg 3: 81–100

9. Brudet J (1989) Ergebnisse des operativen Gelenkersatzes mit dem zementfreien Hüftendoprothesen-System Spotorno-Weill (CLS-CLW). Eine mittelfristige Verlaufskontrolle an 100 CLS-CLW-Prothesen. Inaugural-Dissertation, Fachbereich Humanmedizin der Justus-Liebig-Universität Gießen

10. Callaghan JJ, Fulghum Ch S, Glisson RR, Stranne S (1992) The effect of femoral stem geometry on interface motion in uncemented porous-coated total hip prostheses. J Bone Joint Surg 4-A: 839–848

11. Carlsson L, Röstlund T, Albrektsson B, Albrektsson T (1988) Implant fixation improved by close fit: Cylindrical implant-bone interface studied in rabbits. Acta Orthop Scand 59: 272

12. Gekeler J (1985) Bemerkungen zur Form und Größe des zweymüller-Hüftendoprothesenschaftes. In: Spranger M, Eder H (Hrsg) Zementfreie Hüft-Endoprothesen-Systeme. Huber, Bern Stuttgart Toronto, S 33–38

13. Götze C, Steens W, Vieth V, Poremba C, Claes LE, Steinbeck J (2002) Primary stability in cementless femoral stems: custom made versus conventional femoral prosthesis. Clinical Biomechanics (in press)

14. Gruber G (1999) Knöchernes Einwachsverhalten von Titan-Hohlschaft-Implantaten im Femur. Eine tierexperimentelle und klinische Unter-

suchung. Habilitationsschrift, Fachbereich Humanmedizin der Justus-Liebig-Universität Gießen

15. Gruber G (2002) Die Adaptiva-Hüftendoprothese – ein robotergefräster Individualschaft. In: Konermann W, Haaker R (Hrsg) Navigation und Robotic in der Gelenk- und Wirbelsäulenchirurgie. Springer, Berlin Heidelberg New York, Tokyo, S 173–177

16. Hartwig CH, Reize P (2001) Die Adaptiva-Individualprothese – Eine Alternative zur robotergestützten Implantation von Hüftendoprothesen. Z Orthop 139: A093

17. Kienapfel H (1994) Grundlagen der zementfreien Endoprothetik. Demeter, Gräfelfing

18. Lewis JL, Nicola T, Keer LM, Clech JP, Steege JW, Wixson RL (1985) Failure processes at the cancellous bone-PMMA interface. 31. Annual ORS., p 144

19. Martini F (2001) Wertigkeit osteodensitometrischer Messungen unter besonderer Berücksichtigung des Verlaufs der periprothetischen Knochendichte der Individualprothesen Evolution-K und Adaptiva in Korrelation zur kortikalen Anlagefläche. Habilitationsschrift, Medizinische Fakultät der Eberhard-Karls-Universität zu Tübingen

20. Martini F, Sell S, Kremling E, Küsswetter W (1996) Determination of periprosthetic bone density with the DEXA method after implantation of custom-made uncemented femoral stems. International Orthopaedics (SICOT) 20: 218–221

21. Mittelmeier H (1974) Zementlose Verankerung von Endoprothesen nach dem Tragrippenprinzip. Z Orthop 112: 27

22. Morscher EW (1987a) Die Entwicklung zementfreier Endoprothesen unter besonderer Berücksichtigung der Oberflächenbeschaffenheit und des Elastizitätsverhaltens. In: Refior HJ (Hrsg) Zementfreie Implantation von Hüftgelenksendoprothesen – Standortbestimmung und Tendenzen. Thieme Stuttgart New York, S 17–26

23. Reize P, Giehl J, Martini F, Hoch S (2002) Die Adaptiva-Individualschaftprothese: Erfüllen die 5-Jahres-Ergebnisse die hohen Erwartungen? JBJS (in press)

24. Ungethüm M, Blömer W (1987) Technologie der zementlosen Hüftendoprothetik. Orthopäde 16: 170–183

22 Computer-Assisted Designed Hip Arthroplasty

J.-N. Argenson, X. Flecher, J.-M. Aubaniac

Introduction

The recent general use of computering technology in the operating room to assist the surgeon during the surgery corresponds to the achievement of a global concept which starts at the time of the stem conception, or at the time of computerized pre-operative planning in case of individual stem solution.

The purpose of this chapter is to describe the elements which will lead to the use of computer-assisted hip arthroplasty according to the ten years experience obtained in computer-assisted pre-operative planning of total hip arthroplasty and computer-assisted designed of custom hip stem.

The Concept of Computer-Assisted Hip Arthroplasty

The concept of individual computer-assisted design (CAD) has been the consequence of the natural evolution of the authors in the field of total hip arthroplasty (THA), facing the unacceptable failure rate of conventional stems as reported in the literature for young and active patients [10–15, 17, 25, 32, 34, 35].

The cementless fixation presented as an alternative to cement fixation has gained a global acceptance on the acetabular side but is still facing some controversies on the femoral side partly due to the poor designs proposed in the early days of cementless stem fixation [23, 25].

Quickly, basic studies showed that successful fixation without the use of cement on the femoral side may be possible but requires some principles which include proximal adaptation and avoidance of micromovements in order to obtain an optimal load transmission to the bone [30]. These principles are advocated in order to avoid stress shielding and thigh pain, the two complications often reported with cementless stems [16, 26].

This adaptation to the proximal femur is only possible when the stem can match the patient femoral anatomy. Several anatomical studies have shown the wide range of proximal femoral anatomy faced in either conventional osteoarthritis or more frequently in congenital or traumatic etiology leading to a narrow, curved and excessively ante or retroverted upper femur [7, 28, 31].

The logic answer to the necessary adaptation to the proximal intra-medullary femur combined to the obligatory corrections in the prosthetic neck for solving extra-medullary deformities was CAD of individual stem geometry. In the author's perception the three-dimensional design of the neck is at least of equal importance than the intra-medullary part in order to restore a correct hip function.

The design of a three-dimensional custom neck allows correction in length, lever arm and anteversion. The clinical consequence of such design is the restoration of leg length, abductor function and proper lower limb rotation. The appropriate anteversion of the neck may also contribute to reduce dislocation rate. The mechanical consequence of such neck design is also to optimize load transmission to bone stem interface and finite element analysis have shown the influence of the extra-medullary parameters on the stem stability and stress transfer [29].

The intra-medullary stem design is a combination of CT-based reconstruction of the proximal femoral anatomy and priority areas of contact to obtain stability in rotation. The distal diameter of the stem is reduced to avoid any cortical impingement distally, possible source of thigh pain with maximal canal filling stems. It is thus of high importance to preserve all the cancellous bone around the whole stem from proximal to distal by the use of a smooth compactor of identical shape than the final prostheses.

This concept of computer-assisted hip arthroplasty leading to individual custom neck and stem design was addressed by Aubaniac and Essinger in 1987 and lead to the development of softwares for cancellous bone density evaluation and three-dimensional custom neck design, which is the rationale of the Symbios custom concept (Symbios Inc, Yverdon, Switzerland). The global concept of computerized preoperative planning and the first applications for osteoarthritis following high congenital dislocation of the hip have been originally published ten years ago [3–5].

The Computer-Assisted Planning of Total Hip Arthroplasty

Preoperative Data

X-Ray Data

The radiographic analysis is based on several X-ray views. A full view of the two limbs using scanography is needed to assess the global pelvis and limb anatomical status, and to evaluate the extent of disturbance of the pelvic balance by assessing bilaterally the position of the hip rotation centers (in the vertical axis). A frontal pelvis view is used to determine the extent of lever arms between the rotation centers and the corresponding femoral axes. Discrepancies are recorded and will be used later in the pre-operative planning to correct the anatomy of the diseased joint such that full restoration of the pelvic balance can be achieved. Finally, frontal and lateral X-ray views of the diseased joint are necessary to complete the X-ray data set.

CT Data

Data obtained from computerized tomography scanner are necessary both for the design of the intra-medullary femoral stem and for the planning of the extra-medullary part of the joint reconstruction. Except in special cases, the CT data acquisition must follow an established protocol elaborated by Symbios. However, in special cases such as for instance very severe congenital dislocations, the radiologist may have to select a modified protocol based on the X-ray status.

The intra-medullary femoral anatomy is assessed by CT views taken every 5 mm from the acetabular summit down to the bottom of the lesser trochanter, then every 10 mm until the femoral isthmus.

The extra-medullary planning requires CT views taken at three different levels:

1. at the base of the femoral neck (assessment of helitorsion axis),
2. at the knee level, across the femoral condyles (assessment of posterior bicondylar axis),
3. at the foot level, by the second metatarsus axis (assessment of foot axis).

Preoperative Planning

Acetabular Cup

If the contralateral hip is healthy, planning the rotation center of the replaced joint and the socket size is performed by reproducing the contralateral geometry on the X-ray frontal pelvis view (◘ Fig. 22-1). In presence of a bilateral lesion and in most high dislocation cases, the position of the rotation center and the size of the acetabular socket are decided together with the surgeon. In certain cases, the size is determined using the CT view passing through the center of the true acetabulum (which allows furthermore assessment of bone stock), then by reporting the result on the X-ray pelvic view.

According Position of the Femur

The future position of the femur (as determined for instance by the location of the greater trochanter) is determined on the frontal view based on the position of the acetabular socket, on the desired lengthening as determined from the scanogram, and on the neck lever arm (see Fig. 22-1). This position will determine the level of the femoral cut and assess the correct neck lever arm on the frontal view. However, osteotomy of the greater trochanter may be necessary in cases where extensive lengthening is required, associated to a wrong anteroposterior position of the greater trochanter due to excessive anteversion.

22

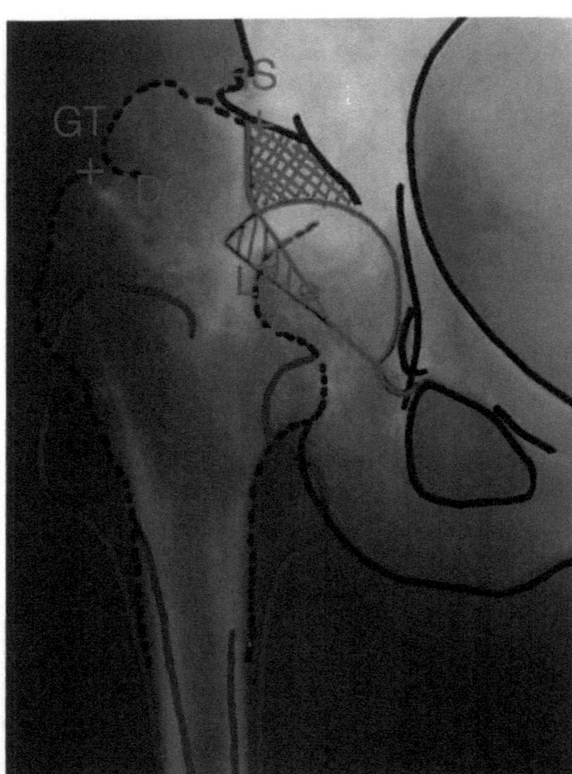

Fig. 22-1. Preoperative planning on the X-ray frontal view with anatomical landmark registration (*in red*), planning of the acetabular socket, and positioning of the greater trochanter

Neck Anteversion

The anteversion angle of the prosthesis neck must be set such that normal gait anatomy can be restored. The normal gait anatomy requires three conditions:

1. foot axis showing 10°–20° of external rotation,
2. posterior bicondylar axis perpendicular to the gait direction,
3. anteversion of the femoral neck between 15° and 20° with respect to the bicondylar axis (**Fig. 22-2**).

It has been shown that in most cases of congenital dysmorphism, the upper femur axis, also called helitorsion axis and defined as the axis passing across the longer diameter at the level of osteotomy, is not aligned with the neck axis [19]. This phenomenon is usually not taken into account in standard prostheses. This results in such cases most frequently in an over- or under-correction of the prosthetic anteversion angle, thus preventing from full

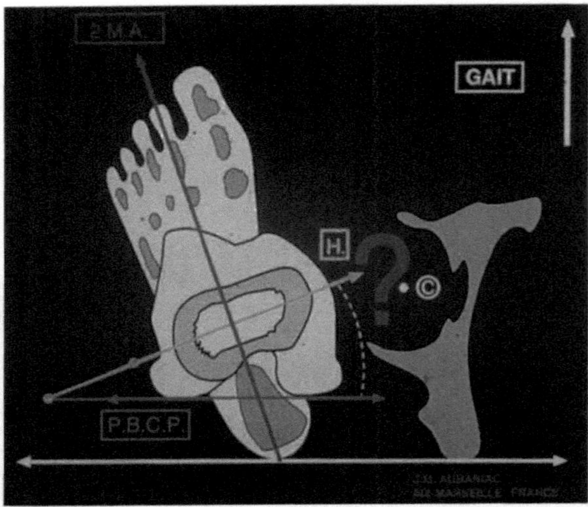

Fig. 22-2. Normal gait anatomy

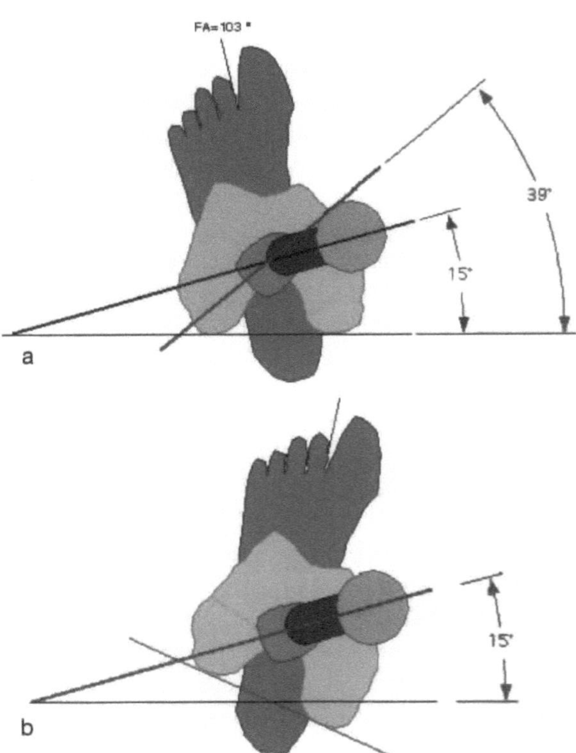

Fig. 22-3a, b. a Restoration of normal gait anatomy based on the correction of the helitorsion angle, **b** same case without this correction

restoration of the normal gait. By superimposing the three CT views of the osteotomy level (usually above the lesser trochanter), and of the knee and foot levels, it is possible to calculate the correction angle to add (or subtract) to the helitorsion angle such that a final prosthetic anteversion angle of 15°–20° is achieved. An example of such a correction is given in ◘ Fig. 22-3a, whereas ◘ Fig. 22-3b shows the same case without the correction for helitorsion.

The Computer-Assisted Design of Custom Hip Stem

The Design of the Intra-Medullary Section

Contouring

Upon their reception, raw CT data is processed by numerical thresholding such that non bony structures are excluded from the images. Following this »image filtering« step, the design engineer runs an image analysis program to select both the internal and external contours of the bone section on each femoral CT slice (◘ Fig. 22-4). This contouring process is normally performed fully automatically, except in the area of the femoral neck and in cases of important artefacts on CT images for which manual intervention is needed.

Matching CT and X-Ray Data

Anatomical landmarks on the diseased joint must be first registered. These landmarks will be used later for the definition of the osteotomy. The summits of the greater and lesser trochanters (GT and LT), the digital gap (DG) and the femoral head summit (HS) are localized and indicated on the X-ray frontal view (see Fig. 22-1).

The next step in the design process consists in superimposing the CT and X-ray data on the same image file. For this, frontal and lateral radiographic views of the diseased hip are first digitalized using an X-ray compatible image scanner. The contouring data obtained during the previous step is numerically added to the digitalized X-ray views. A manual fitting of the two types of images is then performed independently on the frontal and lateral view.

Definition of Osteotomy Orientation

Once merging of CT and X-ray data is completed, osteotomy directions are calculated and added to the image file. The level of the osteotomy is defined such that neck length, optimized stability in rotation and optimized bone stock preservation are taken into account.

Generation of the Initial Stem and Extraction

Based on the internal contouring data, the design software uses then numerical interpolation procedures to generate a first stem shape limited to the intra-medullary

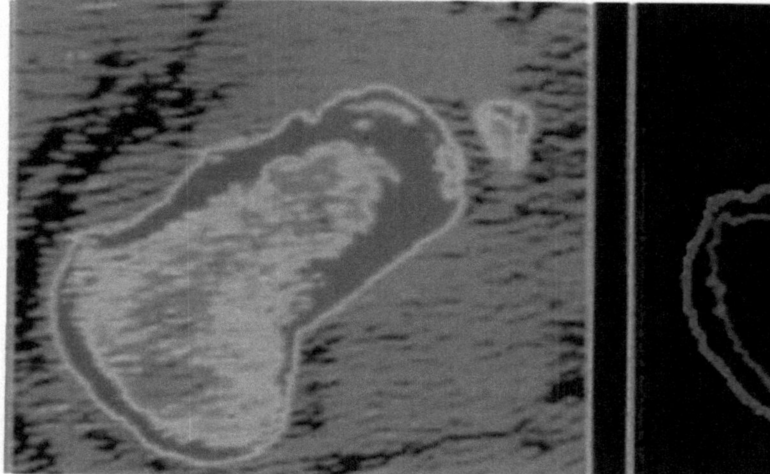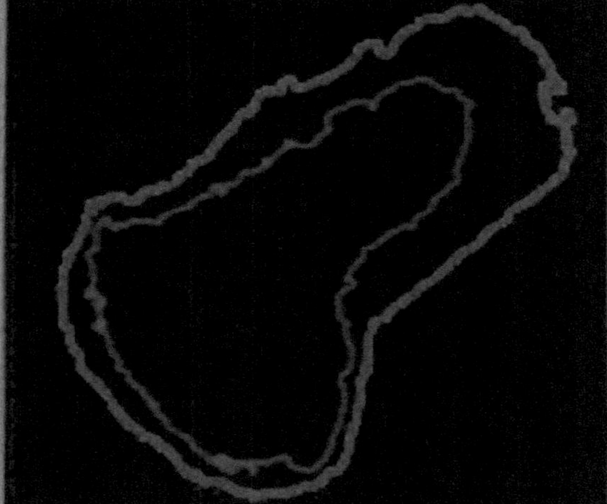

◘ **Fig. 22-4.** Extraction of internal and external femoral contours from CT data

zone. However, the very precise reproduction of the femoral internal contour on this first draft makes it most often useless without modifications, as local protrusions and depressions at the bone surface would prevent any movement of the stem within the femur. It is therefore necessary to simulate numerically the extraction of the stem from the femur. This is done by successive iteration steps during which the stem is extracted incrementally by rotations and translations in the three main orthogonal axes. During each iterative step, incremental stem shape modifications are performed by the software in order to allow the extraction while maintaining the contact zones necessary for an optimized mechanical support of the stem in the femur. Optimized support is sought in medial, lateral, and anterior metaphyseal areas. At the end of the simulation, a new, modified version of the stem is obtained that can be implanted into the femur with a very restricted degree of freedom for the insertion path.

Final Adaptations

At the end of the extraction process, numerical integration of the new stem shape in the CT data is performed. It enables the design engineer to view each CT section together with the corresponding stem section (»composite« view). By switching to the editor mode of the software, the engineer can also perform a final design »tune up«, during which he can still implement slight modifications on each stem section to further optimize bone-prosthesis adjustment.

Stem Insertion and Resistance Simulation

The final step in the design of the intra-medullary part of the femoral stem consists in simulating a subsidence of the stem in the femoral canal in order to be sure that the stem is at worst in contact with the cortical bone in this shifted position.

A numerical 3-point bending simulation test is then performed to validate the mechanical resistance of the stem.

The Design of the Extra-Medullary Section

The design of the extram-edullary part of the stem is performed as well in the frontal and lateral as in the sagittal plane. The determination of the anteversion angle of the prosthesis neck taking into account the correction for helitorsion, has already been explained earlier (see Fig. 22-3). With the intra-medullary stem integrated in the X-ray frontal view, the design engineer calculates the optimized combination of CCD angle, neck length and head offset such that the planned rotation center and lever arm are respected (see Fig. 22-5).

The Prosthesis Validation

The pre-operative planning of a custom made prosthesis is performed together by the surgeon and the design engineer at Symbios.

Following the planning, the design of the stem is done entirely by the design engineer. Therefore the final design must be validated by the surgeon before the fabrication of the prosthesis can be launched. A complete patient file is provided to the surgeon including the CT composite view, the normal gait restoration scheme (see Fig. 22-3a), and the X-ray frontal (with osteotomy parameters, ■ Fig. 22-5) and lateral view with the designed stem.

The Stem Manufacturing

Stem Machining

Upon validation of the stem design and pre-operative planning by the surgeon, the fabrication of the prosthesis can proceed. For this, the stem CAD data is transferred into a computer-assisted machining (CAM) software that pilots a 5-axis milling machine. In parallel, a compactor with a smooth surface is machined with the same design as the stem itself. It is used for compaction of the cancellous bone before the stem itself is introduced (■ Fig. 22-6).

Materials and Coatings

Wrought Ti6Al4V titanium alloy is used most of the time for the fabrication of the stem. In very few cases, stainless steel stems are produced upon request of the surgeon. The rasp itself is made out of wrought stainless steel. After machining, the prosthesis stem undergoes a surface plasma spray coating procedure which can vary from one

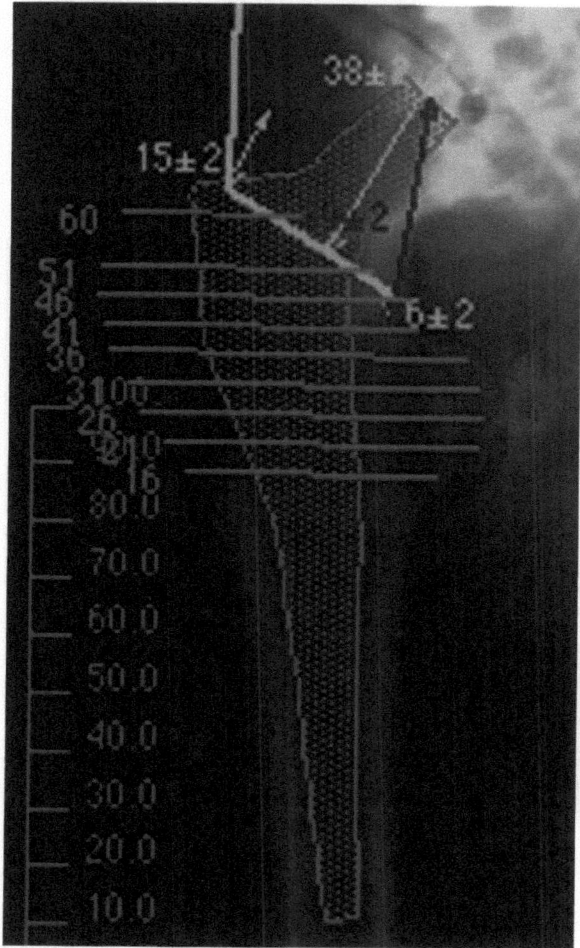

Fig. 22-5. Composite X-ray frontal view with integration of intra- and extra-medullary stem sections

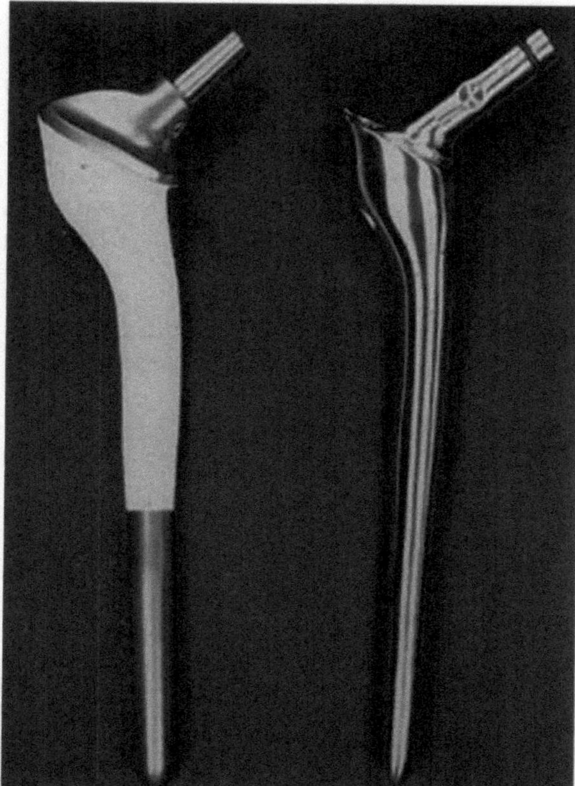

Fig. 22-6. Example of porous coated custom made prosthesis together with the corresponding »rasp« for compaction of cancellous bone and implant preparation

stem to the other, depending again on the surgeon's request. In most cases a first layer of ~300 μm of porous titanium followed by a ~80 μm layer of porous hydroxyapatite (HA) are coated on the intra-medullary section of the stem, from the osteotomy level down to the distal level at which the transition from an elliptic to a circular section takes place.

Sterilization and Packaging

The final steps in the production of the prosthesis are the gamma sterilization and the final packaging procedure which is performed in clean room conditions.

The Ten-Years Clinical Use of Individual CAD for Cementless Hip Arthroplasty

The Rationale for the Use of Custom CAD for Hip Arthroplasty

The self-preservation of the dense cancellous bone compacted towards the inner cortical femur is obtained by the use of a smooth compactor of identical intra and extra-medullary shape than the final prostheses. The preservation of this cancellous bone is mandatory for secondary biologic fixation to the hydroxyapatite (HA) covering the final prosthesis. Both the clinical and the radiological evaluation of different stem coatings lead us to move from a proximal HA to a full HA coating [6].

The solution provided by three-dimensional designed custom neck to face excessively anteverted upper femur often encountered in dysmorphic or dysplasic hips was a retroversion of the custom neck. to restore an appropriate anteversion of 15° to 20° on the knee condylar plane [2, 8]. In such situations some authors have described the association of a derotational osteotomy to a conventional stem or the use of modular necks [26].

The Authors Indications for Custom CAD in Cementless Hip Arthroplasty

The dysmorphic and dysplasic hips in which conditions of normal hip anatomy cannot be restored by a standard neck and a standard stem.

The young and active patients for whom full and quick recovery of hip function is required. In the future the increasing lifetime expectancy will emphasize this need of long standing solution for highly sollicited hips [24].

The Clinical Results of Computer-Assisted Designed Stems in THA

The experience of such concept of computer assisted planning and computer-assisted designed hip stems (Symbios, Yverdon, Switzerland) started clinically in January 1990.

We report on a group of 726 hips concerning only patients aged 65 years or less with a mean age group of 52 years (range 17–65 years). The mean weight was 72 kg (range 49–147). The etiologies included: osteoarthritis in 273 cases (38%), avascular necrosis in 101 cases (14%), congenital dislocation of the hip in 200 (18%) and dysmorphy in 152 hips (20%).

After a two to 10-years follow-up and excluding cases for patient death, lost, or with inadequate follow-up we ended up with a group of 680 hips studied at an average of 6.2 years of follow-up. The clinical Harris hip score averaged 99 points (range 84–100) for the 387 enthusiastic patients and averaged 95 points (range 83 – 100) for the 279 satisfied patients. At the time of follow-up 98% of the patients ranked their result as excellent or good, eight

patients (1.2%) found no change with a mean objective Harris score of 12%, and six patients were disappointed (0.8%) with a mean Harris score of 80 points.

Seven hips were revised for sepsis (1%) and eleven for aseptic failure (1.6%). These revisions for aseptic failure consist in nine loosening, one fracture and one persistent pain. Nine of these eleven aseptic failure occurred with the proximal HA coating used originally. Considering stem revision for aseptic failure, as an end point, the Kaplan-Meier survivorship analysis showed a 96.7% survival at 10 years, with a 95% confidence interval. The dislocation rate for all etiologies was 1.7% (12 cases) and considering only patients with primary osteoarthritis 0.04% (3 cases).

The Basis for Computer-Assisted Hip Arthroplasty

This global concept of computer-assisted pre-operative planning and CAD for THA represents in the authors perception the ideal basis for the use of computer assisted surgery in THA. The clinical results obtained at 10 years are encouraging, and are at least similar or better to the one previously reported with conventional cemented implants in young age groups using modern cementing technique [1, 9, 13, 14, 18, 21, 22, 27, 33, 34], or with standard cementless prosthesis [16, 26]. The goals fixed in 1990 seem to be reached in 2000 with an increased stem longevity for patients under 65 years old, a reduced dislocation rate regarding the 0.6% to 15% reported in the literature [20], and a return to full social and sport activities. The challenging problems remain the choice of the ideal bearing surface in order to minimize wear with options like ceramic on ceramic, metal on metal or the promising highly cross-linked polyethylene.

However the remaining problems for the current use of CAD custom stems are: higher price, delay for conception, and surgeon adaptation. The price difference regarding conventional implant moved from a factor to five to a factor to two during the ten last years and this process must continue in the coming years. The 5 weeks delay for stem fabrication may be significantly reduced to 3 weeks in the short future with the regular use of teleradiology. Finally the orthopaedic surgeon used to have a large number of size in the operating room has to deal with one compactor and one final prosthesis with the CAD concept. This requires a learning curve, quickly achieved by the full computerized pre-operative planning helpful during surgery and once this adaptation is achieved this custom concept may be able to solve a number of surgical difficulties previously encountered with conventional implants.

Finally, the logical following step is the use of computer-assisted technology for improving the positioning of the implants, specially on the femoral side since the optimal final position of the stem has been determined by the computerized pre-operative planning. Indeed the simulation of penetration –extraction realized during the stem conception will be highly helpful to provide the correct information for guiding the CAD-designed custom rasp. This will ideally prepare the intra-medullary femoral cavity ready to receive the final implant. Since the rotational stability will have been determined during the proximal femur reconstruction based on density data this step will be much more precise than the usual manual rasping. Additionally, the three-dimensional design of the custom neck combined to the possibilities offered by the computer-assisted technologies will allow the surgeon to evaluate intraoperatively the global range of motion achieved with such socket location and neck offset orientation.

The Hip-Pilot (Symbios) allows to navigation of both cementless anatomical stems and cementless acetabular components with the Surgetics navigation platform (Praxim) for primary osteoarthritis.

The objective of the system is to reconstruct the original anatomy of the patient in a reproductible way. The system guides the surgeon in order to reproduce the acetabular center of rotation, as decided during the planning, while reaming the acetabulum and implanting the cup. It also measures the rasp and stem position and orientation during implantation. Finally, the Hip-Pilot simulates a virtual reduction of the joint in order to compute the optimal neck design that will best reconstruct the hip joint.

The system works with passive rigid bodies. It does not require a preoperative CT scan examination. The anatomy is acquired preoperatively with palpation of landmarks and utilization of the bone morphing technology (Praxim).

The main measurements provided are:

- the distance between the acetabular center of rotation and the initial dynamic center of rotation;
- the angles of varus valgus and the torsion of the stem measured in relation to the bicondylar axis;
- the final offset and leg length after reduction.

Stability tests can be performed and include range of motion angles, as well as maximum piston distance. All measurements are recorded on a CD ROM per patient.

We believe this system will help the surgeon to routinely improve the accuracy of the hip joint arthroplasty. Our experience with custom CAD stems leads us to believe that precise repositioning of the joint contributes to faster recovery of the patient.

Furthermore, the Hip-Pilot system is fully compatible with a mini invasive technique. When the visibility and access are reduced, the navigation technology may bring additional help to the surgeon.

Conclusion

Computer-assisted hip arthroplasty is certainly a step forward in the future of hip arthroplasty for restoring function and improve implant longevity for patients with high activity and/or modified anatomy. The experience obtained after ten years of computer-assisted planning and CAD for custom stem will logically provide the natural basis for the use of the computer in the operating room since all the previous steps will have been managed in the planning and during stem conception.

Further research in the biomechanical field including the expected bone remodeling around the stems by finite element analysis and the evaluation of the patient hip function after total hip arthroplasty using gait analysis, fluoroscopy, or accelerometry during everyday activities will be also necessary in order to assess step by step such emerging technology.

References

1. Amstutz HC, Markolf KL, McNeice GM, Gruen TA (1976) Loosening of total hip components: cause and prevention. The hip: proceedings of the fourth open scientific meebog of the hip society. Mosby, St Louis, pp 102–16

2. Argenson JN, Hostalrich FX, Essinger JR, Aubaniac JM (1992) Preoperative planning in designing custom made hip prosthesis. J Bone Joint Surg [Br] 74-B [Suppl 2]: 180

3. Argenson JN, Pizzetta M, Essinger JR, Aubaniac JM (1992) Symbios custom hip prosthesis: Concept, realization and early results. J Bone Joint Surg [Br] 74-B [Supp2]: 167

4. Argenson JN, Simonet JY, Aubaniac JM (1993) The indications for cementless custom prostheses in congenital hip dislocation. J Bone Joint Surg [Br] 75-B [Supp1]: 113

5. Argenson JN, Aubaniac JM (1994) Preoperative planning of total hip reconstruction for congenital dislocation of the hip using custom cementless implants. J Southern Orthop Assoc 3: 11–18

6. Argenson JN, Ettore PP, Aubaniac JM (1997) Revêtement des tiges fémorales non cimentées. Etude comparative clinique et radiographique. Rev Chir Orthop 83 [Suppl 2]: 44–45

7. Argenson JN, Aubaniac JM, Flecher X, Ryembault E (2002) The three-dimensional anatomy of the hip in congenital hip dysplasia: radiographic and CT-scan analysis of 312 cases (presented at the 69th annual meeting of the AAOS, Dallas, February 2002)

8. Aubaniac JM, Argenson JN, Pizzetta M (1990) Addressing the anteversion problem in severe CDH and primary or secondary dismorphic, with Egoform and Symbios custom made prosthesis. 3rd Annual International Symposium of Custom Made Prosthesis, 3–5 October

9. Ballard WT, Callaghan JJ, Sullivan PM, Johnston RC (1994) The results of improved cementing techniques for total hip arthroplasties in patients less than fifty years old. J Bone Joint Surg (Am) 76-A: 956–964

10. Boeree NR, Banister (1993) Cemented total hip arthroplasty in patients younger than 50 years of age. Clin Orthop 287: 153–159

11. Chandler HP, Reineck FT, Wixson RL, Mc Carthy JC (1981) Total hip replacement in patients younger than thirty years old: a five years follow-up study. J Bone Joint Surg (Am) 63-A: 1426–1434

12. Collis DK (1984) Cemented total hip replacements in patients who are less than fifty years old. J Bone Joint Surg (Am) 66-A: 353–359

13. Collis DK (1991) Long-term (twelve to eighteen-year) follow-up of cemented total hip replacements in patients who were less than fifty years old. A follow-up note. J Bone Joint Surg (Am) 73-A: 593–597

14. Dorr LD, Luckett M, Conaty JP (1990) Total hip arthroplasties in patients younger than 45 years. Clin Orthop 260: 215–219

15. Dorr LD, Takei GK, Conaty JP (1983) Total hip arthroplasty in patients less than forty five years old. J Bone Joint Surg (Am) 65-A: 474–479

16. Glassman AH (1990): Porous coated total hip replacement in young patients. Read at the annual meeting of the American Academy of Orthopaedic Surgeons, New Orleans, Louisiana, Feb. 8.

17. Halley DK, Wroblewski BM (1986) Long term results of low-friction arthroplasty in patients 30 years of age or younger. Clin Orthop 211: 43–50

18. Harris WH, McCarthy JC, O'Neill DA (1982) Femoral component loosening using contemporary techniques of femoral cement fixation. J Bone Joint Surg (Am) 64-A

19. Husmann D, Rubin PJ, Leyvraz PF, DeRoguin B, Argenson JN (1997) Three-dimensional morphology of the proximal femur. J Arthroplasty 12: 444–450

20. Huten D (1996) Luxation et subluxation des prothèses totales de hanche. In Cahiers d'Enseignement de la SOFCOT: 19–46. Expansion Scientifique Française, Paris

21. Indong OH, Carlson CE, Tomford WW, Harris WH (1978) Improved fixation of the femoral component after total hip replacement using a methacrylate intramedullary plug. J Bone Joint Surg (Am) 60-A: 608–613

22. Joshi AB, Porter ML, Trail IA, Hunt LP, Murphy JC, Hardinge K (1993) Long term results of Charnley low-fraction arthroplasty in young patients. J Bone Joint Surg (Br) 75-B: 616–623

23. Judet R, Siguier M, Brumpt B, Judet T (1978) A non cemented total hip prosthesis. Clin Orthop 137: 76–84

24. Kerjosse R, Tamby I (1999) La situation démographique en 1999. Mouvement de la population. Démographie société in INSEE. Résultats 1999

25. Malchau H, Herberts P (1998) Prognosis of total hip replacement in Sweden. Proceedings of the 65th annual meeting of the American Academy of Orthopaedic Surgeons

26. Mont MA, Maar DC, Krackow KA, Jacobs MA, Jones LC, Hungerford DS (1993) Total hip replacement without cement for non-inflammatory osteoarthritis in patients who are less than forty-five years old. J Bone Joint Surg (Am) 75-A: 740–751

27. Mulroy RD, Harris WH (1990) The effect of improved cementing techniques on component loosening in total hip replacement. An 11 year radiographic review. J Bone Joint Surg (Br) 72-B: 757–760

28. Noble PC, Alexander JW, Lindahl LJ (1988) The anatomic basis of femoral component design. Clin Orthop 235: 148–165

29. Ramaniraka N, Rakotomanana L, Rubin PJ, Leyvraz PF (1998) Influence of the extramedullary parameters on the stem stability and the stress transfer. Proceedings of the 11th annual symposium of the International Society for Technology in Arthroplasty

30. Robertson DD, Walker PS, Hirano SK (1988) Improving the fit of press-git stems. Clin Orthop 228: 134–140

31. Rubin PJ, Leyvraz PF, Aubaniac JM, Argenson JN, Esteve P, Deroguin B (1992) The morphology of the proximal femur: a three dimensionnal radiographic analysis. J Bone Joint Surg (Br) 74-B: 28–32

32. Sharp DJ, Porter KM (1985) The Charoley total hip arthroplasty in patients under age 40. Clin Orthop 201: 51–56

33. Solomon MI, Dall DM, Learmonth ID, Davenport MD (1992) Survivorship of cemented total hip arthroplasty in patients 50 years of age or younger. J Arthroplasty 7 [Suppl]: 347–352

34. Stauffer RN (1982) Ten-year follow-up study of total hip replacement with particular reference to roentgenographic loosening of the components. J Bone Joint Surg (Am) 64-A: 983–990

35. White SH (1988) The fate of cemented total hip arthroplasty in young patients. Clin Orthop 231: 29–34

23 Navigation and Robotics in Joint and Spine Surgery
Computer-Assisted Orthopadic Surgery – Difficulties and Prospects

J. Hassenpflug, M. Prymka

Introduction

We seem to be at the beginning of an entire new development in the field of orthopaedic surgery, the climax of which appears impossible to imagine. Over decades treatment options and improvements of both implant materials and design lead to considerable change for the better in joint arthroplasty. For the first time we face a chance to focusing on precision and technique with the view to standardize and optimize surgical procedures. With the use of computer-assisted surgery improved long-term outcomes over decades are expected.

Computer-assisted design (CAD) and robot-guided manufacturing (CAM) are standards in today's quality of surgical implants. Computer-assisted three-dimensional planning in orthopaedic surgery allows so far a not known precision. There are numerous details worth discussing when robots will operate on humans, particularly logistics of particulate steps and ethics. In general, exact positioning of surgical tools may be accomplished both by computer navigation and robots.

Some details in the field of robot surgery alter when comparing with conventional techniques and may possibly be of increased risk such as prior reference screw fixations in hip surgery. Therefore, hip implantation is to be considered a »revision« procedure potentially adding risk of infection. However, there are no reports in the literature indicating that risk. Addition surgery time decrease with the learning curve, but remains compared with an implantation of a cementless hip prosthesis [1, 2].

Intraoperative alterations of reference points were observed despite the use of heavy femoral bone clamps leading to time consuming re-referencing (⬛ Fig. 23-1).

Since clean conditions are always a problem in crowded (personal and equipment) operating rooms, we endeavor a spinal anesthesia in the mornings with pin placement and consequent CT scan followed by the hip replacement operation at lunch time in general anesthesia. This requires intense logistics to all departments involved and are, therefore, difficult to realize in most hospitals. Due to high quality thin cut CT scans radiation is increased. The surgical approach has the disadvantage of putting the greater trochanter in danger when straight stems are desired, whereas curved or anatomically shaped stems

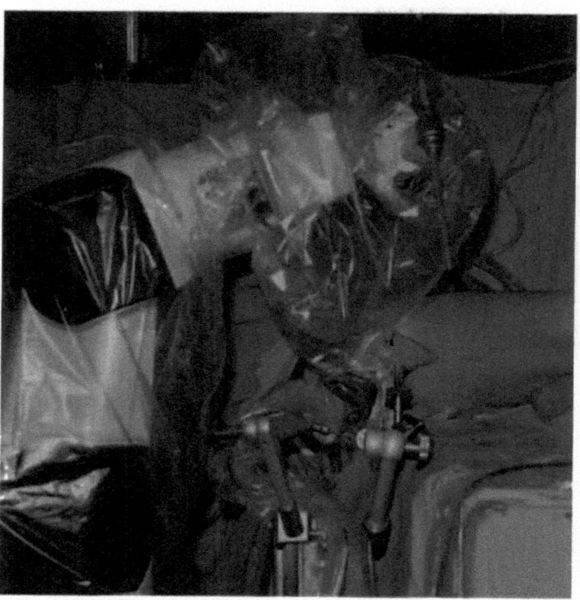

⬛ **Fig. 23-1.** The robot is positioned near the patient and is engaged to the femur via a clamp in an external and adducted position

are reducing that hazard. There is limited place for robotic milling of the femur, particularly in overweight patients and may be associated with considerable soft tissue trauma. There are different hip stems with different fixation principles. The desired shape of implant type, size, fixation principle (cortical or cancellous), and position can be planned and executed very precisely. The current situation is comparable to the technical advances of personal computers a decade ago when digital possibilities in text editing showed a breakthrough with what you see is what you get (WYSIWYG). Furthermore, we could extend this to »WYSIWYG, but what do you really want to see?« Due to the accuracy of the system one question arises: what is the perfect implant position in detail? Close communication amongst the team members of new technology and prostheses is crucial for avoiding repetitive errors in patient's treatment.

We were able to collect considerably helpful experience and better results with the robotic stem implantation in severely distorted posttraumatic or post-osteotomy femora (◘ Fig. 23-2). Although the accuracy of this method was more precise than compared with manual technique, it was still inferior to CAM techniques [5].

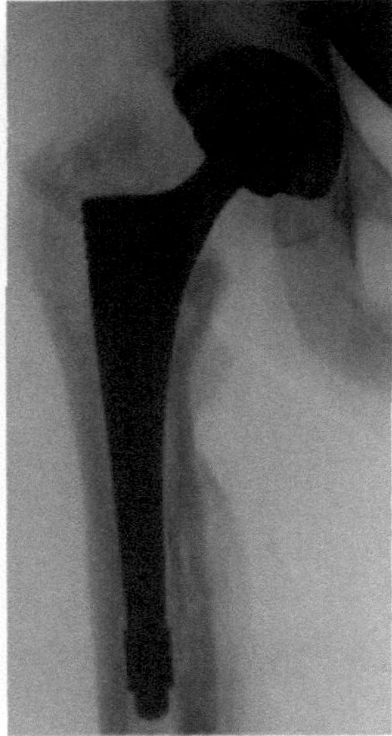

◘ **Fig. 23-2.** Severe damage of the proximal femur and hip joint post multipart fracture. Prosthetic implantation was difficult due to considerable bone deformity and intra-medullary cancellous trabeculae. The right side shows perfect position of an Ostelock prosthesis after CASPAR robotic implantation

Longitudinal stem position was perfect in 11 of 16 trial components only. Mediolateral deviation measured 0.4 mm laterally, dorsoventral deviation 0.75 mm, and antetorsion angle measured an increase of 1.1 degrees anteriorly.

The main advantage of robotic implantation comes to play when bone resections must be highly accurate. Mechanically speaking, this is true for prosthesis-bone interfaces [3, 4, 7]. We found in cadaver studies a significant difference in bone-prosthesis femoral fit when milling was performed by robots compared with annual techniques, furthermore, complications such as fissures, fractures, gaps, and bone damages were not encountered with robots (◘ Fig. 23-3) [8]. The clinical implications remain to be seen. A further question is whether interface gaps or bone damage zone actually improve or deteriorate both primary and secondary stability and biological healing response of the prosthesis. Another issue is the fact that continuous lavage during milling eliminates vital bone cells important for ingrowth.

Correction of increased anteversion in dysplastic hip femora into »proper« version may have a negative effect at the stem shaft with regards to elevated pressure zones [4,6], however, this problem can be calculated with the computer prior to implantation. Manual rasping has the advantage of positive feedback that avoids cortical damage due to the fact of increased bone resistance, which drives a manual rasp automatically home. This sensory information can only be seen at the monitor, but is not appreciated by the robot arm. In cases where a non-physiologic torsion of the stem is desired, this would have significant implication on the acetabular alignment. A subsequent positioning of the acetabulum in inclination and anteversion will have to be defined by navigation tools.

Current perspectives for robotic implantation of hip stems include:
- good planning facilities,
- acceptable accuracy of positioning and fit,
- requirement of two anesthetics, CT scans and additional OR time,
- increased staff, costs, and radiation,
- advantages in femoral deformities.

Because conventional hip implantation technique lead to acceptable long-term outcomes, the advantages of robots

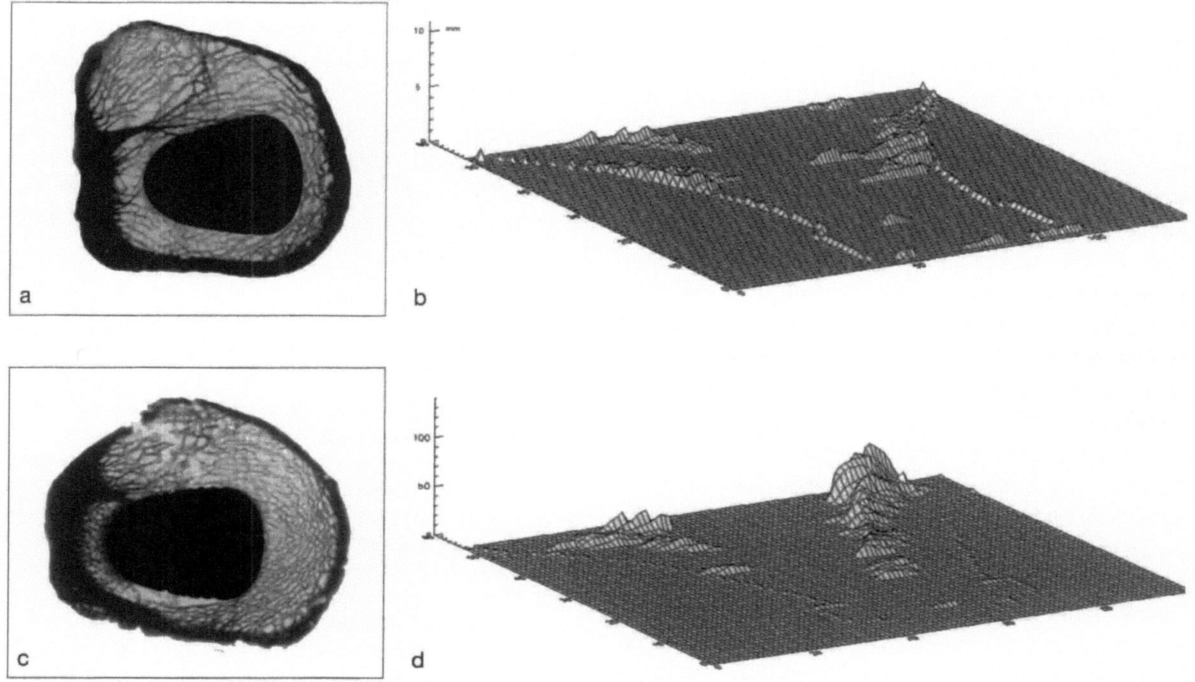

Fig. 23-3a–d. a, b Prosthetic fit after robotic preparation. On the *left side* demonstration after plastination and surface mapping. **c,d** Cross-section of an implanted femoral stem after manual rasping shows considerable destruction of interfacial bone with increased periprosthetic gaps reducing the total area of bone contact compared with robotic preparation

will have to counterweigh the disadvantages with this new technology. Data from our **Orthopedic Department at the University of Kiel**, Germany, have shown a hip replacement survival rate of 98% after 10 years [9].

First long-term results of robotic hip implantations will demonstrate a possible advantage of the concept. Until then in vitro investigations of primary stability and micromotions will help in understanding the accuracy and possible long-term implication at the bone-implant interface. Computer-assisted orthopaedic planning and robotics stand at the beginning of a new area. (Amongst the many advantages this technology is the first that increases partly surgical accuracy superior to surgeon skills (**Fig. 23-4)). Careful prospective documentation of the positives and draw-backs will have to prove whether computer-assisted surgery and robotics actually improve results and reduces complication in the field of endoprosthetics, osteotomies, ACL reconstructions, and cancer surgery. The current development in this field shows similarities with the beginnings of minimally invasive surgery and arthroscopy. Careful and precise documen-

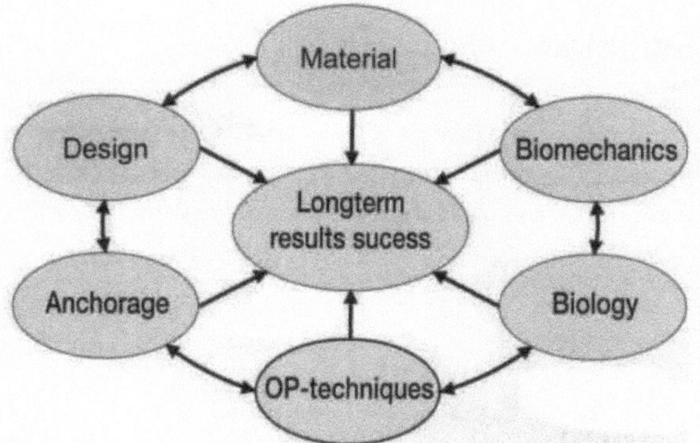

Fig. 23-4. Multifactorial influence of success or failure in orthopaedic surgery. Computer enhanced surgical techniques promote the surgery itself to a higher level of interest

tation of clinical experience and basic science as well as improved results compared with conventional techniques are required for establishing CAS and robotics as a standard tool. Risks, developmental potential, and complications must be discussed in a realistic but not enhanced manner in order to decrease unnecessary fear and scepticism for this technology.

A variety of advantages with computer-assisted surgery include the three-dimensional planning and prediction of the surgical result. Detailed parameters such as stem rotation, interface preparation and relation to the implant, and leg length can be calculated and predicted. CAS allow for an execution of precise surgical planning. However, these accuracies require additional scientific answers to unknown questions. With regards to total hip replacements there are posing questions; what is the optimal rotation of the stem, the optimal position of the acetabulum, what is the best relationship between them, and should one reconstruct the original anatomy?

At the end it is still the surgeon, who independent of all fascination for modern technology and tools, has to be aware and knowledgeable about the concept of total hip arthroplasty. Together with the individual patient he or she must find the optimal solution with regards to longterm outcomes, postoperative function, patient's satisfaction, and prevention of immobility or dysfunction. European centers demonstrate a comprehensive interest and experience in this field and should not neglect these scientific advantages.

Summary

Computer-aided design (CAD) procedures and computer-aided manufacturing (CAM, robotics) are transferred from industrial utilization to medical treatment. The application of robotics in the medical field has evolved to a reliable and precise procedure. Prosthetic fit can be planned with a high 3D precision and reproduced accurately to a fraction of a millimeter during surgery. Interface fit has improved in comparison to manual preparation. Clinical application of robots show increased utilization, however, there are gaps within the basic knowledge and longterm outcomes.

References

1. Bagar WL, Bauer A, Birner M (1998) Primary and revision total hip replacement using the Robodoc system. Clin Orthop 354: 82–91

2. Birner M, Bauer A, Lahmer A (1997) Rechnerunterstützter Robotereinsatz in der Hüftendoprothetik. Orthopäde 26: 251–257

3. Engh CA, Glassman AH, Suthers KE (1990) The case for porous-coated hip implants. The femoral side. Clin Orthop 261: 63–81

4. Harris WH, Mulroy RD Jr, Maloney WJ, Burke DW, Chandler HP, Zalenski EB (1991) Intraoperative measurement of rotational stability of femoral components of total hip arthroplasty. Clin Orthop 266: 119–126

5. Knoch von M, Wiese K, Hahne HJ, Prymka M, Gehrke T, Hassenpflug J (2000) Vergleich von Planung und Implantationsergebnis bei roboterunterstützter Hüftschaftimplantation. Z Orthop 138: S60–S61

6. Otani T, Whiteside LA (1992) Failure of cementless fixation of the femoral component in total hip arthroplasty. Orthop Clin North Am 23: 335–346

7. Pilliar RM, Cameron HU, Welsh RP, Binnington AG (1981) Radiographic and morphologic studies of load-bearing porous-surfaced structured implants. Clin Orthop 156: 249–257

8. Prymka M, Hahne HJ, Koebke J, Hassenpflug J (2000) Roboterunterstützte Implantation von Hüftendoprothesenschäften. Eine mikroradiographische Untersuchung. Z Orthop 138: S56

9. Traulsen FC, Hahne HJ, Hassenpflug J (2001) Langzeitresultate von zementfreien Hüftvollprothesen (Zweymüller). Z Orthop 139: 206–211

III Total Knee Arthroplasty

24 Total Knee Arthroplasty

F. F. Buechel, J. B. Stiehl

History

Knee replacements have evolved from the single-axis fixed-hinge devices of the 1950's (Walduis, Shiers) [23] to the unlinked fixed-axis devices of the 1960's (Geomedic, Polycentric) [3, 13], both of which had a limited clinical use because of loosening and wear problems.

In the early 1970's incongruent contact fixed-bearing prostheses (UCI, Marmor, Townley, Total Condylar) [8, 16, 19, 20] improved the outlook for replacements is by enhancing fixation and improving kinematics to the point where pain relief and kneereasonable function was the usual outcome. However, the price for incongruent contact was higher than allowable contact stresses of the polyethylene, which was subjected to accelerated wear in heavy or active patients.

By the late 1970's, a »renaissance in total knee development« occurred. A more congruent contact fixed-bearing with an intercondylar posterior-stabilized post (Insall-Burstein) [21] was developed to improve upon the successful Total Condylar device which had limited flexion and dislocation problems. An important advance in the late 1970's, however, was the introduction of mobile-bearings (Oxford, New Jersey LCS) [5, 10] to improve congruent contact during walking, while eliminating constraint forces. By using metallic components for fixation, these wear resistant implants could be implanted with methyl methacrylate (bone cement) or be used with biological fixation (Porocoat) to improve wear properties and minimize loosening.

Another important feature of mobile bearings, aside from ease of bearing exchanging in case of necessity, was their ability to self-adjust the tibia rotation and patella rotation position to optimize knee kinematics, thus allowing the collateral ligaments and extensor mechanism to physiologically balance during flexion-extension and rotary motion of the knee.

The 1980's brought an increasing number of poorly designed fixed-bearing knee replacement implants (PCA, Ortholoc I, Miller-Galante I, AMK) [9, 11, 26, 27] that overloaded the tibial and patellar polyethylene surfaces and also created »backside wear« from poorly connected modular trays. These fixed-bearing implants were developed to broaden the commercial total knee market while avoiding the overly burdensome requirements of the United States Food and Drug Administration (FDA) by use of the 510 k equivalence process. These devices avoided a formal clinical trial by claiming to be substantially equivalent to knee replacement devices sold prior to 1976, when the FDA Medical Device Act came into existence. Without substantial mechanical or clinical data to support their efficacy, these devices became widely used and developed significant failures, mostly because of premature, accelerated wear. The Anatomic Graduated Component (AGC) total knee [17] was a »bright spot« for fixed bearings of the 1980's, as it successfully used compression molded polyethylene on the metal tibial component to avoid the wear seen in other fixed bearing designs.

Current total knee designs from the 1990's and beyond the year 2000 are generally modifications of previous designs, trying to optimize the fixed-bearing surfaces and eliminate metal-backed fixed-bearing patella components. Most of these designs have developed a mobile bearing alternative, to take advantage of the wear reduction potential offered by this concept, especially since the New Jersey LCS mobile-bearing design has shown such outstanding 20 year total knee results in a rotating platform that is still available in its original form [6].

Mechanical Axis

Proper limb alignment or mechanical axis alignment in total knee replacement is of paramount importance for long-term successful outcome. Normal mechanical axis alignment is defined as a line that passes and through the center of the femoral head, the center of the knee and the center of the ankle (Fig. 24-1). This normal limb alignment provides even load distribution on the medial and lateral bearing surfaces during walking and other activities of daily living (ADL). Excessive wear is avoided when bearing surfaces are well-designed and well-aligned (see Fig. 24-1).

Deviations from mechanical axis alignment will cause excessive loads on the medial polyethylene bearing surface if varus alignment occurs and excessive loads on the lateral polyethylene bearing surface if valgus alignment occurs (Fig. 24-2). Additionally, in valgus malalignment, the lateral border of the patella bearing may be overloaded (Fig. 24-3), and cause excessive wear leading to failure and the need for revision. Lateral retinacular release may be needed to restore central patellar tracking during flexion and extension.

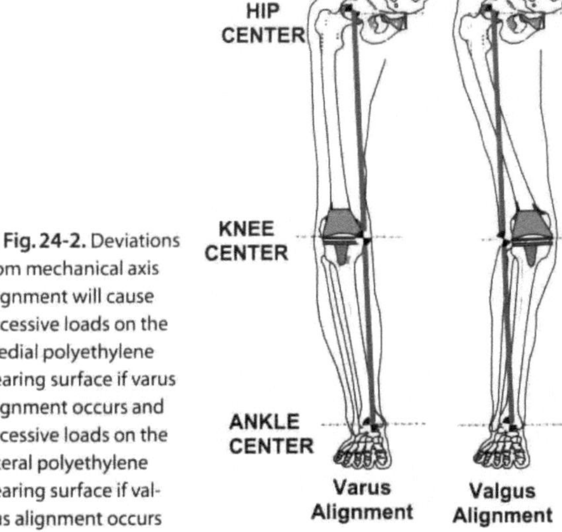

Fig. 24-2. Deviations from mechanical axis alignment will cause excessive loads on the medial polyethylene bearing surface if varus alignment occurs and excessive loads on the lateral polyethylene bearing surface if valgus alignment occurs

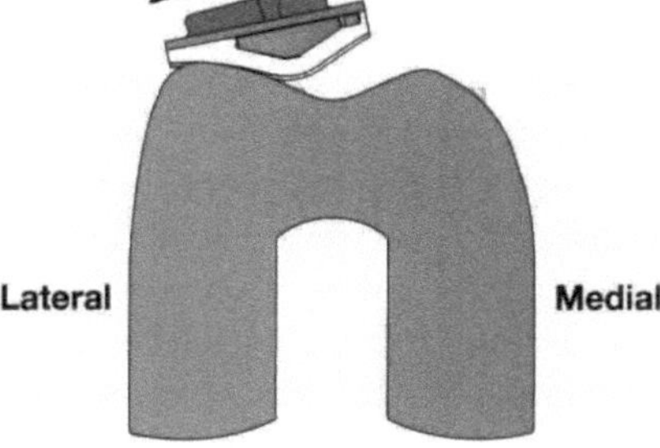

Fig. 24-3. In valgus malalignment, the lateral border of the patella bearing maybe overloaded

Soft Tissue Balancing

To gain proper alignment, soft tissue balancing has become the »art form« of total knee replacement. Strictly making bone cuts to fit the prosthetic parts will not provide stable function if the collateral ligaments are not balanced. Proper ligament balance requires that the flexion-extension arc of knee motion proceeds without impingement and with complete medial-lateral stability in both flexion and extension.

The posterior cruciate ligament (PCL), if retained and properly balanced, should not pull the femur posteriorly beyond the middle one-third of the tibia in the lateral plane during flexion (too tight), nor should it allow forward translation of the femur beyond the middle third of

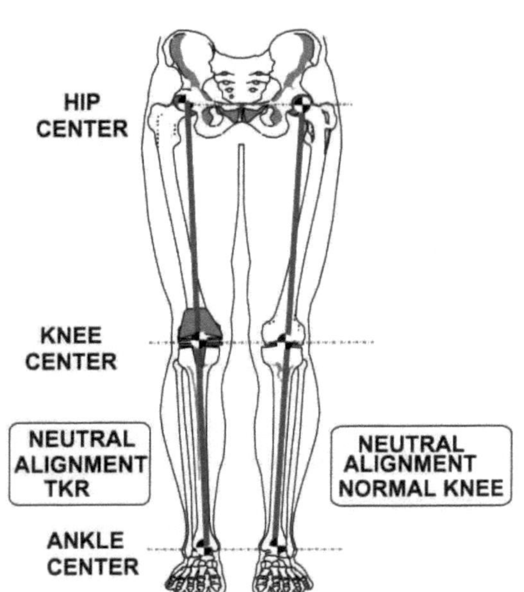

Fig. 24-1. Normal mechanical axis alignment is shown along with proper implant alignment

the tibia during flexion (too loose). Recessing the PCL from its femoral or tibial attachment by incising the tightest fibers can loosen a tight PCL. A loose PCL should not be tolerated, but rather a well-designed PCL sacrificing knee replacement, such as an LCS rotating platform or an IBII should be used.

To gain proper collateral ligament balance, the most logical and »time-tested« way is to perform a proximal medial tibial sleeve release in extension for fixed varus deformities [14] to gain neutral alignment (5° femoral-tibial valgus) with a 5° spring back to 0° during valgus stress prior to resecting the proximal tibia. In fixed valgus deformities, a sequential three-step lateral release approach [4] is recommended to gain neutral alignment with varus stress (0°) with a spring back to 5° femoro-tibial valgus prior to resecting the proximal tibia.

Once the varus or valgus deformity has been corrected and the proximal tibia has been resected perpendicular to the ankle axis in the AP plane, the femoral rotation alignment and the flexion gap can be established in one step by using a **femoral resection guide positioner.**

This U-shaped instrument develops the collateral ligament tension in flexion and rotates the femoral resection guide into proper axial alignment to give equal collateral ligament tension in flexion (◘ Fig. 24-4). Usually this rotation coincides with the femoral epicondylar axis, which can be used for navigational purposes. With the collateral ligaments »fine tuned« to be equal in flexion, the AP femoral resections can be performed with assurance that the flexion gap has a balanced rectangular space (◘ Fig. 24-5).

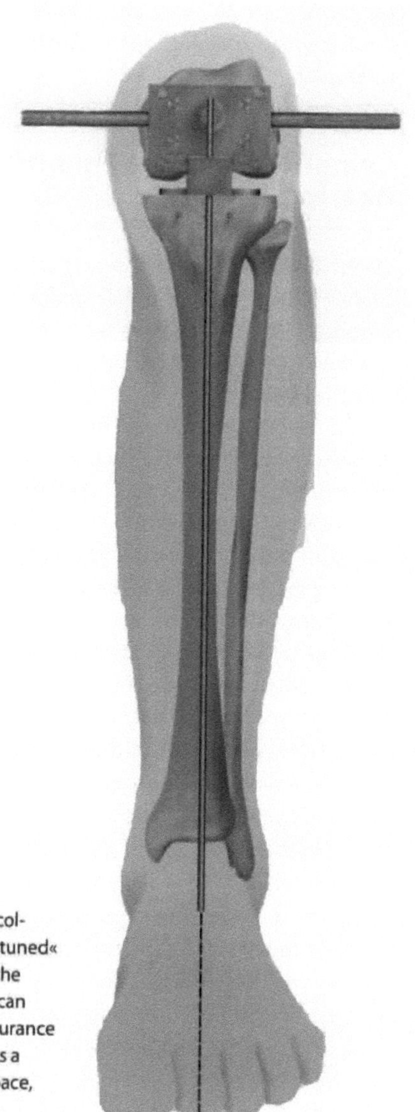

◘ **Fig. 24-4.** The femoral guide positioner develops the collateral ligament tension in flexion and rotates the femoral resection guide into proper axial alignment to give equal collateral ligament tension in flexion

◘ **Fig. 24-5.** With the collateral ligaments »fine tuned« to be equal in flexion, the AP femoral resections can be performed with assurance that the flexion gap has a balanced rectanglar space, along with the correct alignment

The knee is brought into extension and the proper valgus angle (3° to 6°) is determined to gain mechanical axis alignment, then the distal femur is resected in an amount to give an extension gap that is equal to the flexion gap. This sequence of flexion gap and extension gap balance provides a reproducible, stable arc of motion during flexion and extension, which works well for either fixed-bearing or mobile-bearing knee replacements. It has been »time-tested« in the Total Condylar [25], Insall-Burstein, [2] and New Jersey LCS [6] total knee systems for more than 20 years and has contributed to greater than 90% survivorship for these devices over that time interval.

Cemented Versus Cementless Mobile Bearing TKA

Twenty-year evaluation of cemented and cementless LCS mobile bearing knee replacement has confirmed the durability of these devices when properly implanted by the mechanical axis and soft-tissue methods previously described [6].

Survivorship of 100 primary cementless posterior cruciate retaining (PCR) meniscal bearing LCS knee replacements, using an endpoint of revision for any reason was 83% at 16 years. Four worn meniscal bearings in this group of patients were successfully revised by simple bearing exchange without removing the well-fixed metallic components, whose survivorship for fixation was 100% at 16 years. Shelf-aged, gamma irradiated in air, poor quality polyethylene was a major contributing factor to the bearing failures seen in this group of patients.

Survivorship of 48 primary cemented rotating platform LCS knee replacements, using an endpoint of revision for any reason, was 97.7% at 20 years. One immediate postoperative bearing dislocation required insertion of a thicker bearing to gain stability and one femoral component loosening required revision to a stemmed femoral component to restore fixation. No wear-related failures were seen in this group of patients.

Survivorship of 118 primary cementless rotating platform LCS knee replacements, using an endpoint of revision for any reason, was 98.3% at 18 years. One rheumatoid patient after 6.8 years sustained a traumatic supracondylar femur fracture that required revision to a long-stemmed femoral component to gain fracture stability. No bearing failures or component loosening was seen in this group of patients.

Rotating Platform Versus Fixed Platform TKA

A review of long-term clinical and survivorship data reveals excellent clinical results for a variety of fixed-platform (fixed-bearing) total knee designs. Most notably, the Total Condylar knee has a reported implant survivorship of 91% at 23 years with a range of motion of 90 to 100 degrees [22]. The Insall-Burstein (I-B) I records an 11 year survivorship of 96.4% and the I-BII (modular) records an 11 year survivorship of 98.1% [2] (not including 3/154, 1.9% patella failures), although John Insall himself, prior to his death in 2000, reported worrisome osteolysis in the modular I-BII design beyond 11 years, driving him to favor mobile bearings over his older I-B devices [15].

The Anatomic Graduated Component (AGC) knee replacement has a reported average range of motion of 110 degrees and survivorship of 98.86% at 15 years [24], although curiously, 62 (1.3%) knees were revised for infection, 180 (4.2%) all-poly-patella components were loose and 28 (9.5%) loose, metal-backed patella components were revised. With this much data confusion, it seems that the survivorship is still good, but probably closer to 90% at 15 years.

The Cementless Natural Knee replacement has a reported survivorship of 88.3% at 14 years with metal-backed patella component failure and tibia bearing wear accounting for most of the mechanical problems [12]. Cementless fixation with this device was exceptionally good as was the cementless fixation of the Ortholoc I knee replacement which noted an 18 year fixation survivorship of 96.1% of femoral and tibial components [28].

The cemented Genesis knee replacement used both cruciate-sparing and cruciate-sacrificing (posterior stabilized) devices that reported 12 year survivorship of 94% and 96%, and average postoperative motion of 117 degrees and 114 degrees, respectfully [18].

The cemented Miller-Galante I knee replacement survivorship of 84.1% at 10 years was improved to a reported 100% survivorship for the Miller-Galante II at 10 years for a cohort of 109 knees. Improvement in femoral trochlear design and change to an all poly patella component are given as reason for this success, even though the contact surfaces remain suboptimal [1].

The success of multiple fixed-bearing knee replacement designs remains noteworthy, but lacks the longer term success of the cemented LCS rotating platform knee replacement which has an average postoperative range of motion of 110° (range 62°–135°) and twenty-year survivorship of 97.7%. This is similar to the results reported by Callahan et al. in which the cemented rotating platform survivorship was 100% at 12 years, with no failures or pending revisions seen in a series of 119 knee replacements [7].

The cementless LCS rotating platform has an average postoperative range of motion of 107 ° (range 55°–125 °) and 18 year survivorship of 98.3% [6]. This device is still being used in original design configuration, as well as improved modifications (LCS Universal and LCS Complete knee systems, DePuy International, Leeds, England). Continued attention to the biomechanical principles of maximizing congruency while minimizing constraint remains the foundation for the LCS family of knee devices. Such principles have stood the »test of time« and should remain part of the evolution of knee replacement surgery in the future.

References

1. Berger RA, Rosenberg AG, Barden RM et al. (2001) Long-term follow-up of the Miller-Galante Total Knee replacement. Clin Orthop Rel Res 388: 58–67

2. Brassard MF, Insall JN, Scuderi GR, Colizza W (2001) Does modularity affect clinical success? A comparison with a minimum 10-year followup. Clin Orthop 388: 26–32

3. Bryan RS, Peterson LF, Combs JJ (1973) Polycentric knee arthroplasty. A review of 84 patients with more than one year follow-up. Clin Orthop Rel Res 94: 136–139

4. Buechel FF (1990) A sequential three-step lateral release for correcting fixed valgus knee deformities during total knee arthroplasty. Clin Orthop Rel Res 260: 170–175

5. Buechel FF, Pappas MJ (1986) The New Jersey low-contact-stress knee replacement system: biomechanical rationale and review of the first 123 cemented cases. Arch Orthop Traum Surg 105: 197–204

6. Buechel Sr FF, Buechel Jr FF, Pappas MJ, D'Alessio J (2001) Twenty-year evaluation of meniscal bearing and rotating platform knee replacements. Clin Orthop Rel Res 388: 41–50

7. Callahan JJ, Squire MW, Goetz DD et al. (2000) Cemented rotating platform total knee replacement. J Bone Joint Surg 82A: 705–711

8. Evanski PM, Waugh TR, Orofino CF et al. (1976) UCI knee replacement. Clin Orthop Rel Res 120: 33–38

9. Flivik G, Ljung P, Rydholm U (1990) Fracture of the tibial tray of the PCA knee. A case report of early failure caused by improper design. Acta Orthop Scand 61: 26–28

10. Goodfellow JW, O'Connor J (1986) Oxford clinical results of the Oxford knee. Surface arthroplasty of the tibiofemoral joint with a meniscal bearing prosthesis. Clin Orthop Rel Res 205: 21–42

11. Hirakawa K, Bauer TW, Yamaguchi M et al. (1999) Relationship between wear debris particles and polyethylene surface damage in primary total knee arthroplasty. J Arthroplasty 14: 165–171

12. Hoffman AA, Evancih D, Ferguson RP et al. (2001) Ten to 14 year clinical follow-up of the cementless natural knee system. Clin Orthop Rel Res 388: 85–94

13. Holman PK, Tyer HD (1975) Proceedings: Early results of geomedic total knee arthroplasty. J Bone Joint Surg May 57B: 249

14. Insall JW (1984) Surgical approaches to the knee. In: Insall JN (ed) Surgery of the knee. Churchhill Livingston, New York, pp 4–54

15. Insall JN (1998) Adventures in mobile-bearing knee design: A mid-life crisis. Orthop 21: 1021–1023

16. Insall J, Ranawat CS, Scott WN, Walker P (1976) Total condylar knee replacement: preliminary report. Clin Orthop Rel Res 120: 149–154

17. Jacchia GE, Gusso MI, Ciampalini L, Civinini R (1991) The AGC 2000 knee prosthesis: observations on the first 35 cases. Arch Putti Chir Organi Mov 39: 231–237

18. Laskin RS (2001) The Genesis Total Knee Prosthesis: a ten-year follow-up study. Clin Orthop Rel Res 388: 95–102

19. Mallory TH, Smalley D, Danyi J (1982) Townley anatomic total knee arthroplasty using total tibial component with cruciate release. Clin Orthop Rel Res 169: 197–201

20. Marmor L (1976) The Modular (Marmor) knee: case report with a minimum follow-up of 2 years. Clin Orthop Rel Res 120: 86–94

21. Patel DV, Aichroth PM, Wand JS (1991) Posteriorly stabilised (Insall-Burstein) total condylar knee arthroplasty. A follow-up study of 157 knees. Int Orthop 15: 211–218

22. Pavone V, Boettner F, Fickert S, Sculco TP (2001) Total Condylar Knee Arthroplasty: a long-term follow-up. Clin Orthop Rel Res 388: 18–25

23. Rand JA, Chao EY, Stauffer RN (1987) Kinematic rotating hinge total knee arthroplasty. J Bone Joint Surgery 69A: 489–497.

24. Ritter MA, Berend ME, Meding JB et al. (2001) Long-term follow-up of anatomic graduated components posterior cruciate-retaining total knee replacement. Clin Orthop Rel Res 388: 51–57

25. Rodrigquez JA, Bhende H, Ranawat CS (2001) Total Condylar Knee Replacement: A 20-year follow-up study. Clin Orthop Rel Res 388: 10–17

26. Rorabeck CH, Bourne RB, Lewis PL et al. (1993) The Miller-Galante knee prosthesis for the treatment of osteoarthrosis. A comparison of the results of partial fixation with cement and fixation without any cement. J Bone Joint Surg Am 75: 402–408

27. Whiteside LA (1989) Clinical results of Whiteside Ortholoc total knee replacement. Orthop Clin North Am 20: 113–124

28. Whiteside LA (2001) Long-term follow-up of the bone-ingrowth ortholoc knee system without a metal backed patella. Clin Orthop Rel Res 388: 77–84

25 Why the Tibia Cut First in Mobile Bearing TKA Technique?

J. B. Stiehl

Introduction

There are three major objectives of surgical technique in total arthroplasty. First is the need to achieve anatomical alignment of 5° to 7° valgus angulation to the mechanical axis. Second is to establish ligamentous balance by achieving careful balance of the flexion and extension gaps within 2 to 3 millimeters of physiological. Finally, is the desire to optimize the potential kinematics of the chosen prosthetic implant. The »Tibial Cut First« technique follows the original idea of Dr John Insall that establishing the flexion gap was the most important variable in successful total condylar arthroplasty [1]. We will discuss why this approach has become an attractive surgical technique for mobile bearing total knee arthroplasty and how surgical navigation will more accurately place the proximal tibial cut in total knee arthroplasty.

Rationale

Insall Method

The goals of surgical technique of mobile bearing total knee arthroplasty are the same as those originally established by Insall for inserting the total condylar prosthesis including balancing the ligaments and resecting the ends of the femur and tibia so that the spaces between the cut ends were the same when the knee was in flexion and in extension. The classic Insall method required resecting the anterior and posterior femoral condyles with a degree of external rotation relative to the posterior condylar axis, resecting the proximal tibia at 90° flexion with the plane of resection perpendicular to the long axis of the tibia, and then resecting the distal femur using the spacer that fits the flexion space dimension with a long rod to determine correct valgus angulation of the knee [8]. The particular innovations of this approach were to preferentially determine the flexion space, to use a perpendicular cut on the proximal tibia, and to cut the extension space based primarily on a tension spacer that matched the flexion space. The principles of preliminary ligamentous balancing and flexion/extension spacing became well established.

Measured Resection of the Distal Femur

From a different point of view, surgeons sought to preserve the cruciate ligaments or at least the posterior cruciate ligament, and the concept of spacer tensioning and cutting the tibia before the femur, became secondary to anatomical preparation of the distal femur. In other words, the focus of the technique was measured resection of bone cuts with the goal of recreating the joint line and alignment of the knee. With the preservation of the posterior cruciate ligament, the primary ligamentous issue was recreating a neutral or 0° mechanical axis in the frontal plane. Balancing of the flexion space was a secondary issue and centered more on recognizing tightness or looseness of the posterior cruciate ligament. If too tight, the posterior cruciate ligament would hold the femur posterior on the proximal tibia causing anterior tibial lift-off. If too loose, there would be flexion space laxity and potential clinical instability. Numerous authors have endorsed balancing the ligaments after all bone cuts have been made focusing on the ligaments that affect primarily extension such as the superficial medial collateral, pes tendons, iliotibial tract and lateral collateral ligament. The posterior cruciate ligament could be recessed off the tibia at the end of the procedure.

More recent improvements of the measured resection technique have been to precisely determine the amount of distal femoral rotation for the posterior condyle cuts such that they parallel the axis of knee rotation. These have included posterior condylar reference with cuts of 3° to 5° external rotation, the Whiteside intercondylar line which utilizes a line from the center of the intercondylar groove bisecting the intercondylar space, and the transepicondylar axis reference which roughly parallels the knee flexion axis (◘ Fig. 25-1). Stiehl et al. developed the tibial shaft axis method which uses a long rod attached to a femoral intra-medullary rod which centers on the ankle mortise [9, 10]. The goal of these methods was to create a bone resection resulting in a rectangular flexion space based on the principle that the transepicondylar axis is

parallel the knee flexion rotation axis and is the target anatomical structure for prosthetic placement (◘ Fig. 25-2).

LPS-High Flex Mobile Bearing Technique

The current LPS-High Flex mobile bearing technique is consistent with the Insall method with »tibial cut first« resection. With older mobile bearing devices such as the LCS total knee, flexion space instability was implicated as a primary cause for complications including mobile bearing »spin out« and dislocation which ranged from 0.5% for the rotating platform to over 3% for meniscal bearings. Perhaps this was best demonstrated by the experience of Bert et al. who through surgical misadventure had a dislocation rate of nearly 50% using the LCS [3]. The problem was so severe that bearings were nearly falling out in the recovery room. Appropriately, focusing on stability of the flexion gap became the primary goal of the surgical technique. With the LPS-High Flex prosthesis, obtaining »perfect« flexion space stability virtually every time is critical to eliminating bearing instability problems.

Tibial Shaft Axis Method

The LPS High Flex tibial shaft axis method determines the proximal tibial cut utilizing either an extra-medullary guide system or a surgical navigated cut of the tibia is

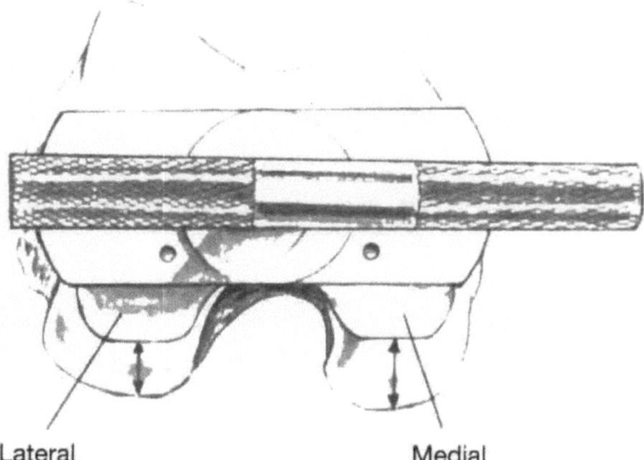

◘ **Fig. 25-1.** Distal femoral measured resection with external rotation using the Whiteside line, transepicondylar axis, or a 3°–4° external rotation

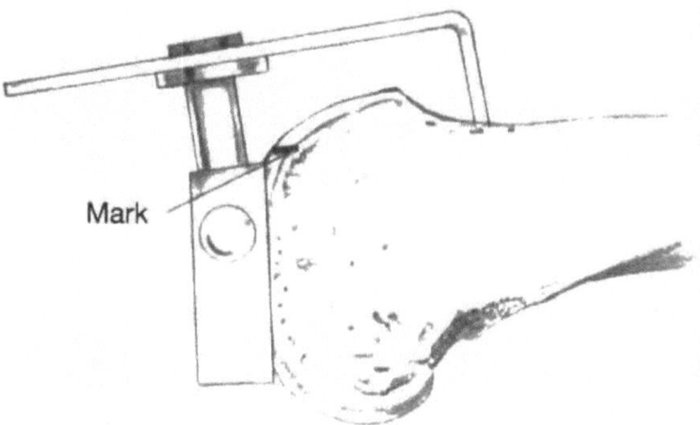

◘ **Fig. 25-2.** Posterior condylar resection based on anterior cortical reference with appropriate measured external femoral rotation

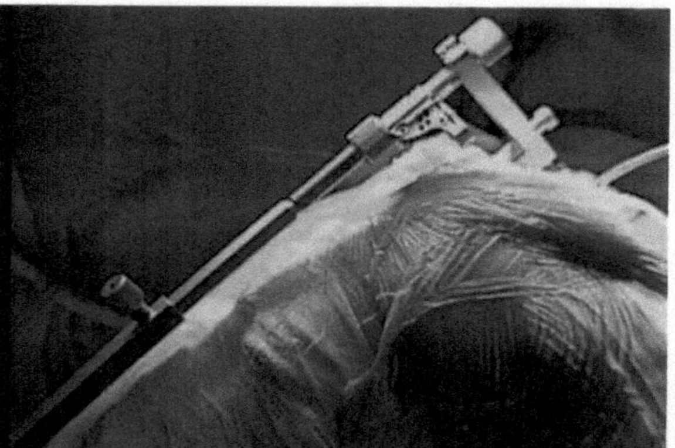

◘ **Fig. 25-3.** LPS High Flex tibial shaft axis method uses extra-medullary guide to cut tibia perpendicular to the limb mechanical axis

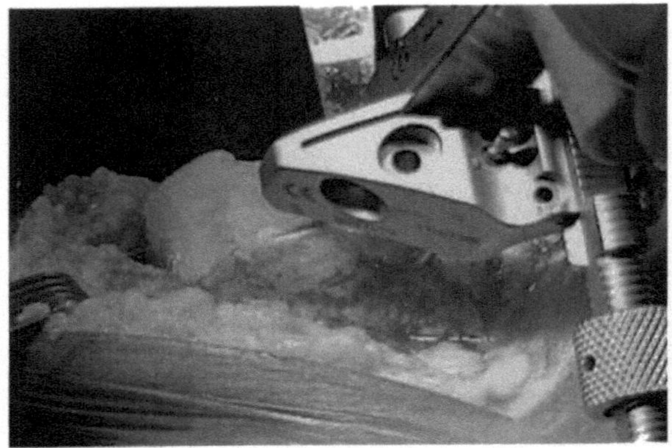

Fig. 25-4. Proximal tibial cut is made perpendicular to the tibial shaft axis

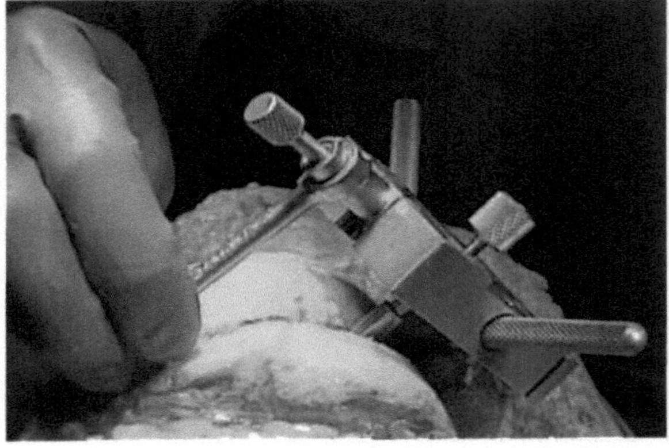

Fig. 25-5. LPS High Flexion blocks are used with the final thickness determined to be 2 millimeters greater than that for the extension space

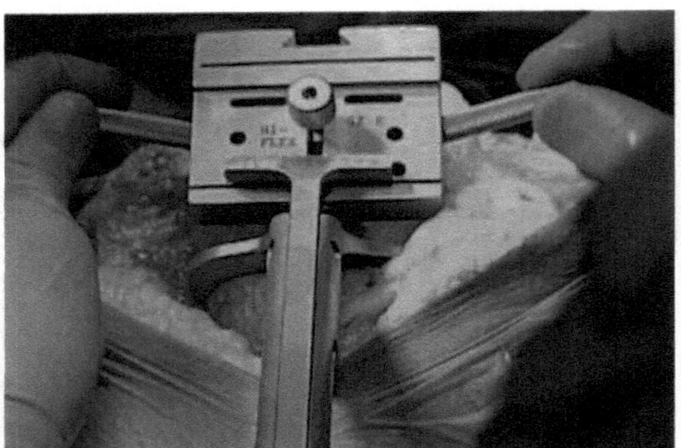

Fig. 25-6. The tensor device used for determining flexion space posterior femoral condylar cuts allows for a rough measurement of the flexion gap

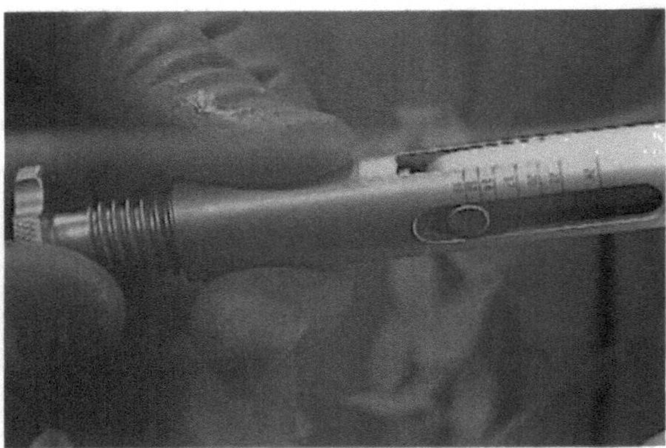

Fig. 25-7. The LPS High Flexion tensor device allows precise measurement of the flexion gap

made perpendicular to the mechanical axis of the leg (■ Fig. 25-3 and 25-4) An intra-medullary femoral rod is placed with the anterior/posterior condylar cutting block. Flexion spacing is done with an anterior/posterior cortical cutting block based off the anterior cortical reference (■ Fig 25-5). The exact dimension of the flexion space is determined with a tensor that precisely tensions and measures a rectangular flexion space (■ Fig. 25-6 and 25-7). The final assessment is done with a spacing block that also allows determination of the tibial shaft mechanical axis (■ Fig. 25-8).

An important step with the tibial shaft axis method is that primary extension ligamentous balancing must be established before the flexion space is created. This is because any ligamentous balancing done after these cuts

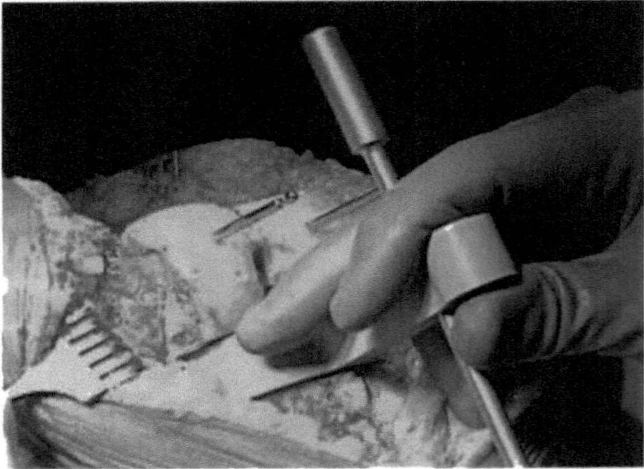

Fig. 25-8. LPS flexion space assessment measures both rectangular space and alignment

are made can result in the creation of a trapezoidal flexion space. Such a problem often results in bearing dislocation or »spinout«. The surgeon must have the knee balanced as his primary step though some releasing such as the posterior capsule may be made after the proximal tibial cut. This can be advantageous as the posterior capsular origin on the distal femur becomes more accessible. With the knee in full extension, the ligaments should be balanced and tense. If not, additional release should be done.

Discussion

The distinct disadvantage of a measured distal femoral resection is the inability to deal with certain outliers such as lateral femoral condylar hypoplasia or severe angular deformities such as proximal tibia vara with a varus joint line. In these patients, ligamentous imbalance occurs commonly and can lead to chronic instability. Berger et al. found the posterior condylar axis to the surgical transepicondylar axis (point of lateral epicondyle to the sulcus of the medial epicondyle) to average 3.5° for males and 0.3° for females which was a highly significant statistical difference. However, the clinical angle using the prominence of the medial epicondyle was 4.7° for males and 5.2° for females. Significantly, the variance could range from 1° to 9.3° [1]. Mantas et al. found in normal femurs that the range of posterior condylar axis reference to the transepicondylar axis ranged from 0.1° to 9.7° [6].

Fehring compared the Insall method with the measured resection method of distal femur resection using a fixed posterior condylar reference guide finding that the measured resection technique resulted in rotational errors of at least 3° in 45% of knees [4]. This means that well balanced flexion gaps would have been distorted to trapezoidal gaps in 45% of cases with potential flexion instability.

Similarly, Olcott and Scott found that the transepicondylar reference most readily determined a balanced flexion space while using 3° rotation off the posterior condyles was least consistent [7].

Berger et al. has shown that internal rotation of the femoral component from the transepicondylar reference combined with tibial internal rotation from the center of the tibial tubercle was a substantial cause of patellofemoral complications. In other words, a group of

patients with patellar subluxation, tilt, dislocation, and prosthetic loosening, all demonstrated the presence of combined femoral-tibial prosthetic internal rotation of up to 17°.

Boldt et al. has studied the tibial shaft axis method with the LCS total knees comparing the resultant posterior condylar axis with the transepicondylar axis. He found the posterior condylar reference of implanted LCS components paralleled the transepicondylar axis (mean 0.3°). Lateral patellar subluxation was seen in two knees where there was femoral component internal rotation of 4° and 6°. In another study, Boldt found a consistent relationship of femoral component internal rotation (average 5° internal to the transepicondylar axis) and arthrofibrosis from a variety of causes [2].

While the flexion space cuts depend primarily on ligamentous tension, one must avoid certain pitfalls that may occur. For example, if the leg is fixed in a leg holder at 90°, it is possible for the weight of an obese leg to place an artificial tension on the lateral side of the joint, distorting the appropriate ligament tension. With the flexion spacing jig, the surgeon should carefully assess this to make certain that tension and position are appropriate. Also if an unusual amount of medial or lateral condyle will be resected, the surgeon must check the primary extension balance to make certain that all is correct.

The advantage of surgical navigation with the tibia cut first approach is accurately determining the proximal tibial cut. This is critical as the remaining operation is based off of this cut. The other particular gains of surgical navigation are to accurately determine frontal and sagittal plane alignment such as whether the not the knee comes to full extension with prosthetic insertion. It is anticipated that navigation will displace the need for intra-medullary determination of the distal femoral cut, typical of most current systems. With evolution, ligamentous balancing may be enhanced by pressure sensitive electronic devices applied to the spacing blocks.

Conclusion

The author's experience using the tibial cut first method with the LPS-High Flex mobile bearing total knee has been highly favorable and not a single case of bearing dislocation has been noted to date. The additional design

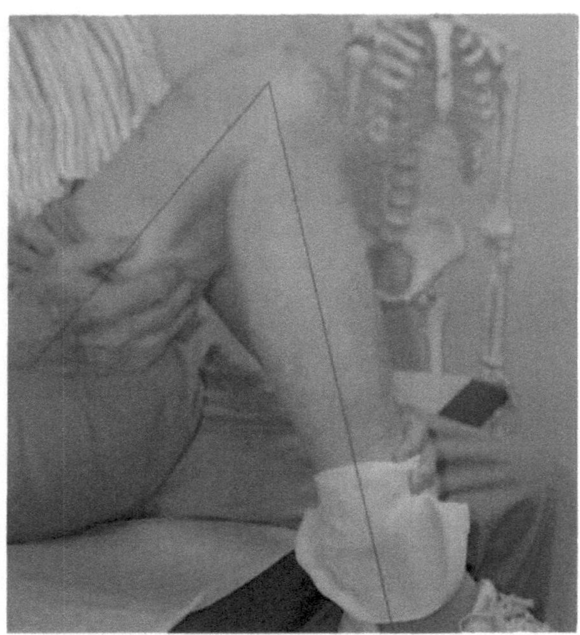

◘ Fig. 25-9. LPS High Flex total knee with early flexsion of 135°

features of the LPS High Flex femoral component with the post/cam articulation and the enlarged prosthetic femoral condyles have allowed extraordinary flexion not found in earlier series. Experience and careful attention to detail can explain this result with a conscious effort of achieving perfect knee flexion/extension balancing and mechanical alignment (◘ Fig. 25-9). The tibial shaft axis method developed for the LPS High Flex surgical technique relies on the anatomical relationship of the mechanical axis of the tibia shaft being virtually perpendicular to the transepicondylar axis in both flexion and extension (◘ Fig. 25-10). Surgical navigation will allow accurate orientation of the tibial cut and confirm anatomical knee alignment during the surgical procedure.

References

1. Berger RA, Rubash HE, Seek MJ, Thompson WH, Crossett LS (1993) Determining the rotational alignment of the femoral component in total knee arthroplasty using the epicondylar axis. CORR 286: 40–47
2. Boldt JG, Munzinger UK, Keblish PA, Drobny T, Varma CL (2001) CT Evaluation of Femoral Rotational Aignment in TKA: Comparison of the Tibial Shaft Axis Method to the Transepicondylar Line. Proceedings of the AAOS Annual Meeting, Feb 13-17, Dallas, Texas, page 438
3. Bert JM (1990) Dislocation/subluxation of meniscal bearing elements after New Jersey low-contact stress total knee arthroplasty. CORR 254: 211–215
4. Fehring TK (2000) Rotational malalignment of the femoral component in total knee arthroplasty. CORR 380: 72–79
5. Insall JA, Binazzi R, Soudry M, Mestriner LA (1983) Total knee arthroplasty. CORR 192: 13–17
6. Mantas JP, Bloebaum RD, Skedros JG, Hoffmann AA (1992) Implications of reference axes used for rotational alignment of the femoral component in primary and revision knee arthroplasty. J Arthroplasty 7: 531–535
7. Olcott CW, Scott RD (2000) A comparison of 4 intraoperative methods to determine femoral component rotation during total knee arthroplasty. J Arthroplasty 15: 22–26
8. Scott WN, Rubinstein M, Scuderi G (1988) Results after knee replacement with a posterior cruciate substituting prosthesis. JBJS 70A: 1163–1173
9. Stiehl JB, Abbott BD (1995) Morphology of the transepicondylar axis and the application in primary and revision total knee arthroplasty. J Arthroplasty 10: 785–789
10. Stiehl JB, Cherveny PM (1996) Femoral rotational alignment using the tibial shaft axis in total knee arthroplasty. CORR 331: 47–55

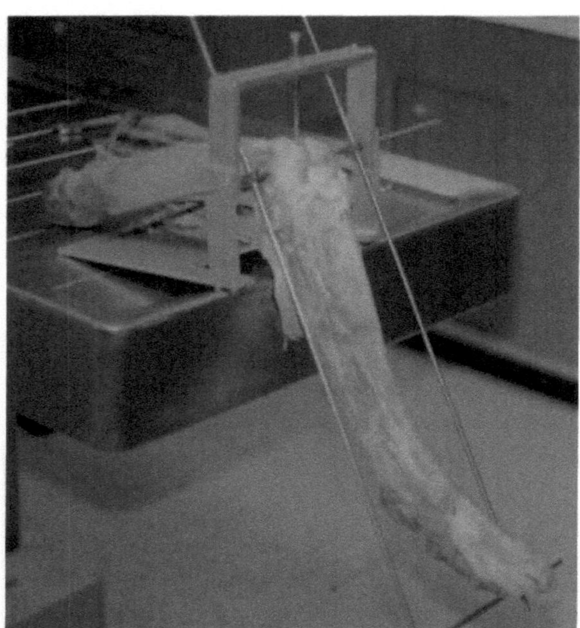

◘ Fig. 25-10. Cadaver specimen demonstrates perpendicular relationship of tibial shaft axis to the transepicondylar axis with transecting pin

26 Femur First Approach in TKA – Surgical Techniques

K. A. Krackow

Background — Evolution

Unquestionably, the era of modern total knee replacement commenced with the production of the Polycentric Knee Prosthesis designed by John Gunston of Canada, in the late 1960's. This prosthesis was soon followed by the Geomedic Knee developed by a design team of five by the prosthesis manufacturer Howmedica. Both prostheses incorporated the technology pioneered by John Charnley in the U.K., combining methylmethacrylate bone cement with cobalt chrome alloy or adequate stainless steel.

The Polycentric design consisted of four separate pieces that had to be properly aligned, while the Geomedic seemed to be so simple, made up of only two pieces, that only two rudimentary instruments were used for its implantation by most surgeons. Certainly in the USA the latter became a popular prosthesis from 1971 through about 1975.

With the development of »condylar« knees, those with a single piece of metal essentially enveloping the femoral condyles, surface contact was enlarged and a desire for more specific cutting guides arose. As well, these designs involved preparation of the anterior bone, because they provided for covering the trochlear groove of the femur. Very importantly, these designs sacrificed both cruciate ligaments and relied upon dishing-camming action to engage the collateral ligaments to block untoward anterior and posterior displacement, i.e. indirectly substitute for the cruciate ligaments.

At this stage, total knee instrumentation was still relatively primitive. The major change evolved with the introduction of the Universal Instrumentation System from Howmedica, which was developed in association with the first three-component, fully uncemented porous ingrowth prosthesis. Such an initially press-fit, uncemented design naturally called for a relatively precise set of femoral bones cuts that clearly had to be made with the help of cutting block jigs. The conceptualization of these jigs introduced the problem of how best to position them, leading to rather more specific cutting jigs. The basic starting point of femoral preparation, and later tibial resection relied upon a new technique whose term this author coined, »measured resection«. The concept then, as well as now, was to remove the amount of bone from each surface which corresponded to the thickness of the prosthesis at that location. Such specific placement of the bone cuts, together with the recognition that malalignment, in terms of varus-valgus deformity, was associated with early failure, led to an interest in associating the placement of cutting jigs correctly to establish proper axial alignment. The first system to accomplish this in an acceptably sophisticated way was probably the Universal Knee Instrumentation System of Howmedica.

Probably because of the emphasis on accurate placement of femoral cuts the Universal Knee Instruments led the surgeon to prepare the femur first, which is the major issue of this chapter. Ever since this change, orthopaedists have always raised questions as to which is better: »femur first or tibia first«, and »what are the differences?«.

Gap Kinematic Differences (Measured Resection vs. Gap Balancing)

In theory, measured resection and equi-replacement reestablish the anatomic relationship of the epicondyles to the femoral joint surfaces. It is clear from cadaver studies addressing ligament attachment positions that to a very good approximation ligaments function properly with the desired »isometry« if their origin position is at or closely related to the epicenters/axes of tibio-femoral, flexion-extension rotation. For essentially circular condylar geometry, and considering relatively conforming or dished tibial plateau geometry, these centers of femoral rotation nearly coincide with the centers of femoral surface curvature.

In contrast, the alternative and pre-existing technique – flexion-extension gap balancing – started with a tibial resection. The knee was next flexed to 90° and the posterior femoral condyles resected, leaving just enough space to equal the thickness of the posterior femoral condyles combined with the thickness at the articular surface of the tibial component. Finally, the knee was taken to full extension and the distal femur was resected at a distance that also matched the combined component thickness. Some attention was directed to the varus/valgus orientation of the distal cut, but with relatively crude instrumentation.

Important as well was the recommendation to perform a relatively shallow resection at the proximal tibial surface so that the remaining interface for the tibial component would be the hardest tibial bone available. One must agree that, in at least a moderate number of cases, this latter consideration leads to »over-replacement« of the tibia. And, such over-replacement of the tibia is likely to move the circular geometry of the distal femur a bit proximal and anterior to the original center of rotation or curvature.

An advantage of the flexion-extension gap technique is that one establishes theoretically equally sized gaps at 90° and 0°. One disadvantage, though, is that isometry and optimal ligament balance may not be achieved elsewhere in the flexion cycle. However, the alternative, measured resection technique, does not survive this analysis unscathed. First, developmental as well as degenerative changes in femoral geometry may make it impossible to achieve ideal ligament attachment position with this technique either. And most notably, the common problem of at least mild flexion contracture is totally unaddressed by measured resection. The gap balancing technique would seem to address automatically the achievement of full extension. Most smaller to even medium-sized flexion contractures are not so bad that the knee cannot be brought to full extension once the upper tibial cut is made.

It seems that the definite positioning of femoral cutting blocks inherent in the measured resection method had great appeal. Not only did one get good fit with the

bone preparation, but the associated alignment rods helped maintain or establish proper alignment better than earlier instruments. As a result, we see the incorporation of measured resection with prosthesis systems such as the Total Condylar and posterior substituting Insall-Burstein, both of which originally called upon gap balancing, again, with minimal tibial resection.

To some degree one could argue that the wide acceptance of measured resection now including the tibial surface as well as all of the femoral ones, made any distinction between femur-first and tibia-first largely moot. For many surgeons using many popular posterior cruciate substituting prostheses however, equi-resection of all surfaces, i.e. all five surfaces of the standard femoral preparation and the upper tibia, does not even theoretically lead to perfect gap balancing. This statement follows from work which shows that PCL resection typically leads to disproportionate enlargement of the 90° flexion gap. This observation and its real-life situation do not create a major problem. One may simply resect a few more millimeters of distal femoral bone to enlarge correspondingly the extension gap.

At this point it is this author's conclusion that there need not be, with most modern instrumentation, a fundamental difference between preparing the femur or the tibia first. The only differences would exist if one did not understand the alterations that are necessary still to achieve equality of the gaps. These steps however do not fundamentally depend upon the order of the cuts. However one further point is necessary or implicit in accepting the validity of the first sentence in this paragraph.

Prior to the more modern instrumentation, the levels or thickness of the distal and posterior femoral resection were not the only features referenced from the previously cut tibial surface. Also, at the femur the varus-valgus position and the internal external rotational preparation were referenced from the tibia. The tibia was held in tension, distracted away from the femur in full extension, and the distal femoral cut was marked and later executed parallel to the tibial surface. With this practice alignment results are accurate if there is no soft tissue varus or valgus deformity or if perfect ligament balancing has been achieved. Again, for the extension situation, when either of these conditions does not hold, one has soft tissue balance but not ideal, perhaps even satisfactory axial alignment.

While very few surgeons follow this method today for the distal femoral cut, at least some follow it for the anterior and posterior femoral cuts. These latter cuts are also the preparation aspect that establishes femoral component internal and external rotation. Another way of describing this is to recognize that altering the anterior and posterior femoral cuts via an internal/external rotation is tantamount to creating a varus or valgus positioning of the tibia with respect to the femur, in flexion. To repeat, we are referring to the practice of distracting the femur away from the tibia, here lifting it up when the knee is at 90 degrees of flexion, and then resecting the posterior, then anterior femoral surfaces parallel to the residual cut surface at the tibia

The greatest material difference between femur-first and tibia-first is based upon the practices described in the last two paragraphs. It is probably safe to say, that the difference actually exists only with regard to femoral component internal and external rotation, or varus-valgus position in flexion. It does not commonly exist with regard to the varus-valgus orientation of the distal femoral cut, hence alignment in extension. Today there are very few surgeons who reference the varus-valgus orientation of the distal femoral cut from the distracted tibial surface. However, the anterior and posterior preparation of the femur, completion of the flexion gap is another thing.

It is properly argued that in many cases, and particularly the non-deformed knee, it is preferable to rotate externally the preparation of the tibial component to »square-up« the flexion space and provide symmetric ligamentous stability at 90° of flexion. One can reasonably accept this as preparation of the anterior and posterior femur parallel to the tibial surface. The real differences and debate arise when there is either unreleased deformity that persists during flexion or extensive collateral and cruciate release, sometimes necessary to achieve full correction and proper varus-valgus alignment in extension. In the former situation with under release and under correction, the femur remains tight on the concave side of the deformity. Preparation of the anterior and posterior femoral cuts parallel to the tibia, places the femoral component in a malrotated orientation – malrotated to the degree of inadequate alignment correction in flexion. Similarly, shown in the cadaver laboratory, analyzed in detail, also recognized non-quantitatively by Insall, when extensive collateral release is necessary in extension, one can see proportionately greater opening of the gap at the released side in flexion.

This excessive opening, only in flexion, can be especially dramatic with lateral collateral release. It is even significant with major medial release, sometimes leading to as much as 9°–10° of excessive external rotation of the distracted femur. That is, with such over-release the femur, distracted from the tibia in flexion, rotates abnormally away from the originally tight side. In valgus cases the femur goes into substantially excessive internal rotation with large lateral collateral and popliteus tendon releases, and starting from varus, the femur can go into excessive external rotation.

Given the abnormal internal or external positioning of the femur that results, placing the femur parallel to the tibia puts it in an opposite, abnormal position. On the externally rotated femoral bone, the femoral component winds up internally rotated. In the valgus case with excessive internal rotation of the femur, the component sits in rather excessive external rotation. Three degrees of external rotation to compensate for the non-anatomicity of the proximal tibial perpendicular cut is okay. But an additional 3, 5, or greater degree of external rotation has not been shown over time to be safe.

It also follows that such potentially non-anatomic rotation of the femoral component, even external, leads to malrotation of the limb from the level of the femoral component to the ankle and foot. This rotation is what one would see in extension. In flexion, the non-anatomic rotation, as mentioned above is seen as persistent or new varus-valgus deformity in flexion.

One may attempt to negate, let us say, the potential external rotation of the distal leg due to a larger than 3 to 5 degree »external rotation« of the femoral component. And, this attempt would most logically involve placement the tibial component with a similar amount of external rotation. One can or may expect, however, a collateral ligament conflict in flexion. And, given the nearly perpendicular cut of the tibia, rotating the tibial component externally does not correct the varus positioning in flexion.

Another way of characterizing these differences in femoral preparation is to say that the original measured resection technique led surgeons to emphasize bony landmark orientation of the components, especially the femoral. The alternative tibial-first and flexion-extension gap balancing methods emphasized or created resulting alignment guided by soft tissue considerations.

When one points out the potential for malrotation by referencing the femur from the tibia in flexion, those of opposite persuasion agree about the potential but say that it is either not frequent, not large, or, if large, recognized and some compensation made. Still, those who follow bony alignment argue that in moving from the tibia to the femur one may not always be able to recognize the existence of a problem. The surgeon, following the dictates of squaring the flexion space moves ahead unknowingly. If that surgeon notices an extreme situation this awareness must come from either sharp observation or specific instrumentation together with judgment about the overall appearance of the distal femur. That surgeon needs then to admit that he or she is leaving the dictum of the rectangular flexion space in favor of staying more normally oriented to bony geometry. Interestingly, those advocates never seem to say anything about this possibility in their writing or lecturing.

Mechanical Instrumentation

Utilizing computer-based navigation techniques ultimately eliminate the need for our current types of mechanical instruments. If bone resection is to be done by a hand-positioned saw, however, a requirement for cutting blocks or jigs still exists. The difference is that in the computer setting these mechanical pieces are positioned according to computer feedback rather than by threading the IM canals or measuring only mechanically from joint surfaces. We have the presumed advantage of not manipulating the intra-medullary canals, which manipulation is known to introduce some degree of fat and bony debris embolization. Furthermore, we eliminate many assumptions inherent in mechanical instrumentation. The computer-based system is aligning with the determined center of femoral head, center or centers in the knee and the center of the ankle. Certainly on the femoral side, great accuracy has been claimed for IM instrumentation. But we never know the exact offset angle, the angle between the course of the IM instrument rod as one ray and the line from the center of the distal femur to the center of the femoral head the other.

Working more directly with the axis of the tibia with navigation technology also eliminates problems of tibial bowing and the difficulty of getting IM instrument rods to travel a sufficient distance in the tibia to indicate the tibial axis accurately.

Wrap up

With regard to the issues of femur first vs. tibia first, mechanical instrumentation developers and users need to be aware of the points and distinctions made throughout this chapter. This statement is true not only for our traditional mechanical instrumentation, but also for the currently evolving mechanical accoutrements still necessary for hi-tech knee navigation.

27 Femoral Component Alignment in TKA

J. G. Boldt

Introduction

Femoral rotation positioning is critical for successful total knee arthroplasty (TKA). There are three generally accepted methods of referencing femoral component rotational alignment. These include the transepicondylar axis (TEA), as advocated by Insall, arbitrary external rotation from the posterior condyles, and the so-called Whiteside line. Another less well recognized method, which has been used for over 25 years is referencing femoral component rotation perpendicular to the tibial shaft axis via a balanced flexion tension gap. Placing the femoral component parallel to the TEA leads to a biomechanically sound knee motion in full flexion and extension. However, this method has potential errors that include any anatomical deviations of the distal femur, which may occur in cases with severe varus or valgus angle deformity, condylar dysplasia, or other rotational pathology of the lower extremity.

Clinical outcomes after TKA are dependent upon multifactorial issues; one of which is femoral component rotational alignment. Prosthetic design and implantation of femorotibial components vary with different total knee systems. The surgeon must evaluate and address variables that include varus-valgus alignment, extra-articular deformities, soft tissue contractions, exaggerated Q angle, patella position, size, and shape as well as femorotibial rotation. Intraoperative variables include surgical approach, femorotibial stability, soft tissue management, extensor mechanism and patella treatment, prosthetic selection and positioning. Femoral component rotational alignment has gained more attention in the recent literature, since component malpositioning »negatively« influences knee kinematics, including patellofemoral tracking and range of motion.

Recent successful navigation of femoral component rotational positioning is usually referenced to either CT data or intra-operative identification of the transepicondylar axis. Both methods lack in appreciation of soft tissue tension in both knee flexion and extension ultimately leading to sound TKA biomechanics. The authors has recently developed a spacer tool able to measure tension of the collateral ligaments in both 90° of flexion and full extension. Raw data collected on one knee cadaver showed that this device appears to deliver valuable pressure information, however, data alterations depending on leg position, leg weight and other factors remain challenging.

The TEA is the most commonly referenced anatomic landmark for rotational positioning of the femoral component in TKA. It is reported as being more predictable than Whiteside's line or the posterior condyle. However, the TEA depends on estimated landmarks and may be altered in both varus and valgus knees and/or other pathological variations that may change lower limb rotational axes. Tibial rotation position, an important consideration in fixed bearing designs, is also a factor that affects gap balance and the patellofemoral joint. Tibial rotational positioning is of lesser concern in mobile-bearing TKA because of the ability (of the bearing) to adapt to tibiofemoral rotation in flexion and extension.

Rotational malpositioning creates a trapezoidal rather than rectangular flexion gap with an altered patellofemoral articulation and unbalanced femorotibial kinematics. Instability in flexion with a tighter medial and more lax lateral compartment occurs when the femoral component is internally malrotated. This is frequently combined with lateral patellofemoral subluxation and instability (lift-off) of the lateral compartment in flexion. In most TKA systems, for a given amount of tibial resection, there is an appropriate amount of posterior condylar resection required to create a symmetric flexion gap. Different opinions of surgical approach

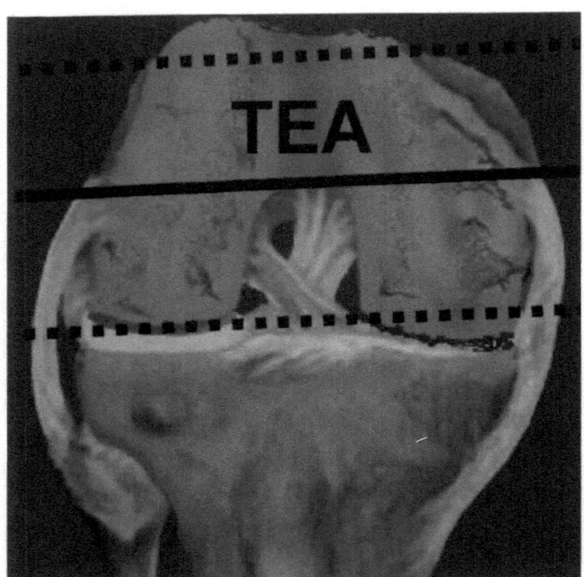

Fig. 27-1. The transepicondylar axis (Insall) is identified after intra-operative identification of both lateral and medial femoral epicondyles. Potential errors are landmark inconsistencies, previous trauma, femoral rotation, and ability to digitally identify both medial and lateral epicondyles

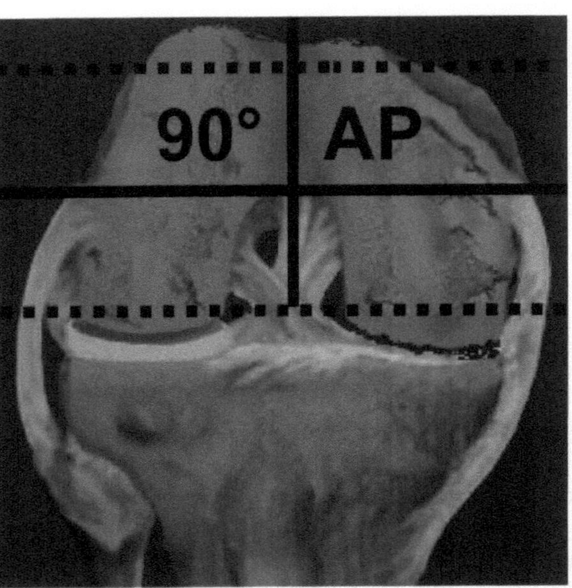

Fig. 27-2. The anteroposterior femoral axis method (Whitesides's line) references femoral rotation perpendicular to that line, which places the component approximately parallel to the transepicondylar line. Potential errors are femoral rotation variables, previous trauma, or patellofemoral diseases that may hinder anatomical identification

exist regarding soft tissue releases, tibia first or femoral first bone cuts, as well as the femoral rotation resection. The most common method of tibial resection is perpendicular to the mechanical axis with some posterior inclination.

The three established methods of determining femoral rotational positioning in TKA consist of: the transepicondylar axis as advocated by Insall (■ Fig. 27-1), Whiteside's line, or a line perpendicular to the anteroposterior femoral axis (■ Fig. 27-2), referencing 3 to 4° external rotation from the posterior condyles (■ Fig. 27-3). The posterior condylar reference as described by Hungerford (■ Fig. 27-4) is seldom utilized since it results in consistent femoral internal rotational positioning, often excessive. The LCS method is based on the tibial shaft axis and balanced flexion gap and has been utilized since 1977 with mobile bearing TKA (■ Fig. 27-5). Potential advantages and errors of each method will be discussed.

Olcott and Scott have recently reported that these three widely accepted methods were consistent in yielding a symmetric, balanced flexion gap within 3°. However, significant variable and inconsistencies were noted.

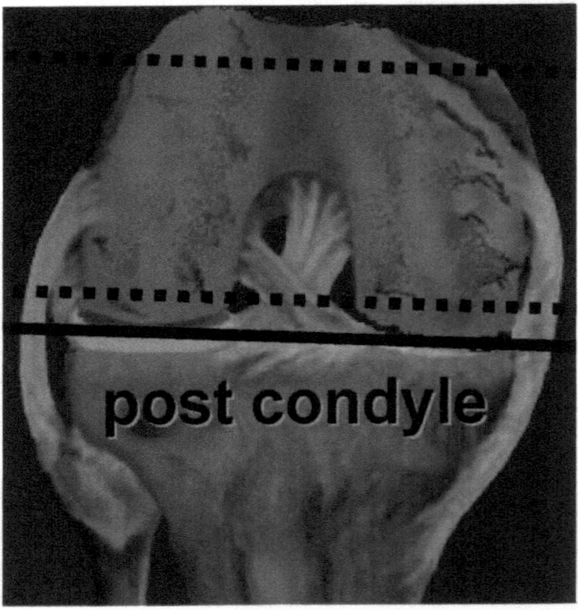

Fig. 27-3. Referencing femoral rotation in 3–4° external rotation to the posterior condylar line leads to an component positioning that approximates to the transepicondylar line, but has a large angular range. This method is arbitrary, based on estimates with variable reference lines in possibly distorted condyles, particularly in valgus or varus deformities

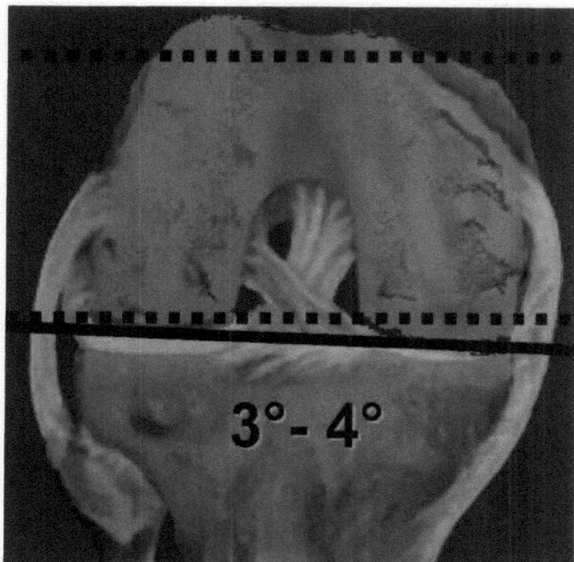

▫ Fig. 27-4. Referencing femoral rotation from the posterior condylar line leads to an internally mal-rotated component positioning with an average of 4–5° to the transepicondylar axis, which requires varus tibial resection and increased valgus femoral resection to achieve a balanced rectangular flexion tension gap. Internal rotation will also have negative impact to the patellofemoral articulation

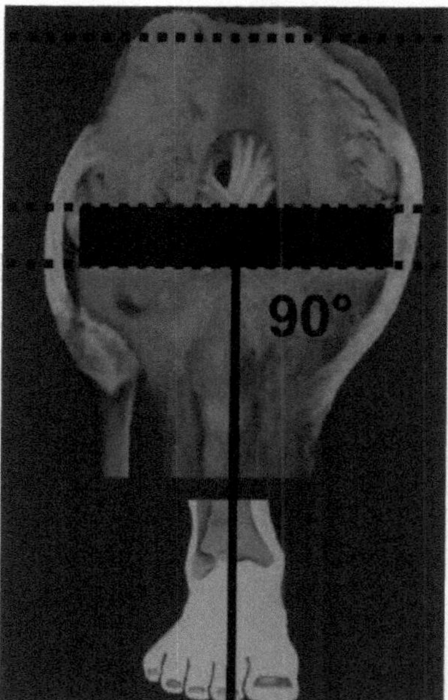

▫ Fig. 27-5. Referencing femoral rotation perpendicular to the tibial shaft axis and a balanced flexion tension gap (LCS method) leads to prospectively predictable alignment parallel to the transepicondylar axis (mean 0.3°)

The transepicondylar axis failed to yield flexion gap symmetry in 10% of neutral varus TKA and 14% valgus TKA, with discrepancies varying from 9° too little to 6° too much external rotation, which is less than desirable. The authors recommended using a combination of these methods to avoid potential malresections.

Clinical studies by Stiehl and Cherveny compared the tibial shaft axis method to other methods for determining femoral rotation in four different fixed bearing knee systems utilizing a femoral first approach. With the post-condylar method, 72% required lateral release with 7% patella fractures reported. When 4 to 5° of external rotation method was used, 28% lateral release were reported. When the tibial shaft axis method was utilized, femoral component placement was reported within 1° of external rotation compared to the TEA. There were decreased number of lateral releases required and no patella complications. Katz et al. showed in a cadaver study of eight knees (a three-surgeon evaluation) that determination of femoral component rotational positioning was more reliable using a balanced flexion gap and the anteroposterior axis. A similar study performed by Jerosch et al. emphasized that the inaccuracy of anatomically identifying the TEA of the femur by eight surgeon in three knee cadavers was 23 degrees. Intra-operative evaluation of the femoral epicondyles and the TEA is less predictable and accurate than previously established methods. The method used to define femoral rotation with the LCS system is referenced on a tibial cut perpendicular to the tibial shaft axis and a symmetrical (rectangular) flexion gap. This method automatically defines the position of the free moveable femoral resection guide (▫ Fig. 27-6), avoiding the need of identifying anatomical landmarks. A rectangular spacer block is then applied to the rotationally unconstrained femoral component and sits flat on the tibial resection. The flexion tension is set and checked for proper balance (▫ Figs. 27-7 and 27-8). The extension gap is balanced to the flexion gap with a distal femoral resection, establishing the mechanical axis. (▫ Fig. 27-9).

Comparison of this tibial axis method with the TEA methods adds to our understanding of this most important technique step in TKA. CT scan evaluation is the most accurate method to objectively assessing femoral component rotational placement compared to a known anatomic landmark post TKA. In order to clinically investigate the accuracy of the LCS method with regard to

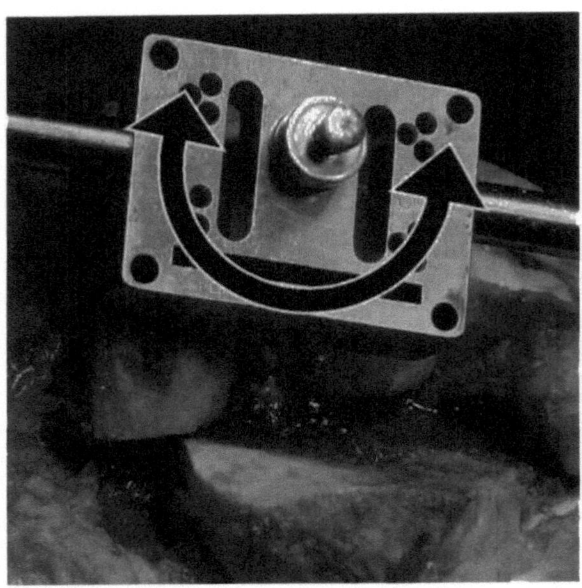

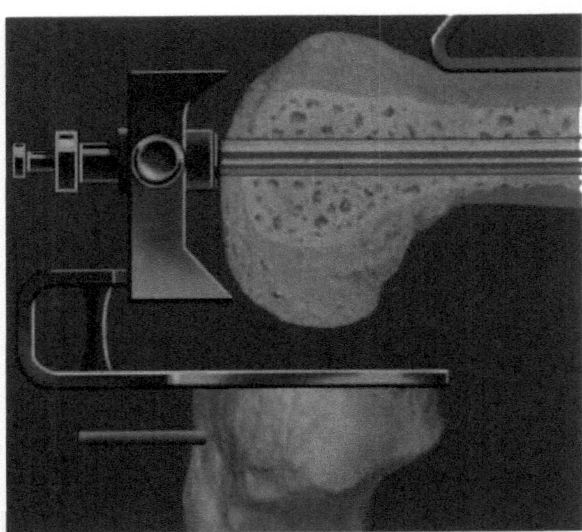

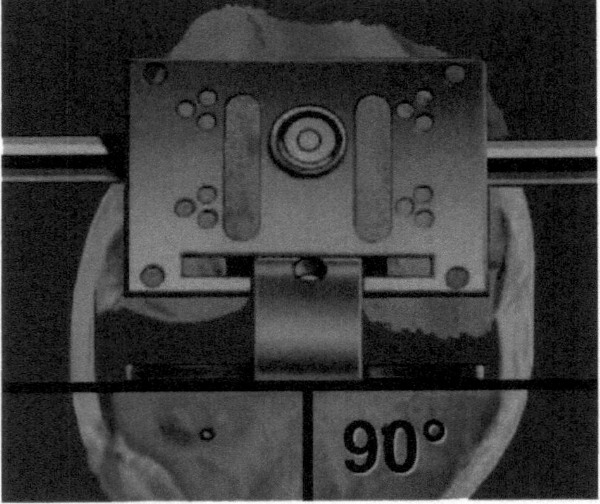

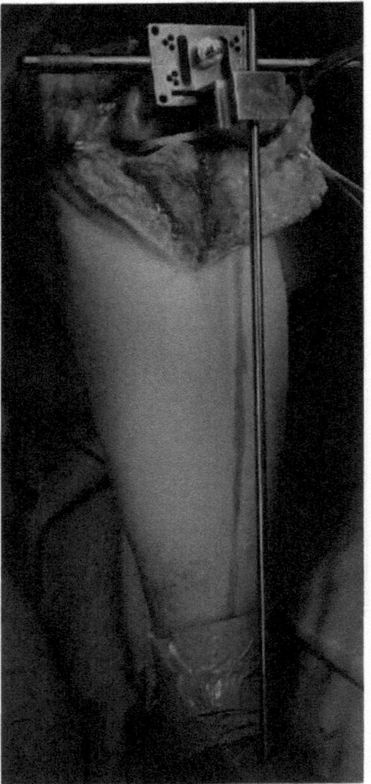

Fig. 27-6. Free moveable femoral resection guide is attached to an intra-medullary femoral rod

Fig. 27-7. Spacer block (perpendicular to the tibial shaft axis) is attached to the femoral component and sits flat on the tibial resection for flexion balance check and determination of femoral rotational alignment

Fig. 27-8. Tibial resection is perpendicular to the tibial shaft axis and femoral resection block parallel to the tibial resection

Fig. 27-9. Spacer block determines rotational alignment of the femoral resection block with a balanced rectangular flexion tension gap setting the guide parallel to the tibial shaft axis

femoral component rotational positioning, we performed a study in which helical CT scan investigation was used referencing the femoral prosthetic placement to the transepicondylar axis. From a cohort of 3058 mobile bearing low contact stress (LCS, Depuy Int, Leeds, UK) TKA, 40 (1.3%) clinically well functioning knees were randomly selected for evaluation of femoral component rotational alignment. All patients with TKA in this center underwent routine clinical examination and follow-up radiographs at 1 week, 6 weeks, 1 year, 5 years, or when complications occurred. Mean age in this cohort was 67 years (range 54 to 77). Inclusion criteria for this subset was range of motion (ROM) over 100 degrees, lack of pre- or postoperative complications, and excellent or good clinical results according to a modified HSS 100-point clinical score with a mean of 91.2 points (81 to 100). One patient had to be excluded because of inability to identify appropriate anatomical landmarks on CT scans, and another patient refused CT investigation. Of the 38 cases available for this study, the patella was left unresurfaced in 36 (95%) cases, one was previously patellectomized, another patella was resurfaced using a metal-backed rotating patella component.

Follow-ups at regular intervals included a clinical evaluation and X-ray protocol. Radiographic analysis was focused on patella tracking, congruency, and patella tilt with comparable pre- and postoperative skyline radiographs. Patella tracking was based on alignment of the femoral trochlear sulcus and the crown of the patella and measured in millimeters of lateral deviation on comparable pre- and postoperative skyline views.

The ultimate 38 cases were randomly selected from patients who were scheduled by a computerized system for 1-, 5-, or 10-year routine follow-up. These patients were invited to participate in the study until the appropriate number was obtained. Of the two cases eliminated one patient refused to participate, another was eliminated for technical reason as noted. Of this group all patients had excellent or good clinical results and no patient refused participation. The local university ethics committee approved the study.

All cases were investigated by one of two consultant musculoskeletal radiologists with CT experience of more than fifteen years. Before the start of the examination, they examined a few patients not included into the investigation in order to use the same criteria, which were identical to those used for everyday examinations. The radiologists were not aware of the patients' knee status (single blinded). They were instructed not to talk with the patients about the status of their knees but about techni-

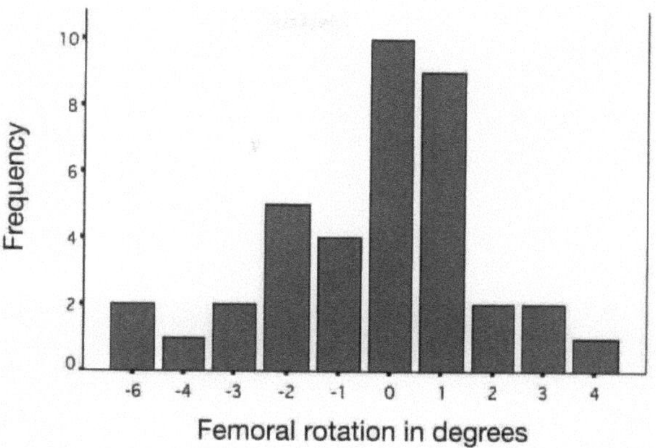

Fig. 27-10. Femoral component alignment parallel to transepicondylar axis ensures optimum patellofemoral tracking

cal CT aspects only. All data for femoral component rotational positioning were analyzed using a helical CT scanner. Femoral component rotational alignment was calculated by referencing the two posterior condyles to the transepicondylar axis, which was a line drawn between the spike of the lateral epicondyle and the sulcus of the medial epicondyle as recently recommended by Yoshino et al. (**Fig. 27-10**). One case was excluded because of inability to identify the medial sulcus despite 2 mm cuts. Angles were calculated utilizing sophisticated helical CT-implemented software.

An independent statistician analyzed all data. The distribution of angles in each group were analyzed using the one-sample Kolmogorov-Smirnov test which indicates whether the number of cases is sufficient and a normal »bell-curve« distribution is demonstrated. A positive Kolmogorov-Smirnov test validates further parametric statistical analyses.

The subset of 38 cases (follow-up: 12 to 120 months) studied in this series had clinical results comparable to a larger cohort group of over 3000 TKA. All cases were well-functioning knees with good or excellent clinical results. The mean ROM was 115° (range 100 to 135). Preoperatively, 3 of 38 cases had documented patella subluxation and tilt of more than 6°. Postoperatively all three achieved perfect patellofemoral tracking. Decreased height and sclerosis of the lateral patella facet was seen in two case without clinical symptoms. There were no fixation failures, no patella failures and no re-operations for any reason in this group.

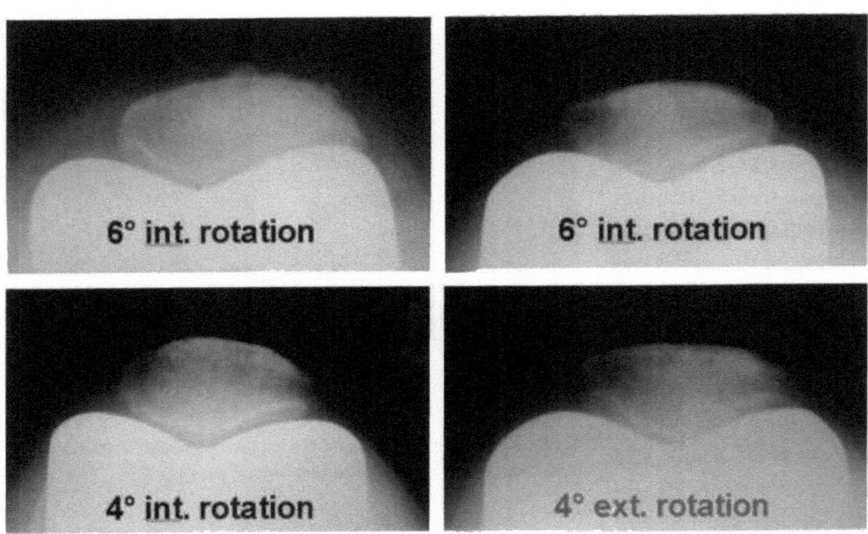

Fig. 27-11. Transversal CT scans are a practical method for accurate determination of femoral component rotational positioning in TKA best referenced to the transepicondylar axis. Example of a well-aligned femoral component parallel to the TEA

Mean femoral alignment was near parallel (0.3° internal rotation) to the TEA with a range of 6° internal to 4° external rotation (**Fig. 27-11**). Standard deviation was 2.2 and standard error 0.4. All angles were normally distributed using one-sample Kolmogorov-Smirnov test, which validates a statistical mean value and outliers. Four

cases fell outside of the predicted mean value (more than 3° internal or external rotation). Three had internal rotation and one case had external rotation. All four cases with maximum internal and external rotation showed perfect patellofemoral tracking on skyline views (**Fig. 27-12**). The data of our study emphasizes that correct femoral component rotational positioning, utilizing the tibial shaft axis method, results in a high level of consistency for accurate patellofemoral alignment and predictable clinical outcome (**Fig. 27-13**). Vice versa internal malrotation of the femoral component is more likely associated with patella maltracking and anterior knee pain (**Fig. 27-14**).

In summary, femoral rotational alignment based on the tibial axis and balanced flexion tension is an instrumented technique that

- avoids relationship to arbitrary landmarks;
- establishes a precise flexion gap which allows for a stable relationship to the corrected biomechanical axis;
- is patient-specific regarding bone and soft tissue variations,
- is reproducible (especially in severe deformities such as the valgus knee), and
- results in predictable patella outcomes in reported series.

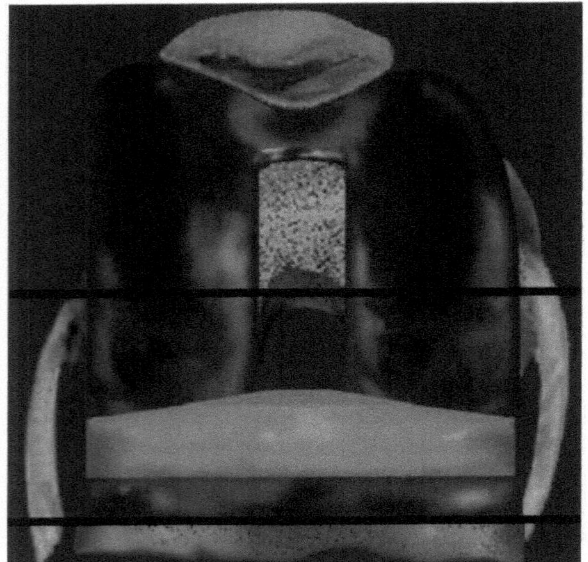

Fig. 27-12. Graph showing normal distribution of femoral component rotational alignment in the subset group. Mean rotation of the femoral component was parallel (0.3°) to the transepicondylar axis, ranging from 6° internal to 5° external rotation

Femoral component rotational alignment is technique- and instrument-dependent and influences patella

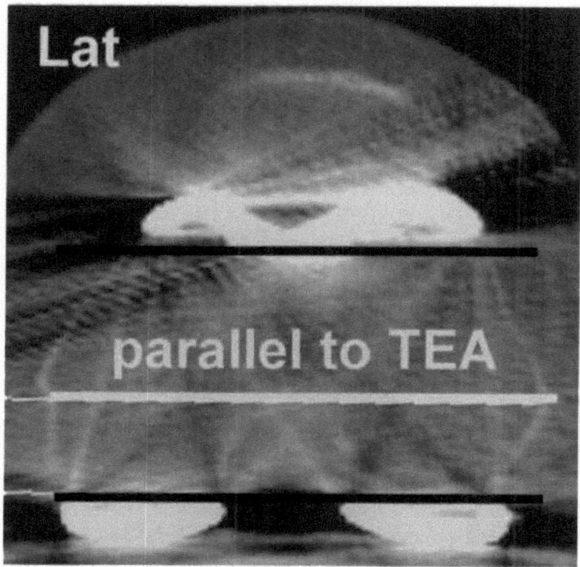

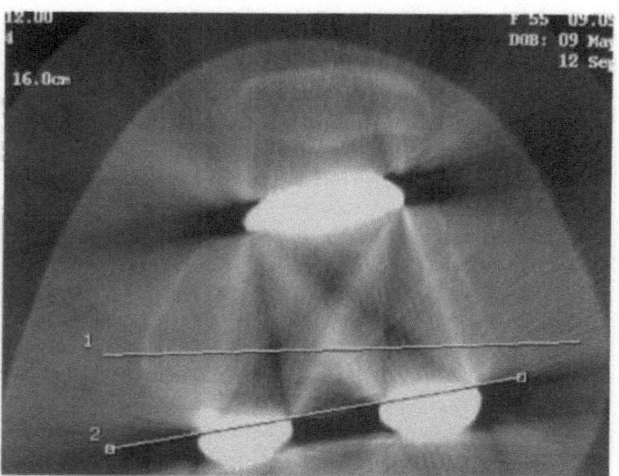

◻ Fig. 27-14. Patello-femoral tracking and flexion gap balancing and tensioning depends on optimal femoral component rotational alignment, which should be parallel to the transepicondylar axis as demonstrated

◻ Fig.27-13. Femoral component internal malrotation leads to a number of potential proplems including primarily pain, functional impairment, reduced ROM, patella maltracking, tight medial and lax lateral flexion gap, and is, as shown in our studies, associated with developing arthrofibrosis

Acknowledgements. U. Munzinger MD for all clinical data and support (Zurich, Switzerland); J. Hodler MD and M. Zanetti MD for CT data (Zurich, Switzerland); P. Keblish MD for manuscript review (Allentown, PA, USA); C. Varma BS for illustrations (Allentown, PA, USA)

tracking, gap balance, and soft tissue kinematics. Deviation into internal rotation results in less than ideal patellofemoral tracking and clinical outcomes. Potential complications, such as the painful and/or stiff TKA (arthrofibrosis) have been shown to correlate with significant internal rotation of the femoral component. The tibial shaft axis method as used with the LCS system provides perfect rotational alignment without anatomical landmark identification, and is, therefore, felt to be more predictable than all other currently practiced methods.

Most navigation and robotic systems do not greatly appreciate the importance of a biomechanically well balanced TKA. We think that our recently developed spacer block will add information to a better understanding of TKA biomechanics with improved soft tissue tension. The concept of implementing tension data in both flexion and extension in knee arthroplasty will certainly enhance TKA function and hopefully clinical long-term outcome. Implementation of knee tension data into existing navigation tools (and proven TKA designs) may represent a perfect symbiosis of all techniques available today.

References

1. Akagi M, Matsusue Y, Mata T, Asada Y, Horiguchi M, Iida H, Nakamura T (1999) Effect of rotational alignment on patellar tracking in total knee arthroplasty. Clin Orthop 366: 155–163

2. Arima J, Whiteside LA, McCarthy DS, White SE (1995) Femoral rotational alignment, based on the anteroposterior axis, in total knee arthroplasty in a valgus knee. A technical note. J Bone Joint Surg Am 77: 1331–1334

3. Berger RA, Crossett LS, Jacobs JJ, Rubash HE (1998) Rotation causing patellofemoral complications after total knee arthroplasty. Clin Orthop 356: 144–153

4. Berger RA, Rubash HE, Seel MJ, Thompson WH, Crossett LS (1993) Determining the rotational alignment of the femoral component in total knee arthroplasty using the epicondylar axis. Clin Orthop 286: 40–47

5. Buechel FF (1982) A simplified evaluation system for the rating of the knee function. Orthop Rev 11: 97–101

6. Churchill DL, Incavo SJ, Johnson CC, Beynnon BD (1998) The transepicondylar axis approximates the optimal flexion axis of the knee. Clin Orthop 356: 111–118

7. Dennis DA, Komistek RD, Walker SA, Cheal EJ, Stiehl JB (2001) Femoral condylar lift-off in vivo in total knee arthroplasty. J Bone Joint Surg Br 83: 33–39

8. Eckhoff DG, Piatt BE, Gnadinger CA, Blaschke RC (1995) Assessing rotational alignment in total knee arthroplasty. Clin Orthop 318: 176–181

9. Engh GA (2000) Orienting the femoral component at total knee arthroplasty. Am J Knee Surg 13: 162–165

10. Fehring TK (2000) Rotational malalignment of the femoral component in total knee arthroplasty. Clin Orthop 380: 72–79

11. Griffin FM, Insall JN, Scuderi GR (2000) Accuracy of soft tissue balancing in total knee arthroplasty. J Arthroplasty 15: 970–973

12. Griffin FM, Insall JN, Scuderi GR (1998) The posterior condylar angle in osteoarthritic knees. J Arthroplasty 13: 812–815

13. Hungerford DS (1995) Alignment in total knee replacement. Instr Course Lect 44: 455–468

14. Katz MA, Beck TD, Silber JS, Seldes RM, Lotke PA (2001) Determining femoral rotational alignment in total knee arthroplasty: Reliability of techniques. J Arthroplasty 16: 301–305

15. Lonner JH, Siliski JM, Scott RD (1999) Prodromes of failure in total knee arthroplasty. J Arthroplasty 14: 488–492

16. Mantas JP, Bloebaum RD, Skedros JG, Hofmann AA (1992) Implications of reference axes used for rotational alignment of the femoral component in primary and revision knee arthroplasty. J Arthroplasty 7: 531–535

17. Nagamine R, Miura H, Bravo CV et al. (2000) Anatomic variations should be considered in total knee arthroplasty. J Orthop Sci 5: 232–237

18. Nagamine R, Miura H, Inoue Y (1998) Reliability of the anteroposterior axis and the posterior condylar axis for determining rotational alignment of the femoral component in total knee arthroplasty. J Orthop Sci 3: 194–198

19. Olcott CW, Scott RD (1999) The Ranawat Award. Femoral component rotation during total knee arthroplasty. Clin Orthop 367: 39–42

20. Olcott CW, Scott RD (2000) A comparison of 4 intraoperative methods to determine femoral component rotation during total knee arthroplasty. J Arthroplasty 15: 22–26

21. Poilvache PL, Insall JN, Scuderi GR, Font-Rodriguez DE (1996) Rotational landmarks and sizing of the distal femur in total knee arthroplasty. Clin Orthop 331: 35–46

22. Scuderi GR, Insall JN, Scott NW (1994) Patellofemoral pain after total knee arthroplasty. J Am Acad Orthop Surg 2: 239–246

23. Stiehl JB, Abbott BD (1995) Morphology of the transepicondylar axis and its application in primary and revision total knee arthroplasty. J Arthroplasty 10: 785–789

24. Stiehl JB, Cherveny PM (1996) Femoral rotational alignment using the tibial shaft axis in total knee arthroplasty. Clin Orthop 331: 47–55

25. Stiehl JB, Dennis DA, Komistek RD, Keblish PA (1997) In vivo kinematic analysis of a mobile bearing total knee prosthesis. Clin Orthop 345: 60–66

26. Stiehl JB, Dennis DA, Komistek RD, Crane HS (1999) In vivo determination of condylar lift-off and screw-home in a mobile-bearing total knee. J Arthroplasty 14: 293–299

27. Whiteside LA, Arima J (1995) The anteroposterior axis for femoral rotational alignment in valgus total knee arthroplasty. Clin Orthop 321: 168–172

28. Yamada K, Imaizumi T (2000) Assessment of relative rotational alignment in total knee arthroplasty: usefulness of the modified Eckhoff method. J Orthop Sci 5: 100–103

29. Yoshino N, Takai S, Ohtsuki Y, Hirasawa Y (2001) Computed tomography measurement of the surgical and clinical transepicondylar axis of the distal femur in osteoarthritic knees. J Arthroplasty 16: 493–497

27

28 Computer-Assisted Ligament Balancing of the Femoral Tibial Joint Using Pressures Sensors

R. C. Wasielewski, D. D. Galat, R. D. Komistek

Introduction

Premature wear of the ultra-high molecular weight poly-ethylene (UHMWPE) tibial insert has been implicated in total knee arthroplasty (TKA) failure [6,7]. Several variables are thought to contribute to polyethylene wear including patient factors, implant design, and surgical technique. While the factors in implant design that optimize implant longevity (such as large contact areas and high conformity) have been defined and implemented, surgical technique has been more difficult to quantitatively evaluate, because it remains more subjective and surgeon-dependent. Therefore, advances in surgical technique that lead to improved implant longevity have been difficult to define.

Soft-tissue balancing requires correct prosthetic alignment with simultaneous release of contracted ligaments about the knee in order to optimize articular geometry, a factor in polyethylene wear. Poor balancing likely contributes to early polyethylene wear. It is hypothesized that when balance is optimized, the pressures in the medial and lateral compartments at TKA should be approximately equal. However, a method of easily and accurately measuring these pressures has been difficult to develop. The purpose of this study is to evaluate a newly developed, intraoperative, computer-instrumented tibial insert trial that measures knee compartment pressures throughout a passive range of motion. Results from this study begin to quantify ligament balancing, thus more clearly illuminating the role that surgical technique plays in polyethylene wear and TKA function. In addition, it is felt that if real-time evaluation of ligament balancing via measurement of compartment pressures could be performed intraoperatively, the surgeon would be more able to optimize implant function and longevity.

Materials and Methods

Thirty-eight patients with knee osteoarthritis (OA) were implanted with a posterior cruciate sacrificing (non-ps) LCS total knee arthroplasty (TKA) by the same surgeon (Dr. Ray Wasielewski, Ohio State University) utilizing a »balanced gap« technique. This technique involves utilizing an extra-medullary alignment jig to cut the tibia perpendicular to its long axis. Afterwards, while simultaneously ensuring normal limb alignment, the knee compartments were balanced in extension with appropriate ligament releases, as determined by the surgeon. After balancing in extension, a rectangular flexion gap was created using a tensor instrument. While equal tension was applied to both knee compartments with the tensor, the femoral cutting guide rotated about a femoral intra-medullary guide until a rectangular gap was created (◘ Fig. 28-1). The gap size in flexion was measured and the distal femoral resection was performed to create an extension gap of the same size. With equal sized and shaped gaps in both flexion and extension, the final femoral and tibial preparations were done to accept the trial implants.

After placement of the femoral and tibial baseplate trial implants on the cut bone surfaces, a computer-instrumented tibial insert trial was placed for trialing (◘ Fig. 28-2). This device, which measures pressures within the compartments of the knee, was developed by modifying an FDA approved pressure sensing matrix array (Novel Electronics, Inc., Munich, Germany) and incor-

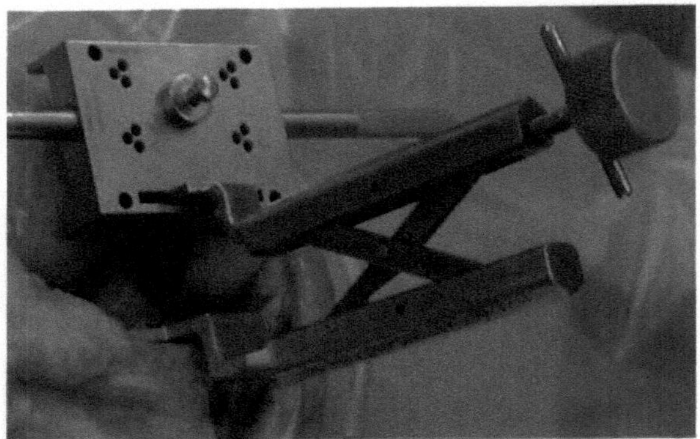

Fig. 28-1. Dynamic tensioning device used to rotate the femoral cutting guide to create a rectangular flexion gap relative to the cut tibial surface. An inter-medullary femoral rod provides the axis about which the guide rotates

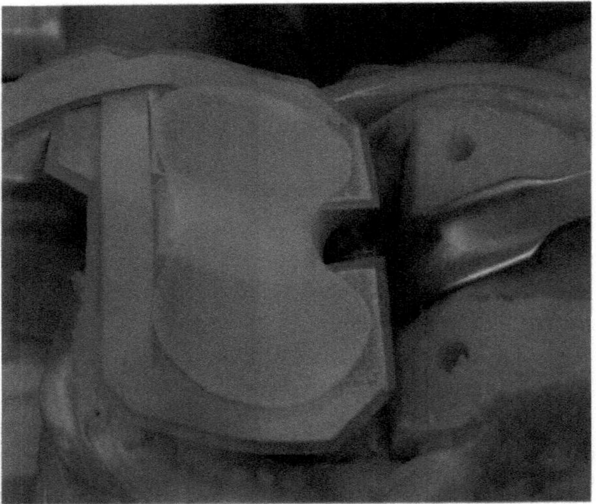

Fig. 28-2. Pressure sensing insert device being placed within the knee joint for trialing

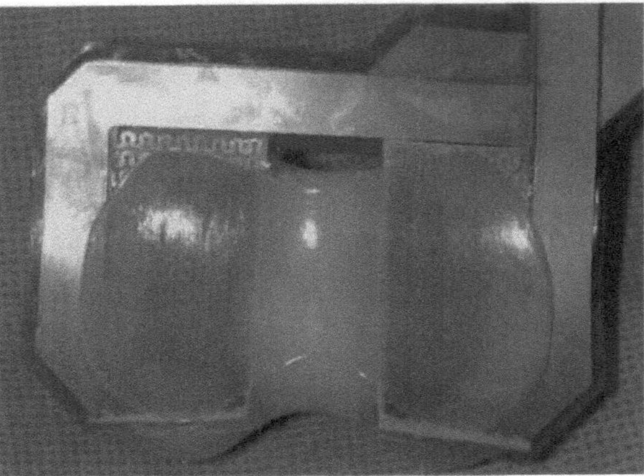

Fig. 28-3. The newly developed pressure sensing device. The device is a modification of a Novel pressure matrix array attached to the upper surface of a tibial polyethylene insert trial. It is sandwiched between the insert trial and a protective low molecular weight polyethylene covering

nism. With trials and sensor in place, the knee was then taken through a passive range of motion from 0–120 degrees. The magnitude and distribution of medial and lateral compartmental pressures was documented throughout this range while video footage was simultaneously gathered (**Figs. 28-4a,b**). Intraoperative stress testing was performed by the surgeon at 0°, 15°, 60°, and 90° to subjectively assess compartment balance, and the results were recorded. After the pressure data was obtained and the stress testing was complete, the device was removed from the knee and the arthroplasty completed. Data from the pressure sensors was compared with stress testing to establish correlations. Normal peri-operative protocols for TKA were instituted, including three to six weeks of physical therapy.

porating it into a TKA trial polyethylene insert (**Fig. 28-3**). The sensor matrix array was glued with silicone adhesive to the trial polyethylene insert, then covered with a protective low molecular weight polyethylene covering. The trial was shaved prior to incorporation of the matrix array so the overall thickness of the instrumented insert would approximate the standard size of the original insert. After the sensor device was placed in the knee, the quadriceps mechanism was re-approximated with three sutures – one directly medial and one each in the infra-patellar and suprapatellar aspects of the extensor mecha-

Results

Computer-generated pressure nomograms were created from data gathered by the intraoperative pressure sensor for all thirty-eight patients enrolled in the study. These nomograms provided information on force (N), area of force distribution (cm^2), and pressure (N/cm^2) in both the medial and lateral knee compartments in flexion and extension (**Figs. 28-5a,b**). Differences in pressure magnitude and distribution between the medial and lateral

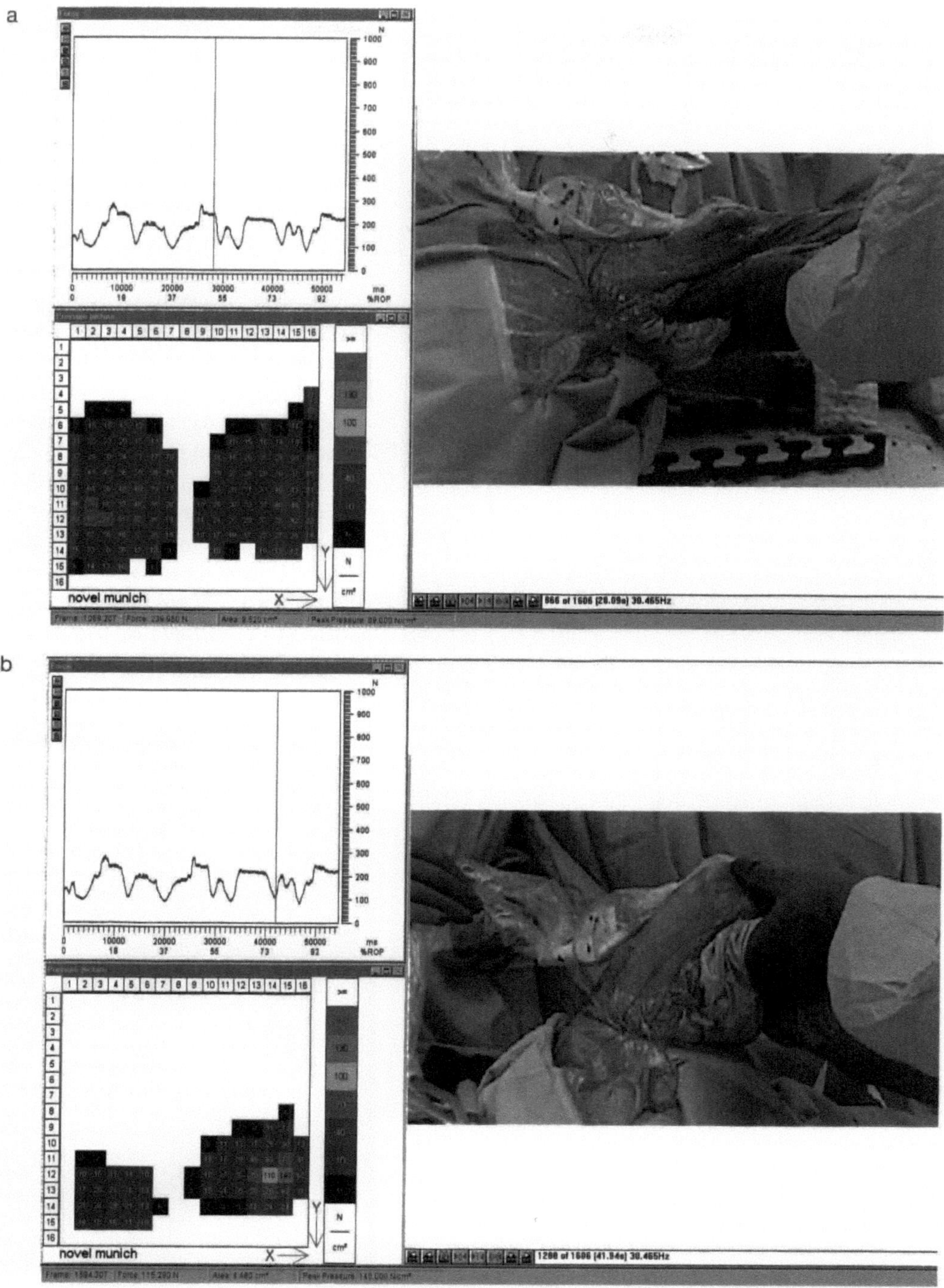

Fig. 28-4a, b. **a** Intraoperative sensor data showing force and pressure measurements and video for patient #4 with the knee in extension. This knee is well balanced in extension, the sensor showing similar pressure and area measurements for both the medial and lateral compartments. **b** Intraoperative sensor data showing force and pressure measurements and video for patient #4 with the knee in flexion. This knee is slightly unbalanced in flexion, the sensor showing slightly dissimilar pressure and area measurements between the medial and lateral compartments

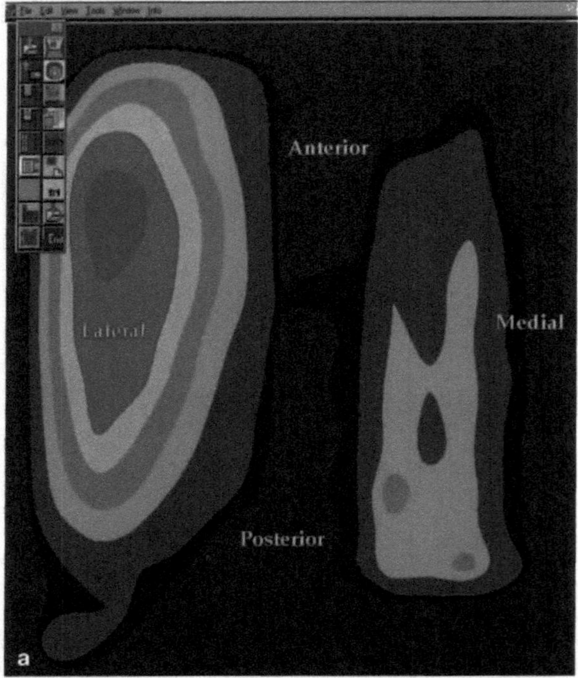

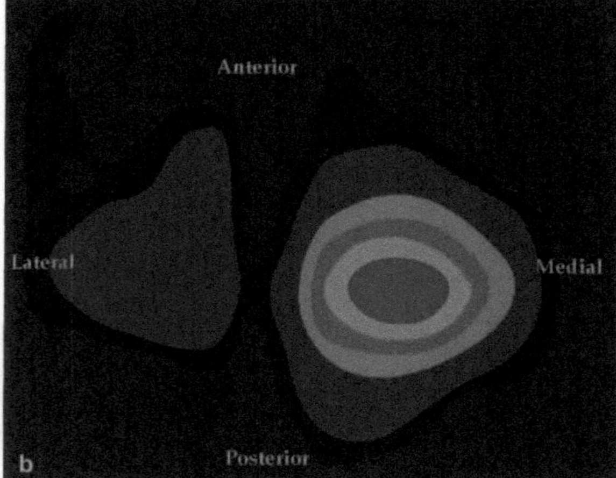

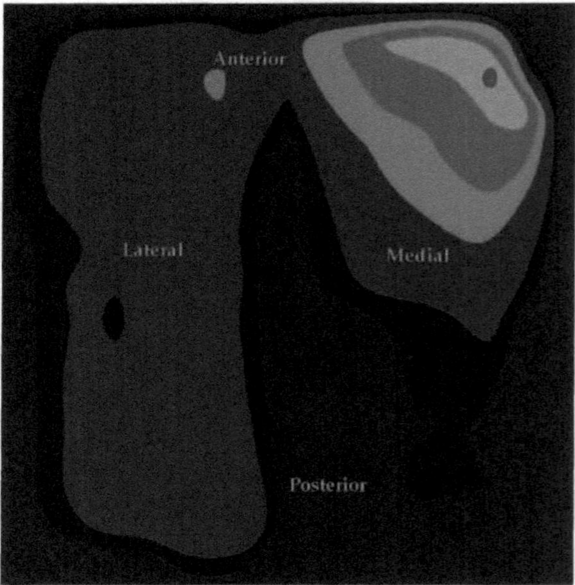

balanced. When pressures were greater in one compartment as compared with the other, or where contact areas were not equal, knees were presumed to be unbalanced.

Compartment pressures between 10–40 N/cm^2 appeared blue on the pressure nomogram and were considered optimal. Of the thirty-eight patients who underwent pressure analysis using the sensor device, nine had maximum pressures in the red and pink ranges (>130 N and >160 N, respectively). Six patients had maximal pressures to these ranges in extension and three in flexion (see Fig. 28-5b). Five patients had a pattern of decreased area of increased pressure in the anteromedial aspect of the medial compartment in extension (◘ Fig. 28-6). All of these patients had extensive surgical release of the medial collateral ligament (MCL) leaving the pes anserinus insertion intact to medially stabilize the knee in extension. All five had pressures greater than 100 N/cm^2 with one patient having a maximum pressure greater than 150 N/cm^2. The contact areas in extension for these five patients averaged 10.9 cm^2. The median pressure with this pattern was 25.3 N/cm^2. No patients with this pattern experienced loss of pressure in one or both compartments

◘Fig. 28-5a, b. a Pressure nomogram demonstrating contact patterns in extension. Note the pressure and contact area differences between the medial and lateral compartments. b Pressure nomogram demonstrating contact pattern in flexion. Note the decreased forces laterally and increased forces medially

compartments were also appreciated from the pressure nomograms. Knees in which both compartments had approximately equal pressures and distributions throughout a passive range of motion were presumed to be well

◘ Fig. 28-6. Example of pressure nomogram in patient having extensive release of the medial collateral ligament, while leaving the pes anserinus insertion intact to serve as the dynamic medial knee stabilizer. Note the high pressures and relatively small contact area in the anteromedial corner of the medial compartment

with early flexion (between fifteen and thirty degrees), nor did any patient enrolled in this study (i. e. no patient enrolled experienced midstance instability).

The average contact area in extension was 11.5 cm^2 (range, 8.33–14.2 cm^2). The average contact area in flexion was 6.2 cm2 (range, 2.80–8.22 cm^2). The average force in extension was 346 N (range, 264–405 N). In flexion it was 143 N (range, 55–247 N). The average pressure in extension was 23.8 N/cm2 (19.8–35.6 N/cm^2) and in flexion was 21.2 N/cm2 (18.7–33.2 N/cm^2).

In all cases of compartment imbalance detected by the surgeon during intraoperative stress testing, the sensors revealed similar compartment pressure imbalance and/or abnormally high pressures. In addition, in twelve instances, the sensors detected subclinical compartment abnormalities not detected by the surgeon – four cases in extension (0 degrees) and eight in flexion (90 degrees).

Discussion

Other attempts have been made to measure knee compartment pressures with some success. Takahashi et al reported improved varus-valgus stability with intraoperative assessment of compartment pressures using pressure-sensitive film and sequential ligament releases based upon the resultant stress pattern [4]. Furthermore, Wallace et al. were able to balance compartment pressures via PCL release after quantifying knee compartment pressures with an electronic pressure transducer [5]. Morris et al. reported the use of an instrumented tibial component with transducing load cells located between the tibial tray and polyethylene insert [3]. The device used in the present study has several advantages over these previous pressure sensing devices. The Novel sensor matrix array was highly conformable to curved surfaces. This enabled placement of the transducers between the articulating surfaces, thus allowing the sensor to be equidistant from the femoral implant counter-surface throughout the range of motion. This increased the sensitivity of this device in measuring contact areas between the femoral and tibial components and the resultant patterns. In addition, the device allowed real-time feedback of both absolute and relative compartment pressure data.

In all cases, the instrumented insert-sensing device successfully measured compartment pressures through-

out the range of motion during trialing of the provisional TKA components. In addition, intraoperative varus and valgus stress testing with the sensing device in place confirmed that real-time increases and decreases in compartment pressures were being detected. In every case that stress testing detected a compartment imbalance, the sensors also recorded compartment pressure imbalance and/or abnormalities. In addition, the sensors detected twelve cases (eight in flexion and four in extension) of subclinical compartment abnormalities not appreciated with stress testing. Thus, we found that the pressure readings were more sensitive than surgeon feel, especially in flexion, where variables including tourniquet placement, patient size, and stability of setup can make qualitative assessment of ligament balance difficult. However, as this device is applied earlier in arthroplasty, its sensitivity may actually be a limitation, if the surgeon attempts to balance the TKA too perfectly. Rather, avoiding pressures in the yellow, red and pink areas, and equalizing and optimizing the size and location of contact areas, should be the objective.

The device and its intraoperative computerized pressure outputs do provide the surgeon some quantitative feedback on gap balance and ligament tension. After calibration, the device was capable of measuring absolute force and pressure values. But, the absolute pressures measured by the device as the knee was taken through the range of motion are likely different than those that will occur with the final insert and components in place. Differences in thickness between the device used to measure pressure and the actual insert implanted in the patient, as well as variations in the thickness of the cement mantle are probable factors accounting for these theorized pressure differences. Ideally, the sensing device should be the same size as the final tibial insert implanted in the knee. During manufacture of the device, variations in thickness of the layer of silicone adhesion and the depth of shaving of the trial insert caused variations in thickness of the device of up to 0.5 mm when compared with the final implanted tibial insert. Additionally, the actual pressures measured by the device as the knee was taken through the range of motion are likely different than those experienced with weight bearing as there is a substantial kinematic difference between the loading conditions during trialing and intraoperative stress testing, and the forces that occur with weight bearing and other activities of daily living [2]. Thus, because of these probable variations, the device likely functions more as a relative – rather than absolute – measure of compartment pressure differences. However, even as a relative measure of pressure differences, the sensor device provides the surgeon with additional insight into the adequacy of knee balance, component position, and alignment. It remains to be seen, however, if this intraoperative information correlates to implant longevity, failure, or patterns of wear at explantation.

The sensors provided important pressure nomogram data depicting contact area patterns and pressure differences between the compartments. In all patients, the contact areas were relatively large, which corroborated the theoretical advantages of the mobile-bearing knee; that is, a highly conforming articulation of large contact areas and low stresses [1]. Decreased contact areas in extension were most commonly due to over-release medially or from pathological medial or lateral laxities (e.g. valgus and varus knees, respectively). The most common cause of decreased area in flexion was over-release medially in extension, which caused a slight concomitant medial laxity in flexion. Additionally, in some cases, slight femoral component over-rotation resulted in decreased area in the medial compartment in flexion. This slight femoral component over-rotation may be attributed to the use of the tensor to balance the knee in flexion. When using the balanced gap technique, the tensor applies pressure to the compartments of the knee in flexion and the AP cutting guide rotates about an intra-medullary guide the appropriate degree in order to create a rectangular flexion gap. We found that when too much tension was applied with the tensioning device, femoral component over-rotation occurred. If the gap was over distracted with the tensioning device greater than 4 mm over the final gap size, too much posteromedial distal femoral bone was resected. Thus, the final flexion gap was not rectangular, but rather slightly trapezoidal. As a result, the trial femoral component was slightly over-rotated, causing a medial laxity in flexion apparent on the sensor nomogram. On the other hand, when just enough tension was applied to distract the flexion gap, the proper amount of bone was resected thus allowing correct femoral component rotation, a rectangular flexion gap, and approximately equal medial and lateral compartment pressures.

Anteromedial tightness was seen in five of the thirty-eight patients. This pattern was characterized by a relatively high-pressure region of low contact area in the anteromedial corner of the medial compartment (see Fig. 28-6). These patients all had severe preoperative varus deformities requiring extensive release of the medial collateral ligament (MCL) while leaving the pes anserinus insertion intact to serve as the dynamic medial stabilizer of the knee in extension. None of these patients experienced midstance instability. The retained pes musculature is presumed to create this pattern of pressures. However, it remains unclear if these anteromedial forces from the dynamic stabilizers will create unacceptable patterns of wear on retrievals. These pressures were almost two orders of magnitude less than the yield point of the polyethylene, so it is unlikely that they will cause accelerated wear. However, these in vivo stresses will likely be amplified by loading conditions. Therefore, the long-term effects will not be known until future insert retrieval studies are performed.

The instrumented insert accurately recorded magnitude, location and dynamic imprint of the pressures in the medial and lateral compartments, intraoperatively. Data from this sensor begins to provide objective evaluation of ligament balancing and confirmed the importance of accurate surgical technique and compartment balancing in achieving good total knee arthroplasty function. Hopefully, the data provided by this sensor will allow the surgeon to better understand those aspects of surgical technique that directly affect implant function and longevity. In addition, as the sensors are employed earlier in TKA, compartment imbalance may be mitigated.

References

1. Heim CS, Postak PD, Greenwald AS (1996) Factors influencing the longevity of UHMWPE tibial components. Instructional Course Lectures 45:303–312
2. Komistek RD, Stiehl JB, Dennis DA, Paxson RD, Soutas-Little RW (1998) Mathematical model of the lower extremity joint reaction forces using Kane's method of dynamics. J Biomech 31:185–189
3. Morris BA, D'lima DD, Slamin J et al. (2001) e-Knee: Evolution of the electronic knee prosthesis: telemetry technology development. J Bone Joint Surg 83A:62–66
4. Takahashi T, Wada Y, Yamamoto H (1997) Soft-tissue balancing with pressure distribution during total knee arthroplasty. J Bone Joint Surg 79B:235–239

5. Wallace AL, Harris ML, Walsh WR, Bruce WJ (1998) Intraoperative assessment of tibiofemoral contact stresses in total knee arthroplasty. J Arthroplasty 13: 923—927

6. Wasielewski RC (2002) The causes of insert backside wear in total knee arthroplasty. Clin Orthop Rel Res 404: 232–246

7. Wasielewski RC, Galante JO, Leighty RM, Natarajan RN, Rosenberg AG (1994) Wear patterns on retrieved polyethylene tibial inserts and their relationship to technical considerations during total knee arthroplasty. Clin Orthop Rel Res 299: 31–43

29 Computer-Assisted Pressure Measurement in the Patellofemoral Joint with Electronic Pressure Sensors

J. Mortier, L. Zichner

Introduction

The patella forms a sesamoid bone in the quadriceps muscle. It has different functions. Apart from force conduction and forming a lever arm for the quadriceps muscle it influences the friction coefficient between quadriceps and femur. A missing patella is last cut not least noted cosmetically. The first developed knee endoprostheses considered the patella only on a peripheral base. Follow-up studies of total knee replacements showed the peripatellar region to be of importance in approximately 10% of the patients complaining about problems [1, 2, 5, 7, 16, 18, 20, 28, 34]. Surgical indication, surgeon and type of endoprosthesis influence the decision for or against patellar replacement during total knee replacement (TKR). Major problems of the patellofemoral region are pain, lateralizing of the patella and rarely soft tissue impingement, patellar fractures and patellar loosening. Literature shows supporters for [6, 21, 26, 29, 33] as well as opponents against patellar replacement [3, 9, 22]. Data are available which speak in favor of both preferences. Although our understanding of the patellofemoral geometry has improved, technical errors continue to play a role in the postoperative course [15, 26, 27]. To function appropriately patella height, patellofemoral contact area and the 3-dimensional position of the patella have to be considered [23]. Walking and squatting differ in the transferred body weight by factor three [19]. In order to achieve an optimal patella position film pressure measurements have been undertaken [10—12, 13, 14, 24, 25]. According to these studies maximal pressures occur between 45° and 60° of flexion. Anatomical patellar variants with maximal contact area show reduced pressure values. Tri-pod patellas show lower intra-osseous maximal tension values compared to single pod patellas [14]. Lateral patellofemoral contact area, femoral external rotation and the lateral femoral placement of the endoprosthesis seem to influence patellofemoral pressure values [8, 17, 18, 28, 31, 32, 34]. Initially favored metal-backed patellas are currently not the first choice due to polyethylen wear followed by possible metal wear [4, 30]. To achieve information about the dynamic joint motion in endoprosthetic knee replacement we performed ex vivo studies and plan in vivo studies with intra-articular pressure sensors.

Material and Methods

The knees were studied in the department of forensic medicine at the University of Frankfurt/Main (Prof. Dr. Bratzke) after obtaining appropriate ethics committee approval. Pressure measurements are performed using the novel pliance system (www.novel.de). The basis for the novel systems are calibrated capacitive sensors (◘ Figs. 29-1 and 29-2). As a result of design and material selection, the sensor pad is flexible and elastic (up to 4% of the original length) and has the ability to conform around highly contoured sites without wrinkling. The individual sensor elements are arranged in a matrix with up to 256 sensors per pad. Maximum sensor resolution is 14 sensors/cm^2, pressure range within 10 kPa and 2 MPa depending on sensor type and sensor thickness is between 0.6 and 1.2 mm. All sensors are individually calibrated and provide pressure data with an accuracy of approxi-

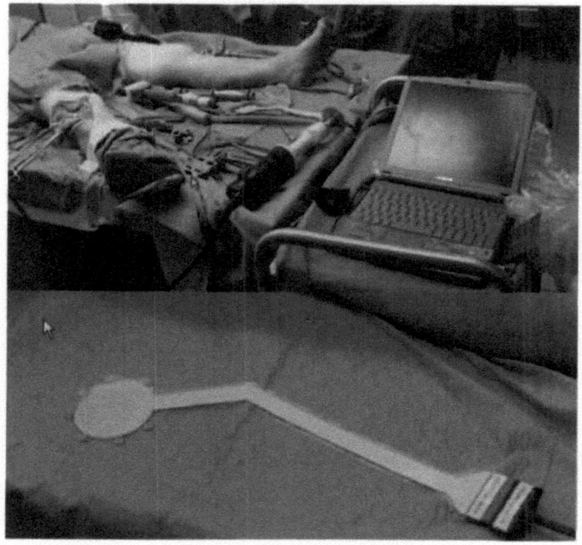

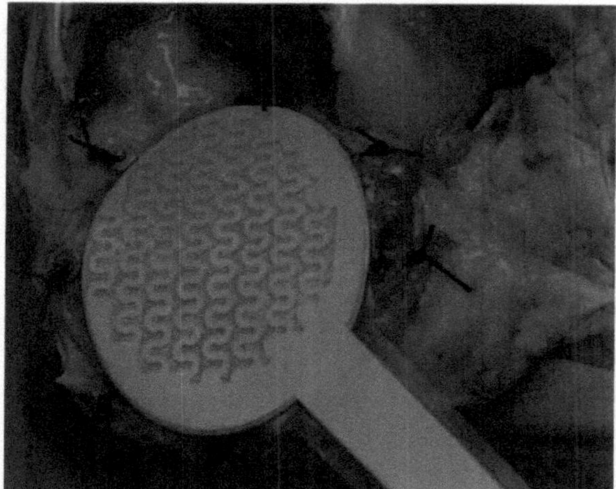

Fig. 29-1. Experimental setup in the department of forensic medicine (*above*) and close up view of the sensor (*below*)

Fig. 29-2. With seven stitches in place sutured sensor (patella everted laterally)

mately 5%. Sensor hysteresis lies between 2 and 7% depending on sensor type. The sensor can be sterilized and utilized in physiological environments in vitro and in vivo during surgical procedure. Pressure data acquisition can be performed on or off-line by a PC, Bluetooth telemetry system or connected to a small pocket PC. Sensors are scanned with a scanning speed of 10,000 sensor signals per second. Fast data collection, analysis and

presentation are performed two- or three-dimensionally via a software package which operates as a Windows application. The sensors are sutured in place in a congruent position to the patella alignment. Ten repeated measurements are made at each flexion angle and then averaged.

Results

Repeated measurements show identical values ensuring validity of the data. Increasing flexion angles corresponds with increasing pressure values (■ Fig. 29-3).

Pressure measurements without any (femoral, tibial or patellar) prosthetic replacement show mean values at 90 degrees of flexion of 80 N/cm^2.

Use of different patellar buttons does not show increased pressure values as compared to no patellar replacement (■ Fig. 29-4).

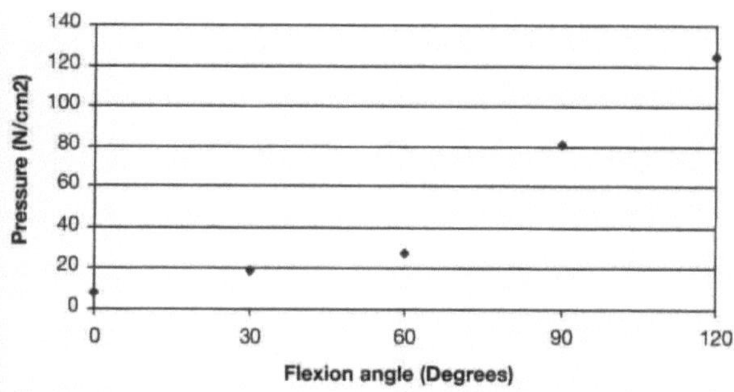

Fig. 29-3. Flexion angle (degrees) versus femoropatellar pressure measurements (N/cm^2; n=12)

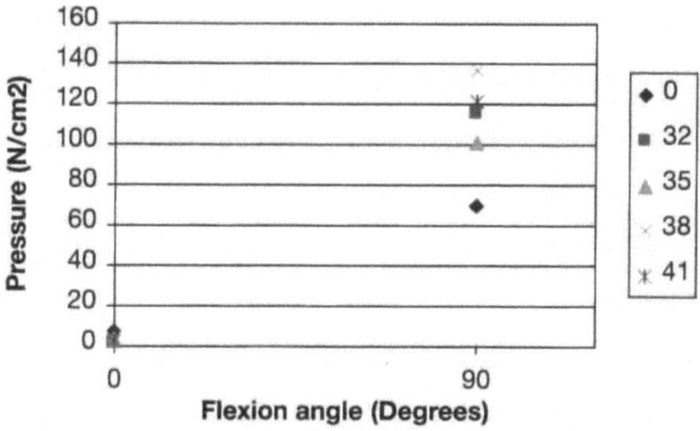

Fig. 29-4. Pressure values (N/mm2) at 0 and 90 degrees of flexion with different patellar button sizes (n=4)

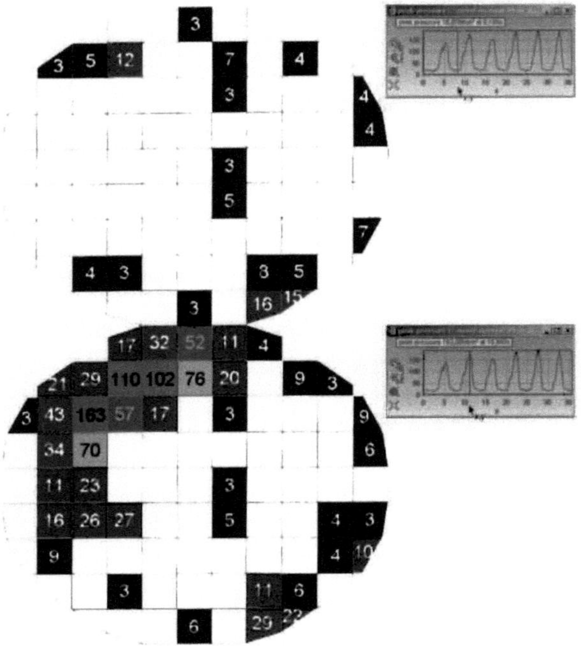

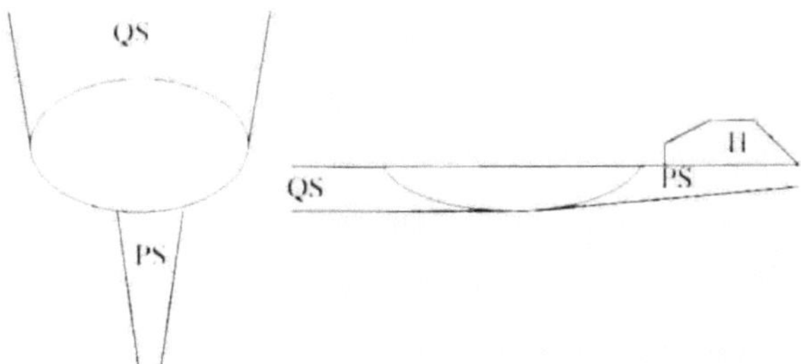

Fig. 29-6. Schematic drawing of the Quadriceps tendon (QS) inserti on and the patellar tendon (PS) insertion in the a.-p. (*left*) and the lateral (*right*) view. The Hoffa fat pad (H) is usually not resected except severe scarring or hypertrophy is noted. The patellar osteotomy should follow the tendon insertions and the patella rest height is usually approximately 12 mm

Fig. 29-5. Repeated measurements at zero (*left*) and ninety (*right*) degrees of flexion prior to patellar replacement. The medial facette is positioned in the righter portion of the ellipsoid and the lateral facette in the left portion of the ellipsoid. The upper portion is proximal and the lower portion distal

Measurements at zero and ninety degrees of flexion are shown in ◻ Fig. 29-5.

Discussion

The measurements show increasing femoropatellar pressure values with increasing flexion angles.

Film studies on the Genesis prosthesis showed no significant difference between the sizes small and medium [12] using a rest patella thickness of 15 mm at 60 degrees of flexion. This conforms with our data. It should be noted that our rest patella thickness was on average 12 mm considering our recommendation of patella resection (osteotomy) from quadriceps insertion to patella tendon insertion (◻ Fig. 29-6). The rest patella thickness does play a role on the pressure and data are currently collected to quantify this relationship.

Knee flexion of 120 degrees shows a 2.5 to 12 time increase in the femoropatellar pressure (on average 5.5 times) compared to 60 degrees of flexion.

Performance of a lateral retinacular release shows more conforming pressures and decreased the maximum pressure 1.2 to 2.5 times (on average 2.0 times).

The influence on the patellar perfusion should always be kept in mind when discussing the necessity of a lateral retinacular release. Literature suggests a 10% reduction of patellar perfusion due to performance of a lateral release.

Femoropatellar pressures as measured by film by McNamara et al. (1994) between 15 and 50 Megapascals correspond with our data.

Same accounts for the film pressure data by Huber et al. (1994) which showed flexion angle dependent values between 0.06 and 1.52 N/mm^2.

At flexion angles above 70 to 80 degrees this group found a decrease of the femoropatellar pressure. Our data do not confirm this finding, as our pressure values without exception increase up to 120 degrees of knee flexion. Also in the study of Huber increased pressure values of the medial facette were measured and differed from our data, where constantly higher values at the lateral facette are found. The antomical patella design is supposed to offer a more evenly spread pressure distribution due to potential area contact between femur and patella. This hypothetical assumption is in reality not always true as follow-up diagnostics (skyline view, Knutsson X-ray view, patella defilee views) suggest and intraoperative findings on revision suggest as well. We currently feel that the Knutsson view (skyline view at 40 degrees of flexion) with ten-

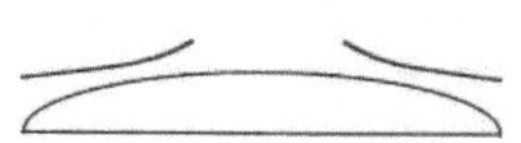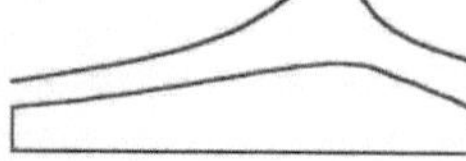

■ **Fig. 29-7.** Comparison of the contact points using the circular versus the anatomic patella. The circular patella (*left*) shows two point contact in the ideal case, while the anatomic patella (*right*) shows area contact in the ideal (hypothetical) case

sion on the quadriceps is reliable in most of the cases. intraoperative findings occasionally show point pressure friction on the patella in cases of revision as opposed to the desired area contact which should not show signs of wear. Simulator studies [18] showed a positive influence on the femoropatellar pressure. Anatomic patella designs are currently offered by most companies (■ Fig. 29-7).

Online patella pressure studies with sensors continue to be performed and will give closer insight on the dynamic femoropatellar relationship and pressure values. This will adapt our understanding of the femoropatellar joint which currently continues to be an issue not only in endoprosthetic knee replacement but also in other orthopedic and traumatologic fields. We hope to be able to produce a sterilizable sensor in the year 2003 to be able to perform in vivo measurements. In the long run we hope to be able to give objective parameters concerning femoropatellar pressure distribution in endoprosthetic knee replacement and other operative procedures.

References

1. Ayers DC et al. (1997) Common complications of total knee arthroplasty. J Bone Joint Surg 79-A: 278–311
2. Barrack RL, Burak C (2001) Patella in total knee arthroplasty. Clin Orthop 389: 62–73
3. Barrack RL, Wolfe MW, Waldman DA, Milicic M, Bertot AJ, Myers L. (1997) Resurfacing of the patella in total knee arthroplasty. A prospective, randomized, double blind study. J Bone Joint Surg 79-A: 1121–1131
4. Bayley JC, Scott RD, Ewald FC, Holmes GB Jr (1988) Failure of the metal-backed patellar components after total knee arthroplasty. J Bone Joint Surg 70-A: 668–674
5. Bindelglass DF, Cohen JL, Dorr LD (1993) Patellar tilt and subluxation in total knee artrhoplasty. Clin Orthop 286: 103–109
6. Boyd AD Jr, Ewald FC, Thomas WH, Poss R, Sledge CB (1993) Long-term complications after total knee arthroplasty with or without resurfacing of the patella. J Bone Joint Surg 75-A: 674–681
7. Brick GW, Scott RD (1988) The patellofemoral component of total knee arthroplasty. Clin Orthop 231: 163–178
8. Chew J, Stewart NJ, Hanssen AD, Luo ZP, Rand JA, An KN (1997) Differences in patellar tracking and knee kinematics among three different total knee designs. Clin Orthop 345: 87–98
9. Feller JA, Bartlett RJ, Lang DM (1996) Patellar resurfacing versus retention in total knee arthroplasty. J Bone Joint Surg 78-B: 226–228
10. Fuchs S, Schutte G, Witte H, Rosenbaum D (2000a) Welche retropatellaren Veränderungen entstehen durch die Implantation einer Oberflächenkniegelenkprothese? Unfallchirurg 103: 972–976
11. Fuchs S, Schutte G, Witte H, Rosenbaum D (2000b) Retropatellar contact characteristics in total knee arthroplasty with and without patellar resurfacing. Int Orthop 24: 191–193
12. Fuchs S, Schutte G, Witte H, Rosenbaum D (2002) Welchen Einfluss haben die Größe und die Platzierung des Patellarückflächnersatzes bei Knieendoprothesen? Unfallchirurg 105: 44–48
13. Glaser FE, Gorab RS, Lee TQ (1999) Edge loading of patellar components after total knee arthroplasty. J Arthroplasty 14: 493–499
14. Goldstein SA, Coale E, Weiss AP, Grossnickle M, Meller B, Matthews LS (1986) Patellar surface strain. J Orthop Res 4: 372–377
15. Gomes LS, Bechtold JE, Gustilo RB (1988) Patellar prosthesis positioning in total knee arthroplasty. Clin Orthop 236: 72–81
16. Grace JN, Rand JA (1988) Patellar instability after total knee arthroplasty. Clin Orthop 237: 184–189
17. Heegaard JH, Leyvraz PF, Hovey CB (2001) A computer model to simulate patellar biomechanics following total knee replacement: the effects of femoral component alignment. Clin Biomech 16: 415–423
18. Hsu HP, Walker PS (1988) Wear and deformation of patellar components in total knee arthroplasty. Clin Orthop 246: 260–265
19. Huberti HH, Hayes WC (1984) Patello-femoral contact pressures. JBJS 66-A: 715–724
20. Johnson DP, Eastwood DM (1992) Patellar complications after knee arthroplasty. Acta Orthop Scand 63: 74–79
21. Kajino A, Yoshino S, Kameyama S, Kohda M, Nagashima S (1997) Comparison of the results of bilateral total knee arthroplasty with and without patellar replacement for rheumatoid arthritis. J Bone Joint Surg 79-A: 570—574
22. Keblish PA, Varma AK, Greenwald AS (1994) Patellar resurfacing or retention in total knee arthroplasty. J Bone Joint Surg 76-B: 930–937
23. Koh JS, Yeo SJ, Lee BP, Lo NN, Seow KH, Tan SK (2002) Influence of patellar thickness on results of total knee arthroplasty. J Arthroplasty 17: 56–61
24. Lee TQ, Gerken AP, Glaser FE, Kim WC, Anzel SH (1997) Patellofemoral joint kinematics and contact pressures in total knee arthroplasty. Clin Orthop 340: 257–266
25. Lee TQ, Budoff JE, Glaser FE (1999) Patellar component positioning in total knee arthroplasty. Clin Orthop 366: 274–281
26. Ranawat CS (1986) The patellofemoral joint in total condylar knee arthroplasty. Clin Orthop 205: 93–99
27. Rand JA (1990) Patellar resurfacing in total knee arthroplasty. Clin Orthop 260: 110—117
28. Rhoads DD, Noble PC, Reuben JD, Mahoney OM, Tullos HS (1990) The effect of femoral component position on patellar tracking after total knee arthroplasty. Clin Orthop 260: 43–51
29. Schroeder-Boersch H, Scheller G, Fischer J, Jani L (1998) Advantages of patellar resurfacing in total knee arthroplasty. Two year results of a prospective randomized study. Arch Orthop Trauma Surg 117: 73–78

30. Stulberg SD, Stulberg BN, Hamati Y, Tsao A (1988) Failure mechanisms of metal backed patellar components. Clin Orthop 236: 88–105

31. Tanzer M, McLean CA, Laxer E, Casey J, Ahmed AM (2001) Effect of femoralcomponent designs on the contact and tracking characteristics of the unresurfaced patella in total knee arthroplasty. Can J Surg 44: 127–133

32. Von Spreckelsen L, Hahne HJ, Hassenpflug J (1998) Patellofemorale Kontaktzonen bei Knieendoprothesen. Z Orthop 136: 560–565

33. Wood DJ, Smith AJ, Collopy D, White B, Brankov B, Bulsara MK (2002) Patellar resurfacing in total knee arthroplasty: a prospective, randomized trial. J Bone Joint Surg 84-A: 187–193

34. Yoshii I, Whiteside LA, Anouchi YS (1992) The effect of patellar button placement and femoral component design on patellar tracking in total knee arthroplasty. Clin Orthop 275: 211–219

30 Patellofemoral Arthroplasty

J.-N. Argenson, X. Flecher, H. Vinel

Introduction

Patellofemoral osteoarthritis is well known by all orthopaedics surgeons. Its expression is variable, from anterior knee pain to classic femoropatellar syndrome when sitting or climbing down stairs. Non-operative treatment is probably the first option to select including medical treatment and physiotherapy. However, non-operative treatment is sometimes insufficient and different surgical techniques can be proposed. These techniques include the articular arthroscopic washing or the section of the lateral retinacular of the patella which efficacy is still debated particulary in the long term despite the low morbidity of arthroscopy. The Maquet procedure [37] (anterior tibial tuberosity advancement), the microperforation of the patella (Pridie procedure) or all kinds of plasty are more invasive techniques, with inconsistent results [24].

Patellectomy has been for a long time considered as the best treatment of patellofemoral arthritis. But it is a non-reversible intervention with a classic loss of quadriceps strength around 30% (◘ Fig. 30-1).

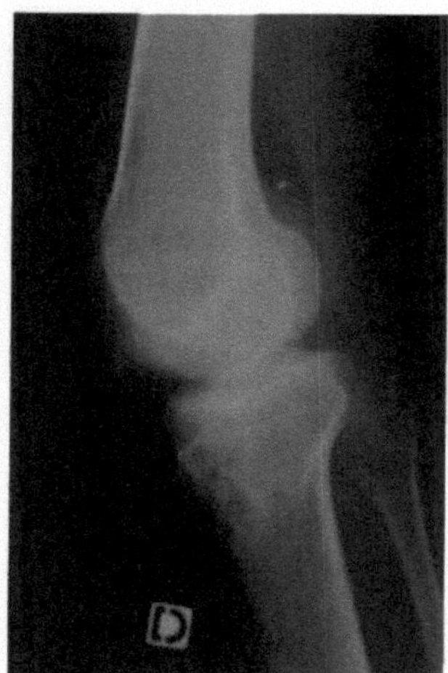

◘ **Fig. 30-1.** Patellectomy

More than that, patellectomy seems to augment the risk of femorotibial arthrosis and deteriorate the results of future total knee prosthesis.

An alternative to patellectomy is represented by the prosthetic resurfacing of the patellofemoral joint, which is an intervention with encouraging short- and mid-term results. Additionally, conversion to total knee arthroplasty is usually an easy procedure.

For us, it is important to preserve the patella in order to maintain its capacity to :
- transfer homogenous load to the knee,
- augment the quadriceps lever arm,
- maintain in appropriate directions the different forces expressed by the quadriceps,
- restraint tibial flexion on femur and stabilize knee rotation,
- protect knee joint,
- keep an esthetic role particularly for women.

History

The first patellofemoral prosthesis was created by Mac Keever in 1949; it was a vitallium patellar coverage fixed by a longitudinal intra patellar screw. In 1955, Mc Keever presented the results of 41 patients with 25 good and very good results [27]. After that, other authors [11, 25, 41] demonstrated the efficacy of this implant on pain and mobility without the need for prosthesis removal.

In 1975, the Insall prosthesis made in chrome cobalt, and without trochlear component was presented, and the outcome showed 2 excellent and 14 good results on 31 patients [1]. It was a spherical dome-shaped patella prosthesis fixed by a cemented peg.

In 1979, the Richards prosthesis was the first with two components. It was a polyethylene patellar implant with a chrome-cobalt femoral prosthesis. Several satisfactory results have been published, some of with 80% of good results [2, 7, 9].

The Lubinus prosthesis [26] is also a femoropatellar prosthesis, with a patellar configuration designed with three rectus edges and a convex lateral edge. The face of the patella which slides on the femoral groove is also convex. The results have been published by different authors [13, 20].

Since the 1980s, the concept of a femoropatellar prosthesis with a polyethylene patellar implant and a chrome-cobalt trochlear implant cemented or not, has received a general agreement: Several designs have then been presented like the Bousquet prosthesis [6], the Grammont autocentric prosthesis [4, 31], the GUEPAR group prosthesis [23, 32, 43], the Rousseau spherocentric prosthesis [28, 33], the Trochleor prosthesis, or the New Jersey low contact stress prosthesis [8].

Prosthesis Conception

Materials

Now, all prosthesis are made of two components: one femoral in metal and one patellar in polyethylene. The trochlear part of the prosthesis is in forged chrome cobalt (50% cobalt, 20% chrome, 10% nickel, 10% molybden, 10% others). This alloy provides a good resistance to corrosion and an excellent acceptance regarding wear and friction.

The patellar implant is made of high density polyethylene (UHMWPE) which confers an excellent friction quality, a resistance to impact, a good biocompatibility, despite a sensibility to cold flow and wear. Metal-backing of the patella has been promoted in order to enhance the area of contact between the femoral and the patellar component at various angles of knee flexion (New Jersey Low contact stress prosthesis). The potential inconvenients are patella bone loss due to osteolysis behind the metallic component and the difficulty at the time of revision for removing the component. In case of well fixed and unworn polyethylene patellar button, metal-backing leaves also less option for the surgeon than a conventional cemented polyethylene patella.

Implant Design

Trochlear Implant

The **proximal extremity** must be high enough to avoid polyethylene on bone contact without the need to be in continuity with the anterior cortex (quadriceps lift up the patella near full extension).

Its **edge** must be tapered to avoid patellar impingement, despite the frequent apparition of a fibrous tissue which lift up the patella and act as a protection for the polyethylene.

The **lateral part** must be larger than the medial part on its superior edge because the patella is essentially located on the lateral side of the trochlea at the beginning of flexion.

The **radius curvature** must match the one the patella describe around the trochlea (24 mm). Some implants are designed to make a smooth transition to the condyles curvature in order to avoid a brutal change of radius bend.

The **angle of the trochlear sulcus** range around 135°. Some prosthesis reproduce this angle while others provide smaller (Smith & Nephew) or bigger (Depuy).

The **distal part** of the trochlear implant must be in perfect continuity with the condyles. The lateral trochleocondylar transition zone is lower than the medial one; the lateral side of the femoral component must be lower, and avoid any contact with the anterior meniscal segment in complete extension.

When this asymmetry is chosen in the design, this requires right and left prosthesis.

Patellar Implant

Difficulty of Bone Resection. Due to the frequent important wear of the lateral side of the bony patella, the endoarticular references are difficult to use. The aim is to reproduce the original thickness of the unworn patella and the bone resection must try to be parallel to the underskin side of the patella.

The Implant Design. It is difficult to obtain a perfect contact between both components during the entire patellar course, as we have observed during in vivo kinematic evaluation using fluoroscopy [3, 12]. However, this is still the remaining goal in order to provide harmonious repartition of loads through the components and to decrease the risk of polyethylene wear.

Thus, various different prosthetic designs have been created to achieve this goal. When biconvex, the implant facilitates the translation movements and helps for control in rotation, but on the other hand may increase the shearing forces with a risk of bone-implant contact at 90°. With a concave-convex (Guepar) design, the congruity is better in the sagittal plane but may be modified during the patellar course (rotation and translation movements).

Finally, the prosthesis with a mobile polyethylene implanted on a metal backed patella have already been described above.

Fixation

Fixation, as for all prosthesis, can be realized with cement or by a porous ingrowth surface like hydroxyapatite coating.

For the femoral groove, the anchorage is secured by some additional pegs proximal or lateral.

For the patella, three fixation modes are possible:
- Cemented inlay patella, but this kind of fixation has a higher risk of patella fracture.
- Cemented onlay patella which is the most frequent fixation mode. The peg(s) location is based on patella fragility and polyethylene resistance.
- Metal backing, but this is less used because of the risk of metallosis when important polyethylene wear induce metal-metal contact. Furthermore, some cases of polyethylene desinsertion or fracture of the peg-plate junction have been described.

Conclusion

The femoropatellar prosthesis must include some criterions for optimal design (◘ Fig. 30-2).

The femoral groove implant must
- conserve the lateral edge and so exist in right and left version,
- have a tapered superior extremity, upper on the lateral side,
- have a radius bend at less equal to 24 mm,
- The trochlean depth should be more or less pronounced according to the mechanical concept (autocentric, spherocentric),

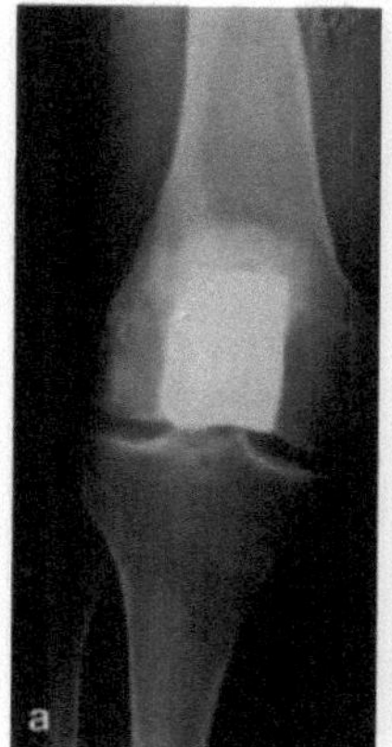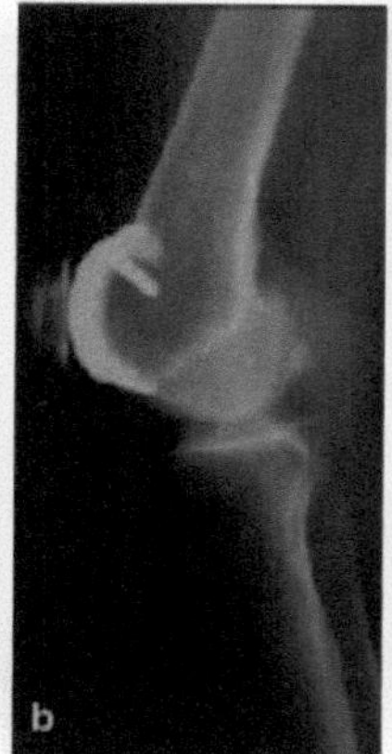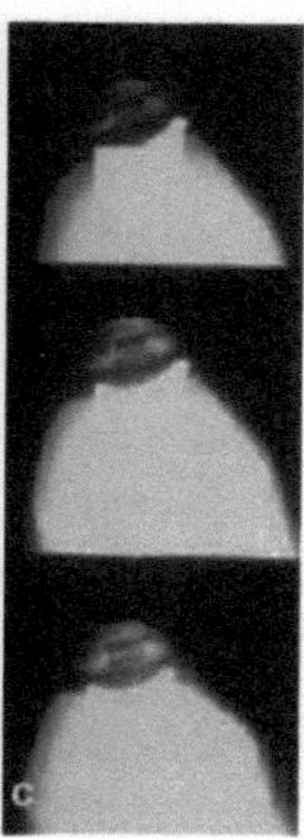

◘ **Fig. 30-2a-c.** Radiographs of patellofemoral prosthesis. **a** a.p. view, **b** lateral view, **c** patellofemoral joint view

- have an inferior extremity which avoid impingement with the condyles.

The patellar implant must
- cover the bone without extend beyond it,
- have a design corresponding to the femoral groove component.

Results of Femoro-Patellar Prosthesis

The literature, as summarized in ◘ Table 30-1, showed some good results, reliable on short and middle term.

◘ **Table 30-1.** Results of femoropatellar prosthesis

Authors	n	Results	Follow-up
Migaud [25]	23	57% satisfactory	–
Krajca Radcliffe [26]	16	85% good and very good	2–18 years
Cartier [10]	75	85% good and very good	4 years
Arciero [8]	36	72% good and very good	5 years
Bauchu [14]	117	56% good and very good	–
Lenfant Et Goutallier [17]	28	79% good and very good	5 years
Witvoet [19]	78	88% satisfactory	5 years
Renard [16]	45	65% satisfactory	6 years
De Cloedt [27]	45	65% satisfactory	6 years
Argenson [15]	70	68% good and very good	2–16 years

In our experience, the results change according to the etiology

- Arthrosis 54%
- Dysplasia 73%
- Post-traumatic 68%

Results seem to be better on pain than gain of mobility. Jouan [20] found an earlier and more important indolence in patellofemoral prosthesis than patelloplasty.

Analysis of Complications and Failures

Fractures

Even rare complications, they are for Goutallier [23] related to some types of »burst fracture« due to an excessive press fit fixation with the uncemented pegs or related to parcellar and peripheric fractures due to an external position of the peg when the bone resection is too large.

For Scott [34, 35], knee mobilization under anesthesia may promote partella fracture.

Lateral Impingement

The second frequent complication is the inadequate patellar implant coverage which can be responsible of pain initiated at 80° of flexion.

We have noticed 8 lateral impingements in our own experience [4] which needed 6 revisions. Hernigou [17] and Goutallier [23] found 15 impingements, and De Cloedt three of them [10].

This complication can be avoided by routine resection of lateral bone in excess, as well as patellar impaction associated to a careful lateral release [4, 10, 16, 17].

The Extension of Osteoarthritis

It is the first cause of failure, and requires conversion to total knee arthroplasty.

We found this type of complication most frequently in primary arthrosis group [4]. This seems to be confirmed by others authors [2, 4, 9, 28, 43].

Loosening

The replacement can be for another femoropatellar prosthesis or a total knee arthroplasty.

When a total knee prosthesis is implanted, it is for the most part because of extension of arthrosis to the others compartments. Loosening of femoropatellar prosthesis seems to be rare, and more frequently limited to the femoral component.

Instability

This is in fact related to some type of conflicts at the beginning of knee flexion or at the beginning of extension when the knee is in hyperflexion. These instabilities are in relation with implant design, but of course also with implant position [7], particularly in case of patella baja.

For Cartier [9], with the Richards prosthesis II and III which has a deep and retentive trochlear groove, only one case of instability was noted, while Witvoet [43] found ten persistent cases of instability of which three needed a revision for total knee arthroplasty.

The second reason is the implant position: the patellar button can be too high, the femoral groove component translated medially or in excessive internal rotation. Patellar button can impinge on the upper extremity of the femoral implant, mainly if the edge is too high [42].

To avoid these instabilities, Mertl [28] proposes a lateral approach with an anterior tibial tuberosity osteotomy and section of the lateral patellar retinaculum.

We found six minor cases of instability, due to implant design. All of them were non-symptomatic, perhaps because of the lateral release associated with the lateral patelloplasty.

Indications

Etiology

Most of the authors have established that femoropatellar arthrosis due to femoropatellar dysplasia or non-traumatic dislocation give the best results. They have also stated that primary femoropatellar osteoathritis can give also good results, but it is necessary to be cautious in case of patella baja [2, 9, 10, 28].

In case of primary arthrosis, some authors prefer a total knee arthroplasty since femorotibial arthrosis may start. So we believe it is important to check the mechanical axis of the knee (total weight-bearing view, stress X-rays).

Age

Femoropatellar arthroplasty is performed in majority of cases for patients close to 60 years of age [2, 4, 21, 30].

It is of course important to preserve the articulation in young patients if possible, this is why resurfacing arthroplasty limited to a single compartment seems more conservative even if for Laskin [22], femoropatellar survival seems to be worse than total knee prosthesis survival.

In Vivo Kinematic Data

Most previous experimental studies of patellar kinematics have involved cadaveric *in vitro* analyses, or have not tested the knee in a weight-bearing mode [14, 15, 18, 36, 39, 40]. Previously, a 2D analysis was conducted at the same institution (RMMRL, Denver, Colorado) under the direction of Richard Komistek, to gain a better understanding of patellofemoral kinematics by determining in vivo patellofemoral contact positions and angular rotations of the patella in the sagittal plane. The overall objective of this project is to derive the in vivo kinematics for subjects having a patellofemoral implant.

Materials and Methods

Patellofemoral kinematics was determined for 20 subjects having a patellofemoral implant. The kinematics that were assessed were:
- Patellofemoral contact positions in the sagittal plane
- Patellotibial tilt angles in the sagittal plane
- Maximum medial/lateral patellofemoral translation determined from a skyline view.

While under fluoroscopic surveillance, each subject was asked to perform two activities:

1. normal gait and
2. deep knee bend.

Only the deep knee bend was analyzed for this study. The fluoroscopic examinations were conducted in our orthopedic department in Marseille and the videos were then analyzed at RMMRL.

Patellar Contact Position

The contact position between the femur and the patella was determined using two-dimensional digitization. Designated points on the femoral, tibial, and patellar components were digitized with respect to the Newtonian reference frame.

The contact point between the patella and the femur was then determined by initially magnifying the fluoroscopic image by a factor of 3.5. The closest distance between the most anterior portion of the femoral component and the most posterior osseous portion of the patella will be denoted as the contact point. The fluoroscopic images were then reduced back to normal size and the distance between the patellar mass center and the patellofemoral contact point was measured. This measured distance was calibrated using a metal ball having a diameter of one inch to obtain the actual amount of patellofemoral translation. This calibrated distance was denoted as Q, the actual distance of the contact point from the patella mass center. A patellofemoral contact point superior to the patella mass center was denoted as positive and contact inferior to the patella mass center was denoted as a negative distance. As knee flexion proceeds, there were actually two contact regions observed:
1. on the lateral condyle, and
2. on the medial condyle.

The patellofemoral contact represents the estimated midpoint of the contact regions in the sagittal plane.

Patellar Tilt Angle

If the most posterior point along the longitudinal axis of the patella is anterior of the longitudinal axis of the tibia, the patella tilt angle was denoted as positive and referred to as patellar extension. If the most posterior point along the longitudinal axis of the patella was posterior of the longitudinal axis of the tibia, the patellar tilt angle was then denoted as negative and referred to as patellar flexion.

Skyline View

Also, we attempted to determine the medial/lateral translation of the patella, relative to the femur in the coronal plane (top view). It was proposed that each subject be fluoroscoped from 30 to 90 degrees of knee flexion, in the plane relative to the tibial plateau (skyline view). As mentioned within the proposal, RMMRL has never conducted an analysis using the skyline view. As previously discussed, this was a very difficult task and we were only able to determine the maximum distance traveled and were unable to correlate this finding with knee flexion angles since the skyline view did not allow for a determination of sagittal plane motion.

Results

Patellar Contact Position

In this present study, on average, subjects having a patellofemoral implant experienced a similar patellofemoral contact pattern compared to the normal knee (■ Fig. 30-3).

Although the average pattern was similar to the normal knee, the patellofemoral contact patterns for each subject having a patellofemoral implant was highly variable. At times, subjects having a patellofemoral implant would experience a significantly inferior contact position, while other subjects would experience a more central contact position. As stated earlier, patella contact patterns were variable and some subjects experienced significant motion.

Patellar Tilt Angles

In this present study, subjects having a patellofemoral implant, on average, experienced a patella tilt pattern and magnitude similar to the TKA subjects from our previous study (■ Fig. 30-4).

At full extension, subjects having a patellofemoral implant experienced an average angle of 1.0 degrees, while the normal knee experienced an average of –7 degrees. Also, on average, the TKA subjects also experienced a negative (flexed angle) patella angle at full extension. Therefore, the subjects having a patellofemoral implant in this present study have been the only group of subjects to experience a positive (extended angle) patella angle at full extension. Similar to the patella contact position data, subjects having a patellofemoral implant experienced highly variable patella tilt angles. Some subjects experienced more normal patella tilt angles, while other subjects experienced significantly larger patellar tilt angles, as large as 48.6 degrees.

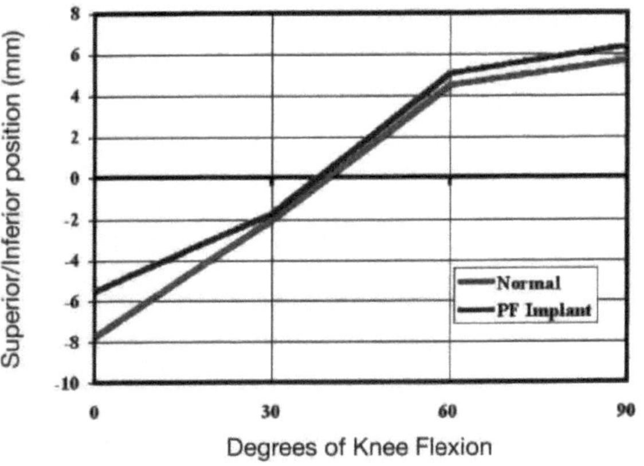

■ **Fig. 30-3.** Patellofemoral contact positions for PF implanted and normal knees

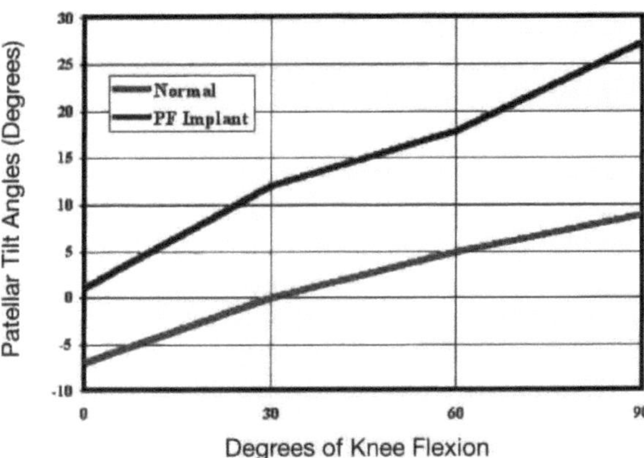

■ **Fig. 30-4.** Patellofemoral tilt angles for subjects having a PF implant and normal knees

Patellar Medial/Lateral Motion

As stated earlier, we attempted to determine medial/lateral motion of the patella relative to the femur using a skyline fluoroscopic view.

Although there were limitations, we were able to determine that the average medial/lateral motion for 18 subjects was only 3.8 mm (0.8 to 9.2 mm). Therefore, we were unable to analyze the fluoroscopic video for two subjects. Five of 18 subjects experienced greater than 5.0 mm of medial/lateral motion, and 14/18 subjects experienced greater than 2.0 mm of medial/lateral motion.

Although the majority of the subjects experienced more than 2.0 mm of medial/lateral motion, some subjects experienced minimal motion with the patella centrally positioned in the patellar grove, other subjects experienced minimal motion but were significantly offset from the patellar grove. Also, some subjects experienced an in-plane tilting motion in the coronal plane.

Discussion

Little attention has been directed to the determination of patellofemoral kinematics in the sagittal plane, especially under in vivo, weight-bearing conditions. Three other studies have concentrated on the determination of patellofemoral contact areas under in vitro conditions and can be used to compare with our patellofemoral contact position data [18, 19, 38].

Huberti and Hayes [19] analyzed patellofemoral contact areas for 12 human cadaver knee joints. They found that the contact area on the patella shifted proximally during knee flexion, similar to our findings. At 20 degrees of knee flexion they reported the contact area to be on the distal portion of the patella, and as the knee flexed this contact area shifted proximally to the most proximal portion of the patella at 120 degrees of knee flexion.

Takeuchi [38] measured patellofemoral contact areas in human cadaver knees after implantation with six different designs of TKA. The contact areas for each of the six implanted knee types were near the mass center of the patella at full extension. During knee flexion the contact areas shifted in the inferior direction for some knee types, but other knee types shifted in the superior direction. In contrast to the normal knee, there was no consistent pattern of proximal-distal migration of the contact areas and flexion angle.

Hsu et al. [18] studied seven unembalmed lower-extremity cadaveric specimens. The femur of each cadaver was rigidly fixed on a test frame with the lower leg free to move. They plotted proximal/distal contact position for each specimen and found that the patellofemoral contact pattern shifted distally during knee flexion. These findings are opposite to our results and those reported by Huberti and Hayes [19].

Comparison of patellofemoral contact patterns and patellar angular rotations in the sagittal plane of normal, ACL-deficient, and knees implanted with TKA was previously performed in an in vivo, weight-bearing fluoroscopic analysis. Translations of patellofemoral contact position from inferior to superior occurred with all implanted and non implanted groups. Abnormal sagittal angular rotation of the patella occurred in all TKA groups and may be related to disturbed femorotibial kinematics previously observed to occur following TKA.

In this present study for patients with patellofemoral implant we determined that the patellofemoral contact positions for subjects in this study were similar in pattern and magnitude to subjects having a normal patellofemoral joint. It was also determined that patella tilt angle for subjects in this study were more similar to TKA patterns than the normal knee. Similar to the normal knee, no subjects having a patellofemoral implant experienced patellofemoral separation. As previously stated, it is hypothesized that the subjects in this study had a normal, functioning ACL which keeps the femur anterior on the tibia in full extension which would eliminate the phenomena of patellofemoral separation. Subjects in this study did experience medial/lateral motion of the patella using skyline fluoroscopy. This was the first study to assess medial/lateral motion using a dynamic, in vivo methodology. Therefore, direct comparisons to normal or implanted knees could not be made at this time. Finally, the weight-bearing range-of-motion for subjects having a patellofemoral implant was significantly less than normal and TKA knees.

Conclusion

Femoropatellar prosthesis represents in our experience less than 5% of knee prosthesis. The indications are still under discussion and it is difficult to avoid failure when appears non-resurfaced compartment degradation.

Improvement in implant design must permit to avoid mechanical complications such as loosening or instability.

Finally, conversion to a total knee prosthesis must remain a straight forward primary surgery.

References

1. Aglietti P, Insall JN, Walker PS, Trent P (1975) A new patella prosthesis. Design and application. Clin Orthop 107: 175–187
2. Arciero RA, Toomey HE (1988) Patellofemoral arthroplasty. A three- to nine-year follow-up study. Clin Orthop 236: 60–71
3. Argenson J, Dennis D, Komistek R, Anderson D, Anderele M (2002) An in vivo determination of kinematics for subjects having a patellofemoral implant. 15th Annual Meeting of the ISTA, Oxford, England
4. Argenson J, Guillaume J, Aubaniac J (1995): Is there a place for patello-femoral arthroplasty ? The Knee Society, 62nd AAOS, Orlando
5. Aubriot J, Levi G (1988) Y a-t-il une place pour la chirurgie dans le traitement des arthroses fémoro-patellaires isolées? Entretiens de Bichat, Paris. Expansion Scientifique Française
6. Bauchu P (1991) Résultats des prothhèses fémoro-patellaires de G. Bousquet. Thèse de Médecine Saint-Etienne
7. Blazina M, Fox J, Del Pizzo W (1979) Patello-femoral replacement. Clin Orthop 144: 98
8. Buechel FF, Rosa RA, Pappas MJ (1989) A metal-backed, rotating-bearing patellar prosthesis to lower contact stress. An 11-year clinical study. Clin Orthop 248: 34–49
9. Cartier P, Sanouiller J, Grelsamer R (1990) Patello-femoral artgroplasty 2–12 years follow-up study. J Arthroplasty 5: 49–55
10. De Cloedt P, Legaye J, Lokietek W (1999) Femoro-patellar prosthesis. A retrospective study of 45 consecutive cases with a follow-up of 3–12 years. Acta Orthop Belg 65: 170–175
11. De Palma A (1962) Reconsideration of lesion affecting the patello-femoral joint. Clin Orthop 18: 63–84
12. D, Komistek R, Scuderi G, Argenson J, Insall JN, Mahfouz M, Aubaniac J, Haas B (2001) In vivo three dimensional determination of kinematics for subjects with a normal knee or a unicompartmental or total knee replacement. J Bone Joint Surg Am 83-A [Suppl II]: 104–115
13. Faraboeuf C (1985) La prothèse de Lubinus. Communication au congrès de la Société Orthopédique de l' Ouest
14. Hefzy MS, Yang H (1993) A three-dimensional anatomical model of the human patello-femoral joint, for the determination of patello-femoral motions and contact characteristics. J Biomed Eng 15: 289–302
15. Hefzy MS, Jackson WT, Saddemi SR, Hsieh YF (1992) Effects of tibial rotations on patellar tracking and patello-femoral contact areas. J Biomed Eng 14: 329–343
16. Hernigou P (1993) Le médaillon rotulien insuffisamment couvrant. Rev Chir Orthop 79 [Suppl I]: 104
17. Hernigou P (1993) Prothèse fémoro-patellaire. In: Langlais F, Delagoutte JO (eds) Conception des prothèses articulaires. Cahier d' enseignement de la SOFCOT N° 43. Expension scientifique Française, Paris
18. Hsu HC, Luo ZP, Rand JA, An KN (1996) Influence of patellar thickness on patellar tracking and patellofemoral contact characteristics after total knee arthroplasty. J Arthroplasty 11: 69–80
19. Huberti HH, Hayes WC (1984) Patellofemoral contact pressures. The influence of q-angle and tendofemoral contact. J Bone Joint Surg Am 66: 715–724
20. Jouan J (1986) La prothèse fémoro-patellaire de Lubinus. Considérations techniques et premiers résultats. Ann Orthop Ouest 18: 45–49
21. Krajca Radcliffe J, Coker T (1996) Patello-femoral arthroplasty: a 2-to 18 years follow-up study. Clin Orthop 330: 143–151
22. Laskin RS, van Steijn M (1999) Total knee replacement for patients with patellofemoral arthritis. Clin Orthop 367: 89–95
23. Lenfant J, Goutallier D (1996) Les prothèses fémoro-patellaires du groupe GUEPAR: Revue d' une série de 28 cas au recul moyen de 5,5 ans. Rev Chir Orthop 87 [Suppl II]: 86
24. Lewallen DG, Riegger CL, Myers ER, Hayes WC (1990) Effects of retinacular release and tibial tubercle elevation in patellofemoral degenerative joint disease. J Orthop Res 8: 856–862
25. Lewit RL (1973) A long term evaluation of patellar prosthesis. Clin Orthop 97: 153–157
26. Lubinus H (1955) Patella glide bearing total replacement. Orthopedics 2: 119–127
27. Mc Keever D (1955) Patellar prosthesis. J Bone Joint Surg Am 37A: 1074–1084
28. Mertl P, Van FT, Bonhomme P, Vives P (1997) Femoropatellar osteoarthritis treated by prosthesis. Retrospective study of 50 implants. Rev Chir Orthop Reparatrice Appar Mot 83: 712–718
29. Migaud H, Limousin M, Chantelot C, Duquennoy A (2000) Analyse des facteurs d' échecs de 23 prothèses fémoro-patellaires explantées. 75eme Réunion annuelle de la SOFCOT, Paris
30. Pickett JC, Stoll DA (1979) Patellaplasty or patellectomy? Clin Orthop 144: 103–106
31. Renard J, Grammont P (1989) La prothèse autocentrique de la rotule. Techniques et résultats après 7 ans de recul. Rhumatologie 41: 241–245
32. Roulot E (1992) La prothèse fémoro-patellaire du groupe GUEPAR. Thèse de Médecine, Broussais, Hôtel-Dieu, Paris
33. Rousseau J (1995) Prothèse partielle sphéro-centrique de rotule, justification du concept et études préliminaires des premiers résultats. A propos d' une série de 45 prothèses fémoro-patellaires, revue avec un recul maximum de 6 ans. Rev Chir Orthop 81 [Suppl II]: 176
34. Scott RD (1979) Prosthetic replacement of the femoro-patellar joint. Clin Orthop 10: 129–137
35. Scott RD, Turoff N, Ewald FC (1982) Stress fracture of the patella following duopatellar total knee arthroplasty with patellar resurfacing. Clin Orthop 170: 147–151
36. Singerman R, Davy DT, Goldberg VM (1994) Effects of patella alta and patella infera on patellofemoral contact forces. J Biomech 27: 1059–1065
37. Solund K, Hvid I (1988) Patello-femoral instability and malalignment surgically treated by the Trillat method. Ugeskr Laeger 150: 2968–2970
38. Takeuchi T, Lathi VK, Khan AM, Hayes WC (1995) Patellofemoral contact pressures exceed the compressive yield strength of UHMWPE in total knee arthroplasties. J Arthroplasty 10: 363–368
39. van Kampen A, Huiskes R (1990) The three-dimensional tracking pattern of the human patella. J Orthop Res 8: 372–382
40. Veress SA, Lippert FG, Hou MC, Takamoto T (1979) Patellar tracking patterns measurement by analytical x-ray photogrammetry. J Biomech; 12: 639–650
41. Vermeulen H, De Doncker E, Watillon M (1973) The Mac Keever patellar prosthesis in femoro-patellar arthrosis. Acta Orthop Belg 39: 79–90
42. Witvoet J (1994) L' état actuel des prothèses fémoro-patellaires. In: Conférences d' enseignement. Cahier d' enseignement de la SOFCOT N° 46, Paris, Expension scientifique Française. pp 79–92
43. Witvoet J, Benslama R, Orengo P, Aubriot JH, Broutart JC, Le Balc'h T (1983) Guepar femoropatellar prosthesis. Description. Initial results. Rev Chir Orthop Reparatrice Appar Mot 69 [Suppl 2]: 156–158

III A Navigation: Total Knee Arthroplasty

31   Postoperative Alignment of Conventional and Navigated Total Knee Arthroplasty

W. H. Konermann, M. A. Saur

Introduction

Total knee arthroplasty (TKA) requires attention to the entire complex of knee joint mechanics, active muscle forces and passive ligament structures. Prosthetic component design must accommodate the patients knee anatomy, biomechanical stability, function, and mobility. It is uniformly reported in the literature that the longevity of a knee prosthesis is patient specific, but depends upon correct component design and alignment, implant fixation, soft tissue balancing and a physiological lower extremity axis [1, 12, 15, 17, 22, 24]. One has to appreciate that minimal mal-positioning of intra- or extramedullary tools may lead to considerable variations of implant positioning. Thus reconstruction of the correct mechanical lower extremity axis as well as soft tissue balancing is vital for good results. TKA Survivorship of 80% to 95% after 10 years are reported [10, 16, 18, 19, 24] but is significantly reduced in cases with more than four degrees of varus or valgus deformity, as Rand and Coventry reported in their series with 71% and 73% respectively compared to 90% in cases, where the component alignment was within the range of 4 degrees [20]. In a similar study of Jeffrey et al. the loosening rate after 12 years was 3% in well-aligned TKA (less than 3 degrees varus/valgus) and 24% less optimal aligned cases (more than 4 degrees varus/valgus) [8].

Alignment of the Lower Extremity

The mechanical axis of the leg (Mikulicz) is defined as a line that passes the femoral head center, the center of the knee and the center of the ankle joint. Any alteration of that line represents a mal-alignment. In cases of varus deformity the mechanical axis deviates medially and in valgus deformity laterally from that line. The femoral angle between anatomical and mechanical axis ranges from 5 to 9 degrees depending of the neck length. The inner angle of the femoral implant is taken from the tangent to the

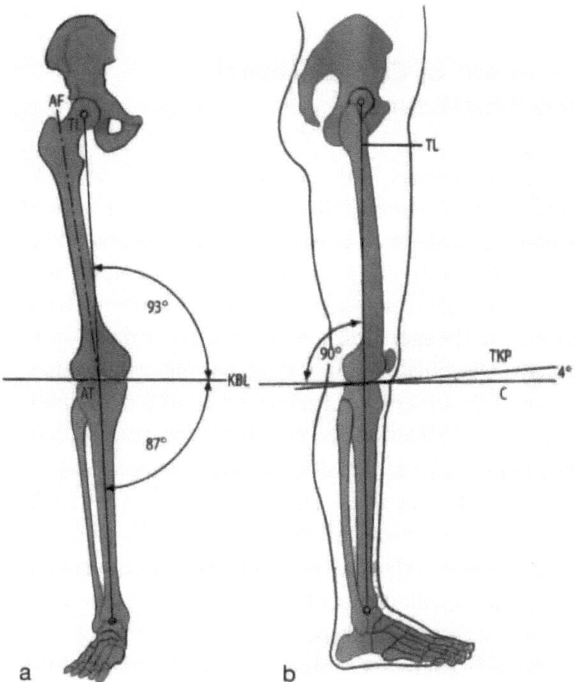

Fig. 31-1a, b. a Anterior-posterior (a.-p.) view of anatomical and mechanical axes and angles [AF anatomical axis of femur, AT anatomical axis of tibia, KBL knee base line, TL weight bearing line (Mikulicz)]. **b** Lateral view with mechanical axis and tibia tangent [TKP Tangent of tibia plateau, TL weight bearing line (Mikulicz), C vertical to TL. (Mod. from [3])

femoral condyles and the mechanical femoral axis. The inner angle of the tibial implant is taken from the tibial shaft axis, which is identical with the mechanical axis and the tibial plateau plane (implant) on a.p. views. In physiological cases the inner tibia angle measures 87 degrees or 3 degrees varus slope, the inner femoral angle measures 93 degrees. On sagittal views tibial and femoral slope can be measured. The femoral slope is taken from the tangent of the implant and mechanical femoral axis, as is the tibial slope (◘ Fig. 31-1). Position of the patella component (central, lateral, medial, superior, inferior) is calculated off axial and lateral patella views.

All axes are subject to computed calculations [3, 6, 14, 20, 21]. In order to minimize potential errors standardized radiographs with one leg stand are required making sure that central beams are crossing the midline of the patella. Lateral views should fall perpendicular to the joint space so that both implant pegs have the same length. Exact radiographs will require fluoroscopic guidance.

Alignment of Conventional Knee Prostheses

Rand and Conventry [20] reported a series of 193 TKA with more than 11 years follow-up (1972–1975) in which 83% had moderate or no pain, the revision rate was 20%, and a survivorship of 69% after 10 years. Components with an increased mal-alignment of 3 degrees varus deformity to the mechanical axis (17 of 53) or more than 4 degrees to the tibial axis (21 of 45) show a higher loosening rate. Revision surgery was performed in 20% (39 of 193) of the cases. Indication for revision surgery included 7 cases with component mal-alignment (6 varus, 1 valgus defomity). Jeffrey et al. [8] reported a series of 115 TKA (1976–1981) with a mean follow-up of 8 years in which an aseptic loosening rate of 24% was significantly associated with mal-alignment of more than 3 degrees. In 11 revision cases only 2 cases had proper alignment. There was no correlation between loosening and preoperative deformity, but high significant correlation between loosening and postoperative deformity.

Ritter et al. [22] observed about 420 TKA's (1975–1983) of which 56% had varus, 31% had neutral, and 13% had valgus mal-alignment postoperatively. Eight cases required revision surgery due to component loosening, of which 5 cases had varus mal-alignment, 3 cases had neutral mechanical axis.

Delp et al. [2] confirmed the importance of accurate implant alignment for optimal outcome. Their complication rate included aseptic loosening, instability, dislocation, fracture, and infection which counted for 5–8%. Complications such as patellofemoral pain and reduced range of motion ranged from 20 to 40%.

Matsuda et al. [13] examined 20 Miller-Galante TKA with a mean follow-up of 87 months of which 17 were implanted in a mean varus angle of 0.9 degrees (4 valgus to 5 varus). However, Matsuda demands a longer follow-up period for more definitive statement to mal-alignment an loosening.

Schwitalle et al. [23] looked at 248 PFC TKA with a follow-up over 5 years. In 15 (4.5%) cases revision was related with mal-alignment and surgical technique. In their series mal-alignment and not well balanced soft tissues increased the incidence of late complications, i.e. 6 cases (2%) with aseptic and 4 cases (1,3%) with septic loosening.

König et al. [11] reported long-term results of 495 PFC TKA after 5 to 10 years with only 2 aseptic loosening of tibial and femoral components after 5 and 6 years, respectively, which were treated successfully with revision surgery. The complication rates of 5.2% after 10 years and revision rate of 2.4% are published [4].

In summary, not all authors consider mal-alignment as a major contributing factor of implant failure. Whereas Jeffrey et al. [8], Rand and Coventry [20], as well as Ritter et al. [22] consider the postoperative angle as a major concern, Tew et al. [25] and Hsu et al. [5] do not. Gomoll et al. [4] investigated a series of 155 PFC TKA after 10 years and found no aseptic loosening and non-progress radiolucent lines of less than 1 mm in 16%. In another series of 235 TKA with PCL retention 90% did not require surgery 8% had aseptic loosening.

Ranawat et al. [19] investigated 112 TKA after 11 years and found radiolucent lines (RLL) in 60% of the cases with BMI being a factor. The mechanical axis ranged from 3 degrees varus to 10 degrees valgus (10 had 0 to 3 degrees varus, 17 had 0 to 4 degrees valgus, the remaining cases had 5 to 10 degrees valgus). Survivorship after 11 years was 94.1%. Ranawat reported no association with age, sex, diagnosis, cement mantle or mal-alignment, but a significant correlation of RLL and BMI.

Comparison of Alignment in Navigated and Conventional TKA: Literature

Miehlke et al. [15] compared results of 60 OrthoPilot (Aesculap, Tuttlingen, Germany) navigated TKA with 30 conventional TKA. Three months postoperatively mechanical, femoral and tibial axes in anterior-posterior and lateral view were evaluated. With regards to the mechanical axis 61,7% were within 2 degrees of varus or valgus angle, 35% cases had a deviation of 3 to 4 degrees, and 3.3% had more than 4 degrees mal-alignment. In the conventional group more than 4 degrees of mal-alignment was observed in 10% of the cases. The authors state a significantly better alignment in the lateral tibial axis when using the OrthoPilot navigation system particularly with less outliers.

Jenny and Boeri [9] implanted 40 Search Prosthesis TKA with the OrthoPilot navigation system and compared this with a matched group of conventionally implanted Search Prosthesis TKA. In 85% of the navigated cases the axis was within 3 degrees with only 72% in the conventional group. Taking all five axis into account, optimal results within 3 degrees were obtained in 62% of the navigated compared with 30% in the conventional group. Janecek et al. [7] using the same system reported 30 cases and compared the results with 30 conventional PFC and T.A.C.K. TKA. Angle of less than 2 degrees were found in 83% of the navigated TKA and only 37% in the other group. Four degrees deviation was found in 17% of the navigated, but in 46% of the conventional group. None of the navigated TKA had more than 4 degrees, but 17% in the other group.

Comparison of Alignment in Navigated and Conventional TKA: Own Series

In the time between 09/1999 and 12/2001, 100 Search Evolution prostheses (Aesculap. Tuttlingen, Germany) were implanted using the OrthoPilot navigation system (Aesculap. Tuttlingen, Germany). A control group underwent conventional implantation using LCS knee prostheses (DePuy Int, Leeds, UK) in the time between 03/2001 to 07/2001. There were 2 surgeons in the navigated group and 6 surgeons in the control group with no significant differences among them. Lateral radiographs in lying position were compared two weeks postoperatively. The error of this method is one degree for individual measurement and two degree for beam position [26]. The following data were reported: sagittal orientation of the femoral component in relation to distal and ventral (slope) as well as sagittal alignment (slope) of the tibial component. The mechanical axis and alignment of both components in relation to it was measured on standardized one-leg stand views. Demographic data include mean age (70 years), with 75% females. There were no differences comparing both groups.

Radiographic results were separated into perfect, optimal, acceptable, and unacceptable. Categories were defined using deviation from ideal values (◘ Table 31-1).

Mechanical Leg Axis, a.p. View

A neutral mechanical axis (0 degree) was achieved in 55% in the navigated group (A) and in 27% in the conventional group (B). Alignment within 3 degrees of varus or valgus was observed in 93% in group A and 77% in group B. Both differences were significant (◘ Fig. 31-2).

◘ **Table 31-1.** Definition of results, deviation from the desired angle

	Coronal mechanical axis	Coronal orientation of the femoral component	Sagittal orientation of the femoral component	Coronal orientation of the tibial component	Sagittal orientation of the tibial component
Perfect	0	0	0	0	0
Optimal	≤3°	≤2°	≤2°	≤2°	≤2°
Acceptable	4°–5°	3°–4°	3°–4°	3°–4°	3°–4°
Unacceptable	>5°	>4°	>4°	>4°	>4°

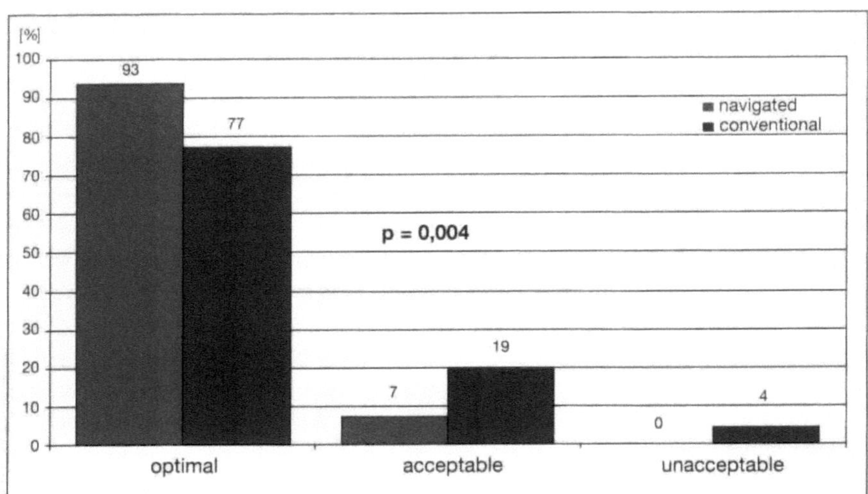

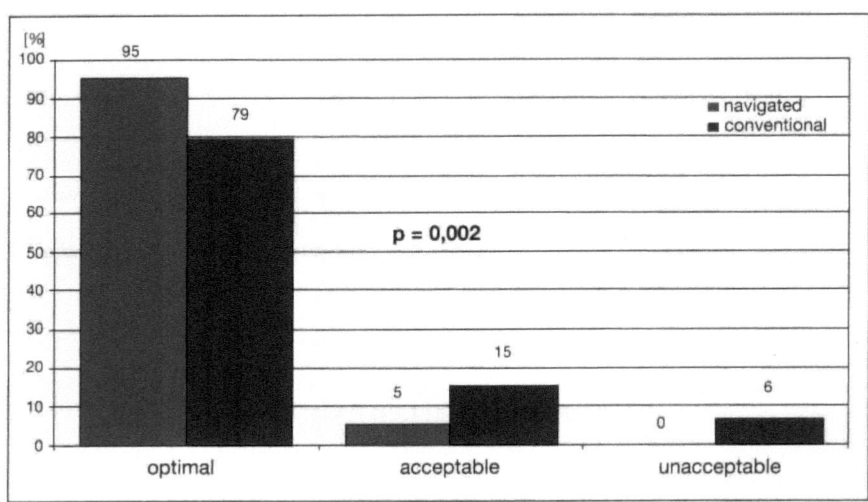

Fig. 31-2. Coronal mechanical leg axis, comparison of both groups

Fig. 31-3. Coronal orientation of the femoral component, comparison of both groups

Femoral Axis, a.p. View

Perfect perpendicular alignment (90 degrees) was obtained in 49% in group A (navigated group) with 95% within 2 degrees varus/valgus deviation. In group B 42% were perfectly aligned with 79% within 2 degrees deviation. Both differences were significant (Fig. 31-3).

Femoral Axis, Lateral View

Perfect slope alignment (0 degree) on lateral views was obtained in 39% in group A (navigated group) and in 65%

within 2 degrees anterior/posterior deviation. Ideal value for posterior slope in this design was defined by the manufacturer with 5 degrees. In group B (5 degrees slope considered perfect) only 10% were perfectly aligned (0 degree) and 45% within 2 degrees deviation. Both differences were significant (Fig. 31-4).

Tibial Axis, a.p. View

Perfect perpendicular alignment (90 degrees) on coronal views was obtained in 53% in group A (navigated group) and in 98% within 2 degrees varus/valgus deviation. In

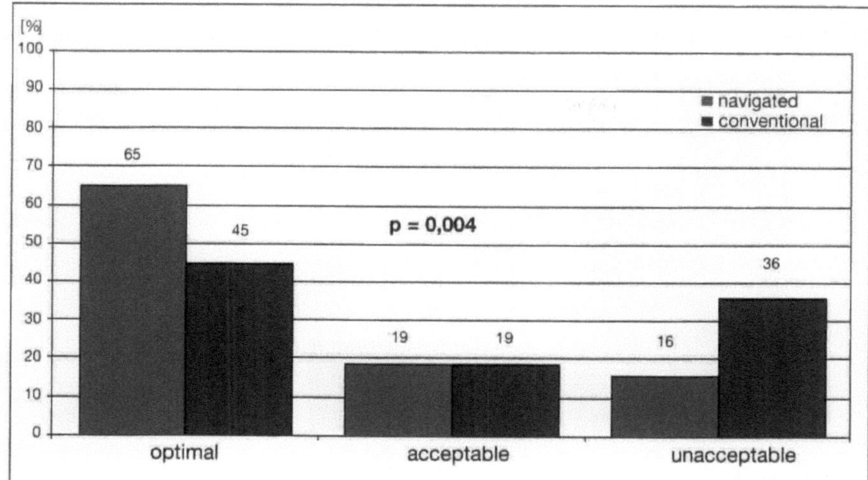

Fig. 31-4. Sagittal orientation of the femoral component, comparison of both groups. Planned posterior slope of 5 degrees in conventional group B

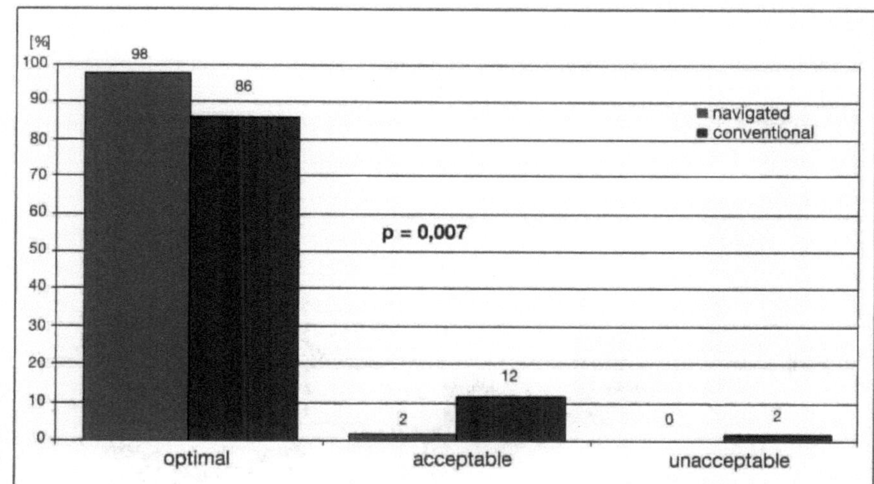

Fig. 31-5. Coronal orientation of the tibial component, comparison of both groups

group B 57% were perfectly aligned and in 86% within 2 degrees varus/valgus deviation. In group B were some outliers. Both differences were significant (**Fig. 31-5).

Tibial Axis, Lateral View

Perfect slope alignment (0 degree in group A) on lateral views was obtained in 55% in group A with 91% within 2 degrees anterior/posterior deviation. As described, 5 degrees posterior slope was defined as ideal angle, however, different angles may have been considered intraoperatively from the surgeon due to individual patients' anatomy.

Taking 5 degrees as ideal angle, we found in group B (5 degrees slope considered perfect) only 14% perfectly aligned tibial components with 65% within 2 degrees deviation. Both differences were significant (**Fig. 31-6).

Summary of All Five Axes

We defined the following criteria as a acceptable result: mechanical axis within 5 degrees and each other of the four axes within 4 degrees. There were 84% in group A (navigated group), that met these criteria and 61% in group B. An optimal result (mechanical axis within 3

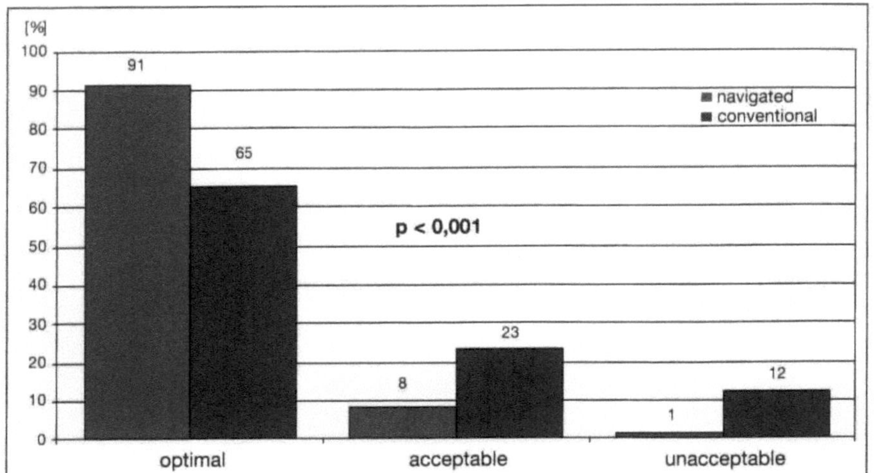

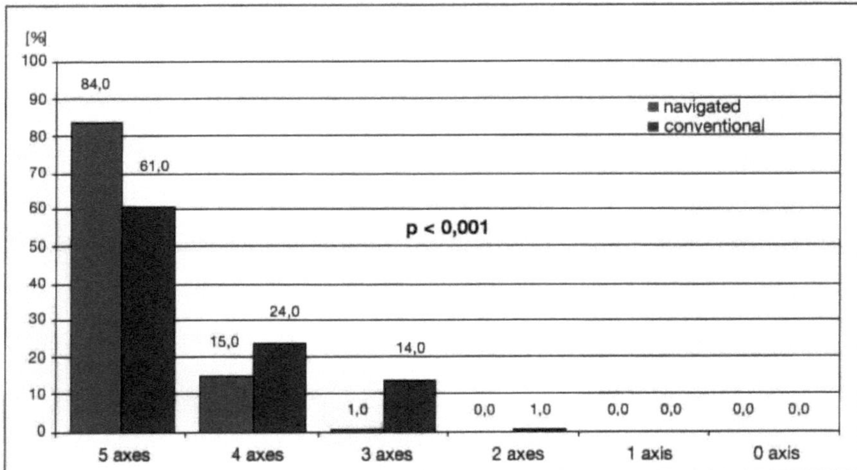

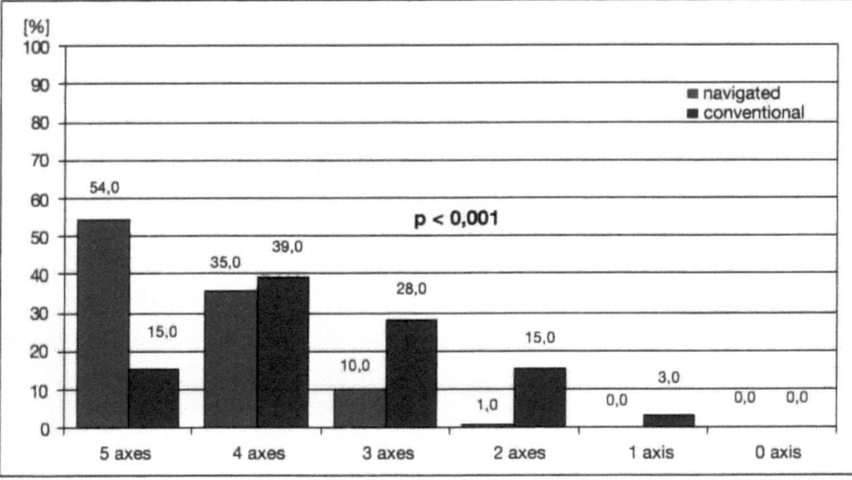

Fig. 31-6. Sagittal orientation of the tibial component, comparison of both groups. Planned posterior slope of 5 degrees in conventional group B

Fig. 31-7. Number of cases with acceptable alignment (mechanical axis: 0 degrees ± 5 degrees, each other axis ± 4 degrees deviation). Planned femur and tibia slope in the sagittal plane in conventional group was 5 degrees

Fig. 31-8. Number of cases with optimal alignment (mechanical axis: 0 degree ± 3 degrees, each other axis ± 2 degrees deviation). Planned femur and tibia slope in the sagittal plane in conventional group was 5 degrees.

degrees and each other of the four axes within 2 degrees) was observed in 54% in group A and 15% in group B (◘ Figs. 31-7 and 31-8).

Statistical Analyses

The Wilcoxon et al. U-Test was employed for statistical significance. Both groups were compared using the Chi-Square-Test.

Summary

Reconstruction of mechanical axis, perfect component alignment/design, and balancing of the soft tissues are major factors that increase survivorship of TKA. The literature states, that TKA components are implanted significantly more accurately and precise when using computer navigation. In this series, we were able to confirm these data. Current comparative studies, however, focus on radiographic data, but not on clinical outcome. Whether or not more precise aligned TKA components will improve the long-term outcome may be expected, but has yet to be confirmed by future trial.

References

1. Bargren JH, Blaha JD, Freeman MAR (1983) Alignment in total knee arthroplasty. Clin Orthop 173: 178–183
2. Delp SL, Stulberg SD, Davies BL, Picard F, Leitner F (1998) Computer-assisted knee replacement. Clin Orthop 354: 49–56
3. Elke R, König A (2001) Präoperative Planung der Knietotalprothese. In: Eulert J, Hassenpflug J (Hrsg) Praxis der Knieendoprothetik. Springer, Berlin Heidelberg New York Tokyo, S 33–41
4. Gomoll AH, Schai PA, Scott RD, Thornhill TS (2001) Das PFC-Modular-System. In: Eulert J, Hassenpflug J (Hrsg) Praxis der Knieendoprothetik. Springer, Berlin Heidelberg New York Tokyo, S 233–243
5. Hsu HP, Garg A, Walker PS, Spector M, Ewald FC (1989) Effect on knee component alignment on tibial load distribution with clinical correlation. Clin Orthop 248: 135–144
6. Insall JN, Binazzi R, Soudry M, Mestriner LA (1985) Total knee replacement. Clin Orthop Relat Res 192: 13–22
7. Janecek M, Bucek B, Hart R (2001) OrthoPilot (Aesculap) – Computer-navigation der Endoprothese des Kniegelenks. Acta Chir Austriaca 33: 175
8. Jeffrey RS, Morris RW, Denham RA (1991) Coronal alignment after total knee replacement. J Bone Joint Surg 73 B: 709–714
9. Jenny JY, Boeri C (2001) Navigiert implantierte Knietotalendoprothesen – Eine Vergleichsstudie zum konventionellen Instrumentarium. Z Orthop 139: 117–119
10. Knutson K, Lindstrand A, Lidgren L (1986) Survival of knee arthroplasties, a nation-wide multicenter investigation of 8000 cases. J Bone Joint Surg 68 B: 795–803
11. König A, Gruss J, Kirschner S (2001) Ergebnisse der Press-Fit-Condylar-Prothese (PFC). In: Eulert J, Hassenpflug J (Hrsg) Praxis der Knieendoprothetik. Springer, Berlin Heidelberg New York Tokyo, S 226–230
12. Lampe F, Honl M, Wieman R, Hille E (1999) Computergestützte Navigation Gelenkerhalt und Endoprothetik bei Gonarthrose. In: Implant 2-1999/Kasuistik. Springer, Berlin Heidelberg New York Tokoy
13. Matsuda S, Hiromasa M, Nagamine R, Urabe K, Harimaya K, Matsunobu T, Iwamoto Y (1999) Changes in knee alignment after total knee arthroplasty. J Arthroplasty 14: 566–570
14. Merchant AC, Mercer RL, Jacobsen RH, Cool CR (1974) Roentgeno-graphic analysis of patellofemoral congruence. J Bone Joint Surg 56A: 1391–6
15. Miehlke RK, Clemens U, Jens JH, Kershally S (2001) Navigation in der Knieendoprothetik – vorläufige klinische Erfahrungen und prospektiv vergleichbare Studie gegenüber konventioneller Implantationstechnik. Z Orthop 139: 109–116
16. Nafei A, Kristensen O, Knudson HM, Hvid I, Jensen J (1996) Survivorship analysis of cemented total condylar knee arthroplasty. J Arthroplasty 11: 7–10
17. Picard F, Saragaglia D, Montbarbon E, Chaussard C, Leitner F, Raoult O (1999) Computer-assisted knee Arthroplasty preliminary clinical results with the OrthoPilot System. 4th International CAOS Symposium, Davos 1999
18. Ranawat CS, Boachie-Adjei O (1988) Survivorship analysis and results of total condylar knee arthroplasty. Clin Orthop Relat Res 226: 6–13
19. Ranawat CS, Flynn WF, Saddler S, Hansraj KH, Maynhard MJ (1993) Long-term results of total condylar knee athroplasty. Clin Orthop 286: 94–102
20. Rand JA, Coventry MB (1988) Evaluation of geometric total knee arthroplasty. Clin Orthop 232: 168–173
21. Rand JA, Ilstrup DM (1991) The accuracy of femoral intramedullary guides in total knee arthroplasty. J Arthroplasty 12: 677–682
22. Ritter MA, Faris PM, Keating EM, Meding JB (1994) Postoperative alignment of total knee replacement. Its effect on survival. Clin Orthop 299: 153–156
23. Schwitalle M, Eckhardt A, Heine J (2001) Ergebnisse der Press-Fit-Condylar-Prothese (PFC). In: Eulert J, Hassenpflug J (Hrsg) Praxis der Knieendoprothetik. Springer, Berlin Heidelberg New York Tokyo, S 217–224
24. Scuderi GR, Insall JN, Windsor RE, Moran MC (1989) Survivorship of cemented knee replacement. J Bone Joint Surg 71B: 798–803
25. Tew M, Waugh W (1985) Tibial-femoral alignment and the results of knee replacement. J Bone Joint Surg 67 B: 551–556
26. Wright JG, Treble N, Feinstein AR (1991) Measurement of lower limb alignment using long radiographs. J Bone Joint Surg 73B: 721–723

32 Computer-Assisted Implantation of Total Knee Endoprosthesis with no Preoperative Imaging: the Kinematic Model

D. Saragaglia, F. Picard

History

Computer-assisted surgery began at the end of the 1980s with stereotactic neurosurgery [13]. The objectives of this new technique were to increase the precision, reduce the invasiveness and improve the validation of the operation.

At the beginning of the 1990s the Medical Information Technology School in Grenoble, under the leadership of J. Demongeot and P. Cinquin, became interested in this promising technology and persuaded a number of surgeons to collaborate in projects on computer-assisted surgery: P. Merloz [16] for spinal surgery in 1991, and in 1992 R. Julliard [11] for anterior cruciate ligament surgery and ourselves for the implantation of total knee endoprostheses.

The history of the computer-assisted implantation of total knee endoprostheses began in 1993, when we formed a working group composed of two surgeons (D. Saragaglia and F. Picard), one medical information technologist (P. Cinquin), two information technologists (S. Lavallée and F. Leitner) and an industrial partner. At that time this was the company I.C.P. France, which was bought in 1994 by Aesculap, Tuttlingen, Germany. In this first meeting we laid down our fundamental requirements as experienced surgeons for a computer-assisted surgical procedure. No preoperative CT should be necessary as the basis for intraoperative navigation, and this was for several reasons: firstly, because at this time this method of examination did not form part of the preoperative planning for knee replacements; secondly, because we intuitively thought that an examination of this kind would only complicate the operating procedure, and finally, because it would cause additional cost as well as substantial radiation exposure for the patient. We needed a permanent reference to the mechanical leg axis from the beginning to the end of the operation, in order to position the cutting blocks at right angles to this axis in both frontal and sagittal planes. It had to be possible to place the cutting blocks »freely« onto the bones, with no intra-medullary or extra-medullary alignment aids. Finally, the operation had to last less than two hours (this was the maximum time we allowed for tourniquet application) and had to be possible for any surgeon to perform, regardless of his or her computer skills.

This project was entrusted to F. Leitner, an information technologist just finishing his course of study, and F. Picard, who made it the object of a study in the context of his scientific research in biological and medical technology. After two years' work the results were as follows: the implantation of a total knee endoprosthesis without preoperative imaging (scanner) is possible simply by establishing the rotational axes in the hip, knee and ankle joints, additional palpation of the knee and ankle joint is recommended to improve the robustness of the system, and finally, according to the current state of knowledge, the best system for spatial localization is not electromagnetic or electromechanical systems but an optoelectronic system based on infrared diodes. We validated the system by implanting ten knee prostheses into ten cadavers, and published the results in 1997 in several national and international meetings (CAOS, SOFCOT, SOBCOT, etc).

After the ethical committee of the University Hospital in Grenoble gave their approval on 04.12.1996, the first computer-assisted implantation of a prosthesis into a living patient was performed on 21.01.1997 (D. Saragaglia, F. Picard, T. Lebredonchel). The operation lasted 2 hours 15 minutes with no major intraoperative problems. A prospective randomized study comparing this procedure with the conventional operating technique was begun in January 1998 and completed in March 1999. The results were published in several national and international journals and as the main article in the Revue de Chirurgie Orthopédique [21].

Operating Technique

Preoperative planning is exactly the same as for a knee endoprosthesis implantation using the conventional procedure: normal X-rays or, better still, pangoniometry under load to evaluate the leg axis and the shape of the femur and tibia. X-rays under load are not necessary, since the computer calculates the reducibility of the deformity through varus and valgus movements.

Equipment

The equipment consists of a navigation system (Ortho-Pilot, Aesculap, Tuttlingen, Germany; 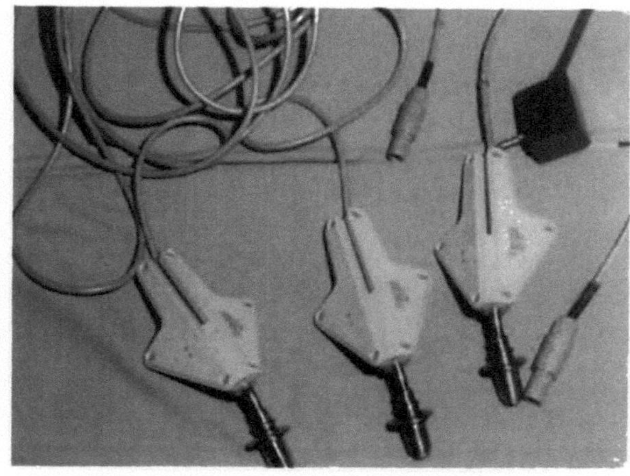 Fig. 32-1) which traces and records the spatial positions of transmitters in real time, together with instruments which are specially adapted for use with this navigation system. The navigation system comprises a personal computer, a Polaris infrared camera (Northern Digital Inc.) and a dual control foot pedal. The course of the operation is defined in the software, and the surgeon controls the procedure via the foot pedal and a dedicated graphic user interface.

This navigation system also includes transmitters and their fixation system. A transmitter, also called »rigid body« (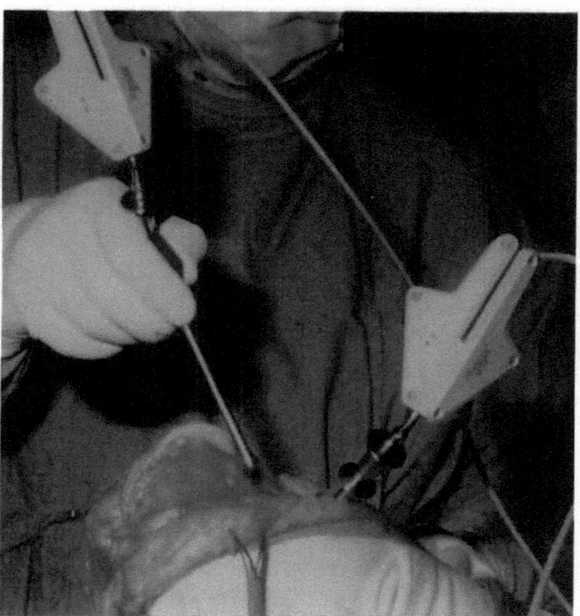 Fig. 32-2), consists of infrared diodes which are fixed rigidly into position. The position of each of these diodes is recorded by the camera, establishing both the position and the orientation of the transmitter. The transmitters can be fixed onto any object whose movements one wishes to trace. In particular, it is possible to establish

Fig. 32-2. Transmitter, also called »rigid bodies«

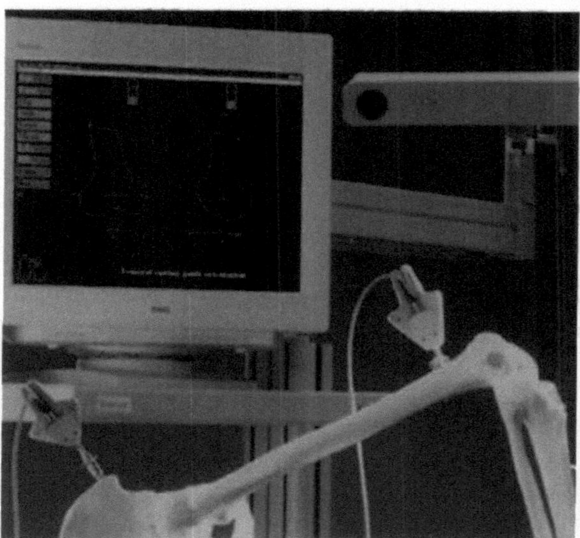

Fig. 32-1. The OrthoPilot system

Fig. 32-3. Transmitter-attached pointer

points in space with the help of a pointer with known coordinates attached to a transmitter (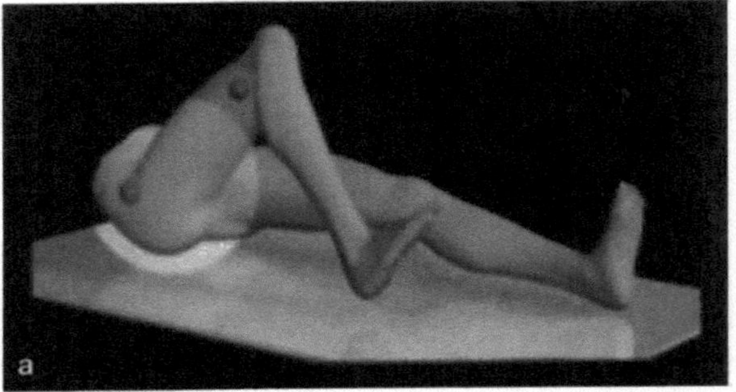 Fig. 32-3). The transmitters are fixed onto the bone using special bicortical screws.

The instrumentation is based on that used with the Search prosthesis (Aesculap, Tuttlingen), but we have mounted transmitter connectors on all the cutting blocks. It seemed important to us to be able to transfer to conventional total knee instrumentation at any time and without affecting the optimal implantation of the prosthesis, should the computer system break down.

Operating Procedure

»Calibrating« the Lower Extremity

The mechanical leg axis is determined through three points: the centers of the femoral head (H), the knee (K) and the ankle (A), respectively. These three points lie on a straight line when the leg is in extension. The leg is calibrated by establishing these three points, which are kinematic points. They are therefore identified through appropriate movements of the hip, knee and ankle joints. To identify the centre of the femoral head it is necessary to fix rigid bodies onto the anterior superior iliac crest and the distal end of the femur. The transmitter on the femur is introduced through the same incision as for the implantation itself. The upper leg is rotated and moved through flexion and extension, allowing the centre of the femoral head to be computed via the camera and the infrared diodes (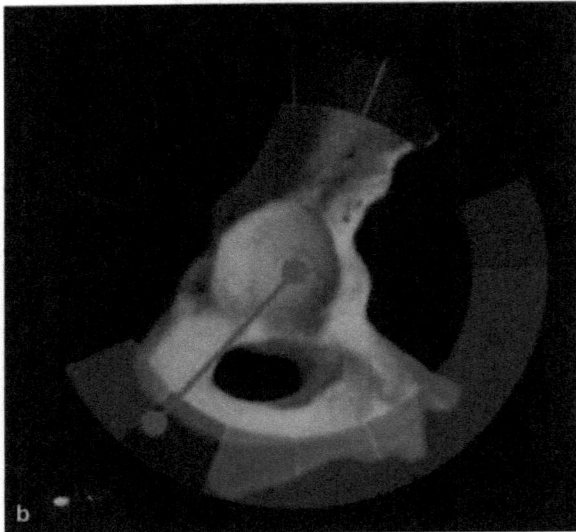 Fig. 32-4a, b).

Since the ankle has only one degree of freedom, identifying its center is more complicated than for the hip joint, since only one rotational axis can be determined. However, with the foot extended it is possible to effect lateral movements which are sufficient to determine the centre of the ankle joint. To do this, one transmitter is attached to the proximal end of the tibia through the implantation approach, and a second transmitter mounted on a metal plate is fixed onto the neck of the talus, thus avoiding an incision on the ankle bone. Flexion and extension and varus and valgus movements are performed to determine the center of the ankle joint via the camera and infrared diodes.

Fig. 32-4a, b. a Rotating movements at the hip joint. **b** Graphic user surface for identifying the rotation center of the hip joint

Determining the center of the knee joint is also relatively complicated, because this is an instantaneous center of rotation which changes position during rotation. Nevertheless, it is essential to identify a midpoint in order to establish the mechanical leg axis. One possibility is to palpate an anatomical point at the level of the femur and the tibia with the knee open. A second possibility is to calculate a rotational center of gravity by looking for the point on the femur which is most equidistant (in the sense of the fewest squares) from a point on the tibia. Flexion and extension movements give the flexion and extension axis, and rotation of the tibia at 90° flexion gives a second axis. The point at which these two axes intersect is taken as the centre of rotation of the knee. To identify this centre, rigid bodies are first fixed onto the distal femur and the proximal tibia. After flexion and extension movements and rotation at 90° flexion, the centre of the knee is computed using the camera and the infrared diodes.

Palpating the Bone Contours

The resection height is established through palpating the healthy tibial plateau. Using the pointer with the mobile rigid body mounted on it that was used on the pelvic crest and the ankle, the healthy tibial plateau is palpated as far towards the back as possible. This allows the posterior slope of the tibia, if there is one, to be calculated into the resection height and also takes account of the resected space at the level of the posterior and not the anterior cruciate ligament, which is a classic trap in conventional surgery.

Palpation of the femur (posterior surface of the medial and lateral condyles and the anterior cortex on the upper margin of the trochlea) determines the size of the prosthesis and establishes the articular centre of the femur.

Palpation of the ankle (◘ Fig. 32-5) includes its midpoint, thus supporting the cinematic identification of the joint center. The medial and lateral malleoli and the midpoint of the ankle joint must be palpated.

Now the points H, K and A have been identified and their coordinates recorded in the rigid bodies reference system of the tibia and the femur. The mechanical leg axis has also been defined (◘ Fig. 32-6) and can be compared with the preoperative pangonometry. The prosthesis size has also been established and is displayed on the screen.

The surgeon can create valgus and varus movements through placing the knee under load, in order to perform gonometry of the knee under load. This tests reproducibility and it can be seen in advance whether it will be necessary to release the peripheral soft tissues. The system also permits a dynamic gonometry, with which the varus or valgus deviation can be assessed at 30° flexion (walking position) and at 90° flexion. This gives an indication of the global femoral rotation – a topic completely ignored todate, particularly when systematic external rotation is applied to a femoral implant in the conventional operating techniques.

Positioning the Cutting Blocks

The tibial cutting block is mounted on a rod, which enables valgus-varus, resection height and posterior slope to be

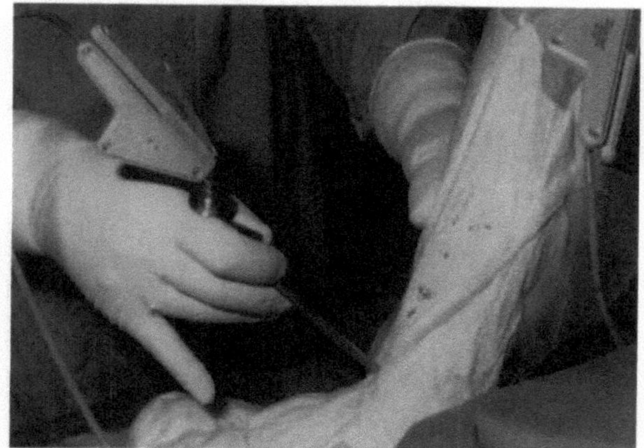

◘ Fig. 32-5. Palpation of the ankle

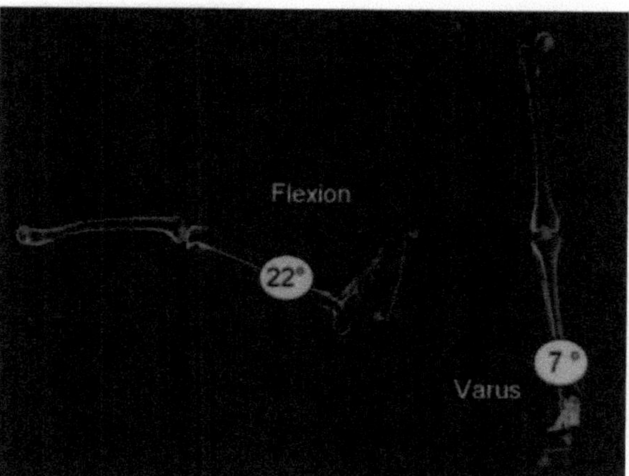

◘ Fig. 32-6. The mechanical leg axis is displayed on the screen. In this case: 7° varus at 22° flexion

adjusted. The cutting block with transmitter attached is positioned in front of the tibia (◘ Fig. 32-7) and fixed onto the bone with four threaded pins as soon as the correct settings appear on the screen (◘ Fig. 32-8). For us that means: 0° valgus-varus, 0° posterior slope and a resection height of 8 or 10 mm, according to the thickness of the plateau of the tibial implant component. After the cutting blocks have been fixed, the rod is removed and the tibia is resected using the oscillatory saw.

The femoral cutting block with transmitter attached is then placed on the distal femur with the knee in 90° flexion (◘ Fig. 32-9). Its position is first adjusted in the sagittal plane without extension or flexion. When the correct position is displayed on the screen (◘ Fig. 32-10)

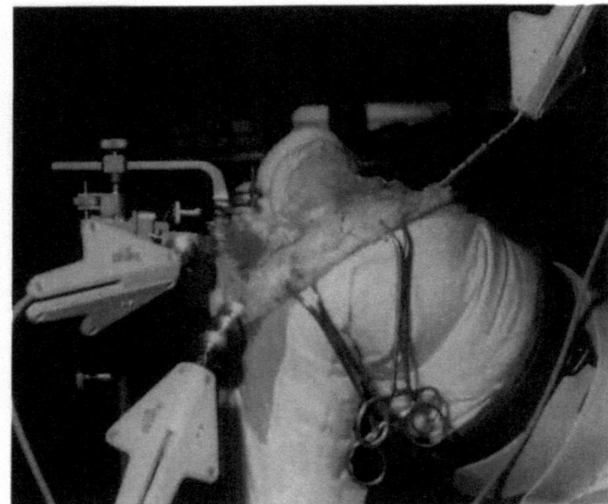

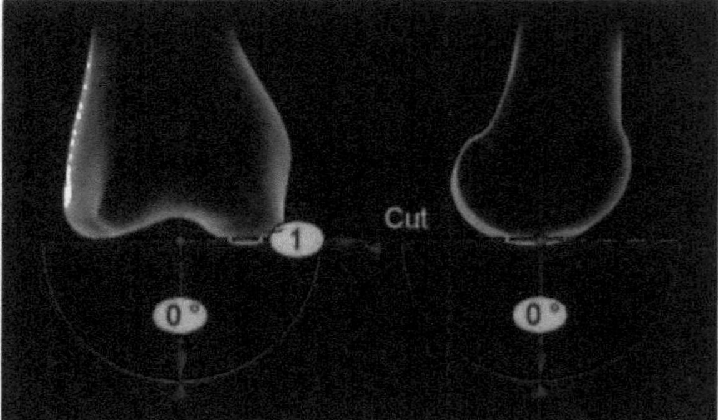

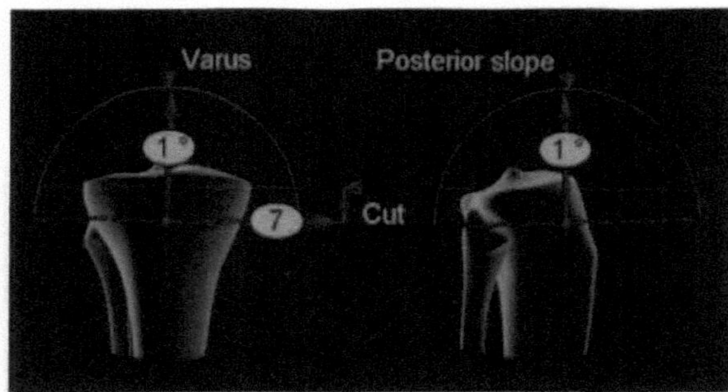

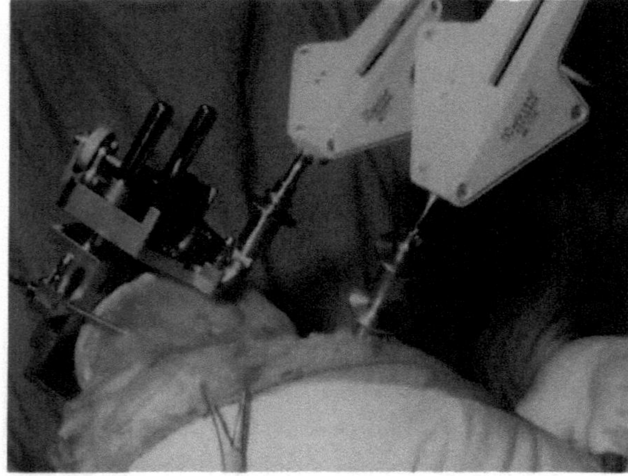

Fig. 32-7. Transmitter-attached tibial cutting block

Fig. 32-8. The settings for the tibia resection appear on the screen. varus-valgus, resection height, tibial slope

Fig. 32-9. Transmitter-attached femoral cutting block

Fig. 32-10. Setting of the varus-valgus and flexion-extension of the femoral component

the cutting block is fixed onto the bone with four threaded pins. The distal resection and alignment in the frontal plane are performed with the help of a distal cutting block mounted on the first cutting block using two movable metal columns.

We normally place the distal cutting block at right angles in the frontal plane and fix it to the bone with four threaded pins, the remaining auxiliary instrumentation is removed and the resection is performed. The bone alignment of the lower extremity has already been calculated by the computer and the prosthesis is implanted using the classical instrumentation, in particular for the anterior and posterior resections and the chamfers. The femoral rotation is easily quantifiable at this stage, based not on the distal epicondylar rotation, which is very difficult to assess with classical operating methods [3], but on the global rotation of the femur (mostly in external rotation in the genu varum). In our opinion, this method is more suited to the biomechanics of the implanted leg.

During trial implantation the computer checks the leg axis in extension, walking position and 90° flexion, the ligamentary balance through loading in varus and valgus and the medial and lateral degree of opening. We regard this balance as equal as long as the medial and lateral sides only differ by 2–3°. If the difference is more than this, progressive release of the ligaments is necessary until the ideal balance (medial opening equal to lateral opening) is attained. The leg axis can also be checked during the definitive implantation. This sometimes permits the removal of excess cement medially or laterally, which can alter the leg axis by 1° or 2° (1 mm cement = 1°).

Results

The results of our prospective, randomized study with the prototype were published in 2001 in the Revue de Chirurgie Orthopédique [21]. They show this system to be fully functional, reliable and reproducible. Even if it has not been able to demonstrate statistically relevant proof of its superiority over the conventional surgical technique (84% of HKA angles = 180° ± 3° as opposed to 75% conventional), it nonetheless assures a better distribution of axes around 180°, as well as more accurate implantation of the condyle and tibial components around 90° in both the frontal and the sagittal plane. It must be emphasized that this study was carried out using a prototype, and that some technical incidents (especially unstable transmitter fixations, imprecise palpation of the ankle joint) probably had a negative effect on the accuracy of some data.

Another study (Jenny [10]) with the OrthoPilot navigation system (latest generation) shows a statistically significant advantage for the computer-assisted operating technique (94% ideal implantations as against 78% conventional). We ourselves recently completed a study of 50 implantations with the OrthoPilot system with the objective of determining femoral rotation through navigation. In this study, which we will publish shortly, 100% of the mechanical leg axes lay between 177° and 183°.

Discussion

The implantation of total knee endoprostheses demands a highly developed instrumentation system, which among other things makes it possible to position the implant at right angles to the mechanical leg axis. The difficulty of this procedure depends on the shape of the femur (e.g. congenital curvature of the femur and coxa vara) and/or possible valgus or varus deformities, as well as callous formations on the femur and tibia. Correct positioning is however crucial for the long term prognosis of the prosthesis, reducing the risks of implant loosening and premature wear [1, 2, 5–9, 12, 17, 19, 20, 22].

Computer-assisted navigation with no preoperative CT can nowadays be regarded as a reliable procedure that allows the surgeon to achieve a mechanical axis between 177° and 183° in the frontal plane and optimal lateral positioning of the femoral and tibial components in more than 95% of all cases.

With this procedure we wish to avoid the use of intra-medullary (femur and tibia) and extra-medullary (essentially on the tibia) centering aids. In view of the highly sophisticated operating systems now available, some of these objectives might be considered to make little sense. However, inserting a stem into the femoral medullary cavity is no harmless procedure, even if incidents occur only rarely, and sometimes this implantation is not easy for various reasons: e.g. incorrect introduction of the implant into the femur (too far forwards or back, too far in a medial or lateral direction), congenital curvature of the femur, callous formations on the femur and a protruding hip prosthesis with a long stem. The use of intra- and extra-medullary centering aids on the tibia is also not without problems: with intra-medullary alignment varus resection, or a narrow or valgus tibia which does not allow the stem to enter; with extra-medullary alignment an incorrect tibial slope or varus or valgus deviation.

Our technique is adapted to a navigation system which assists the surgeon in carrying out the implantation. This computer-assisted system, orientated to the mechanical leg axis, differs from the two other newly developed systems for implanting knee prostheses, namely image-based or robotic-operating techniques [4]. To date we do not know of any published study containing results from these two computer-assisted methods, let alone prospective, randomized studies comparing these methods with the conventional operating techniques. Disadvantages of the image based procedure are on the one hand the use of a scanner for the 3D representation of the leg (100 sections 1 mm apart are necessary to depict the articulation of the knee [4]), and on the other hand the use of magnetic sensors (Navitrack, Sulzer Medica), which can interfere with the metal components of a surgical unit as well as with electrocardioscopes or respiration equipment. As far as the robotic technique is concerned, this appears to guarantee remarkable accuracy in bone resections (although this is not yet proven). This could lead to a more frequent use of cement-free prostheses – the question is whether this is of fundamental importance. However, we see here the same reasons for criticism as with the image-based procedure, with the addition that the robotic technique involves prohibitive costs (more than 500,000 dollars [4]). This must certainly be weighed against the effectiveness of the system, if one wishes to see such a system developed further in future. However, to date the interests of the industry have lain certainly partly in improved precision and reproducibility, but principally in increased production and higher profits, which are far removed from the concerns of surgery.

The technique we developed is however open to criticism in some respects. In the first place, the access for fixing the transmitter onto the pelvic crest was an additional surgical procedure which could lead to complications (hematoma, infection, residual pain, scar). Apart from the almost invisible scar on older patients, no such complications have actually arisen so far, either in this series or in the total number of 150 cases we have operated on to date. Nevertheless, we now use the software version 3.0, which permits us the same level of reliability while omitting the referencing procedure on the pelvic crest.

Apart from this, one could criticize the longer operation time. With the navigation system we currently use (OrthoPilot, Aesculap, Tuttlingen) and with second generation accompanying instrumentation, we can more than halve the average time lost (between 10 and 15 min). We consider this lengthening of the overall operating time (75–90 min for the experienced surgeon) to be completely acceptable.

One could also criticize the difficulties which arise in identifying a »midpoint« of the knee where there is severe gonarthrosis with ruptured anterior cruciate ligament and loose peripheral conditions as well as posterior-medial or posterior-lateral wear. The trials with cadavers showed that the resection of the anterior and/or the posterior cruciate ligament had little effect on the rotational centre of the knee (establishing a rotational centre of gravity by looking for the point on the femur which is most equidistant, in the sense of the fewest squares, from a point on the tibia). This realization is also confirmed by the clinical results from our series, in which we were able to correct substantial deformities with ruptured anterior cruciate ligament perfectly with computer assistance (two cases with HKA angle 162°, end result 177°, and one case with HKA angle 210°, end result 181°).

The advantages of our operating technique should also be emphasized. In the first place, the absence of any complicated imaging procedures (2D and 3D scanners) and in future also of pangonometry (except for callous formations or traumatic secondary conditions which are difficult to classify) gives this technique a not inconsiderable economic advantage (only normal X-rays could be required) and leaves the responsibility with the surgeon, which can make sense, for instance when the quality of the images is not of the standard required. Apart from this, permanent orientation to the mechanical leg axis and identification of the rotational centers of the hip, knee and ankle are classic and familiar concepts for the orthopaedic surgeon; the surgeon remains in control of the tools and can check the correct functioning of the system at any time through a classical procedure. Even with such a system, however, an experienced surgeon is absolutely essential. The height of the tibial resection, ligament balancing, patella tracking and patella surface replacement are procedures that cannot be improvised, but demand experience.

Finally, the direct intraoperative determination of the mechanical leg axis opens up new horizons. Thanks to this system we can achieve the mechanical axis by the end of the operation in real time without pangonometric checking. We can check whether the knee has a normal orientation (residual valgus or varus deformity). We can establish the tautness of the peripheral conditions medially and laterally and establish varus or valgus deformity up to 90–100° flexion. In the classical techniques, all these methods were either approximate, subjective or impossible (varus or valgus deformity in flexion).

Conclusion

Computer-assisted surgery heralds the start of a new era. This procedure should now become part of the technical equipment of the surgeon, as it already has in many other areas. Its use in implanting knee endoprostheses has validated the system and concluded the trial phase. Future studies with mature equipment should confirm the solid foundation of computer-assisted surgery. Its use in other orthopaedic operations (among others high tibial osteotomy, unicondylar knee replacement) offers very interesting prospects with regard to the accuracy, reliability and reproducibility of surgical procedures.

References

1. Aglietti P, Buzzi R (1988) Posteriorly stabilized total condylar knee replacement: three to eight years follow up of 85 knees. J Bone Joint Surg 70B: 211–216

2. Bargren JH, Blaha JD, Freeman MAR (1983) Alignment in total knee arthroplasty: Correlated biomechanical and clinical observations. Clin Orthop 173: 178–183

3. Boisrenoult P, Scemama P, Fallet L, Beaufils P et le groupe BIOMED (2001) La torsion épiphysaire distale du fémur dans le genou arthrosique. Etude tomodensitométrique de 75 genoux avec arthrose médiale. Rev Chir Orthop 87: 469–476

4. Delp SL, Stulberg, SD, Davies B, Picard F, Leitner F (1998) Computer assisted knee replacement. Clin Orthop 354: 49–57

5. Ecker ML, Lotke PA, Windor RE, Cello JP (1987) Long term results after total condylar knee arthroplasty. Clin Orthop 216: 151–158

6. Hood RW, Vanni M, Insall JN (1981) The correction of knee alignment in 225 consecutive total condylar knee replacements. Clin Orthop 160: 94–105

7. Hsu H, Garg A, Walker PS, Spector M, Ewald FC (1989) Effect of knee component alignment or tibial load distribution with clinical correlation. Clin Orthop 248: 135–144

8. Insall JN, Scott W, Ranawat CS (1979) The total condylar knee prosthesis. A report of two hundred and twenty cases. J Bone Joint Surg 61A: 173–180

9. Jeffrey RS, Morris RW, Benham RA (1991) Coronal alignment after total knee replacement. J Bone Joint Surg 73B: 709–714

10. Jenny JY, Boeri C (2001) Implantation d'une prothèse totale de genou assistée par ordinateur. Etude comparative cas-témoin avec une instrumentation traditionnelle. Rev Chir Orthop 87: 645–652

11. Julliard R, Lavallée S, Dessenne V (1998) Computer-assisted reconstruction of the anterior cruciate ligament. Clin Orthop 354: 57–64

12. Laskin RS (1984) Alignment in total knee replacement. Orthopaedics 7: 62–72

13. Lavallée S (1989) Geste médico-chirurgicaux assistés par ordinateur: application à la neurochirurgie stéréotaxique. Thèse, génie biologique et médical, Grenoble

14. Leitner F, Picard F, Minfelde R, Schultz HJ, Cinquin P, Saragaglia D (1997) Computer-assisted knee surgical total replacement. In »lecture note in computer science«: CURMed-MRCAS'97. Springer, Berlin Heidelberg New York Tokyo, pp 629–638

15. Lotke PA, Ecker ML (1977) Influence of positioning of prosthesis in total knee replacement. J Bone Joint Surg 59A: 77–79

16. Merloz Ph, Cinquin P (1994) Geste médico-chirurgical assisté par ordinateur: application à la visée automatisée du pédicule vertébral. Etude expérimentale. Rev Chir Orthop 80 [Suppl I]: 124–125

17. Peterson TC, Engh GA (1988) Radiographic assessment of knee alignment after total knee arthroplasty. J Arthroplasty 3: 67–72

18. Picard F, Leitner F, Saragaglia D, Cinquin P (1997) Mise en place d'une prothèse totale du genou assistée par ordinateur: A propos de 7 implantations sur cadavre. Rev Chir Orthop 83 [Suppl II]: 31

19. Ranawat CS, Boachie-Adjei O (1988) Survivorship analysis and results of total condylar knee arthroplasty. Clin Orthop 226: 6–13

20. Ritter MA, Faris PM, Keating EM, Meding JB (1994) Postoperative alignment of total knee replacement: its effects on survival. Clin Orthop 299: 153–157

21. Saragaglia D, Picard F, Chaussard C, Montbarbon E, Leitner F, Cinquin P (2001) Mise en place des prothèses totale du genou assistée par ordinateur: comparaison avec la technique conventionnelle. A propos d'une étude prospective randomisée de 50 cas. Rev Chir Orthop 87: 18–28

22. Tew M, Waugh W (1985) Tibial-femoral alignment and the results of knee replacement. Bone Joint Surg 67B: 551–556

33 Computer-Assisted Navigation with the *OrthoPilot* System Using the Search Evolution TKA Prosthesis
Results of a MultiCenter Study

U. Clemens, W. H. Konermann, S. Kohler, H. Kiefer, J.Y. Jenny, R.K. Miehlke

New evolving technology usually lacks sufficient data indicating clear advantages to conventional methods. We, therefore, performed a five-center study in order to demonstrate the consistency and superiority of the OrthoPilot navigation system in TKA.

Background

The survivorship of total knee arthroplasties (TKA) have improved up to 95% after ten years of surgery [10, 15]. Long-term results are influenced by various factors including optimal physiological component alignment. Therefore, the accuracy of component positioning during surgery is a crucial factor for long-term outcome [1, 9, 21].

Rand and Coventry [20] reported a survivorship of 90% after ten years when the mechanical axis was within 0 to 4 degrees of valgus, but was reduced to fewer than 73% when the mechanical axis was above 4 degrees of valgus. Computer navigation tools were merely evolved in order to improve the accuracy and reproducibility of the surgical technique. Various computer navigation systems were developed recently [4, 12, 14], but published data are limited and usually represent small series [8, 19]. Our hypothesis of this study was to demonstrate the superiority of implant positioning when computer navigation was used during surgery in comparison to conventional implanted TKA.

Patients and Methods

We report a five center, prospective, randomized study in the time period between 1999 and 2001. Of 821 patients that underwent primary TKA (SEARCH, Aesculap, Tuttlingen, Germany), 555 cases were implanted using the OrthoPilot navigation system (group A; ◘ Fig. 33-1) and 266 TKA were implanted using conventional instruments (group B). In group A, 514 TKA were fully cemented, 35 TKA hybrids, and 6 TKA uncemented. In group B 238 TKA were fully cemented, 8 hybrids, and 20 TKA uncemented. The accuracy of implant positioning with regards to all four planes and views were compared on single leg stance radiographs 3 months postoperatively by an independent reviewer. Operating time (skin to skin) and parameter of the excellent results in both groups were compared. Results for excellent, good, and poor data were

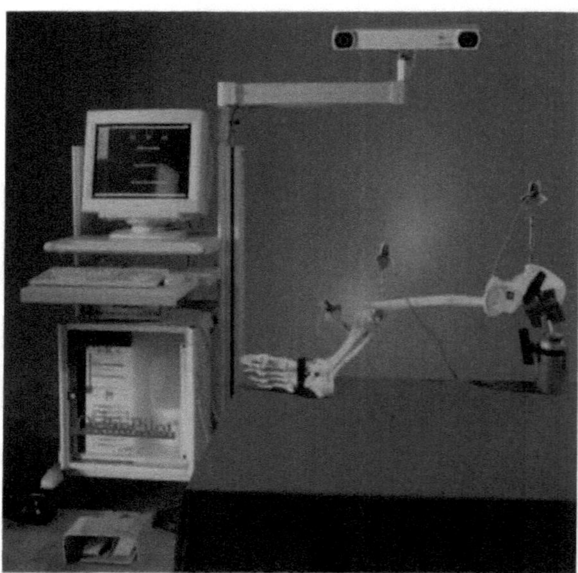

◘ Fig. 33-1. OrthoPilot navigation system.

Table 33-1. Definition of radiographic results (deviation from ideal values)

	Mechanical axis	Other axes
Excellent	0°–3°	0°–2°
Good	4°–5°	3°–4°
Poor	>5°	>4°

defined according to recommendations from the literature (■ Table 33-1).

Group A (with navigation): There were 142 males and 413 females with a mean age of 71 years (42 to 91). Preoperative mechanical axis ranged from 22 degrees valgus to 42 degrees varus (mean 5.2 degrees varus, SD: 8.5).

Group B (without navigation): There were 63 males and 203 females with a mean age of 69 years (24 to 95). Preoperative mechanical axis ranged from 30 degrees valgus to 30 degrees varus (mean 5.5 degrees varus, SD: 10.3). There were no statistical differences in both groups with regards to gender, age, sex, and diagnosis.

Surgical Technique

All knees were approached from a mid-line skin incision, a medial or lateral parapatellar retinacular arthrotomy was performed according to the preoperative deformity. Two different prosthetic TKA implants were used: the SEARCH classic and the SEARCH evolution system. No semi-constraint systems were used. The patella was resurfaced in 59 cases in group A and in 117 cases in group B. Patelloplasty was performed in some cases including partial denervation. The femoral component was positioned with 3 degrees external rotation to the posterior condylar axis in 607 knees and between 0 to 3 degrees in 214 knees according to the surgeon's preferences.

Navigation

The OrthoPilot navigation system (Aesculap, Tuttlingen, Germany, see Fig. 33-1) consist of a 3D infrared camera (Polaris, Northern Digital) tracing six infrared diodes mounted on a rigid body, which is connected to either a tool, a finger pointer, or a cortical bone screw. One rigid

body each is connected to the ilium, to the distal femur and the proximal tibia. An ankle strap is used for connecting a rigid body to the distal tibia. Rigid bodies also home in to the resection blocks of tibia and femur.

The individual mechanical leg axis is calculated using mathematical algorithms and intraoperative kinematics analysis with surface matching of key anatomical structures. Resection blocks are positioned »on-line« comparing images on a monitor. Resections are performed manually. The navigation system additionally suggests implant size and tibial resection height. The position of all rigid bodies is monitored continuously in a 3D space and to one another. All navigation steps are calculated by a Windows-NT-Workstation and are guided by the surgeon via a foot switch. This particular system does not require CT or MRT data, therefore, both pre- or intraoperative data matching and planning is not required.

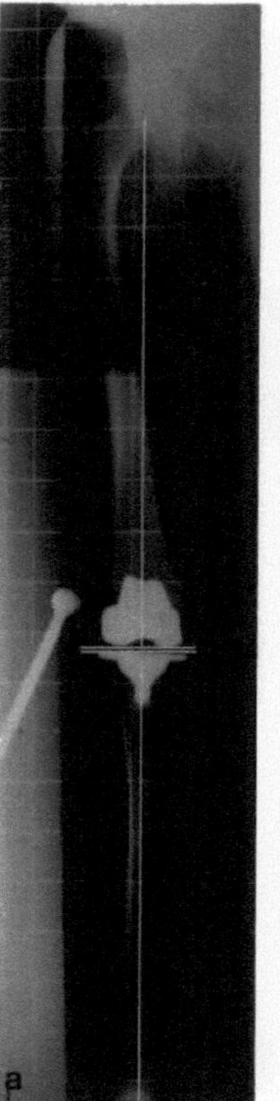
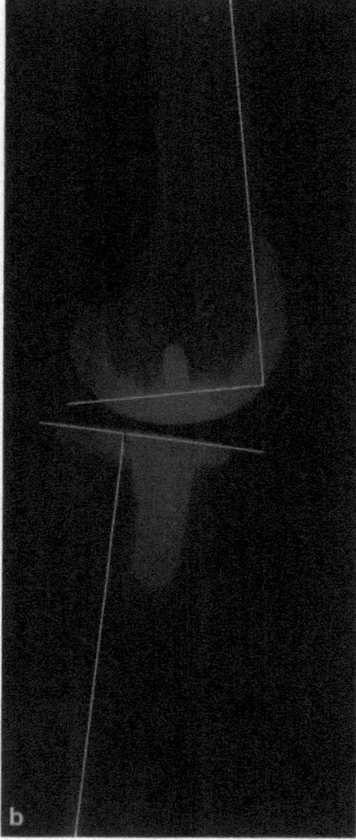

■ **Fig. 33-2a, b.** Radiographic evaluation tools. a Single leg stance view, b lateral radiograph

Conventional Implantation

Manually implanted TKA in this series were performed using the SEARCH classic and SEARCH evolution instruments with intra-medullary guides for femoral resection and extra-medullary guides for tibial resection.

Radiographic Evaluation

Standardized radiographs after three months with one leg stand are required making sure that central beams are crossing the midline of the patella. Lateral views should fall perpendicular to the joint space so that both implant pegs have the same length (□ Fig. 33-2). On sagittal views tibial and femoral slope are measured. The femoral slope is taken from the tangent to the anterior cortex and the distal cut. The tibial slope is taken from the tangent to the dorsal cortex and the tibial cut.

Statistical Analyses

For all five angles the Wilcoxon et al. U-Test was employed for statistical significance ($p<0.05$). Both groups were additionally compared using the Chi-Square-Test.

Results

Single Parameter

There were significant differences with better results in the OrthoPilot group A for the mechanical axis a.p.,

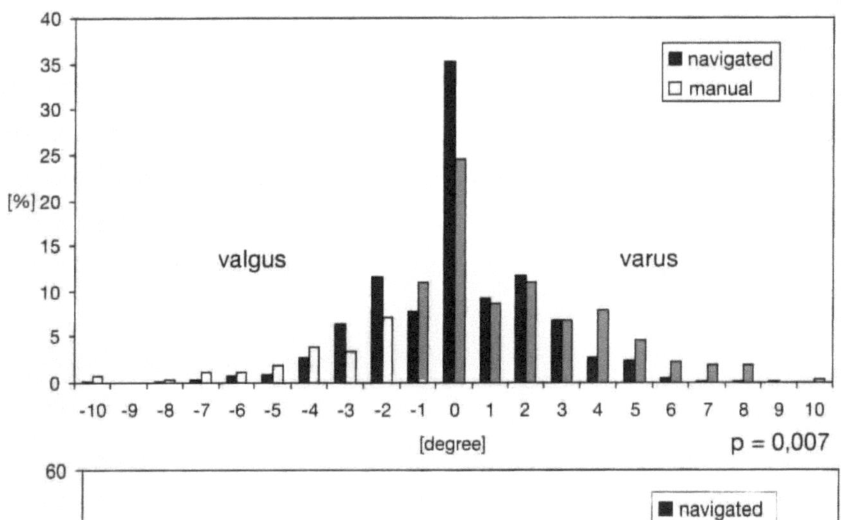

□ **Fig. 33-3.** Postoperative mechanical axis a.p.

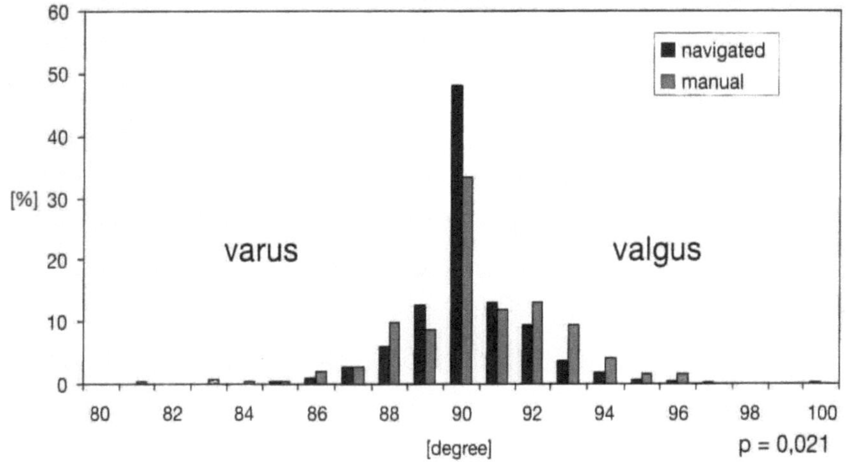

□ **Fig. 33-4.** Postoperative femoral axis a.p.

the femoral and tibial axis a.p. and the femoral axis lat. (■ Figs. 33-3 to 33-7). Looking at the distribution to the categories (■ Table 33-2) with the Chi-Square-Test there are significant differences for the mechanical axis a.p., femoral axis a.p., tibial axis a.p. and lateral.

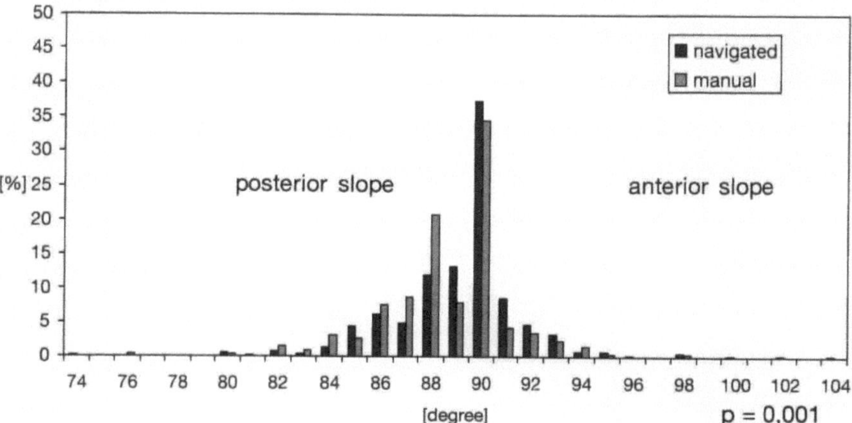

■ **Fig. 33-5.** postoperative femoral axis lateral

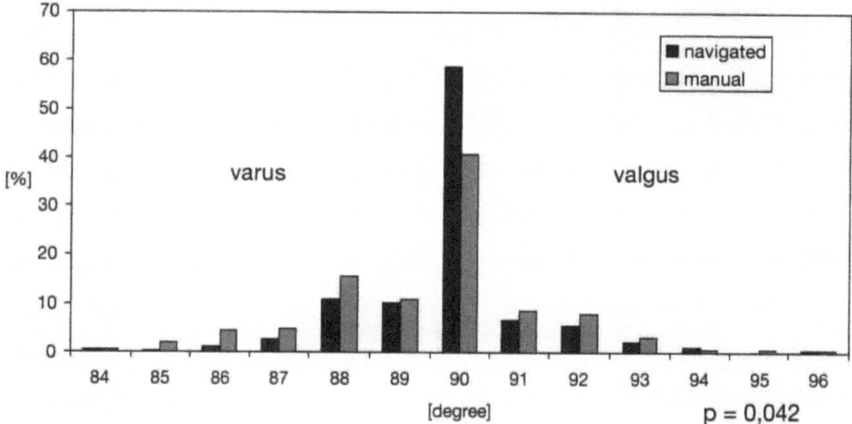

■ **Fig. 33-6.** postoperative tibial axis a.p.

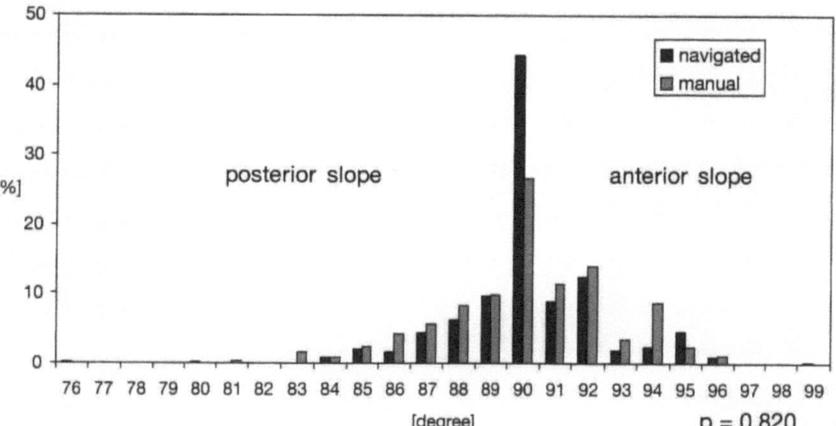

■ **Fig. 33-7.** postoperative tibial axis lateral

Table 33-2. Distribution of results and significances

	Mechanical axis		Femur a.p.		Femur lateral		Tibia a.p.		Tibia lateral	
	Navigated	Control	Navigated	Control	Navigated	Control	Navigated	Control	Navigated	Control
Excellent	88	72	89	77	76	71	92	84	81	70
Good	9	18	9	18	15	20	7	13	10	22
Moderate	3	10	2	5	9	9	1	3	9	8
Significance	$p<0{,}001$		$p<0{,}001$		$p=0{,}197$		$p<0{,}001$		$p<0{,}001$	

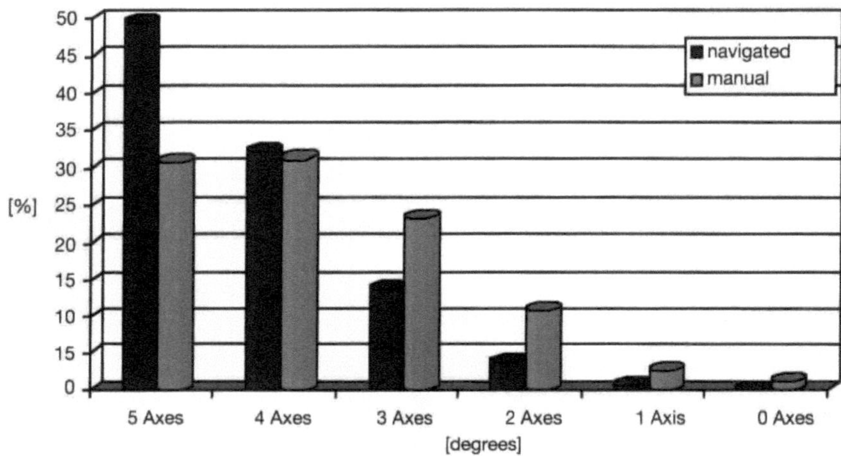

Fig. 33-8. Distribution of excellent results in navigated and manual group

Number of Excellent Axes

The results were excellent in 49.6% for all five axes in the navigated group A compared with 30.8% in the conventional group B (**Fig. 33-8**). When four axes were compared, group A had a higher number with 32.3% (A) to 31.2% (B), both differences were significant.

Skin to Skin Operating Time

The mean time in the navigated group A was 107.8 min (70–193, SD:22) and, therefore, 8.7 min longer compared with group B, which took a mean of 99.2 (56–165, SD:22).

Complications

There were fewer complications in the navigated group A with 6.1% compared with 21.8% in group B (**Table 33-3**).

Intraoperative fractured occurred in group A and B one each. In group A one drill broke in the ilium and one navigation screw was left in the femur.

Table 33-3. Complications

	Manual		Navigated	
	n	%	*n*	%
Total *n*=	58	21.8	34	6.1
Thrombosis	12	4.5	8	1,4
Pulmoembolism	2	0.8	5	0.9
Hematoma	11	4.1	4	0.7
Skin necrosis	6	2.3	0	0.0
Deep infection	3	1.1	1	0.2
Wound problems	3	1.1	0	0.0
Poor mobility	8	3.0	8	1.4
Others	13	4.9	8	1.4

Discussion

The accuracy of the measuring angles on single long leg views is 2 degrees and is, therefore, more precise than short knee films - 5 degrees [2]. Further disadvantages of short leg views include errors from 1.6 to 1.9 degrees [16, 18], oblique errors, as well as rotational errors up to 2 degrees, which mimic increased valgus in internal rotation and increased varus in external rotation [11, 22]. Inter-observer error is reported with 1.1 degree and intra-observer error with 0.9 degrees [3].

Mechanical Axis

The a.p. mechanical axis was significantly more accurate in the navigated group A and represented a calculated angle of both the femur and tibia axes, but depends on the right size inlay as well as correct soft tissue balancing, since all radiographs were single leg weight bearing views. Excellent radiographic results can be achieved, when bone resections are precise or in cases with mutual alignments. Implanting the components correctly in all planes also increases overall accuracy.

What caused poor results in the navigated group, since the accuracy of the infrared diodes and software algorithm lies in less than 1 degree [18]? The largest factor appeared to be the learning curve in all five centers. In one center, the rigid body kept rotating, causing considerable errors of all resection planes, which was noted only after case 15 and was subsequently changed. However, the poor results were not excluded from this study. All resection planes were created using a manual oscillating saw with its known inaccuracy, particularly at both soft and sclerotic bone qualities. We, therefore, recommend a navigational double check of all resection planes. However, this has not been applied in the current study. The cementing technique represents a further error regarding finite component alignment.

Femoral Axis a.p.

The mean results were significantly more accurate in the navigation group (89.4% compared with 77.1%). Intra-operative identification of the femoral axis is difficult because of soft tissues and tourniquet. Laskin reported a 4 cm error of the surgeon identifying the femoral head center [13]. This could be optimized using intraoperative fluoroscopy, with its downsides of radiating and added operating time [6]. Intra-medullary alignment was the preferred method in this study [6, 7]. However, potential errors with this method include a wide or deformed femur and a correct entry point [7]. With navigation, the femoral head is calculated more precisely as is demonstrated in our results: 1.6% compared with 4.9% in the poor results.

Femoral Axis Lateral

Lateral radiographs were non-weight bearing as recommended in the literature. Component alignment on sagittal views were less accurate than on anteroposterior films, but with 75.5% excellent alignment in the navigated group A better than in the manual group B with 70.7% excellent results. Antecurvation of the femur is a problem for both manual component positioning during surgery and postoperative radiographic evaluation. Intra-medullary tools generally tend to place the femoral component into increased flexion [17] with the positive side effect of anterior femoral cortex non-notching. Navigated femoral implants have a bigger tendency for anterior notching because they do not respect the antecurvation. This could be prevented with the femoral component flange being more open. Thus, experience from navigation may influence component design.

Tibial Axis a.p.

Frontal tibial component alignment was most accurate in both groups, but alignment in the navigated group A was better (91.9% excellent results), compared with the manual group B (83.5%). Both groups showed a trend to varus positioning according to the natural slope of 3 degrees [3]. The surgeon tends to resect the tibial head with similar mediolateral thickness, rather than oblique. However, accurate resection of the tibia is facilitated due to less soft tissue coverage [13].

Tibial Axis Lateral

Group A had significantly more excellent results (81.3%) compared with the manual group B (69.9%). Poor results were equally distributed due to the fact discussed above.

Number of Excellent Results

Most data in the literature focus on one or two a.p. planes only, however, consideration of all axes and perfect positioning of both components in all planes will ultimately improve the long-term outcome and vice versa. When looked at TKA with all five axes being excellently implanted a significantly higher number was observed in the navigated group A (49.5%) compared with the conventional group B (30.8%).

Surgery Time

Although an increased surgery time was expected in the navigated group, only a mean of 8.7 minutes additional time was encountered including the learning curve of five different centers. Therefore, the additional time required with this procedure is expected to decrease. Further improvements include the non-necessity of the ilium rigid body, which will certainly gain more time in future. The operating time will be increased, when femoral component rotation/a.p. positioning and soft tissue tension in both flexion and extension are navigated, however time is saved due to decreased need of considerable time consuming correcting maneuvers. All participating surgeons reported a decreased necessity of correcting soft tissues when navigation was used.

Complications

There were significantly less complications in the navigated group A (6.1%) compared with group B (21.8%), possibly due to the fact, that the protocol included a considerable number of alignment data and that two centers contributed navigation data only. However, fewer complications in the navigated group are expected because of reasons that include a non-hollowed femoral canal (decreased bleeding, hematoma, wound healing) and less fat embolism. Further parameters will have to be included in future study designs in order to show these effects more precisely. There were less manipulation under anesthesia required and better mobility of the TKA due to improved implant positioning in the navigation group A. Complication in the navigated group A such as one screw left in the ilium and one broken drill in the femur are now technically abandoned..

Conclusions

TKA navigation using the OrthoPilot system led to significantly increased precision of component positioning compared with manually implanted TKA in our study. Continuous improvements on both the software and hardware tools will further compliment this technique. There will be an increased number of patient specific information, which can be implemented to this system. However, more data from the patient and the prosthetic components are needed to further improve the quality. Fluoroscopy and ultrasound are another source of additional information. The resection technique can be optimized with more sophisticated instruments (cutting guides, milling). Navigation of TKA with the OrthoPilot system is an important step to a superior and more precise component implantation and will ultimately influence prosthesis design.

References

1. Bargren JH, Blaha JD, Freeman MAR (1983) Alignment in total knee arthroplasty. Clin Orthop 173: 178–183
2. Bonnici AV, Allen PR (1991) Comparison of long leg and simple knee radiographs in assessment of knees prior to surgery. J Bone and Joint Surg (Br) 73-B [Supp 1]: 65
3. Coull R, Bankes MJK, Rossouw DJ (1999) Evaluation of tibial component angles in 79 consecutive total knee arthroplasties. Knee 6: 235–237
4. Delp SL, Stulberg SD, Davies BL, Picard F, Leitner F (1998) Computer assisted knee replacement. Clin Orthop 354: 49–56
5. Dorr LD, Conaty JP, Schreffier R, Mehne DK, Hull D (1985) Technical factors that influence mechanical loosening of total knee arthroplasty. In Dorr LD (ed) The knee. Baltimore University Park Press, Baltimore, pp 121–135
6. Ischii Y, Ohmori G, Bechthold J, Gustilo RB (1995) Extramedullary versus intramedullary alignment guides in total knee arthroplasty. Clin Orthop 318: 167–175

7. Jeffery JA (1999) Accuracy of intramedullary femoral alignment in total knee replacement: intraoperative assesment of alignment rod position. Knee 6: 211–215

8. Jenny JY, Boeri C (2001) Computer-assisted implantation of total knee prostheses: a case control comparative study with classical instrumentation. Computer Aided Surg 6: 217–220

9. Jonsson B, Astrom J (1988) Alignment and long-term clinical results of a semi-constrained knee prosthesis. Clin Orthop 226: 124–128

10. Knutson K, Lindstrand A, Lidgren L (1986) Survival of knee arthroplasties, a nation-wide multicenter investigation of 8000 cases. J Bone Joint Surg 68B: 795–803

11. Krackow KA, Pepe CL, Galloway EJ (1990) A mathematical analysis of the effect of flexion and rotation on apparent varus/valgus alignment at the knee. Orthopaedics 13: 861–868

12. Krackow KA, Serpe L, Phillips MJ Bayers-Thering M, Mihalko WM (1999) A new technique for determining proper mechanical axis alignment during total knee arthroplasty: Progress toward computer assisted TKA. Orthopedics 22: 698–702

13. Laskin RS (1984) Alignment of total knee components. Orthopaedics 7: 62

14. Leitner F, Picard F, Minfelde R, Schulz HJ, Clinquin P, Saragaglia D (1997) Computer assisted knee surgical total replacement. In: Troccaz J, Grimson E, Mösges R (eds) CVRMed-MRCAS. Springer, Berlin Heidelberg New York Tokyo, pp 630–638

15. Nafei A, Kristensen O, Knudson HM, Hvid I, Jensen J (1996) Survivorship analysis of cemented total condylar knee arthoplasty. J Arthroplasty 11: 7–10

16. Patel DV, Ferris BD, Aichroth PM (1991) Radiological study of alignment after total knee replacement. Int Orthop 15: 209–210

17. Petersen TL, Engh GA (1988) Radiographic assessment of knee alignment after total knee arthroplasty. J Arthroplasty 3: 67–72

18. Picard F, Leitner F, Raoult O, Saragaglia D (1999) Computer assisted total knee arthroplasty. In: Jerosch J, Nicol K, Peikenkamp K (Hrsg) Rechnergestützte Verfahren in Orthopädie und Unfallchirurgie. Steinkopff, Darmstadt, S 461–471

19. Picard F, Saragaglia D, Montbarbon E, Chaussard C, Leitner F, Raoult O (1999) Computer assisted knee arthroplasty – preliminary clinical results with the OrthoPilot System. In: Proceedings, 4th International CAOS Symposium, Davos

20. Rand JA, Coventry MB (1988) Ten-year evaluation of geometric total knee arthroplasty. Clin Orthop 232: 168–173

21. Ritter MA, Faris PM, Keating EM, Meding JB (1994) Postoperative alignment of total knee replacement its effect on survival. Clin Orthop 299: 153–156

22. Swanson KE, Stocks GW, Warren PD, Hazel MR, Janssen HF (2000) Does axial limb rotation affect the alignment measurements in deformed limbs? Clin Orthop 371: 246 – 252

34 The *OrthoPilot* Navigation System in Total Knee Arthroplasty: Version 4.0

R. K. Miehlke, R. G. Haaker, W. H. Konermann

Introduction

Following its development period from 1993 to 1997 [12] in joint and spinal surgery, the OrthoPilot system has proved its technical efficiency from 1997 onwards in a cadaver study [9] and in subsequent clinical trials [7]. Moreover, the OrthoPilot navigation system has also shown substantially better results compared with the use of manual instrumentation [2– 4, 8, 11]. It was reported in a multicenter study [1] that a statistically significant improvement in the alignment of the knee prosthesis components in respect of the mechanical leg axis and the femoral and tibial individual axes could be achieved with the OrthoPilot system as opposed to the manual technique. It should be noted here that the »learning curve« of all the centers taking part was included in the results. The superiority of the navigated implantation technique became particularly obvious when the five set parameters of $0° \pm 3°$ for the mechanical axis and $90° \pm 2°$ for the individual axes were observed. Such results, which are to be considered very good, were achieved in 49.6% of cases with the navigated technique, whereas the attainment rate with the manual implantation technique was only 30.8%. In a comparative investigation between 100 navigated cases with the Search Evolution knee and the manually instrumented LCS knee system, Konermann and Saur [5] showed even clearer differences in favor of the navigated technique using the same criteria. With the navigation technique they observed very good results in respect of all five axes in 54% of the cases, whereas this was the case in just 15% of the patients treated with manual implantation technique.

In software versions 1.0 to 2.2 the OrthoPilot system simply navigated the tibial resection and the distal femoral resection planes of a total knee arthroplasty.

Versions 3.0 and 3.1 included, in addition, the rotational alignment of the femoral component through acquisition of the transepicondylar axis via the medial and lateral femoral epicondyle. The inaccuracies in defining the femoral epicondyles must be taken into account here.

The goal in total knee replacement is not only to create an accurate axis of the leg within $\pm 3°$ of the Mikulicz' line, but also to balance the soft tissues. This is necessary to prevent unequal polyethylene wear and early implant failure as well as to achieve stability of the knee during the whole range of motion.

Exact positioning of the femoral component in relation to the tibial component in both extension and flexion may be facilitated by recording the data of the flexion and extension gaps.

A first step in this direction had already been made with the SurgiGATE system [14]. The Galileo system [12] and the VectorVision system (see chapter 36) also integrate the measurement of extension and flexion gaps. The Stryker Leibinger navigation system [6, 13] uses the distance between femoral epicondyles and the resection on the proximal tibia to arrive at two curves for the medial and lateral side of the knee joint over the entire range of movement. These curves provide information about contractures on the one hand or instability on the other, and in this way make soft tissue management possible. However, inaccuracies exist in the difficulties in exactly determining the femoral epicondyles.

Version 4.0 of the OrthoPilot system uses a special gap spreader to achieve accurate recording of flexion and extension gap data. This allows conclusions to be made about a necessary soft tissue release, and thus soft tissue management as a whole.

Surgical Technique with Version 4.0

There are no differences from the previous software versions 3.0 and 3.1 in respect of the distal femoral entry point, intraoperative kinematic analysis with circumduction of the hip to determine the femoral axis which runs through the centre of the femoral head, the definition of the centre of the ankle and knee joints and the acquisition of the knee joint line, the deepest defect point of the dorsal femoral condyles, the anterior cortex on the distal femur and the malleolar triangle. When the leg axis has been established and displayed on screen following kinematic analysis, the first qualitative information about a necessary soft tissue release is provided.

But Version 4.0 goes further than this limited possibility of performing soft tissue release.

In addition, the more modern system employs a universal alignment guide for both tibial head and distal femoral resection. This guide can be adjusted in all three degrees of freedom, allowing the valgus/varus position, slope and resection height to be adjusted. Only the resection blocks for the tibial and femoral sides are different.

The tibial resection block is first fixed into position provisionally on the head of the tibia using the universal alignment guide. Next follows the precise alignment in all planes and final fixation of the block, after which the tibial resection is performed. The tibial resection plane data are subsequently recorded using a tibial template and the accuracy of the resection is checked.

When this has been completed, a femoral plate is placed on the distal femoral condyles, positioned at right angles to the defined femoral axis, and used to record the distal femoral condyle plane, which is important for determining the extent of the distal femoral resection. The potential size of the femoral component, established by the acquisition of the femoral data, is also continuously displayed on the screen.

The next step is to make precise measurements of first the flexion gap and then the extension gap using a special spreader. The measurements are brought together and also indicated on screen. Then the universal alignment guide is provisionally fixed onto the distal femur and aligned in all planes, including the resection height, before being finally fixed into position on the distal femur. The femoral alignment always takes account of the medial and lateral sides simultaneously in their relation to the tibial resec-

tion. The respective value with reference to the resultant height for the tibial polyethylene component is also given.

This is followed by distal femoral condyle resection. The data of the distal femoral condyle resection are recorded with the femoral navigation template (■ Fig. 34-1).

Now the femoral template is laid onto the distal femoral resection and the femoral component is brought into rotational alignment with the tibial resection plane. During this procedure the effects of the rotation of the femoral component on the flexion and extension gaps can be directly observed, as can the effects on the flexion and extension gaps of changing the size of the femoral component. In addition, the system informs the surgeon on screen about the anterioposterior position of the component, to avoid notching of the anterior femoral cortex (■ Fig. 34-2).

When properly balanced conditions of the medial and lateral side in flexion and extension have been achieved, after the correct size of femoral component has been selected and rotational alignment performed, the locating points for the four-in-one resection template are drilled through the femoral template. Then the remaining femoral bone resection is carried out using the four-in-one cutting block.

In practice, a difference of more than 5–6 mm should not be tolerated between the medial and lateral side of the knee joint when measuring the flexion and extension gaps with the spreader. If the differences between the medial and lateral side are too great, additional soft tissue release on the more contracted side should be performed at this point, after which the flexion and extension gaps should be re-measured. This procedure helps to ensure that no unrealistic values for the femoral component occur during subsequent rotational alignment.

Version 4.0 of the OrthoPilot system also contains a module that, following tibial resection, gap measurement and distal femoral condyle resection, permits the surgeon to simulate the conditions that would exist if potential femoral and tibial components were used.

After all the bone resections have been completed, the trial components are implanted and the final axial conditions achieved are displayed on screen. The bones are prepared for the femoral and tibial anchoring mechanisms and the knee endoprosthesis is implanted, including a patella component if required. After implantation the data for the definitive position of the endoprosthesis components are recorded (■ Fig. 34-3).

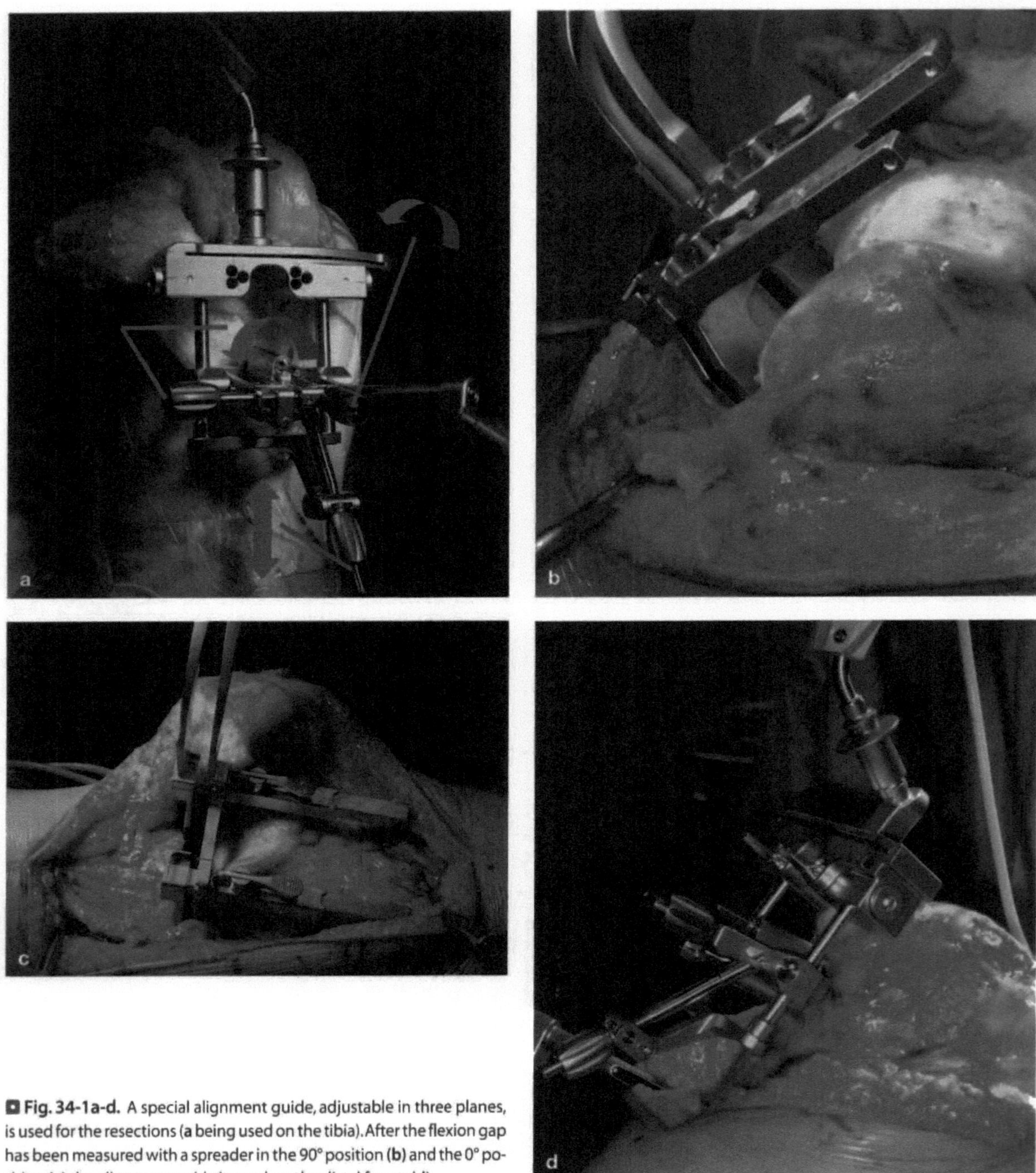

◘ Fig. 34-1a-d. A special alignment guide, adjustable in three planes, is used for the resections (**a** being used on the tibia). After the flexion gap has been measured with a spreader in the 90° position (**b**) and the 0° position (**c**) the alignment guide is used on the distal femur (**d**)

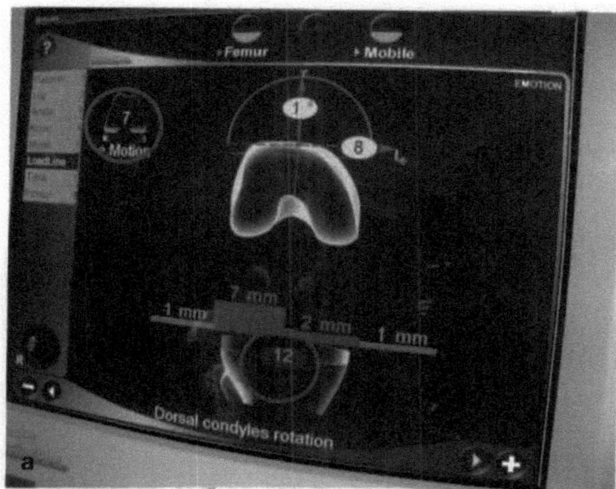

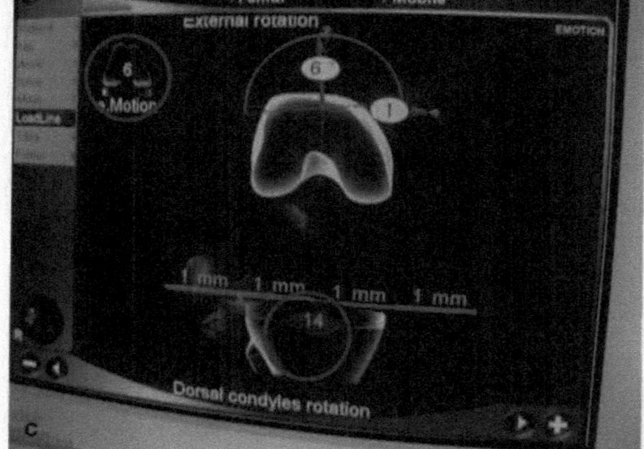

◘ Fig. 34-2a-c. Example of the final matching of medial and lateral flexion and extension gaps as well as rotation of the femoral component and height of the tibial component, **a** balanced extension gap, flexion gap laterally 7 mm, medially 2 mm, femoral component size 7 with 1° external rotation, tibial height 12 mm, **b** balanced extension gap, balanced flexion gap but still too wide, femoral component size 7 with 6° external rotation, but still too large (as in a), tibial height 12 mm, **c** femoral component correct size 6 with 6° external rotation, tibial height 14 mm, flexion and extension gaps now completely balanced

Preliminary Results

Version 4.0 of the OrthoPilot knee navigation system is used in combination with the e.motion[1] and Columbus[1] knee prostheses (see chapter 35).

The e.motion knee endoprosthesis system offers a prosthesis that maintains a high surface congruence between the femoral component and the tibial polyethylene component between 5° hyperextension and 90° flexion, with the help of a rotational gliding platform.

The first authors' clinical experience was gained using the e.motion knee endoprosthesis system. 150 navigated implantations of e.motion knee endoprostheses have been carried out to date. Complete data records are available for the first 25 cases.

Using the same assessment criteria cited by Clemens et al. [1] (see chapter 33) and Konermann and Saur [5] (see chapter 31), the results were as follows: a very good result was achieved for the mechanical axis in 22/25 cases (88%), for the femoral axis a.p. in 23/25 (92%), for the femoral axis in the lateral plane in 16/25 (64%), for the tibial axis a.p. in 22/25 (88%) and for the tibial axis in the lateral plane also in 22/25 (88%). Outliers were present in 1/25 (4%) in respect of the mechanical axis, in 0% in respect of the femoral axis a.p., in 7/25 (28%) in respect of the femoral axis in the lateral plane, and in 0% in respect of the tibial axis a.p. and the tibial axis in the lateral plane. Certain weaknesses can still be found in the femoral alignment in the lateral plane.

To sum up, the latest OrthoPilot software version, integrating soft tissue balancing, shows excellent overall results.

---

[1] Manufactured by (BBraun Aesculap)

34

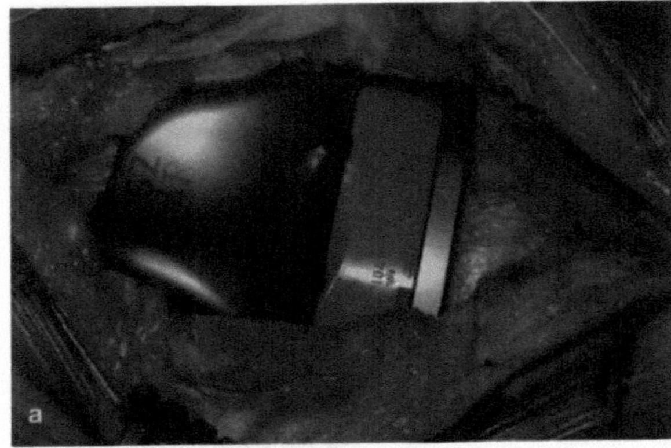

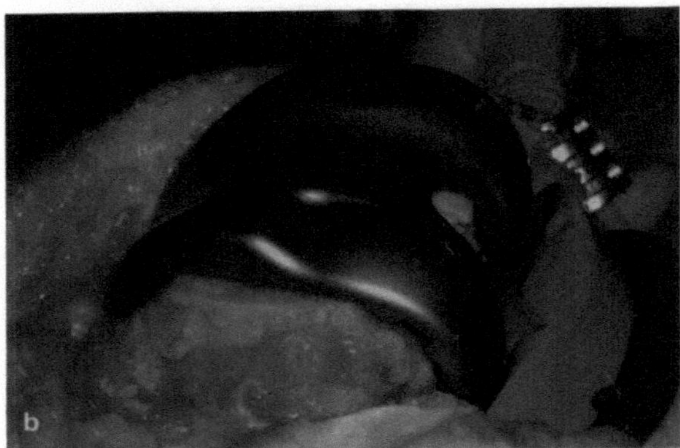

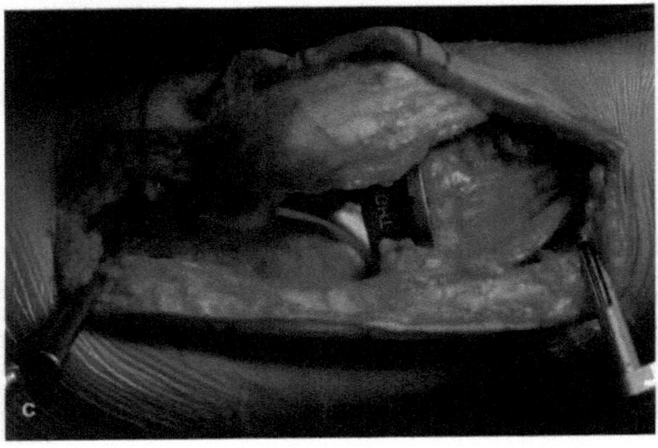

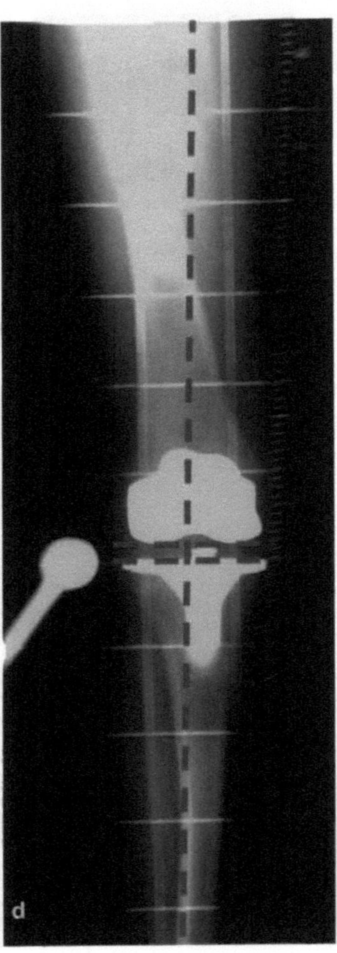

Fig. 34-3a-d. Final check on leg axes in extension (**a**), flexion (**b**) and with repositioned patella (**c**), postoperative x-ray measurement in optimum range (**d**)

References

1. Clemens U, Miehlke RK, Kohler S, Kiefer H, Jenny JY, Konermann W (2002) Computerassistierte Navigation mit dem OrthoPilot-System und der Search-Evolution-Knieendoprothese -Ergebnisse einer Multicenter-Studie. In: Konermann W, Haaker R, (eds) Navigation und Robotic in der Gelenk- und Wirbelsäulenchirurgie. Springer, Berlin Heidelberg New York Tokyo, 207–216

2. Delp SL, Stulberg, SD, Davies B, Picard F, Leitner F (1998) Computer assisted knee replacement, Clin Orthop 354: 49–57

3. Jenny JY, Boeri C (2001) Computer-assisted implantation of total knee prostheses: a case control comparative study with classical instrumentation. Comp Aided Surg 6: 217–220

4. Jenny JY, Boeri C (2001) Implantation d´une prothèse totale de genou assistée par ordinateur: étude comparativ cas-t´moin avec une instrumentation traditionelle. Rev Chir Orthop 87: 645–652

5. Konermann W, Saur MA. Postoperatives Alignment von konventionell und navigiert implantierten Knietotalendoprothesen, in: Konermann W, Haaker R, (eds) Navigation und Robotic in der Gelenk- und Wirbelsäulenchirurgie. Springer, Berlin Heidelberg New York Tokyo, 189–199

6. Krackow KA, Serpe L, Philips MJ, Bayers-Thering M, Mihalko WM (1999) A new technique for determining proper mechanical axis alignment during total knee arthroplasty: Progress toward computer assisted TKA. Orthopedics 22:698–702

7. Leitner F, Picard F, Minfelde R, Schultz HJ, Cinquin P, Saragaglia D (1997) Computer-assisted knee surgical total replacement. In »lecture note in computer science«: CURMed-MRCAS`97. Springer, Berlin Heidelberg New York Tokyo, 629–638

8. Miehlke RK, Clemens U, Jens J-H, Kershally S (2001) Navigation in der Knieendoprothetik – vorläufige klinische Erfahrungen und prospektive vergleichende Studie gegenüber konventioneller Implantationstechnik. Z Orthop 139:109–116

9. Picard F, Leitner F, Saragaglia D, Cinquin P (1997) Mise en place d´une prothèse totale du genou assistée par ordinateur: A propos de 7 implantations sur cadavre. Rev Chir Orthop 83 [Suppl II]:31–36

10. Ritschl P, Machacek Jun F, Fuiko R (2003) Das Galileo-System – Eine integrierte Lösung aus Navigation und Robotic zur Implantation von Knietotalendoprothesen. In: Konermann W, Haaker R (Hrsg) Navigation und Robotic in der Gelenk- und Wirbelsäulenchirurgie. Springer, Berlin Heidelberg New York Tokyo, S 225–229

11. Saragaglia D, Picard F, Chaussard C, Montbaron E, Leitner F, Cinquin P (2001) Mise en place des prothèses totale du genou assistée par ordinateur: comparaison avec la technique conventionelle. A propos d´une étude prospective randomisée de 50 cas. Rev Chir Orthop 87:18–28

12. Saragaglia D, Picard F (2003) Computergestützte Implantation von Knietotalendoprothesen ohne präoperative bildgebende Verfahren: Das kinematische Modell. In: Konermann W, Haaker R (Hrsg) Navigation und Robotic in der Gelenk- und Wirbelsäulenchirurgie. Springer, Berlin Heidelberg New York Tokyo, S 199–206

13. Sparmann M, Wolke B (2003) Knieendoprothesennavigation mit dem Stryker-System. In: Konermann W, Haaker R (Hrsg) Navigation und Robotic in der Gelenk- und Wirbelsäulenchirurgie. Springer, Berlin Heidelberg New York Tokyo, S 250–255

14. Strauss JM, Rüther W (2003) Freihandnavigation mit dem SurgiGATE-System unter Berücksichtigung der computerassistierten Weichteilbalance. In: Konermann W, Haaker R (eds) Navigation und Robotic in der Gelenk- und Wirbelsäulenchirurgie. Springer, Berlin Heidelberg New York Tokyo, S 218–224

35 Navigated Implantation of the *Columbus* Total Knee Arthroplasty with the *OrthoPilot* System: Version 4.0

F. Lampe, E. Hille

Authors' Experience with the OrthoPilot Navigation System in Total Knee Arthroplasty

We started the OrthoPilot-assisted implantation of the Search Evolution knee endoprosthesis (Aesculap, Tuttlingen, Germany), which was the implant available for use with navigation at the time, in our hospital in June 1999 [1]. Stulberg, Saragaglia and Miehlke have already described the OrthoPilot navigation system in detail in various chapters in this volume, and reported on the good prosthesis alignment they were able to achieve. In our own patients we have compared the radiological results in 110 cases. 55 patients were treated with **navigated** Search Evolution knee replacements and 55 with **conventionally** implanted Press Fit Condylar (PFC) knee endoprostheses (DePuy, a Johnson&Johnson Company). It should be borne in mind that the navigated cases constituted our first patient series, and were therefore affected by the learning curve, whereas for conventional implantation of the PFC system we already had years of experience in our hospital to draw on. In spite of this, looking at the so-called alignment index, which makes it possible to consider as a whole the five relevant parameters for evaluating prosthesis alignment – the mechanical leg axis and the four femoral and tibial component angles in the anterior and the sagittal plane – we could already record significantly better results in the navigated group, even though the differences compared with the conventionally treated patients in our series were not quite so pronounced as in other comparable studies (◻ Table 35-1) [2, 3].

Based on our positive experiences with the OrthoPilot system, we started navigated implantation of the new Columbus knee endoprosthesis (Aesculap, Tuttlingen, Germany) in December 2002. This implant has a convincing concept and design and in our opinion satisfies all the criteria of a modern surface replacement. Furthermore, the new Version 4.0 of the OrthoPilot system promises adequate support in balancing the soft tissues in order to achieve congruent and symmetrical gaps, so that the combination of the Columbus knee with the OrthoPilot navigation system appears very promising.

Concept and Design of the Columbus Knee Endoprosthesis

The foundations for the design of surface knee replacements were laid in the 1970s. The experiences gathered in the subsequent decades led to growing convergence in the requirements concerning implant design. Today, new developments have to be orientated towards and assessed according to these requirements. For this reason we should first give a short summary explaining some particular aspects of the Columbus design concept which have persuaded us to introduce this implant as first users in our hospital (◻ Fig 35-1).

◻ **Table 35-1.** Radiological alignment index[a] – authors' own results

Deviation from optimum	Navigated [% of cases]	Conventional [% of cases]
0–10° (very good – good)	72	50
11–20° (satisfactory)	25	45
21–30° (poor)	3	5
>30° (unacceptable)	0	0
Average deviation [°]	8.5 ± 4.4[b]	10.8 ± 5.3[b]

[a]Sum of the 5 individual angle deviations. [b]Significance $p<0.05$

— The implant geometry guarantees the greatest possible femorotibial congruence in the frontal and sagittal plane to maximize the contact surfaces and minimize contact stresses. This reduces polyethylene wear and improves the intrinsic stability of the implant.

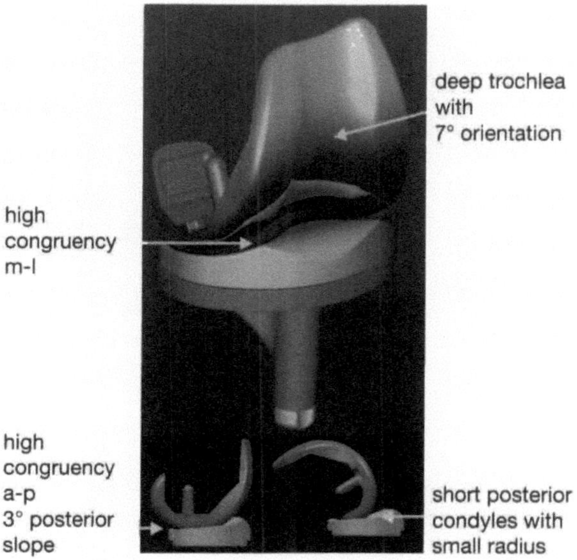

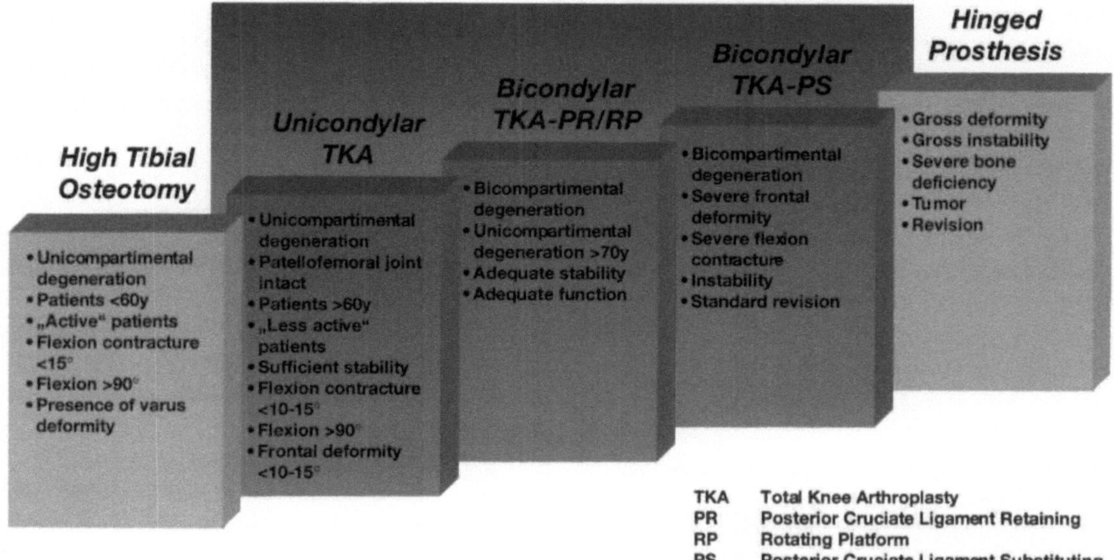

◘ Fig. 35-1. Columbus Knee Replacement (Aesculap, Tuttlingen, Germany)

— The anteroposterior and mediolateral geometry of the femoral components has been optimized. There are 7 femoral sizes and 5 tibial sizes (of which sizes 1–4 each have an additional plus variation with a larger sagittal diameter) available. Femoral and tibial components of all dimensions can be combined with each other freely. This means that optimum consideration can be taken of the individual anatomical and biomechanical conditions.

— The femoral geometry has a deepened and retropositioned trochlea in the kinematically favorable 7° position. This improves femoropatellar congruence and kinematics, which has a positive influence on flexion ability and polyethylene wear after patellar resurfacing.

— The radius and length of the posterior condyles in the sagittal plane have been reduced, improving the intrinsic flexion ability of the implant.

— Polyethylene components with a 3° posterior slope are available in posterior cruciate ligament retaining (PR) versions. Furthermore cruciate ligament substituting (PS), »rotating platform« (RP) and »deep dish« versions are provided. The components have modular heights up to 20 mm.

— The conventional instrumentation is highly advanced. The possibility of navigation with the new OrthoPilot Version 4.0 exists as an alternative.

◘ Fig. 35-2. Histogram of differential indications in the treatment of degenerative knee joints in our hospital. The three central columns (green) correspond to the indication spectrum for the Columbus system with OrthoPilot navigation.

— The system will shortly be enlarged with stem extensions and augmentations. A unicondylar and revision system will also be available.

The Columbus System can cover most indications in the treatment of degenerative knee joints or revision surgery thanks to its modular structure and the possibility of using PR, PS and RP components. The surgeon is able to choose between conventional instrumentation and the OrthoPilot navigation system, which has proved itself in routine use in many hospitals (❑ Fig. 35-2).

In our hospital, OrthoPilot-navigated implantation of the Columbus knee prosthesis is now a standard treatment. To date, we have performed around 40 implantations using this system. We will now focus on the special aspects of navigated implantation and report on our first clinical experiences.

OrthoPilot Navigation of the Columbus Knee Replacement

Following a median longitudinal skin incision, approach to the knee joint is via medial parapatellar arthrotomy. After subperiosteal exposure of the anteromedial tibia and lateral eversion of the extensor mechanism the tibia can be subluxated in front of the femoral condyles (❑ Fig 35-3). In this way the joint is exposed so that all the steps required for navigation (including acquisition of the anatomical landmarks, alignment of the navigated templates and resection blocks) can be carried out safely and reproducibly. The screw for the femoral transmitter is fixed into place within the arthrotomy, the tibial screw is fixed somewhat more distally via a small additional skin incision (see Fig 35-3).

After recording the anatomical and kinematical data by navigation, the OrthoPilot system provides the surgeon on screen with a graphic and numerical display of the individual leg axis of the patient in the frontal and sagittal plane, enabling an objective, dynamic assessment of the deformity, function and stability to be made. We then perform the tibial resection in the frontal and sagittal plane perpendicular to the mechanical tibial axis. Here it must be remembered that a 3° posterior slope has already been integrated into the polyethylene components. A larger slope can of course also be chosen in the bone resection,

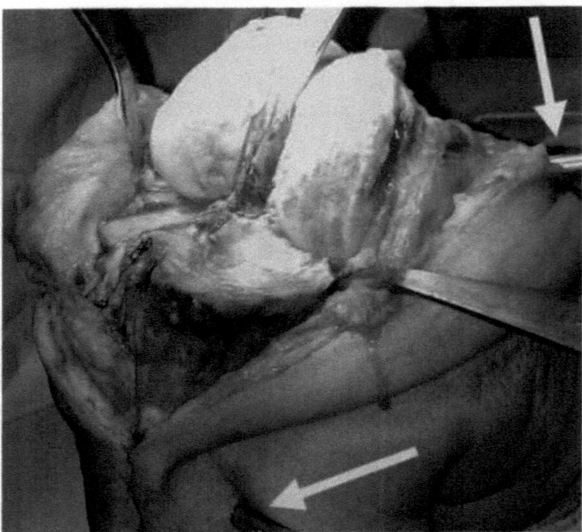

❑ **Fig. 35-3.** Exposure of the joint for navigated implantation of a knee endoprosthesis. The arrows indicate the position of the fixation screws for the transmitters on the tibia and femur

but this must then be added on to the pre-set slope of the polyethylene components. A special universal alignment device is available for three dimensional alignment of the tibial resection block. This guide is fixed onto the bone (femur or tibia) and permits the spatial positioning of the cutting blocks via thumb screws. However, we prefer freehand navigation for both tibia and femur, which with some practice is reliable and in particular quick to perform. After the bone resection the actual resection plane achieved is checked by navigation with the help of a template and any resection errors (e.g. through saw-blade drift in subchondral sclerosis) are corrected.

In our opinion, one crucial innovation in the OrthoPilot Version 4.0 is the navigated measurement of the flexion and extension gap using a spreader that now follows. This means that, at an early stage in the operation, the surgeon has information available about the mediolateral soft tissue balance and the congruence of the flexion and extension gaps, which can be used in later planning calculations. Here is a typical example:

The extension gap measures 11 mm laterally and 9 mm medially. Thus it corresponds to around the thickness of the thinnest tibia component (10 mm). In this case the extension gap can be expected to present an adequate width after the distal femoral resection has been performed and, if necessary, it will be perfectly possible to balance it with a medial release. The measurement of the flexion gap in this example is 12 mm laterally and 9 mm medially. Here it can be expected that, through the later external rotation of the femoral component, a symmetrical flexion gap will be formed which will be wide enough to accommodate the tibial component. If the flexion gap is clearly too narrow in relation to the extension gap, it can already be assumed that this will have to be widened through an appropriate release (e.g. posterior cruciate ligament release), a corrective tibial resection with increased posterior slope or the selection of a smaller femoral component. If the opposite is the case, and the flexion gap is too wide, a larger component would be appropriate in order to reduce the flexion gap in relation to the extension gap.

As this example shows, the surgeon has quantitative data available for flexible intraoperative planning, which can be made more concrete and implemented by navigation as the operation proceeds.

The following step serves to navigate and record the posterior condyle tangent (relevant for femoral rotational alignment and establishing size) and the distal femoral joint line (relevant for defining the distal femoral resection plane) with the help of a corresponding template. Subsequently the distal femoral resection block is navigated, taking the resection height into consideration, orientated into frontal and sagittal alignment and fixed into place (either using the universal alignment aid or freehand). The surgeon can again follow the effect of the positioning of the cutting block on the size and symmetry of the extension gap graphically and numerically on screen, and for example decide in narrow conditions (as long as the flexion gap has already been measured as wide enough) whether to resect 11 mm from the distal femur (with slight proximalization of the joint line) instead of the required 9 mm (distal component thickness). Alternatively, the surgeon can increase the extension gap later through a posterior capsule release to match it to the flexion gap. After resection, the result is again checked by navigation and the resection plane is corrected if necessary.

In the step that now follows, a navigation template is used to determine the position of the resection block for the remaining femoral resections, thus establishing the rotational and translational alignment of the femoral component. During this process, the system informs the surgeon on screen about the anteroposterior position of the component to prevent notching of the anterior femoral cortex (we position the component so that it finishes 1 mm in front of the anterior cortex). The rotation of the component in relation to the posterior condyle line is also displayed. As a rule we turn the component externally until the system shows a symmetrical flexion gap. Additional soft tissue release might have to be performed if an unrealistic rotation of the femoral component would otherwise have to be made to balance the flexion gap. In addition, the system shows for orientation purposes the deviation of the posterior condyle tangent from the transepicondylar axis established by palpation. Here the limited reliability and objectivity of epicondyle palpation should be borne in mind. The navigation template has after all been designed to allow visual assessment of its alignment in relation to the Whiteside line. The important thing is to keep looking at the symmetry and width of the gaps during this procedure. If the flexion gap is too narrow, the surgeon can reduce the size of the femoral component suggested by the system. After re-aligning the navigation template, the effect on the width of the flexion gap can be seen on the screen. In the opposite case, if the flexion gap is too wide, a larger femoral component is suggested to the system. Thus, the final size of the femoral component is established at this point, as part of balancing the flexion gap. The seven very close component sizes represent a clear advantage here. A further example:

The system suggests a femoral size 4. The template is moved anteriorly until the value –1 for the femoral notching is shown on the screen. The template is now rotated externally until the flexion gap measures 2 mm medially and laterally (corresponding to the distance between the components), and is thus symmetrical and congruent to the extension gap. In this example, this occurs at 4° external rotation in relation to the posterior condyle line. At 6°, the transepicondylar axis deviates only by 2° from the orientation of the components. Visually, the template is optimally aligned in relation to the Whiteside line. The system proposes a 10 mm thick tibial component. In this case optimum conditions exist for all navigated parameters, so that the position of the size 4 resection block is now established. If in this example the flexion gap would be too large at 6 mm, the surgeon calls up the size 5 in the system instead of the size 4. The system now virtually defines the decreased flexion gap with a correctly positioned navigation template as only 1–2 mm. In this case the size 5 resection block is selected.

In general, the surgeon will tolerate a gap asymmetry of maximum 2–3 mm. Above this the situation has to be corrected, for example through further soft tissue balancing. After final positioning and fixing of the femoral resection block, the remaining resections are performed. Trial components of the appropriate dimensions are fitted and then function, stability, gap symmetry (ligament balancing), gap congruence (gap balancing) and patella tracking are checked both by navigation and clinically (plausibility check). After obligatory jet lavage the definitive components are implanted; we cement both the femoral and the tibial components. Apart from a few exceptions we leave the surface of the patella native, merely removing osteophytes and performing denervation to the margin by electro-cauterisation. After placement of intra-articular and subcutaneous drainage connected to an autotransfusion system, the wound is closed in the usual way.

The patients who have been treated in this manner are mobilized on the first day postoperatively. Additionally, continuous passive motion is prescribed from the first day postoperatively. If possible, in order to increase the efficiency of the physiotherapy, pain is treated for 5–7 days via a peridural catheter placed during surgery. When the patients have attained free extension and at least 90° of flexion they are discharged into the rehabilitation clinic.

First Clinical Experiences with the Columbus Knee Endoprosthesis

We have now been using the Columbus knee for about 3 months. As we had already gained sufficient experience using the previous OrthoPilot versions in combination with the Search Evolution prosthesis since 1999, the changeover to the new implant system and the OrthoPilot software version 4.0 did not cause any problems. The operation is already being routinely performed by two surgeons experienced in navigation. The experiences to date with the implant and the new software can be described as thoroughly positive, especially with regard to the new aspects of gap and soft tissue balancing. It has been confirmed once again that the OrthoPilot system can be reliably used in everyday clinical practice. Because of the as yet short period of use of the first Columbus series, we cannot present any follow-up data on this at the current time. Instead, two case reports are used to illustrate the possibilities of navigated treatment with Columbus. One case concerned a 75 year old man with osteoarthritis and pronounced varus deformity. Function was limited significantly to 0/25/60° (extension/flexion; ◘ Fig. 35-4). The X-rays show the preoperative status and the resection planning. Despite the high grade function limitation, after adequate exposure of the joint (see Fig 35-3) it was possible to treat the patient with an OrthoPilot-navigated Columbus knee. The intraoperative

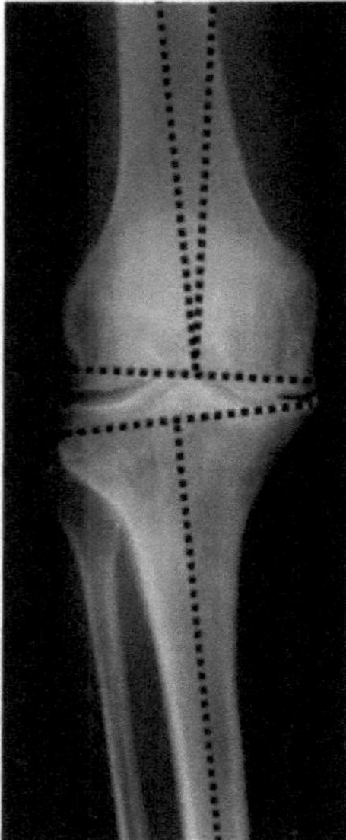
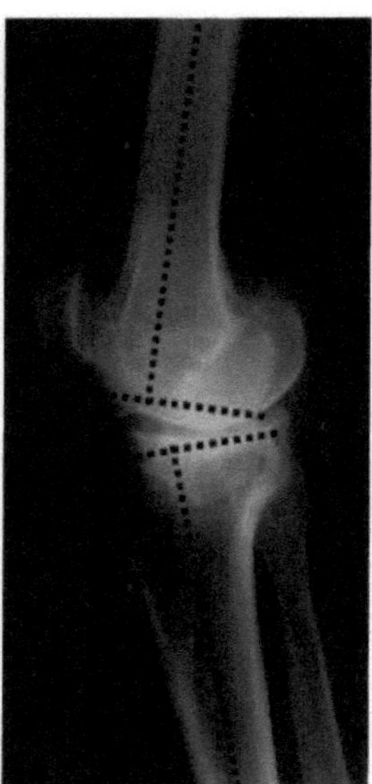
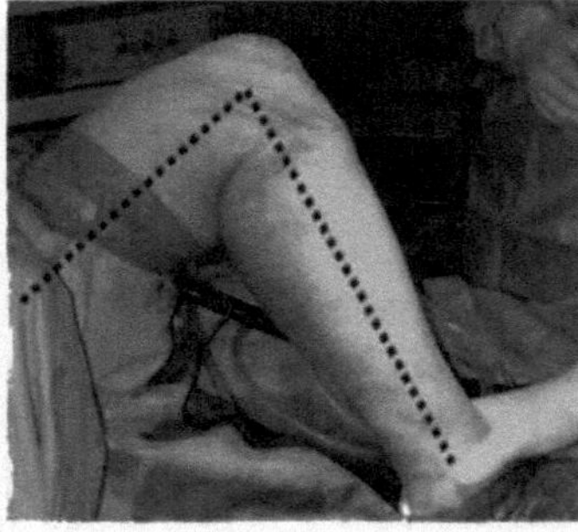
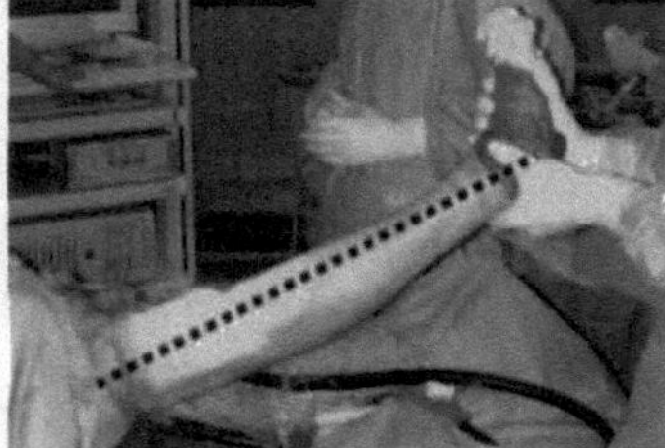

◘ **Fig. 35-4.** Case 1

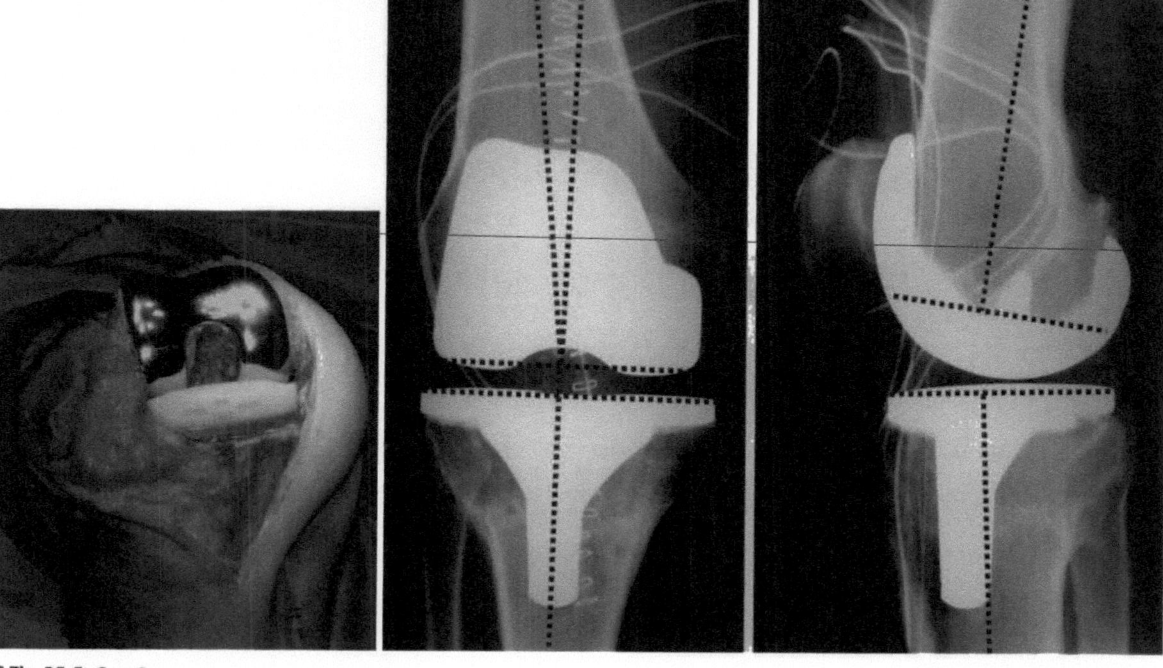

◗ Fig. 35-5. Case 2

images show a restoration of function with stable ligaments after implantation of the prosthesis. The second case concerned a 76 year old man with osteoarthritis of the knee after high tibial osteotomy with a function of 0/10/100° (extension/flexion; ◗ Fig 35-5). Displayed is the operating site after implantation of the prosthesis and the postoperative X-ray status showing correctly aligned components.

This year will see the beginning of an international prospective multicenter study with regard to the Ortho-Pilot-navigated implantation of the Columbus knee replacement.

References

1. Hille E, Lampe F (2000) Erste praktische Erfahrungen mit einem Navigationssystem. In: Eulert J, Hassenpflug J (Hrsg) Praxis der Knieendoprothetik. Springer, Berlin Heidelberg New York Tokyo, S 91–96
2. Konermann W, Saur MA (2003) Postoperatives Alignment von konventionell und navigiert implantierten Knietotalendoprothesen. In: Konermann W, Haaker R (Hrsg) Navigation und Robotik in der Gelenk- und Wirbelsäulenchirurgie. Springer, Berlin Heidelberg New York Tokyo, S 189–199
3. Miehlke RK, Clemens U, Jens JH, Kershally S (2001) Navigation in der Knieendoprothetik – vorläufige klinische Erfahrungen und prospektive vergleichende Studie gegenüber konventioneller Implantationstechnik. Z Orthop 139: 109–116

36 CT-Free Navigation Including Soft-Tissue Balancing: LCS-TKA and *VectorVision* Systems

W. H. Konermann, S. Kistner

Introduction

The specific challenges in total knee replacement surgery are sufficiently well known. In order to obtain excellent long-term results, the following criteria have to be considered:

- General criteria
  - Selection of the right patient
  - Correct determination of indications for use
  - Peri-operative management
- Specific criteria
  - Design of the prosthesis
  - Surgical techniques, implantation techniques
  - Reconstruction of the mechanical leg axis
  - Reconstruction of the joint line
  - Ligament balancing

Mal-alignment of the mechanical leg axes, the prosthesis and the imbalance of the soft tissue, reduce the life span of knee implants [4,7].

The advantages of navigated surgery compared to the conventional technique were presented in the largest multi-center study worldwide [3] (see chapter 33). The results were based on an optimal alignment of the prosthesis in respect to the reconstruction of the mechanical leg axes.

F. Buechel [1, 2] (see chapter 24) reported on specific data relevant for the LCS knee implant, e.g. the optimal ligament balancing and an equal flexion and extension gaps. Besides the correct alignment of the prosthesis, an optimal ligament balancing is of utmost importance for excellent long-term results.

Konermann and Saur based their prospective study on 100 patients with a conventionally implanted LCS prosthesis compared to 100 patients with the Search Evolution prosthesis placed using the OrthoPilot navigation system. The authors found an optimal alignment with a maximal aberrance of 3° from the mechanical leg axis (varus, valgus) in 77% of conventional cases versus 93% in navigated cases [5] (see chapter 31).

Concept of the VectorVision CT-free Knee Navigation System

The VectorVision CT-free knee navigation system (Brain-LAB AG, Germany) assists in achieving correct alignment of the prosthesis, the reconstruction of the joint line as well as in implementing an optimal balance of the ligaments and equal extension and flexion gaps.

The camera arm and computer workstation are integrated into the VectorVision compact navigation system. The navigated instruments are tracked passively via reflective marker spheres. The spheres reflect the infrared-light, emitted by the cameras, which enable the tracking of surgical instruments in the operating room. There are no bothersome cables in the surgical field. The system is controlled by the surgeon via the touch screen monitor. Reference arrays are attached to both the femur and tibia using a bicortical Schanz pin.

Steps in a Navigated Procedure

The points, acquired through pivoting of the hip joint and with the pointer, are utilized for the patient registration and are at the same time the basis for the planning of the

---

implant position. After the acquisition of the registration points, a generic model from the database is morphed to the acquired points. This model then has to be verified using relevant points on the tibia as well as the femur. It has to be taken into consideration that this model can only offer an additional 3D orientation. The correct planning of the implant position is based on the collected points and clouds of points, which are acquired by dragging the tip of the pointer along defined areas of the bone surface.

Registration

1. The first step is to define the center of the femoral head by pivoting the femoral head in the acetabulum. The center is defined as the average value of three calculated rotational centers. The indicated error value is the deviation of these centers to each other (■ Fig. 36–1).

2. In the next step the center of the distal endpoint of the mechanical tibia axis is defined by identifying the medial and lateral malleolus with the pointer.
3. Definition of the proximal point of the tibia mechanical axis (■ Fig. 36-2).
4. Definition of the tibia size:
   - The tibia size is defined by defining the most medial, lateral, and anterior points on the tibia with the pointer. The points should be acquired in the area where the resection level is planned to be and will be utilized to define the size of the tibial implant component (■ Fig. 36-3).

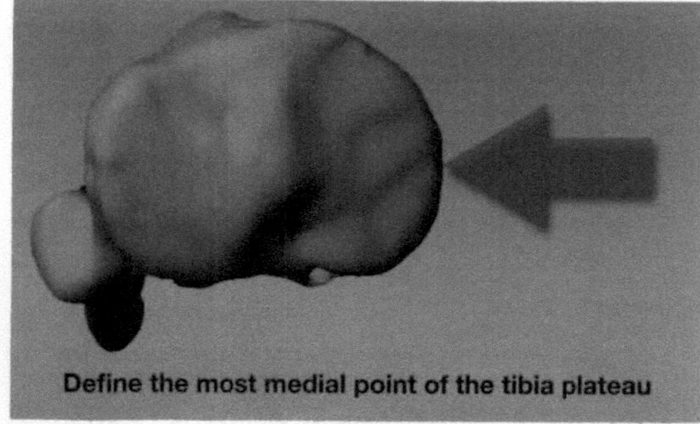

■ **Fig. 36-3.** Define tibial implant component

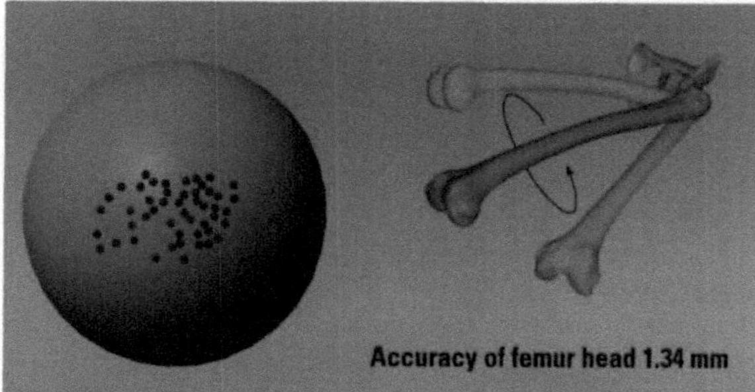

■ **Fig. 36-1.** Femoral head calculation

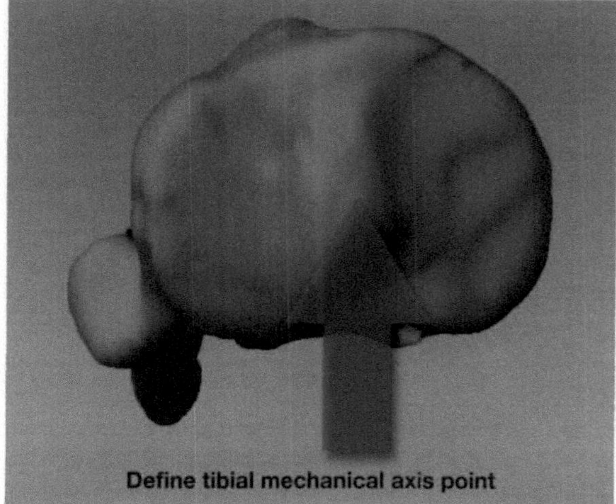

■ **Fig. 36-2.** Define tibia mechanical axis

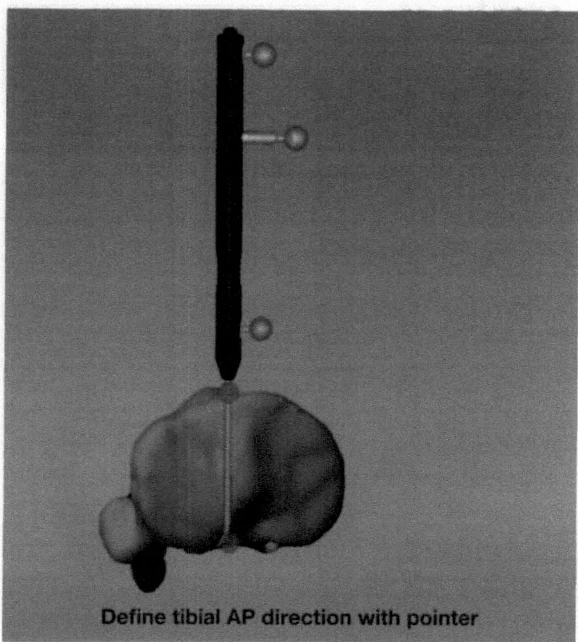

■ **Fig. 36-4.** Define a.p. direction of the tibia

5. Definition of the A-P direction of the tibia:
   - The A-P direction of the tibia is defined with the VectorVision pointer as it is essential to define the neutral rotational alignment of the tibia implant component. The A-P direction is also the basis for the alignment of the posterior slope, which is defined along the mediolateral direction (90° to the a.p. direction) (Fig. 36-4).

6. Acquisition of landmarks on the tibia:
   - A series of landmarks are collected on the tibial bone surface by dragging the tip of the pointer along three defined areas: the anterior cortex, and the medial and lateral tibia plateaus. The deepest point is calculated from the points acquired on the medial and lateral tibia plateaus, which is then used as the reference for the resection level (Fig. 36-5).

7. Epicondylar femur axis:
   - The most medial and lateral point of the epicondyles are acquired on the bone surface. The line connecting these two points is the reference for the femoral rotation and influences the implant position accordingly (Fig. 36-6).

8. Definition of the femoral sulcus
   - The femoral sulcus determines the exit point of the anterior cutting plane and has an important impact on the sizing of the prosthesis. A correct definition avoids anterior notching (Fig. 36-7).

9. Femur mechanical axis:
   - The most distal end point of the femur mechanical femur axis is defined, which influences the varus and valgus position (Fig. 36-8).

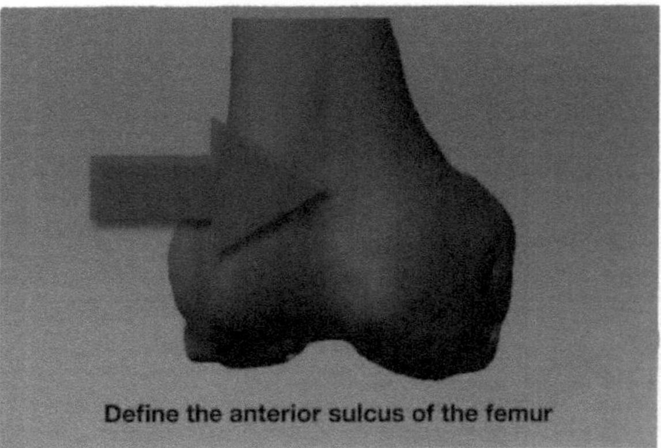

Fig. 36-7. Define femoral sulcus

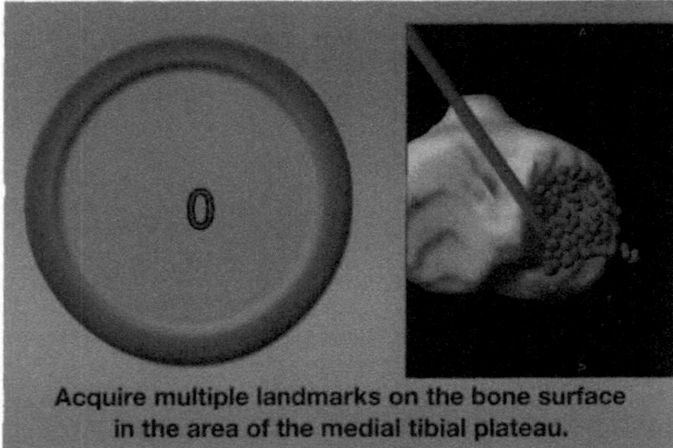

Fig. 36-5. Define medial tibia plateau

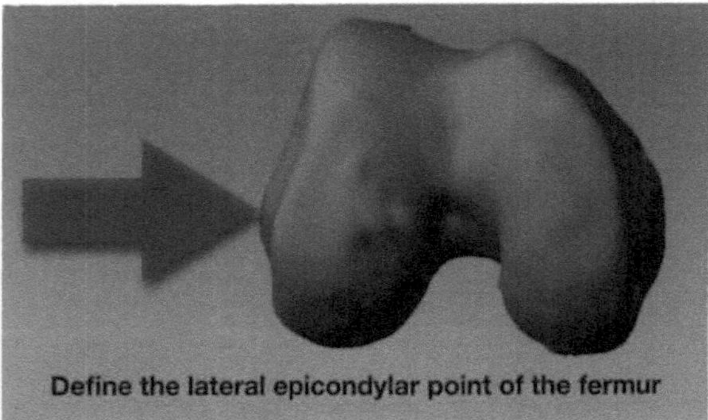

Fig. 36-6. Define lateral epicondyle

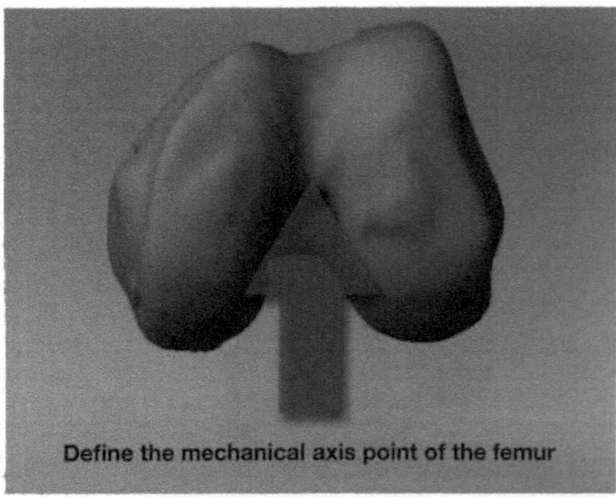

Fig. 36-8. Define femoral mechanical axis

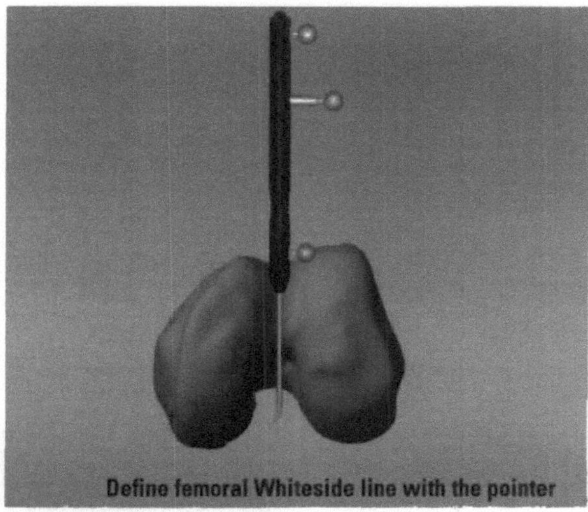

◘ Fig. 36-9. Whiteside line

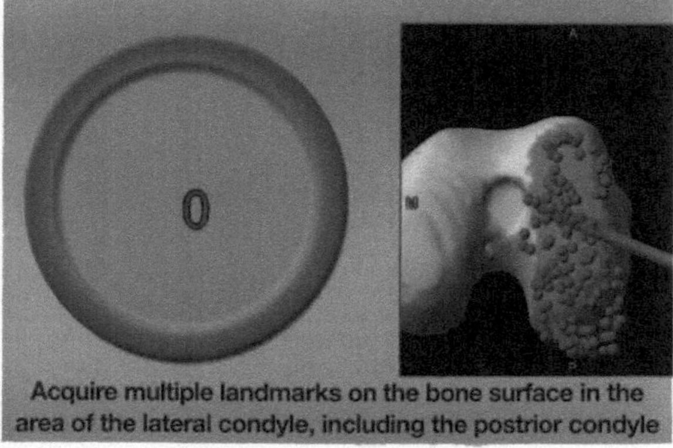

◘ Fig. 36-10. Define lateral femur condyle

10. Whiteside line:
    - The Whiteside line is defined with the VectorVision pointer (◘ Fig. 36-9).
11. Acquisition of landmarks on the medial and lateral femoral condyles:
    - Multiple points are acquired on the medial and lateral femur condyles. The resection level of the distal femur will be calculated from the most distal point. The system automatically calculates the posterior condylar axis as a rotational reference. This has an impact on the implant size as well (◘ Fig. 36-10).

12. Model morphing:
    - An integrated anatomical knee joint database enables a generic 3D model to be morphed to the actual patient anatomy.
13. Verification of the model:
    - The calculated 3-D model has to be verified by identifying various points on the patient's knee joint with the VectorVision pointer. The distance between the tip of the pointer and the model is displayed on the VectorVision monitor. This is how exact deviations of the model and the patient´s anatomy can be identified. If the deviation is too big, additional points or clouds of points can be acquired for a re-registration (◘ Fig. 36-11).

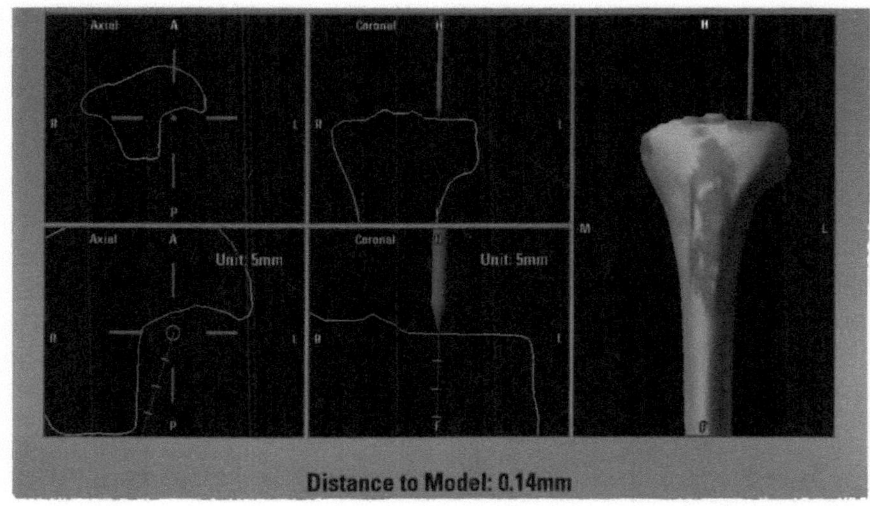

◘ Fig. 36-11. Verify adapted tibia model

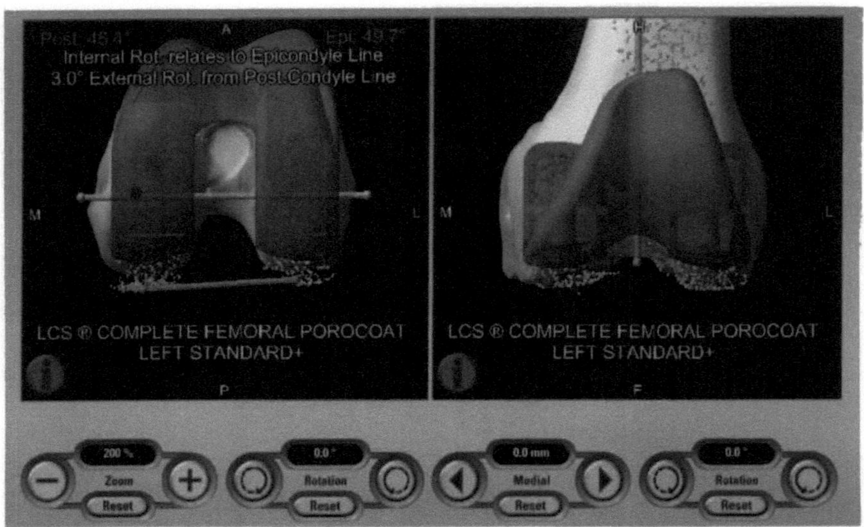

Fig. 36-12. Confirm position of femoral implant

Planning

Based on the data acquired intraoperatively, the system automatically calculates an initial optimal implant position. The implant position is displayed on the monitor in a comprehensive planning overview.

Fine-Tuning of the Femoral Implant

After the implant size and position are calculated by the system, the implant components can be fine-tuned by the surgeon. The following fine-adjustment features are provided:

1. Resection level
2. Anterior-posterior alignment of the implant
3. Medial-lateral alignment of the implant
4. Anterior-posterior slope
5. Medial-lateral slope
6. Internal and external rotation
7. Implant size (◗ Fig 36-12)

Fine-Tuning of the Tibial Implant

The same adjustments can be applied to the tibia:

1. Resection level
2. Anterior-posterior alignment of the implant
3. Medial-lateral alignment of the implant
4. Anterior-posterior slope
5. Medial-lateral slope

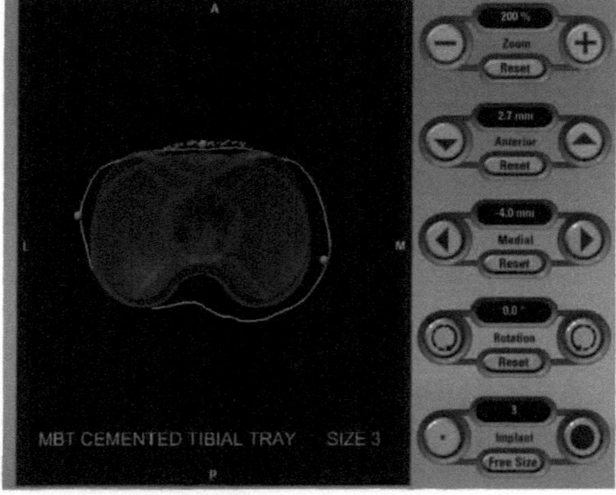

Fig. 36-13. Confirm position of tibial implant

6. Internal and external rotation
7. Implant size (◗ Fig. 36-13)

The system's toolbox enables the calculation process to be influenced. The treatment planning allows basic alignment parameters to be pre-defined, such as:

1. Determination of tibia resection (in relation to the deepest point on the affected or healthy plateau)
2. Selection of the rotational axes (posterior condylar axis, epicondylar axis)
3. Selection of the implant alignment (posterior alignment, anterior alignment)

Additionally, the toolbox provides the possibility for:
1. A re-registration
2. The acquisition of additional reference points
3. The selection of the implant (cemented, non-cemented, rotating platform, a.p. glide inlay, etc.)

Navigation and Verification

The ligament balancing function as well as the navigation and verification of the bone cuts enable a continuous adaptation and optimization of the LCS implant position. Tibia and femur are not adapted one after the other, but alternating step by step. Adhering to the conventional surgical technique, the distal femur cut and the tibia resection level have to be parallel when the knee joint is in full extension.

The VectorVision software determines the tibia slope based on the antecurvature of the anterior femoral cortex and therewith against the femur implant position. The limits of the slope range from a maximal 10° to a minimal 5°.

1. Calculation of the angle between the femoral anatomical axis and the mechanical axis from lateral
   - To define the femoral antecurvature the LCS-yoke is placed on the anterior cortex of the distal femur. The angle between the femur mechanical axis and the tangent on the distal anterior femur is defined. The position of the LCS-yoke is navigated using the LCS navigation adapter and stored (◨ Figs. 36-14 and 36-15).
2. Calculation and verification of the tibia slope
   - Within a specific range (5°-10° posterior slope) the software recommends a tibia slope depending on the calculated antecurvature of the femur. The value of the tibia slope – regardless of the recommendation – can be adjusted by the user (◨ Fig. 36-16).
3. Navigation of the tibia resection
   - The resection level can be referenced either from the highest or lowest tibia plateau. The slope is defined through the previous calculation. The tibial cutting block is navigated to the planned position

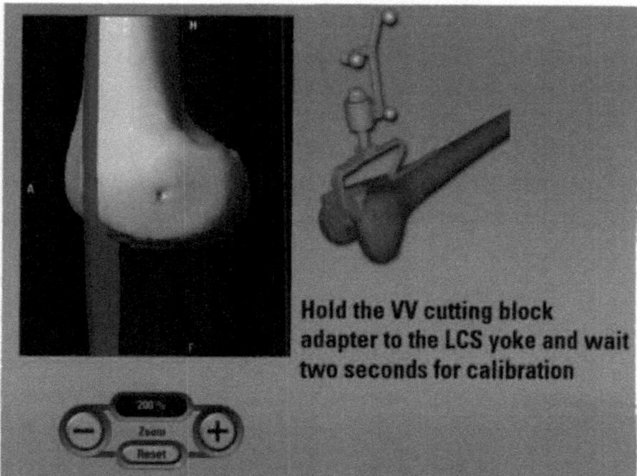

◨ **Fig. 36-14.** Calculate anterior alignment

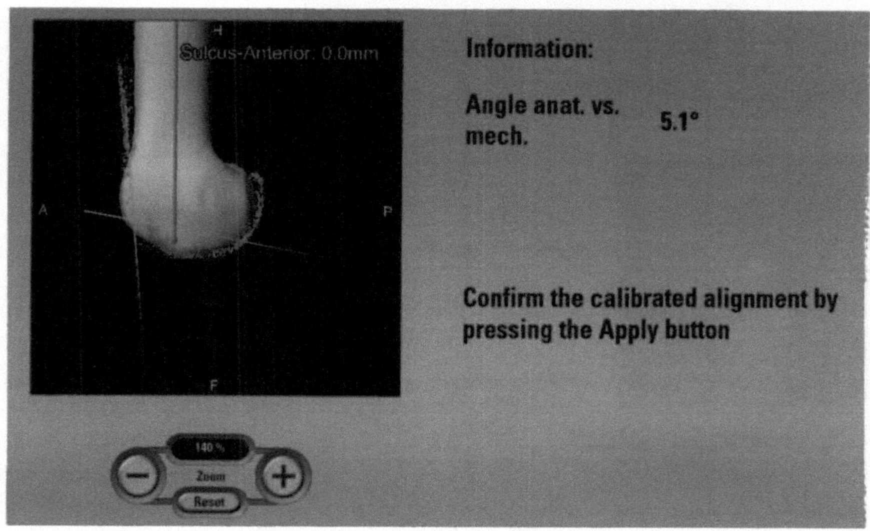

◨ **Fig. 36-15.** Confirm anterior alignment

36

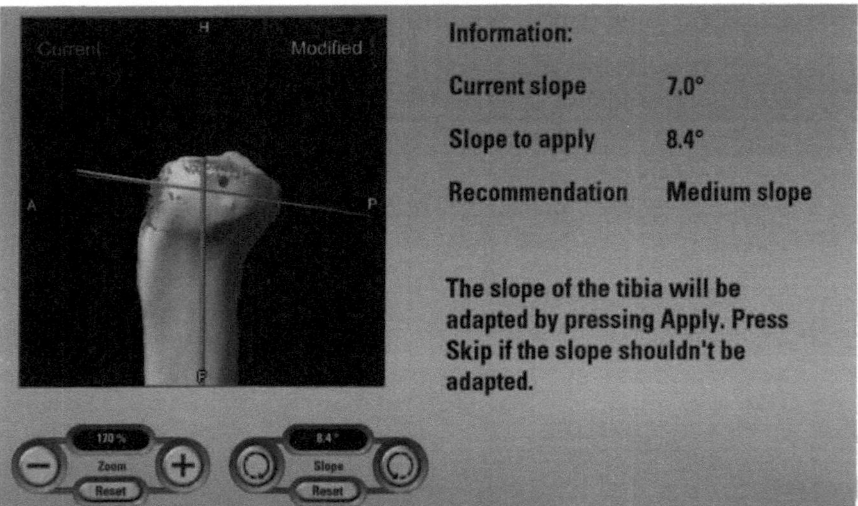

Fig. 36-16. Verify tibia slope

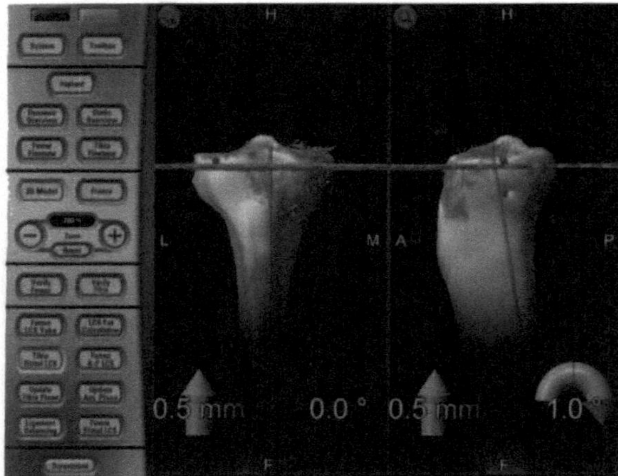

Fig. 36-17. LCS tibia plane navigation

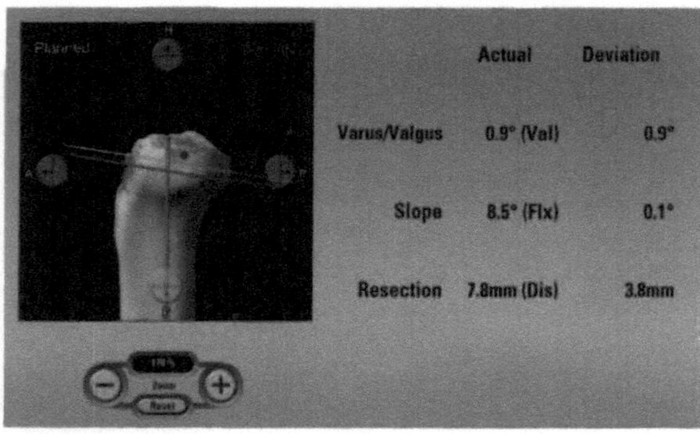

Fig. 36-18. Verify tibial plane

and fixed with pins. The bone cut is performed and verified. The performed cut is updated and displayed. Deviations to the planned resection level on the tibia (varus/valgus, slope) are displayed allowing for additional navigation and resection if necessary (**Figs. 36-17 and 36-18**).

4. Ligament balancing in extension
   - In extension a defined force is transferred to the joint with a specific spreader tool. Flexion, extension and the size of the joint gap are calculated by the navigation system and displayed. If deviations (varus/valgus) from the mechanical leg axis (0°) are displayed on the monitor, an optimal ligament balancing can be achieved by an appropriate release of soft tissue to achieve the proper mechanical axis. The system recalculates and displays the actual ligament values and the extension gap in extension. For further calculation of the LCS implant position the extension gap is essential (**Fig. 36-19**).

5. Ligament balancing in flexion
   - In flexion the same forces are transferred to the ligaments and the maximal internal and external rotation as well as the flexion gap is calculated. The system automatically displays the actual data of the ligament tensions and the flexion gap. The rotational alignment of the femur is then calculated so that the posterior femur cut and tibia cut are parallel (**Fig. 36-20**).

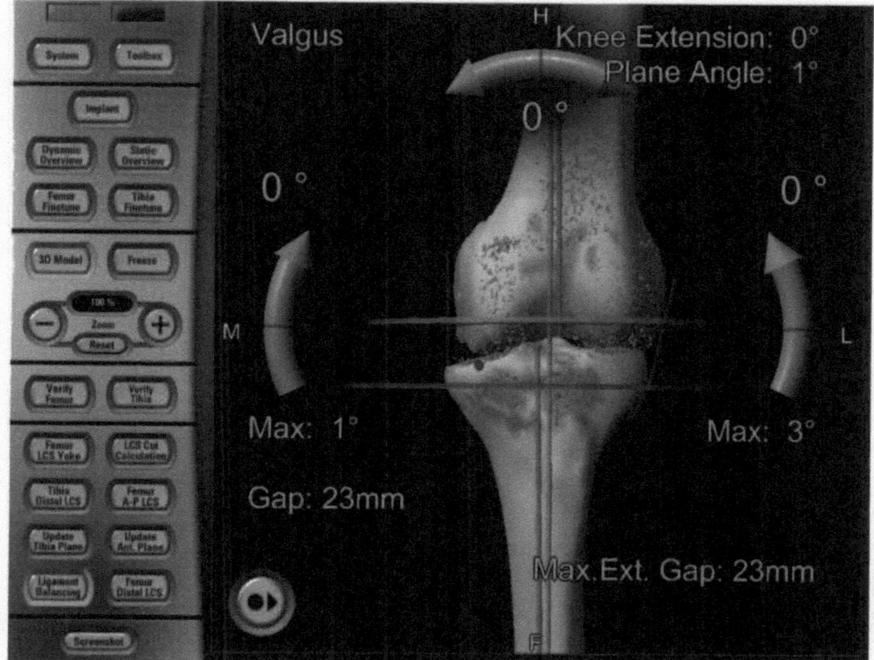

Fig. 36-19. Ligament balancing in extension

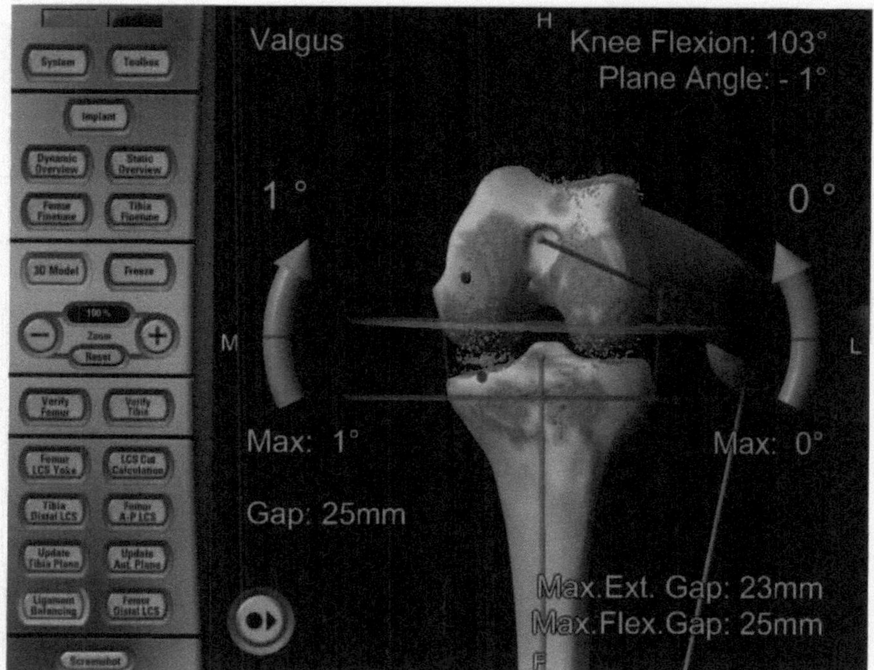

Fig. 36-20. Ligament balancing in flexion

36

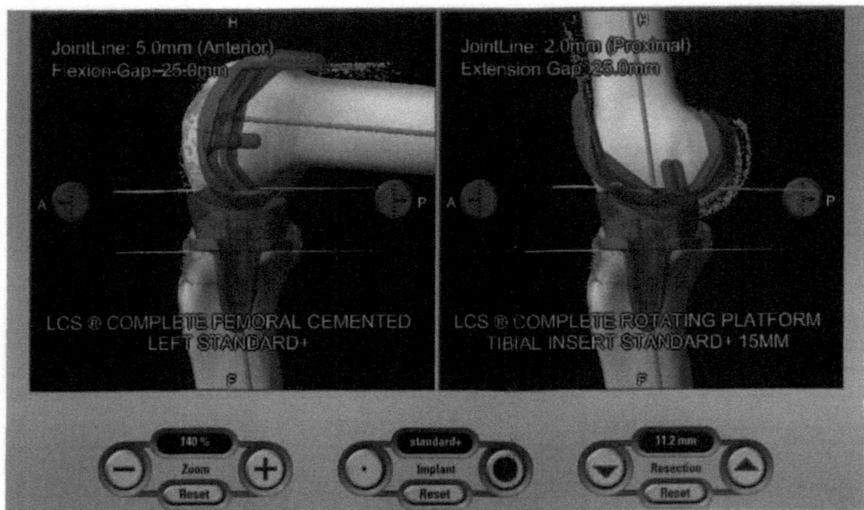

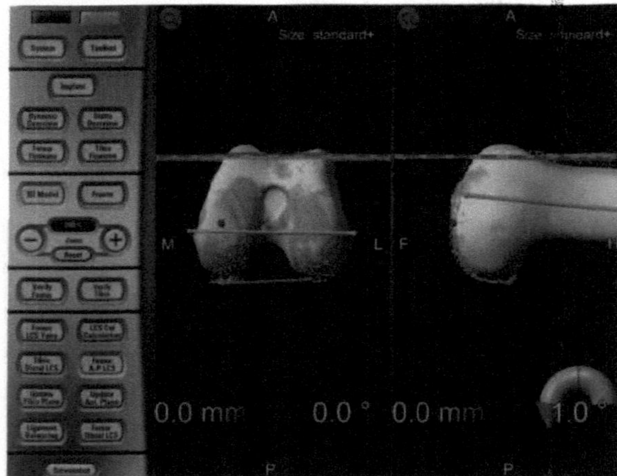

Fig. 36-21. Confirm LCS optimization

Fig. 36-22. Navigate LCS anterior cutting block

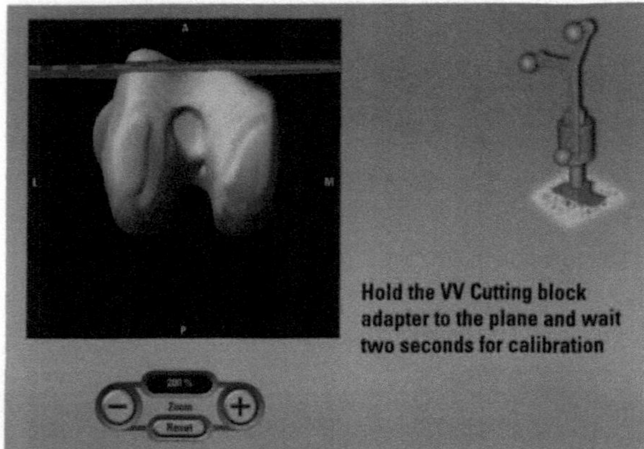

Fig. 36-23. Verify femoral anterior cut

6. Calculation of the femoral LCS position
   - Based on the information stored from the ligament balancing, the VectorVision system can calculate the ideal position and size of the femoral component as well as the required size of the inlay, so that flexion and extension gap will be identical. The surgeon can find a compromise between retaining the joint line and having an equal flexion and extension gap by modifying the distal resection level or changing the implant size (Fig. 36-21).
7. Navigation of the anterior and posterior femur cut
   - The rotation and the position of the anterior and posterior resection level are defined by the previous calculations. The a.p. femoral cutting block is navigated to the planned position and fixed with pins. The anterior and posterior cuts are performed. By verifying the performed cuts the femoral data are

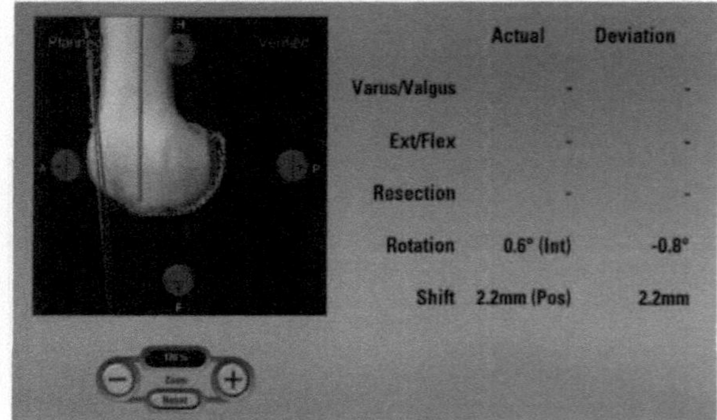

Fig. 36-24. Femur plane deviations

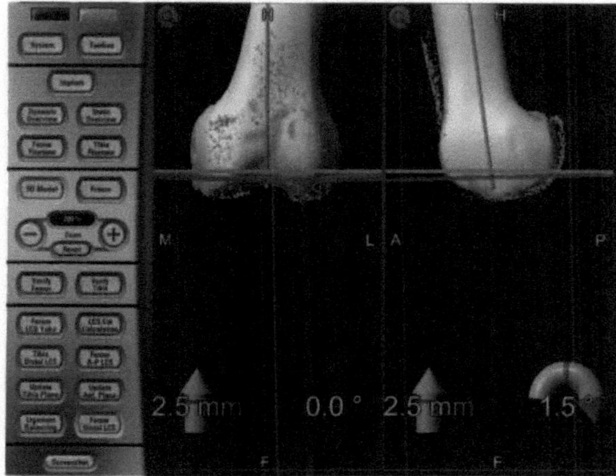

Fig. 36-25. Navigate LCS femur distal cut

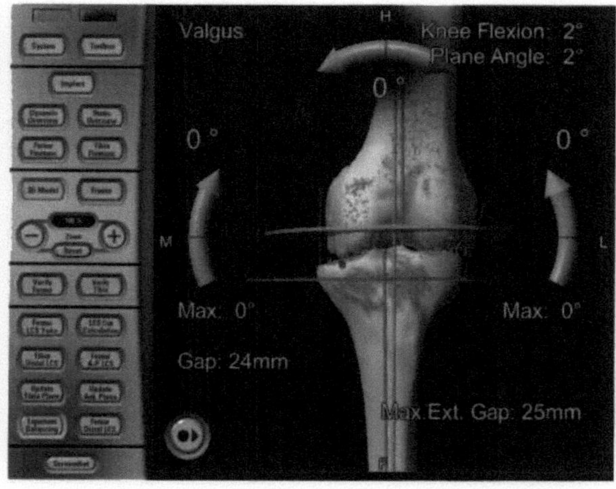

Fig. 36-26. Documentation of the implanted LCS Prosthesis in Extension

updated. If the actual cuts deviate from the planned femoral cuts (rotation, slope) the surgeon has the opportunity to perform additional navigated cuts (**Figs.** 36-22 to 36-24).

8. Navigation of the distal femoral cut and additional cuts
   - The distal femoral cut is performed based on the verified anterior cut. This ensures an ideal preparation of the bone and results in an ideal fusion of the implant with bone. The distal femoral cutting block is navigated to the planned position, fixed with pins and the cut is performed. By verifying the cut, the information on the femur is updated and visualized on the monitor. Any deviations to the treatment plan can be intraoperatively detected and immediately corrected. The final preparation (angled cuts) of the femur is performed using the conventional cutting template (**Fig.** 36-25).

Implantation

After performing the cuts, assisted by the navigation system, the components of the prosthesis are implanted in the same way as during a conventional surgery. In this step a correct rotational alignment of the tibial component in respect to the tibial resection level is essential.

Documentation of the Navigated Surgery

During navigation every phase of the surgical procedure can be documented with screenshots. All performed cuts are automatically documented by the VectorVision system. After the implantation the achieved leg axis can be checked with support of the navigation system. The stability of the leg can be controlled by bringing the leg in full flexion and extension as well as positions in-between. The documentation of the displayed values is performed with screenshots (**Fig.** 36-26). A navigation report includes all parameters of the patient and the screenshots are copied onto a CD-ROM. The reference instruments for navigation (two reference stars and Schanz pins) are removed and the wound is closed conventionally.

Results

The first 50 protheses presented were placed with navigation by three surgeons, who are experienced in computer-assisted surgery. Within the group of surgeons no significantly diverse results were achieved. Measurements were made two weeks after surgery based on a lateral fluoroscopy with the patient lying supine. The slope of the femoral component was defined in relation to the distal, anterior femur cortex. The slope of the tibial component was defined in relation to the proximal posterior tibial cortex.

The mechanical leg axis was measured using an AP long leg X-ray. The frontal orientation of the femoral component in relation to the femur mechanical axis and the frontal orientation of the tibia component in relation to the tibia were measured as well. The long leg X-ray images were acquired in a strictly standardized method, the central X-ray was adjusted to the patella, which is defined as centric between the femoral condyles.

The values determined using the X-ray images contain a human error of 1° and a positioning error of 2° for the radiological measurements. It should be taken into consideration that a more accurate method, the navigation system, is currently being evaluated with the X-ray measurement technique, which has a total inaccuracy of 3°.

Mechanical Leg Axis

The mechanical leg axis was measured as 0° in 26% of the cases. If a deviation of ≤3° varus/valgus for the mechanical leg axis is defined as a very good result and the potential radiological measurement error is taken into consideration, then 94% of the navigated prostheses were placed with good results.

Femoral a.p. Axis

The inner angle of the femoral prosthesis in the frontal plane was measured to be the ideal 90° in 30% of the navigated cases. 92% achieved a good result when considering a deviation of ≤2° varus/valgus.

Lateral Femoral Axis

In 24% of all navigated cases the desired 0°-slope was achieved and 90% of the measured prostheses were within a range of ≤2° anterior/posterior slope.

Tibial a.p. Axis

In 38% of all navigated tibia prostheses an exact alignment to the frontal tibial axis, defined as having an inner angle of 90°, was achieved. Good results were achieved for 92% of all navigated knee joints accepting a ≤2° deviation in varus/valgus alignment.

Lateral Tibial Axis

The navigated ideal value for the lateral tibial axis was achieved in 26% of all cases. A good result with a deviation of ≤2° anterior/posterior slope can be seen on 80% of all cases.

Comprehensive Overview on 5 Axes

Summing up the result for all 5 axes and by defining a ≤5° deviation of the mechanical axis and ≤4° for the other 4 axes (frontal and sagittal orientation of the femoral and tibial implant component) as an acceptable result, then 93% of all navigated prostheses meet this goal. An optimal result, defined as ≤3° deviation from the mechanical axis and ≤2° deviation to all other axes, was achieved in 45% of all cases (see chapter 31).

Conclusions and Visions

Based on our actual experiences the VectorVision CT-free knee navigation system in conjunction with the LCS prosthesis enables an optimization of:
- the reconstruction of the mechanical leg axis,
- the implant position,
- the ligament balancing,
- the flexion and extension gap,
- the reconstruction of the joint line.

Another advantage is the user-friendly workflow of the VectorVision software. This can be considered easy to use for surgeons who are not enthusiastic with new technology. The navigation system is adapted to the surgical technique and the surgeon does not have to change his conventional handling for example with the spacer or cutting blocks. The disadvantage of all navigated methods is the extension of the surgery time (5-10 min).

The inaccuracy of the cuts, e.g. caused by the bending of the saw plates treating slcerotic bones, initially are not taken into account by navigation. The verification of the bone cuts after sawing with navigation now provides relevant data on the accuracy of the cuts and they can be intraoperatively corrected by re-sawing. However surgeons need new sawing and milling systems or possibly new minimally-invasive robots.

Once again it has to be stated that the navigation system, as a more accurate technology, is currently being evaluated in conjunction with a measuring instrument, fluoroscopy, that is accompanied with an inaccuracy of 3°.

For the future the integration of pressure sensors (see chapters 28 and 29) has to be demanded. These should be inserted during different surgical steps and being integrated in the trial prosthesis as well as the implanted inlay as well. Utilizing the data further, optimization of ligament balancing can be achieved. Pressure on the medial and lateral implant components can be measured in full extension and different flexion levels. The surgeon would be able to create a navigated fine tuning release to achieve perfect ligament balancing in any stage of the surgery.

Navigation has opened new horizons and shown new directions to take in the last five years. The constant, worldwide interchange of ideas on from both surgeons and engineers will enable the development of minimally-invasive surgical techniques in the near future providing innovative approaches and new designs of the prosthesis.

Thanks to the navigation we are stepping into a new age of total knee replacement surgery. Primarily this will bring decisive advantages for our patients.

References

1. Buechel FF (2003) Die Knieendoprothese. In Konermann W, Haaker R (Hrsg) Navigation und Robotic in der Gelenk- und Wirbelsäulenchirurgie, Springer, Berlin Heidelberg, New York, Tokyo, S 182–186
2. Buechel FF, Pappas MJ (1986) The New Jersey low-contact-stress knee replacement system: biomechanical rationale and review of the first 123 cemented cases. Arch Orthop Traum Surg 105: 197–204
3. Clemens U, Miehlke RK, Kohler S, Kiefer H, Jenny JY, Konermann W (2003) Computerassistierte Navigation mit dem OrthoPilot-System und der Search-Evolution-Knieendoprothese. In: Konermann W, Haaker R (Hrsg) Navigation und Robotic in der Gelenk- und Wirbelsäulenchirurgie, Springer, Berlin Heidelberg New York Tokyo, S 207–216
4. Jeffrey RS, Morris RW, Denham RA (1991) Coronal Alignment after total knee replacement. J Bone Joint Surg 73B: 709–714
5. Konermann W, Saur MA (2003) Postoperatives Alignment von konventionell und navigiert implantierten Knietotalendoprothesen. In: Konermann W, Haaker R (Hrsg) Navigation und Robotic in der Gelenk- und Wirbelsäulenchirurgie, Springer, Berlin Heidelberg New York Tokyo, S 189–198
6. Mortier J, Zichner L (2003) Computerassistierte Druckmessung im patellofemoralen Gelenk mit elektronischen Drucksensoren. In: Konermann W, Haaker R (Hrsg) Navigation und Robotic in der Gelenk- und Wirbelsäulenchirurgie, Springer, Berlin Heidelberg New York Tokyo, S 425–428
7. Rand JA, Coventry MB (1988) Evaluation of Geometric total knee athroplasty. Clin Orthop 232: 168–173

37 Navigation and Soft-Tissue Balancing of LCS Total Knee Arthroplasty

J.M. Strauss, W. Rüther

Introduction

Of all orthopedic surgical procedures, endoprosthetic total joint replacement today is the most frequent one. While the frequency of total knee replacements in Europe is on a constant rise, in the US total knee replacement has already become more frequent than total hip procedures.

However, the primary success of total joint replacements is compromised by two main factors, namely unprecise intraoperative implant positioning and, as a long-term complication, aseptic loosening of implant components. Today, aseptic loosening is very rare as a early or mid term complication. It is rather observed later due to wear, which is frequently associated with mal-positioning.

In case of the knee joint, exact positioning of the prosthesis relative to the ligamentous structures of the knee is of highest importance and essential for optimal implant function. Even slight flaws in positioning the implant components will increase the mechanical stress on the implant fixation manifold. This may lead to a chronic overload of the interface and ultimately result in loosening of the implant.

A meta-analyis of 9879 patients [2] revealed the need for revision surgery (after only 4 years) in 4% of cases, stressing the importance of exact initial positioning as the failure rate corresponded to the radiological evidence of mal-positioning. The correlation between mal-positioning and premature loosening of the implant was underlined in several different studies. In a study of 421 patients, Ritter [8] (using a flat on flat design) showed that implantation in a varus position resulted in a threefold increase of the loosening rate (15%) as compared to positioning in correct alignment (5%). These results have been confirmed by other authors [1, 4].

The attempt to improve the positioning of the prosthesis by help of navigation systems or robots is not a new

concept. Kienzle et al. [5] developed a computer- and robot-assisted system to plan and carry out tibial and femoral cuts. Using a three-dimensional reconstruction of CT data, the surgeon can plan the placement of the tibial and femoral components. The matching of CT data and surgical object is achieved by use of fiducial markers on tibia and femur. During the operation patient and robot are tightly connected to the operating table. A different robot system [3, 6] retrieves information about the appendage and origin of the knee ligaments from the CT data source and employs them to simulate the kinematics of the prosthesis.

Another group [7] proposes a different concept: Instead of tightly connecting patient and robot, an opto-electronic navigation system follows the movements of the patient, made possible by light emitting diodes (LED) which are fixed to tibia and femur. As a basis for the component implantation, the axis of tibia and femur as well as the mechanical supporting axis of the limb are determined by various technical processes (direct digitalization of anatomical landmarks, determination of the center of rotation in the hip and ankle by »pivoting«). Without the aid of further CT data, the osseous base for the prosthesis can then be formed using an LED-equipped cutting jig and a simple navigation interface.

However the above mentioned existing concepts have however important limitations:

The postoperative outcome after total knee arthroplasty depends to a considerable degree on the soft tissue tension after implantation of the components. Today there is wide agreement among surgeons that TKA is mainly a soft tissue operation. Fadda et al. [3] carried out a cinematic analysis which is based on the length of ligaments. This method, however, is very prone to error because the ligaments are not directly visible in the CT and other essential soft tissue structures such as tendons and capsules are not taken into account. What is more, at the time of CT registration, osteophytes were still present and therefore soft tissue registration was not reliable. Algorithms published by Leitner et al. [7] for the determination of articular centers do not have sufficient reliability. In addition, the system is limited to a specific type of prosthesis because of its special cutting jigs. The user-interface does not contain individual visualization on the basis of standard X-rays.

Up to date, the use of robots requires the fixation of the patient to the robot, inadvertently leading to a larger approach and more soft tissue damage. With current techniques, the employment of robots does allow fitting of the interface with highest precision, but soft tissue balancing cannot be influenced, which, in our opinion, represents the most important aspect of total knee replacement. What is more, a CT, which is an essential requirement for robot-assisted surgery, is time-consuming and not routinely available in the OR setting.

Due to the above mentioned disadvantages of the existing navigation- and robot-systems, a new freehand navigation system for the implantation of LCS prostheses was developed in cooperation of the Maurice E.Mueller Institute in Bern, Switzerland (Chair L.P. Nolte) and the Department of Orthopedics, University Hospital Hamburg-Eppendorf, Germany (Chair W. Rüther). This system was designed to fulfill three requirements:

1. An exact reproduction of the relevant anatomical structures and given statics. This was to be achieved rapidly and efficiently by the digitalization of anatomical landmarks, thereby serving two purposes: exposure to additional CT radiation is not necessary and »matching«, i.e. the intraoperative comparison between the real anatomy and the CT anatomy, which is difficult and prone to error, is not needed any more.

2. A high enough degree of openness and complexity. It was demanded that the surgeon should have complete visual control over each degree of freedom of the implant during any given timepoint throughout the procedure. Valgus/varus, flexion/extension and rotation of both femoral and tibial components should be controllable and the surgeon should be able to manually change them at all times, including the prospective postoperative joint line.

3. Most importantly, a computer-assisted soft-tissue balancing in flexion and extension allowing optimal

functional positioning of the LCS implant. It is problematic to measure soft tissue balance with a computer without specialized sensors. In lack of such sensors, soft tissue balance can only be gauged by indirect measurement using distractors. In addition, it is difficult for the surgeon to translate the figures given by the computer to the intraoperative situation because the release in extension influences the release in flexion and vice versa. Furthermore, the tibial resection level is an important denominator of soft tissue tension. What is more, the optimal position of the bone cuts needed to obtain an ideal balance between the axis of the extremity and the resulting ligamenteous tension is not known to date. Therefore, we intended to design a system that allows the integration of desirable future developments, such as sensors for pressure and tension, at a later timepoint.

Description of the System

A newly created software module, designed to meet the criteria outlined above, was integrated into the optoelectronic navigation system »SurgiGATE« (Medivision; ◘ Fig. 37-1).

The setup consists of an optoelectronic camera (Optotrak, by Northern Digital) with which the motion of the instruments relative to a coordinate system of tibia and femur are monitored. To achieve this, so-called dynamic reference bases (DRBs) are attached to tibia and femur. The coordinates of these DRBs as well as all instruments (◘ Fig. 37-2) connected to the so-called stroberbox (pointer, stillhook, virtual keyboard, navigation clamp) are transferred to the computer system (Sun Ultrasparc III). Thus anatomical data of hip, femur, tibia and ankle can be read via the so-called pointer and visualized. Within this virtual anatomy, the motion of the instruments can then be monitored and calculated (◘ Fig. 37-3).

A so-called virtual keyboard is placed on the OR table under sterile conditions. All relevant navigational options are represented on the virtual keyboard as seen on the computer screen. The virtual keyboard is used to pilot the entire navigation program intraoperatively (◘ Fig. 37-4).

Except for some minor modifications, we could use the conventional »LCS Complete« instruments with the current navigation system. Only the cutting jigs had to be slightly modified by drilling three scanning points into

37

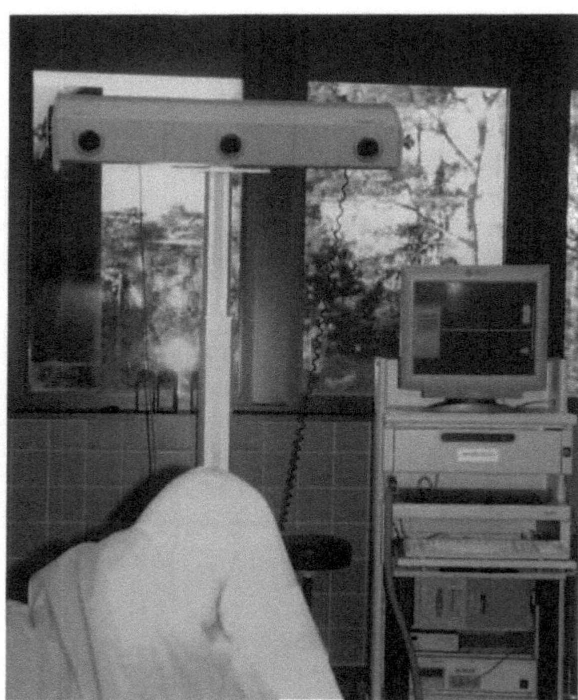

Fig. 37-1. SurgiGATE navigation system (Medivision): LED equipped instruments are tracked by an optoelectronic camera (Optotrak). Calculation and visualization is carried out by a SUN Ultrasparc III computer system

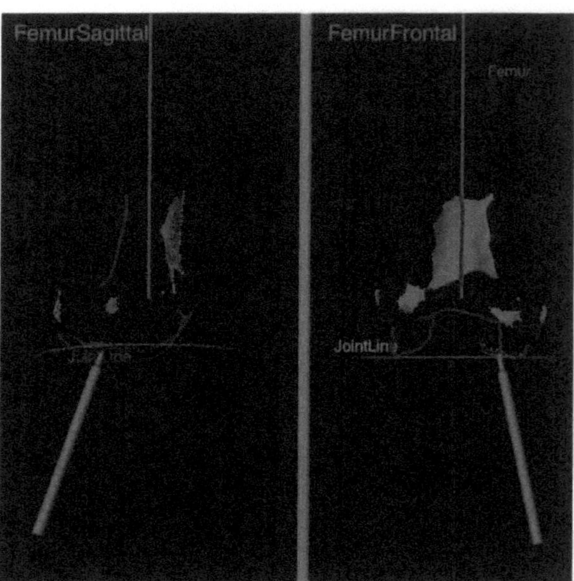

Fig. 37-3. Capture of anatomical landmarks using a Pointer. The screenshot shows the virtual anatomy already registered (mediolateral, *left*, and a.p., *right*, views of the knee joint) and a 3D visualization of the instrument in real-time

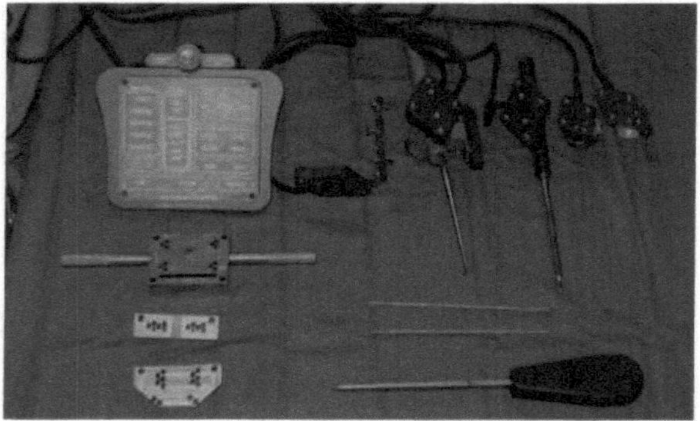

Fig. 37-2. LED equipped instruments for navigation *(background from left to right)*: virtual keyboard, navigation clamp, still hook, pointer, dynamic reference base for femur and tibia. *Front:* standard cutting jigs, K-wire, screwdriver

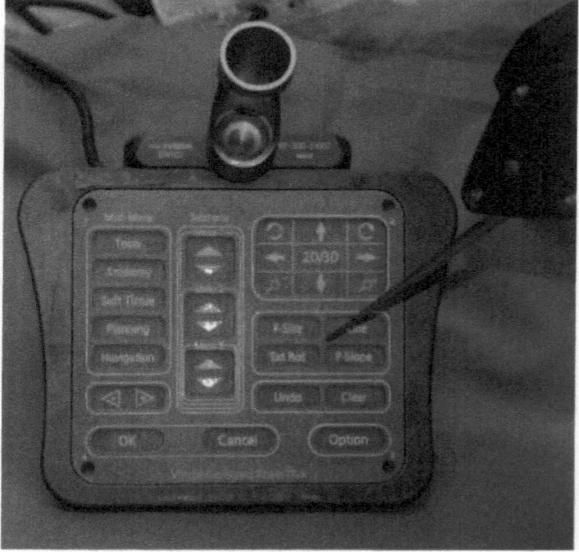

Fig. 37-4. Virtual keyboard: All relevant navigational options are represented on the virtual keyboard as seen on the computer screen. The virtual keyboard is used to pilot the entire navigation program intraoperatively. Action is performed by bringing the tip of the pointer close to the button on the virtual keyboard

each jig to allow registration of the jigs for calibration. The navigation of the cutting jig as such is made possible by the fixation of a navigation clamp (see **Fig. 37-4**) that can be attached to any of the three cutting jigs (tibia, femur a.p., distal femur).

Operative Procedure and Navigation

The computer-assisted operation is performed in five steps guided by the user: Tools, Anatomy, Soft tissue, Planning, Navigation.

Tools

First, the calibration of all instruments is checked for accuracy to rule out that potential mechanical damage leads to erroneous reading of anatomical data. In addition, the camera position as well as the presence of all instruments on the monitor is checked during this step.

Anatomy

In order to define the mechanical axis of the lower extremity, it is required to determine the center of the hip, knee and ankle joints. For the knee, this determination is complex as two relevant anatomical centers account for the relative motion that exists between femur and tibia. This aspect is of importance e.g. when using an a.p.-glide inlay or in order to detect potential problems like the roll back phenomenon. Therefore, it is reasonable to determine one center at the distal femur and another at the proximal tibia.

Hip Joint

The center of the hip joint is defined by the so-called »Pivot Algorithm«: The pointer is attached to the anterior superior iliac spine to define a fixed reference.

The invasive fixation of an additional hip DRB, as commonly required by other systems, is not needed. Now the femur, with the attached femoral DRB, is pivoted, producing a cloud of points as a result of the relative motion of the femoral DRB to the fixed hip reference. The computer calculates the hip joint center from this cloud of points, the other joint centers (distal femur, proximal and distal tibia) are calculated from pre-read anatomical landmarks. Sequential readings of each landmark are averaged, so that by increasing redundancy of the system, the calculation of the center is again based on a cloud of points. Due to the pathological changes of the knee, the Pivot Algorithm should not be used for the joint in question which is to be replaced.

Knee Joint

The anatomical landmarks of the distal femur are the medial and lateral epicondyle, the anterior and posterior cortex, the contour of the femoral condyle in the horizontal and sagittal plane both anteriorly and posteriorly, bony defects and the femoral joint line. These data are used to calculate the distal center of the femur, the size of the femoral implant component and the relative position of the jointline. The landmarks of the proximal tibia are used to calculate the proximal center of the tibia and the jointline (which, in the standing position, is identical to the femoral joint line) and include the following: anterior rim of the tibia, intercondylar tibial spine, tibial tubercle, bony defects and the tibial joint line. In order to determine the degree of rotation of the lower leg, the tibia is brought into the desired postoperative rotation in extension, if necessary after a soft tissue release. In this position the femoral transepicondylar axis is projected onto the tibial plateau, thereby defining the mediolateral axis.

Ankle Joint

The center of the ankle is defined by digitalization of both the lateral and medial malleolus as well as the tendon of the tibialis anterior muscle. Given these centers (3.2.1–3.2.3), the anatomical axis of the extremity is determined and deviations from the mechanical axis (Mikulicz line) can be defined as varus/valgus, flexion/extension and rotation (◘ Fig. 37-5).

Now the »joint play« can be visualized and quantified. Evaluation of soft tissue can only be done after exposure, excision of all osteophytes and release of adhesions. After this first registration of relevant soft tissue, tests are carried out to see if correct alignment through the whole range of motion can be achieved. If not, capsuloligamentous procedures may have to be performed and the soft tissues must be reevaluated for final validation. At this point, the bone cuts can be planned.

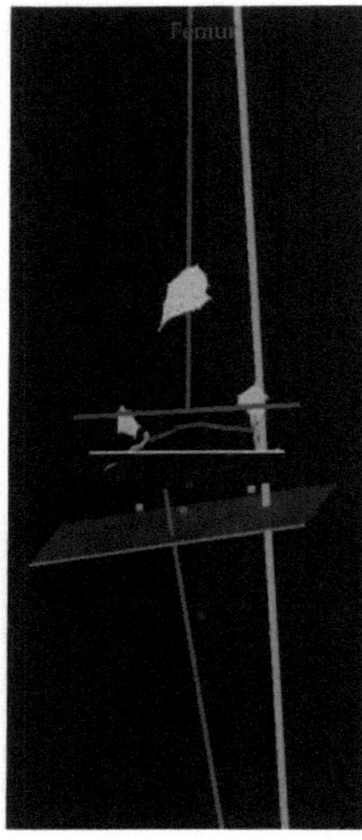

◘ Fig. 37-5. A.p. view of the virtual anatomy of a left knee with a combined valgus and flexion deformity: the screenshot shows the femoral and tibial axis, the mechanical axis (Mikulicz line, *yellow*), anatomical landmarks and preliminarily calculated cuts to restore the mechanical axis. Soft tissue behavior is not yet registered

Soft Tissue

Next to the given axis deviation, the following criteria are essential for the calculation of the bone cut positioning:

- resection level 2 mm below the deepest articular defect,
- conservation of the joint line,
- small inlay size,
- balanced soft tissue in flexion and extension, and
- identical joint gap width in flexion and extension.

The first tibial resection is carried out minimally and preliminary, navigated with default 6 mm below the joint line and with 7° slope, in order to obtain a good approach to the soft tissue, in particular to the dorsal capsule and the popliteus muscle. Next, a distractor is placed into the joint gap first in extension, then in flexion. The resulting ligament tension should correspond to the desired postoperative situation. Now the computer displays the residual axis deviation in varus/valgus, flexion/extension, rotation in extension and the external rotation of the femur in flexion. A conventional soft tissue release is performed until the desired alignment is achieved in flexion and extension.

Planning

The position of femur and tibia are registered in flexion and extension with the distractor in place (◘ Fig. 37-6a,b) and the corresponding bone cuts are calculated with the so-called autoplaner (◘ Fig. 37-6e) according to the criteria described above. If the surgeon does not intend to correct the axis deviation completely (e.g. in cases of a consolidated dislocated femoral fracture or tibial plateau fracture), or if complete alignment cannot be achieved by soft tissue manipulation, all implantation parameters can be changed manually for each component (e.g. flexion or external rotation of the femoral component or changes of the femoral implant size in order to vary the relation of the extension to the flexion gap). Based on the changed parameters, the computer recalculates the optimal cuts for a new planning (◘ Fig. 37-6c,d).

The resulting data (e.g. level of distal femoral resection, tibial re-cut, achieved correction) are processed for navigation.

Navigation

After such planning, the cuts can be performed in a quick sequence (tibial re-cut, a.p. and distal femoral resection). Each time the corresponding cutting jig is calibrated with the navigation clamp. At this point, the monitor displays the planned and actual resection plane for each jig (◘ Fig. 37-7), and, when a perfect match is obtained, the block is attached to bone with pins in this position. It is not necessary to open the marrow cavity. A quality control can now be carried out with conventional spacer blocks to check the extension and flexion gaps. After implantation of the original components, the axis is checked by lifting off the leg hold by the big toe. Finally, the motion of the prosthetic joint is recorded from full extension to maximal flexion with and without the application of varus/valgus stress.

Early Results

Analysis of Precision (Cadaver Study)

To obtain an idea of the precision of the system before clinical application, we tested the exactness of the calcu-

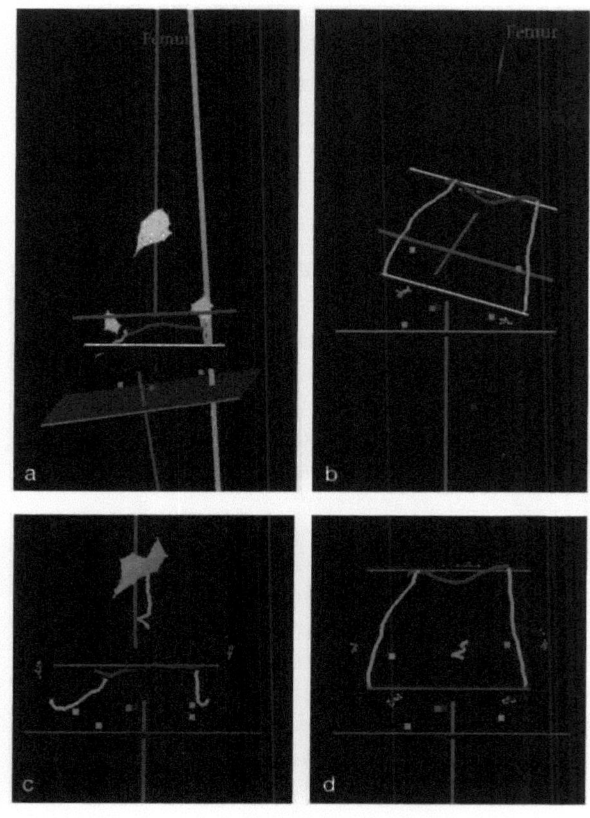
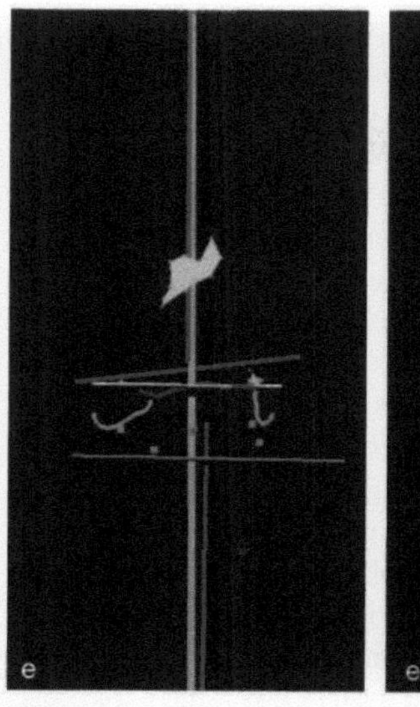
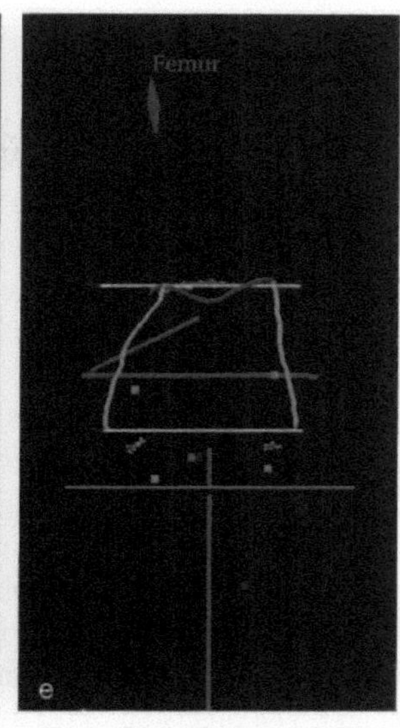

■ **Fig. 37-6a-e.** Soft tissue balancing: The position of femur and tibia is registered in flexion and extension with the distractor in place. Screenshot **a** (extension gap) and **b** (flexion gap) show the unbalanced situation before the soft tissue release. The release can be performed either manually- which allows correction of the orientation of tibial and femoral components - (**c** and **d**) or automatically (**e**). The screenshot shows the aligned situation after a successful soft tissue release. The bone cuts are calculated with the so-called »auto-planner« according to the criteria described in the text. Tibial and femoral resection height, joint line deviation and component size are also listed on the screen

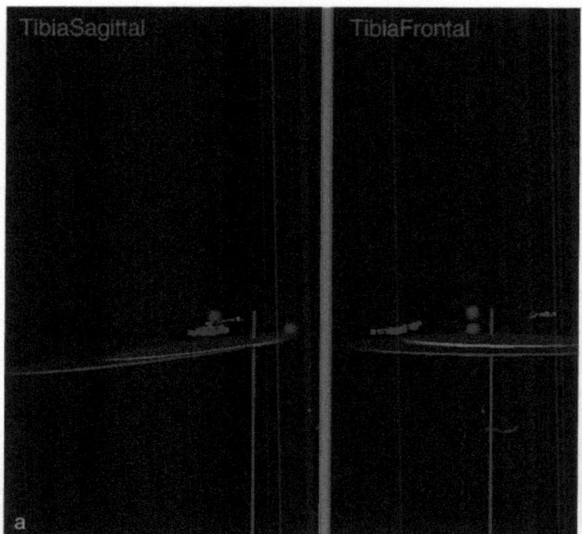
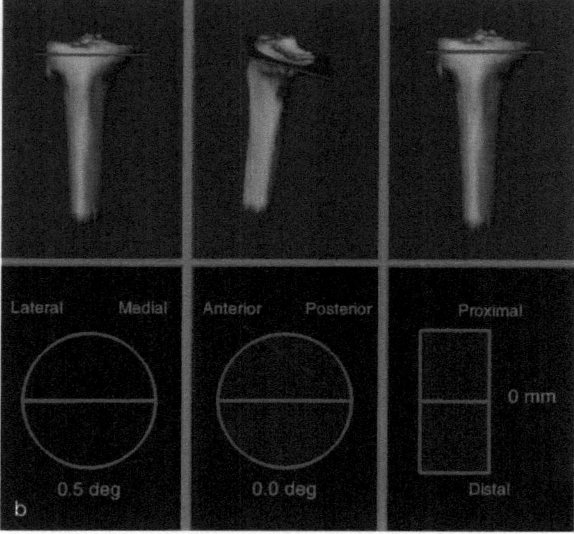

■ **Fig. 37-7a,b.** Navigation of the tibial cut: After calibrating the tibial cutting jig with the navigation clamp, the monitor displays the planned (*yellow*) and actual (*red*) resection plane for the tibia while the surgeon tries to fix the jig to the bone. **a** 3D visualization **b** 2D visualization

lation of the centers of hip, distal femur and ankle in CT-controlled intra- and interobserver cadaver studies. The matching of the CT data with the coordinates of the navigation system was made possible by the implantation of three so-called »fiducial markers« into femur and tibia before the CT was done. The intraobserver study [one surgeon, five readings of the anatomical landmarks with the navigation system for each cadaver ($n=6$)] yielded a mean deviation of the center as defined by CT of 0.7 mm at the hip, 1.1 mm at the knee and 1.8 mm at the ankle. The interobserver study [five surgeons, single reading of landmarks for each cadaver ($n=6$)], resulted in slightly higher deviations: 1.1 mm at the hip, 1.2 mm at the knee and 2.4 mm at the ankle. To put this into perspective, it should be kept in mind that a 1° deviation of the axis of the extremity corresponds to a 7 mm dislocation of the knee center. The precision of the system was influenced more significantly by the manual skills of the surgeon with regard to the resection as such. For instance, the difference between the planned and real resection planes of the distal femoral cut was 1.6° in the frontal plane and 1.9° in the sagittal plane.

First Clinical Results (Preliminary)

A first study, done with 30 gonarthritis patients, resulted in a postoperative axis deviation from the ideal line (measured by X-ray a.p. and lateral of the entire extremity in standing position) of 1.7° in the frontal plane and 3.9° in the sagittal plane for the navigated group ($n=15$). The control group ($n=15$), operated without navigation, yielded a 1.9° deviation in the frontal plane and 4.4° in the sagittal plane. The differences between the navigated and the control group were not statistically significant. However, the range in the non-navigated control group was clearly wider and it comprised the cases with the largest postoperative axis deviation of all (occurring in two cases of extreme obesity and in one valgus deformity of more than 30°). Such extreme deviations were not found among similar patients of the navigation group. The quality of the ligament stability (varus/valgus stress) was comparable in both groups, but the imbalance (difference between medial and lateral stability) was smaller in the navigated group. After analysis of all data including a power-analysis, a prospective randomized study will be performed to look

for statistically significant differences in axis deviation as well as positioning of both tibial and femoral components. In particular such a study will reveal whether the quality of the component positioning achieved by this navigation system is equal for all the implantation criteria outlined above.

Summary and Future Perspective

The disadvantage of the current system is that it takes longer to perform the operation (19 minutes on average, range: 12 to 62 minutes) and that the setup is more complex compared to a non-navigated standard procedure. However, compared to other existing navigation systems, the advantages are apparent:

- The system is minimally invasive thanks to the percutaneously applied reference bases.
- While the surgeon does not have to give up his familiar handling, he receives extra information online about the optimal bone cuts, joint line displacement and the current ligament tension.
- As all degrees of freedom of each component can be manually manipulated and the consequences of these changes for the postoperative situation are displayed in the planning module, the optimal result for the patient can be found **before** the cuts are carried out.
- The precision of the system is sufficient (cadaver study) and first clinical results are promising.
- Last but not least the navigation system can be used by the surgeon to document the quality of his work.

The lack of statistically significant postoperative differences between the navigated and the control group in the clinical study was found with another navigation system as well [9]. This can be explained by the small number of patients in the clinical studies and the relatively small percentage of complex deformities within the cohort, because it is this particular subgroup of patients that is expected to profit from a navigated procedure. The lack of statistical power can also be accounted for by the limited precision of the post-op X-ray measurement which includes up to 3° deviation due to rotational effects. In the future, a standardized and more precise way of evaluating the operative results will be needed.

The quality of soft tissue handling will be improved by the introduction of objective measurements (pressure sensors) and the quality of the bone cuts (the major limiting factor within the present system) may be further optimized by the introduction of a minimal robot system for milling the cuts.

References

1. Bargren, JH, Blaha JD, Freeman MA (1983) Alignment in total knee arthroplasty. Correlated biomechanical and clinical observations. Clin.Orthop 173: 178–183
2. Callahan CM, Drake BG, Heck DA, Dittus RS (1995) Patient outcomes following unicompartimental or bicompartimental knee arthroplasty. A meta-analysis. J Arthroplasty 10: 141–150
3. Fadda M, Bertelli D, Martelli S et al. (1997) Computer assisted planning for total knee arthroplasty. In: Troccaz J, Grimson E, Moesges R (HRSG) CVRMed-MRCAS'97. Springer, Berlin Heidelberg New York Tokyo, pp 663–671
4. Feng EL, Stulberg SD, Wixson RL (1994) Progressive subluxation and polyethylen wear in total knee replacements with flat articular surfaces. Clin Orthop 299: 60–71
5. Kienzle TC III, Stulber SD, Peshkin M, Quaid A, Lea J, Goswami A, Wu C-H (1996) A computer assisted total knee replacement surgical system using a calibrated robot. In: Taylor RH, Lavallée S, Burdea GC, Moesges R (eds) Computer integrated surgery: Technology and clinical applications. Mit Press, London, pp 409–423
6. La Palombara PF, Fadda M, Martelli S, Marcacci M (1997) Minimally invasive 3D data registration in computer and robot-assisted total knee arthroplasty. Med Biol Eng Comput 35: 600–610
7. Leitner F, Picard F., Minfelde R, Schulz H-J, Cinquin P, Saragaglia D (1997) Computer-assisted surgical total knee replacement. In: Troccaz J, Grimson E, Moesges R (eds) CVRMed.-MRCAS'97. Springer, Berlin Heidelberg New York Tokyo, pp 629–637
8. Ritter MA, Faris PM, Keating EM, Meding JB (1994) Postoperative alignment of total knee replacement. Its effect on survival. Clin Orthop 299: 153–156
9. Miehlke RK, Clemens U, Jens J.-H, Kershally S (2001) Navigation in der Knieendoprothetik – vorläufige klinische Erfahrungen und prospektiv vergleichende Studie gegenüber konventioneller Implantationstechnik. Z Orthop 139: 109–116

38 CT-Free Navigation with the LCS Surgetics Station: A New Way of Balancing the Soft Tissues in TKA Based on Bone Morphing

J.L. Briard, E. Stindel, S. Plaweski, F. Dubrana, P. Merloz, C. Lefevre,
J. Troccaz, F. Bertrand, N. Begoc, P. Solodky, M. Breysse

Introduction

Total knee arthroplasty (TKA) aims at achieving a pain-free, stable, mobile and durable knee. With proper selection and good technique, pain relief should be obtained. Obtaining mobility, with a full range of motion, without instability is rather more challenging. Both mobility and stability are very important for implant longevity.

A full range of motion will be achieved if the spaces between the tibial and femoral cuts are equal throughout the flexion-extension, and if good patellofemoral tracking and tension have been obtained.

Stability is a more complex phenomenon, as shown in recent fluoroscopic studies [4, 12]. Even with the most appropriate surgical technique, femoral condylar lift-off is present in more then 30% of the LCS operated with conventional instrumentation. The phenomenon is greatest in the lateral compartment at 90° of flexion. It is probably due to the difficulty of assessing properly the transepicondylar axis and the flexion gap with the patella in proper position during the surgical procedure. Because of this lift-off, patients may feel unsteady, polyethylene wear may increase, and, worst of all, the implant may equire revision.

To increase the survivorship of the prosthesis, several precautions have been taken for the design of the LCS knee. The LCS Mobile Bearing knee looks for a large contact area throughout the gait cycle. These large contact areas (900 mm^2) between 0° and 35° are due to the distal spherical shape of the implants. This large contact is available through a large distal radius (50 mm) which rules out the use of a PS system. In flexion beyond 35°, this stability is even more critical for the LCS as the contact area is a circular coronal line. Therefore, a stabilizing design feature was needed. This is provided by the cup shape of the polyethylene insert. The jump height to dislocate over the rim of the polyethylene is between 6 and 9 mm. However, the stability with the mobile-bearing LCS is critical and relies very much on the soft tissues, which share the loads for stability with the prosthetic design.

Obtaining good soft-tissue balancing and a good orientation of the implants with respect to the mechanical axis is critical with this kind of unconstrained prosthesis. For the past 25 years, a conventional system of instruments has been used to achieve balancing and alignment. However, mal-alignment has been reported following the use of both intra- and extra-medullary systems [5, 17].

For these reasons, computer-assisted instrumentation has been developed recently. Dozens of papers have been published on the subject of computer-assisted knee surgery. The literature to date is too vast for a detailed and exhaustive review in this chapter. Readers who are interested in the taxonomy of computer-assisted TKA systems may find further information in a paper by the authors of the present chapter [15].

In this chapter, we present the LCS Surgetics Application running on the PRAXIM Surgetics Station. This system is a CT-less navigation system that provides geometric and morphologic 3D data without any preoperative or intra-operative imaging (no CT, no MRI, no fluoroscopy). The method relies mainly on data collected with a 3D optical localizer in relative coordinate systems attached to the bones, which is the Bone Morphing technology on the Surgetics Station (PRAXIM patent pending).

Materials and Methods

The LCS Surgetics Application was designed to:

- control the alignment of the implants with respect to the mechanical axis. It enables the surgeon to control and plan any tibial and femoral cuts in 3D (level and orientation),
- control stability, which requires a soft-tissue registration algorithm, in correct alignment, which may necessitate soft-tissue release,
- perform automatic and efficient sizing of the implants,
- navigate the cutting guides,
- control each step.

Moreover, we wanted a surgeon-friendly interface (S.F.I.). Going beyond a user-friendly interface, the concept of an S.F.I. includes the idea that the computer-assisted surgical protocol (CASP) must be surgeon-friendly and displayed on the screen through a user-friendly interface.

Since the principles of the technology are not described in this chapter, readers who wish to obtain further information may wish to study the overview by Lavallée et al [8].

The standard hardware of the LCS-Surgetics station includes:

- A Surgetics Station equipped with a passive optical sensor (PRAXIM, Grenoble, France).
  - There is no cable in the operative field between the patient and the station as this technology uses 3 passive sterile reflective and disposable markers.
- A rigid body »F« attached to the femur with 2 pins.
- A rigid body »T« attached to the tibia with 2 pins.
- A probe »P« equipped on both faces with markers. It features at its end a 2-mm diameter spherical tip to slide smoothly on bone surfaces.
- A rigid body »G« equipped on both faces with markers, to be attached to cutting blocks during navigation.

The software was developed specifically by PRAXIM for DePuy, France. This was made possible through close collaboration between the two companies, allowing the optimization of the implantation of the LCS implant according to its specific philosophy.

The software relies on 3D geometric and morphologic data. Geometric data may be sufficient for controlling an alignment of the components [6, 7, 10, 11]; however, they do not provide a complete representation of the knee, and the most important drawback is that they provide only an approximate knee center, by direct digitization or by kinematic analysis of the pathological knee joint, which is rather controversial. Conversely, 3D morphologic data obtained by the Bone Morphing technique are very useful for the visualization, in real time and in 3 dimensions prior to any actual bone cut, of the bone defects, the planned surgical cuts, the choice of the implant size, position and rotation with respect to the bone cortical surfaces, and the flexion and extension gaps. Each one of these parameters affects directly the implant position during the planning stage, and all of these parameters are linked. Thus, changing the size of the implant will have an immediate impact on implant position and knee balancing, which is why only a global planning strategy makes a sense. The morphologic data also provide much information that helps to control or even automate the location of the points digitized by the surgeon. Therefore, the challenge is really how to obtain geometric and morphologic data. 3D morphologic data are also very important for the concept of S.F.I introduced above. In fact, the visualization of the 3D real morphology of the epiphysis is an important part of the system, designed to allow the surgeon to control the planning, to achieve and to simulate different options in alignment, bone cuts, and their impact on stability. In previous systems, 3D data were collected through CT acquisition followed by 3D reconstructions. Apart the problem of the accuracy of the reconstruction, the CT scan option is very time-consuming and expensive, and raises the issue of irradiation. Thanks to the Bone Morphing technology introduced by PRAXIM, there is no longer any need for CT scans. Bone Morphing, patented by PRAXIM, serves to acquire, intra-operatively, the 3D morphology of the bones. The technology appears to be very well suited to this kind of surgery. For more information on the technical approach, the reader is referred to the specific chapter on Bone Morphing, elsewhere in this book.

Computer-Assisted Surgical Procedure (CASP)

The first step in any CASP is to fix a reference system to each bone or tool that will need to be tracked during the procedure. For TKA, one reference system (DRB) is fixed to the tibia, and one to the femur. The fixation to the bone must be perfectly rigid and stable, even in osteoporotic patients, since the reference systems will be used to build the global geometry of the limb of the patient undergoing surgery.

The second step consists in collecting 3D locations of points in order to build the mechanical axis and to create some reference planes such as the coronal, axial, or sagittal plane.

The Hip Center

During TKA procedures, the hip is outside the operating field; therefore the detection of the center of the joint (H) is based upon a kinematic method. There is no need for a rigid body on the iliac crest. Once the femoral rigid body has been placed, the surgeon imparts a circular motion to the patient's lower limb (with the knee in full extension). During this motion, the successive positions of the femoral rigid body are stored by the computer in the localizer reference system. Since nothing is perfect, there will be some noise because of the non-spheroid shape of the femoral head, the motion of the pelvic bone, and the limits of the accuracy of the optical localizer. Therefore, the hip center is not unique, and is always in motion. Any method of detection that does not take this fact into account will be inaccurate. In our approach, the algorithm searches a point of the 3D space C_h that optimizes some criteria based on the minimum of a function

$$F(c) = \sum_{i=1}^{i=100} \left\| c_{i-1} - c_i \right\|^2$$

where i is the position of the femur at time t and c_i is the corresponding calculated center. The resulting point can be seen as the point of the 3D space attached to the femur with the smallest trajectory during the acquisition motion [13, 15].

The Knee Center

During TKA procedures, the knee joint is wide open, so the digitization of geometric points (landmarks) is easy. Accurate determination of the knee center is difficult, because there is no accurate definition that applies to the pathological knee [1, 2, 9]. However, the direct localization of an approximation of the center of the pathological knee (Ko) is straightforward using the optical probe. Such a point will **not** be used to define the HKA angle during the planning stage; it is only an indication to compute an approximation of the pathological axes in the patient preoperatively. In the Surgetics approach using Bone Morphing the knee center (Kp) is the center of the knee prosthesis that is planned along each step of the CASP. This definition corresponds exactly to what we expect postoperatively. Planning the implant position on the bone is therefore the only way to define an accurate knee center.

The Ankle Center

The purely morphologic approach chosen by us is based on the digitization of two points on the bones. Using the same probe used for the knee joint, the surgeon digitizes one point on the lateral malleolus and one point on the medial malleolus. The system computes the midpoint of the segment defined by these two points. This choice relies upon an accuracy study presented in [14] and partially published in [15]. Our choice has been found to allow a quick and accurate determination of the ankle center.

A number of other points are recorded, such as two points on the anterior femoral cortex, in order to compute the ideal anteroposterior location of the femoral implant. Some points will then be used to build the femoral and the tibial axis. This step depends strongly on the chosen Computer-Assisted Surgical Protocol (CASP) running on the Surgetics Station and adapted to the prosthesis and to the surgical technique. Thus, in the Surgetics CASP applied to the DePuy LCS prosthesis, we have chosen to use two points on the posterior condyles to define the coronal plane (in combination with the hip center to define the 3D plane). The tibial sagittal plane, which is probably one of the most important to define, is defined by the ankle center and two points digitized on the tibia. The first one is on the tibial tuberosity, while the second one is between the medial and the lateral tubercle of the intercondylar eminence. Importantly, for any point for which a mathematical definition exists, the system uses the Bone Morphing surfaces and geometric axes to compute a new point that is more precise than the surgeon-selected point. The surgeon-selected point is then used only to check any (unlikely) gross errors of the automated and refined Bone Morphing points. This is an iterative and complex process that depends on each point and which benefits from the Bone Morphing described in the next sections.

Next, data are collected using the Bone Morphing technique. These data provide a complete and accurate 3D shape of the epiphysis.

Bone Morphing

From the surgical point of view, the Bone Morphing technique consists in collecting two clouds of points with the probe (one for the femur, and one for the tibia). These points are gathered by sliding the probe over the articular surfaces. During this sliding motion, the localizer records the iterative 3D locations of the probe tip. This process takes about 1 minute and 30 seconds for each volume. This cloud of points is then matched to a unique deformable model included in the system. (For a more technical description, see [3,16], or the specific chapters in this book.) The output of this deformation process is an accurate representation of the epiphysis of the bone being operated on. Its accuracy can be checked intra-operatively by the surgeon. The mean error between the model and the actual bone is usually below 0.5 millimeters.

Based on these geometric and morphologic data, the system is able to
- optimize the tibial cut,
- register and validate the soft-tissue envelope,
- optimize and guide the femoral cuts.

Optimization of the Tibial Cut

This is the first step of the planning process. The level of the tibial cut is important in order to have sound and long lasting fixation of the implant and to avoid an unnecessary increase in tibial insert thickness. This level is computed after recording the relative position of the tibia with respect to the femur at 97° of flexion. The level of the joint line is optimized to fit an implant with the smallest polyethylene component (10 mm) and to obtain the best-fitting implant

for the femoral side based on data collected from bone morphing. The tibial cut is then performed as a horizontal cut in the coronal plane, with a 7° slope in the sagittal plane, and centered at the computed level.

Bone morphing allows visualizing the cut and a possible bone defect due to wear. Once the tibial cut has been performed, its accuracy is registered and will be used for further planning.

Registration and Validation of the Soft-Tissue Envelope

Before going further in the CASP, all the osteophytes must be removed to prevent impingement and tethering over the capsule and ligaments. Then the surgeon will assess the capsuloligamentous envelope length between the femur and the tibia. The main object is to collect enough data to optimize the femoral cuts in order to obtain excellent stability at 0° and 97° without any tendency for the knee to go into recurvatum. In osteoarthritic knees, the situation is much more complex, owing to the frequent presence of a fixed flexion deformity. Virtually all orthopaedic companies have tried a distraction device; however, most of them have ended up with spacer blocks. We have chosen to abandon fixed spacer blocks, and developed a spacer called AVS (adjustable variable spacer), which helps monitoring the distances between the components in order to ensure that there is no laxity at 0°, 1 mm at 20°, and 1 mm at 97°.

The first step involves getting rid of the fixed flexion deformity. The collateral ligaments are placed in correct tension at 20°, then at 0° of flexion. A significant difference in the HkpA axis displayed on the screen between 20° and 0° of flexion will indicate a retraction of the posterior capsule, which is tight at 0° (leaving the collateral ligaments slack) and becomes loose at 20°(the collateral ligaments are »taking the tension« now). In such a case, a posterior release will be necessary.

In the second step, we use the AVS at 0° of flexion (◘ Fig. 38-1) to place the collateral ligaments in correct tension. The goal is to try to obtain a good compromise between the HKpA (monitored by the computer) and the balance of the collateral ligaments.

If such a compromise cannot be achieved, then a release of the collateral ligament must be performed. Note

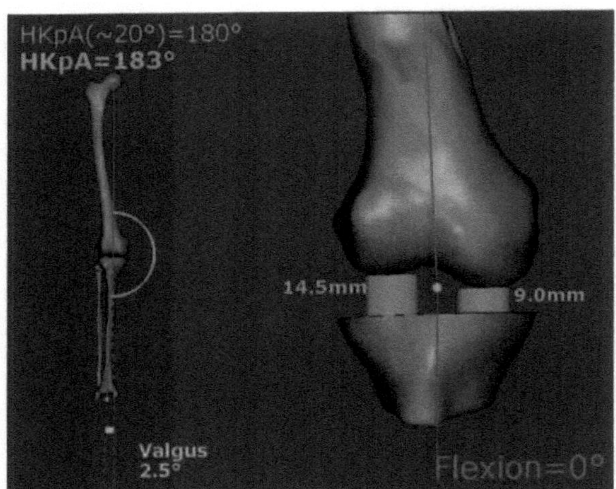

Fig. 38-1. Validation of the soft tissue envelope at 0° extension. With the collateral ligaments in correct tension and well-balanced, the system gives information on mechanical axis and helps to pre-position the distal cut so that flexion and extension gaps are later equivalent

that the surgeon is perfectly free to accept a mechanical axis HKpA that is not strictly 180°. A few degrees of residual varus/valgus is commonly accepted if it occurs in a well-balanced knee in which no release has to be performed. The system helps to make this tradeoff quantitatively. If the compromise between balance and axes cannot be obtained, a concomitant osteotomy may have been indicated by the preoperative planning. However, this situation and specific problem are beyond the scope of this chapter, and will not be discussed further here.

When this has been done, the transformation matrix of the tibia and femur are stored by the computer. Know-

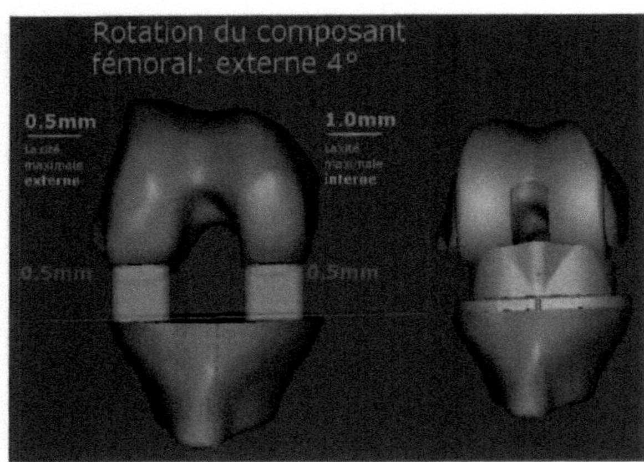

Fig. 38-2. Validation of the soft tissue envelope at 97° flexion

ing that the perception of a »correctly balanced knee« may vary from one surgeon to another, the system is then able to quantify and display the resulting laxities on the medial and lateral side when the knee is stressed in valgus or varus.

The third step consists in the use of the AVS at 97° of flexion (**Fig. 38-2**).

At this stage, the system monitors in real time the angle of external rotation of the femoral implant with reference to the posterior condyles. Again, this helps to accept a given rotation and to make a tradeoff between balance and rotation. Again, the system then measures the residual laxity on the medial and lateral side when the knee is stressed in valgus or varus.

All of the above goes to show that complete preoperative planning is impossible, and that soft-tissue validation can be done only intra-operatively.

The issue of the patella is also very important. The validation of the soft-tissue envelope is achieved with the correct spacer blocks at 0° and at 97°. When placing collateral ligaments in tension, the patella should sit in its original position in the trochlear groove, in order to avoid the »noisy« traction stresses which pulls the femur and the tibia laterally in obese, muscular or stiff multi-operated patients with patella baja. This is also important when using a lateral approach.

Femoral Planning

For each of the three above-mentioned steps, the transformation matrix of the tibia and femur are stored by the computer. Based on these data, femoral planning can then be achieved. An optimization loop is used, and a set of femoral cuts is proposed where the planning gives a flexion gap equivalent to the extension gap (**Fig 38-3**).

Therefore, one can say that the priority of the LCS Surgetics CASP is soft-tissue balancing. Only when this criterion has been satisfied will the other parameters be optimized.

If the surgeon disagrees with the proposition, he or she may use the touch screen of the Surgetics Station and adjust the implant size and positions in all planes. The way in which these changes may be made follows the customary train of thoughts of the operating surgeon.

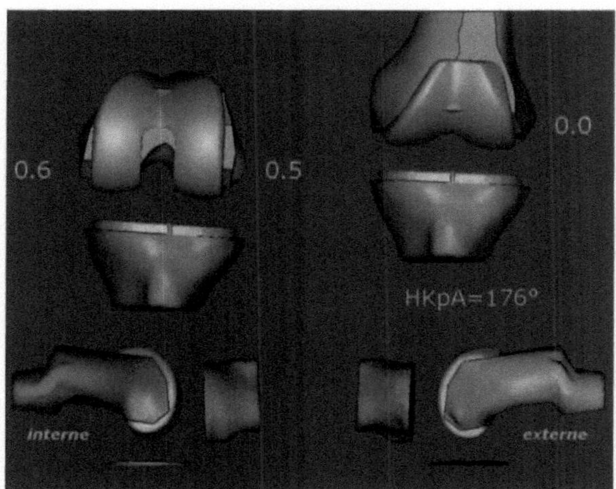

Fig. 38-3. Femoral planning. The system optimizes component placement to match flexion and extension gaps. Priority is given to the extension position

Performing the Cuts: the Action Steps

The navigation of the cutting guides for the tibial cut, as well as for the femoral cuts, is not specific to this application. A rigid body is fixed on each cutting guide, and a calibration of each cutting guide is performed. Each cutting plane must be aligned to the plane displayed on the screen using a few specific jigs, screws and holders that loosely hold the guide on the bone. When the two planes are aligned, the cutting guide is firmly fixed to the bones using standard pins, and the cuts are performed in customary fashion. This technique dispenses with the need for an intramedullary guide, and thereby reduces the risk of subsequent pulmonary embolic events.

When all cuts have been made, the prosthesis is inserted, and tibiofemoral alignment is checked, as is the 1-mm laxity medially and laterally throughout range of motion.

Operative Record-Keeping

All data, steps, and actions are recorded on a patient CD-ROM, for automated patient reporting and further investigations.

Conclusion

The strong points of the LCS Surgetics application developed by PRAXIM and DePuy France are

- a CT-free accurate, fast and easy-to-perform Bone Morphing technology,
- a surgeon-friendly interface (S.F.I.), which provides an easy-to-use system made by surgeons for surgeons, based on a clear linear protocol. Navigation into the different steps of the protocol is made with the help of a simple double pedal, and of a touch screen to modify some default parameters, in the rare cases where there is a need for such modification.
- The registration and validation of the soft tissues are certainly a major aspect of this program; this is in line with the universally accepted view nowadays that total knee arthroplasty is more a soft-tissue than a bone-cut operation.
- The femoral planning calculations and the associated displays are of the utmost importance for the surgeons, who can use and build upon all of their previous experience and know-how when performing a total knee arthroplasty.
- »Flexion gap first« or 'extension gap first' is no longer an issue.
- Finally, the operative record is outputted with precise data concerning bone cuts and soft tissues, which is a real step into the 21st century.

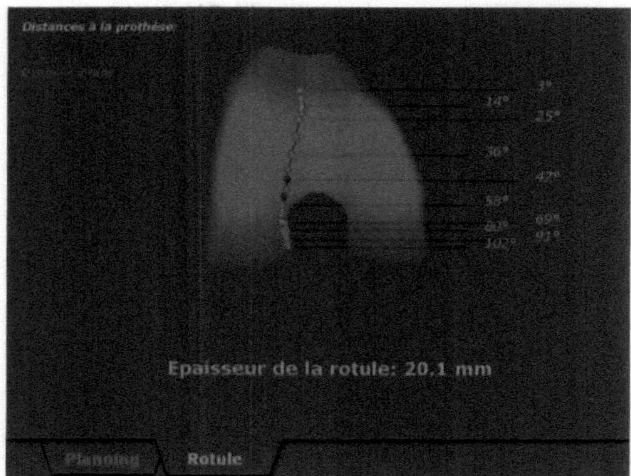

Fig. 38-4. Patella tracking simulation on the pre-positioned femoral component during the femoral planning phase

The Shape of Things to Come (Soon)

Today, a specific module of the LCS Surgetics Station allows navigation of the patella, with a specific light-weight rigid body. It enables to record patella tracking before surgery, and compare the recorded data on the planned femoral component before any cut is made.

■ Figure 38-4 shows the trajectory of the patella before and after surgery. The data collected during the three balancing stages are stored and used for further scientific studies, in order further to improve our knowledge of the biomechanics of the knee after TKA. As developers, all of these topics are of immediate and current concern to us. With the LCS Surgetics, the future is already with us. And looking further into the future, we are working on the revision of TKA.

References

1. Bonnel F (1988) Organisation architecturale et biomécanique de l'articulation fémoro-tibiale. In: Bonnel F (ed) La gonarthrose. Masson, Paris, pp 1–11
2. Cazalis P (1994) Diagnostic et traitement d'un genou douloureux. Editions techniques – Encycl. Méd. Chir. (Paris France), Appareil locomoteur, 14–325-A-10: 1–16
3. Fleute M, Lavallée S, Julliard R (1999) Incorporating a statistically based shape model into a system for computer-assisted anterior cruciate ligament surgery. Medical Image Analysis 3: 209–222
4. Hoff W, Komisteck R, Dennis D, Sarojak M (2000) An interactive fluoroscopy-based system for in vivo kinematics analysis of total joint arthroplasty, Annual Meeting. Orthopedic Research Society, Orlando
5. Jefferry RS, Morris RW, Denham RA (1991) Coronal alignment after total knee replacement. J Bone Joint Surg 73-B: 709–714
6. Jenny JY, Boeri C (2001) Computer-assisted implantation of total knee prostheses: a case-control comparative study with classical instrumentation. Comput Aided Surg 6: 217–220
7. Kunz M, Strauss M, Langlotz F, Deuretzbacher G, Rüther W, Nolte LP (2001) A non-CT based total knee arthroplasty system featuring complete soft-tissue balancing. MICCAI 2001, LNCS 2208, pp 409–415
8. Lavallée S, Bainville E, Bricault I (2000) An overview of computer-integrated surgery and therapy. In: Udupa (ed) 3D imaging in medicine. CRC Press, Boca Raton, pp 207–263
9. Mansat CH (1988) Indications chirurgicales de la gonarthrose. In: Bonnel F (ed) La gonarthrose. Masson, Paris, pp 56–61
10. Miehlke RK, Clemens U, Jens JH, Kershally S (2001) Navigation in knee endoprosthesis implementation – preliminary experiences and prospective comparative study with conventional implementation technique. Z Orthop Ihre Grenzgeb 139: 109–116
11. Saragaglia D, Picard F, Chaussard C, Montbaron E, Leitner F, Cinquin P (2001) Mise en place des prothèses totales de genou assistée par ordinateur: comparaison avec la technique conventionnelle. Résultats d'une étude prospective randomisée de 50 cas. Revue de Chirurgie Orthopédique 87 : 18–28
12. Stiehl JB, Dennis DA, Komistek RD, Crane HS (1999) In vivo determination of condylar lift-off and screw-home in a mobile-bearing total knee arthroplasty. J Arthroplasty 14: 293–299
13. Stindel E, Gil D, Briard JL, Merloz P, Dubrana F, Lefevre C (2002) Detection of the center of the hip in ct less based system for tka navigational guidance. An evaluation study of the accuracy and reproducibility of the surgetic's algorithm. CAOS Symposium, International Society for Computed Assisted Orthopedic Surgery, Santa Fé
14. Stindel E, Gil D, Briard JL, Plaweski S, Dubrana F, Lefevre C (2002) The center of the ankle in CT less based navigation system. What is really important to detect? CAOS symposium, International Society for Computed Assisted Orthopedic Surgery, Santa Fé
15. Stindel E, Briard JL, Merloz P, Plaweski S, Dubrana F, Lefevre C, Troccaz JL (2002) Bone morphing: 3D morphological data for total knee arthroplasty. Computer Aided Surgery 7: 156–168
16. Szelisky R, Lavallée S (1996) Matching 3-D anatomical surfaces with non-rigid deformations using octree-splines. Int J Computer Vision 18: 171–186
17. Tetter KE, Bergman D, Colwell CW (1995) Accuracy of intramedullary versus extramedullary tibial alignment cutting systems in total knee arthroplasty. Clini Orthop Rel Res 321: 106–110

39 The *Galileo* System for Implantation of Total Knee Arthroplasty
An Integrated Solution Comprising Navigation, Robotics and Robot-Assisted Ligament Balancing

P. Ritschl, F. Machacek jun., R. Fuiko, R. Zettl, B. Kotten

Introduction

The following factors are essential for the long-term success of knee implants:

- Correct three-dimensional placement of the implant [1, 4, 5, 8, 10, 12].
- Exact ligament balancing to ensure equal-sized, rectangular flexion and extension gaps [7].

The Galileo system is a modern, practical navigation system with an integrated mini-robot. A ligament tension measuring device additionally permits ligament tension to be measured in flexion and then applied to the extension gap using a computer-controlled mini-robot.

A description is given of the equipment, its mode of operation, preoperative planning and surgical technique, and data from clinical experience. Intraoperative measurements of accuracy in reconstructing the mechanical axis demonstrate that precision is a necessary requirement for the long-term success of an implant.

Patient and Method

Equipment

The Galileo system consists of a navigation unit, a mini-robot and an integrated ligament tension measuring device, here called a ligament tensioner.

Navigation is carried out using an infra-red optical system (Polaris NDI). Active (light-emitting) and passive (retro-reflecting) locators permit communication between the object and the measurement system. These locators are fixed to the bone in the area to be operated or attached to the instruments.

The autoclavable mini-robot has two linear axes driven by servo motors (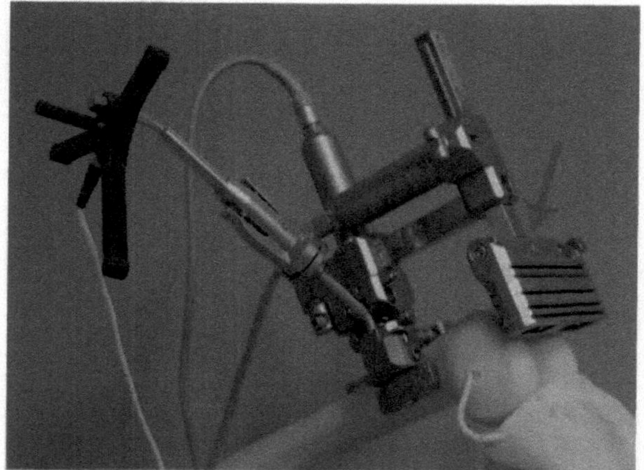 Fig. 39-1). Due to its size and weight it can be directly used on the patient as a sterile unit.

The ligament tensioner (Fig. 39-2) has three scales:

- Force measurement in Newton,
- Measurement of distance in mm,
- Information regarding the polyethylene thickness to be selected.

Fig. 39-1. The mini-robot and the femoral locator of the Galileo system are mounted on the femoral clamp. The femoral clamp is fixed flush to the ventral femoral cortical bone (rigid body). The »one in five« cutting jig is coupled to the inverse T of the robot (*arrow*)

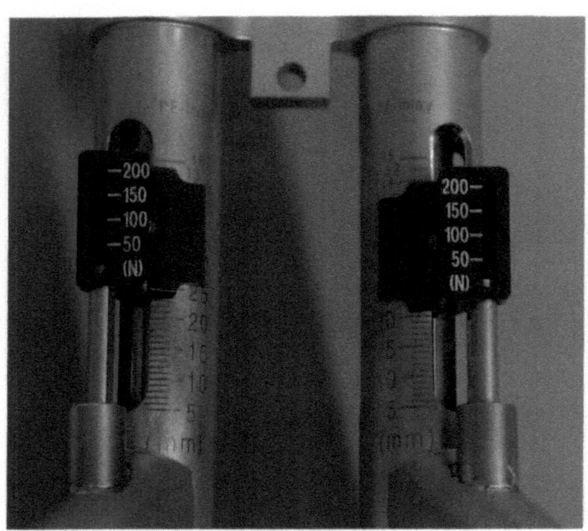

Fig. 39-2. The ligament tensioner is used to achieve balanced and rectangular flexion and extension gaps, characterized by equal force (Newton) and equal distance (mm)

Operating the Galileo System for Total Knee Replacement

Registration of skeletal geometry is carried out by **kinematic analysis** or by **direct palpating** of landmarks relevant for the operation.

The center of the femoral head is determined kinematically by the method of system rotation without using an additional pin on the pelvis. Relative movement of the pelvis is compensated mathematically. In the palpating method definite landmarks and/or directions are registered.

The computer-controlled **mini-robot** moves the femur-cutting block in pre-calculated positions. The unit does not itself actively perform any cutting operations, but positions the saw guide for a conventional oscillating saw. The calculated femoral implant size proposed by the system can be accepted or overridden by the surgeon.

Optimisation of ligament balancing in flexion and extension can be done in two ways.
- By moving the cutting block in a ventral-dorsal and cranial-caudal direction in 0.5 mm steps.
- By using an integrated ligament tensioning system with tension and distance measurements. This allows the system to apply an equal tension from the balanced flexion gap to the extension gap.

Preoperative Planning

Preoperative planning involves carrying out conventional radiographs. Templating or preoperative determination of axes and angles is unnecessary.

Surgical Technique

A step-by-step description is given for registration, instrument alignment (tracking) and robot use. Special consideration is given to the integration of the ligament tensioner into the system.

Step 1: Registration of Skeletal Geometry

Registration of Femur and Sizing of Femoral Components. For registration of the femur, a femoral clamp is first positioned and fixed to the ventral cortical bone of the distal femur (see Fig. 39-1). The flush fit of the clamp with the cortical bone represents the subsequent alignment of the femoral component in the sagittal plane [6]. After fitting a locator to the femur clamp the kinematic determination of the rotational centre of the hip is done. Further registration is carried out by touching procedure. The following are touched and calculated: epicondylar axis [2], AP axis [14], posterior condylar line and distal intersection point of the mechanical axis according to Stiehl [13] and the femoral condyles for the implant size of the femur.

Registration of Tibia. After fixing a tibial base plate (**Fig. 39-3**) to the medial proximal tibial facet, a locator is connected to the tibia and registration of the tibia is carried out. The following landmarks are palpated: proximal point of the mechanical axis of the tibia according to Yoshioka [15], the joint line, the lowest point of the tibial defect, medial and lateral malleolar point, and also three redundant reference points for tibial rotation [9].

Step 2: Axial Alignment of Instruments (Tracking)

In order to align the instruments to the calculated skeletal axes, the cut-controlling instruments must be fitted with a locator.

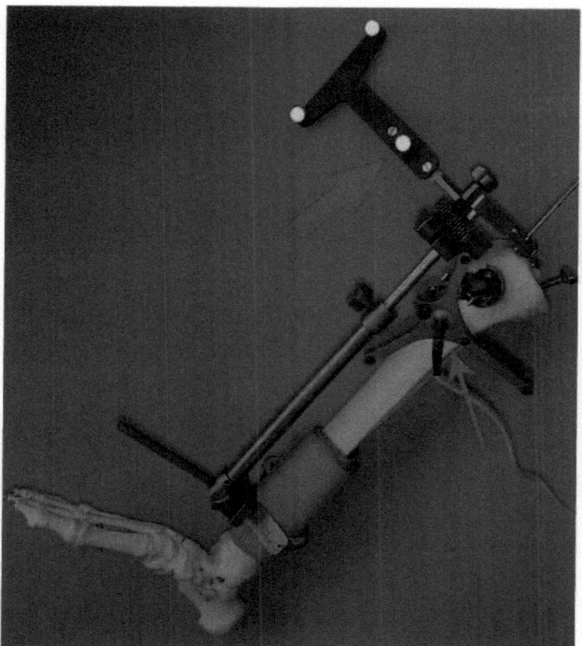

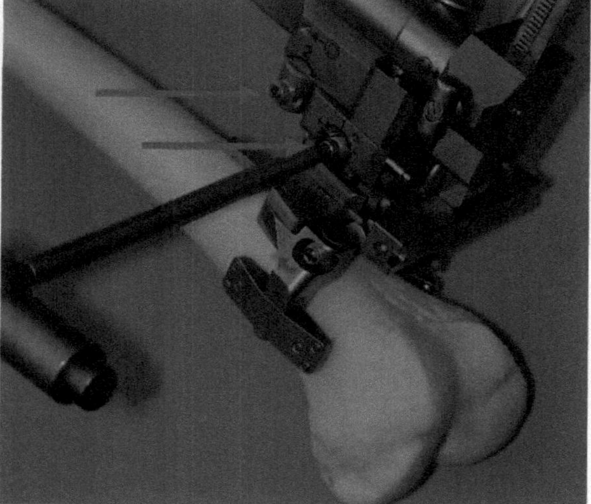

Fig. 39-4. The robot can be aligned to the calculated femoral axes in the frontal (varus/valgus) and the transversal (rotation) plane by using the adjustment screws indicated in the diagram (*arrows*). The angles are shown on the display

Fig. 39-3. Shows the construction of a modified alignment guide. The active locator (*small* arrow) is fixed to the bone and shows the bone geometry. A passive locator (*big* arrow) is mounted on the cutting block. This locator enables matching to the pre-calculated axes of the tibial geometry

Tibial Instrument Tracking. For resection of the tibia, a modified tibial alignment guide is first fixed to the leg and a passive locator fitted to the cutting block (see Fig. 39-3). The real-time position of the instrument in the space is displayed on the monitor and adjusted to the 3D represented skeletal axes. The dorsal slope of the cut and the resection height – measured from the articular plane or lowest point on the tibial plateau – can be individually set by the surgeon. After alignment of the cutting block, the osteotomy is carried out.

Tracking of the Mini-Robot on the Femur. After mounting the mini-robot on the femoral clamp, it is fitted with a passive locator. The monitor displays the real-time position of the robot to the mechanical axis in three planes. The robot can be moved to the calculated axial positions in the rotational and varus/valgus directions by using two adjustment screws (■ Fig. 39-4). The sagittal plane was already determined when the femoral clamp was fixed flush to the bone.

Step 3: Mode of Operation of the Mini-Robot

After correct alignment of the mini-robot on the axes, the cutting program is started, femoral sizing determined and a »one-in-five« cutting jig fitted (see Fig. 39-1).

In the case of a straightforward knee, without ligament deformations and without need for the ligament tensioner technique, the cutting sequence begins distal femoral, followed by ventral, dorsal and the chamfer cuts.

If the ligament tensioner is used (see Fig. 39-2), the tibial and dorsal femoral cuts are first carried out. After removal of all the dorsal osteophytes the ligament tensioner is inserted into the flexion gap with 90° flexion.

The objective is now to achieve equal ligament tension on both sides of about 100 Newton while maintaining a rectangular flexion gap (same mm measurement medially as laterally). If it is not possible to achieve a rectangular flexion gap at 100 Newton, then appropriate soft tissue release techniques must be performed on the ligaments.

The ligament tensioner is then inserted into extension. The distal cut of the femur has not yet been performed at this point. An accessory T-shaped device with a vertical and a horizontal arm is placed on the ligament tensioner (see Fig. 39-5). The objective is now to position both arms of the T parallel to the T of the robot with 100–150 Newton maintained both medially and laterally (■ Fig. 39-5). If the

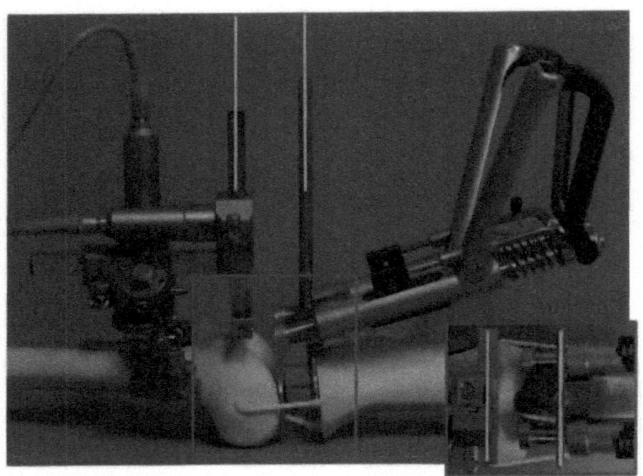

Fig. 39-5. The ligament tensioner is inserted into the extension gap. The inverse »T« on the ligament tensioner is placed parallel to the »T« of the robot, in order to achieve a fully extended and rectangular extension gap

vertical arms are parallel it means there is complete extension of the knee, if the horizontal arms are parallel it means the gap is rectangular. If the gap is not rectangular, appropriate soft tissue release must again be performed.

Since the distal femoral cut has not yet been carried out, there will be unequal mm values on the distance scale of the ligament tensioner. These mm values are now entered into the computer as »variable medial« and »variable lateral« (Fig. 39-6). The robot then guides the cutting

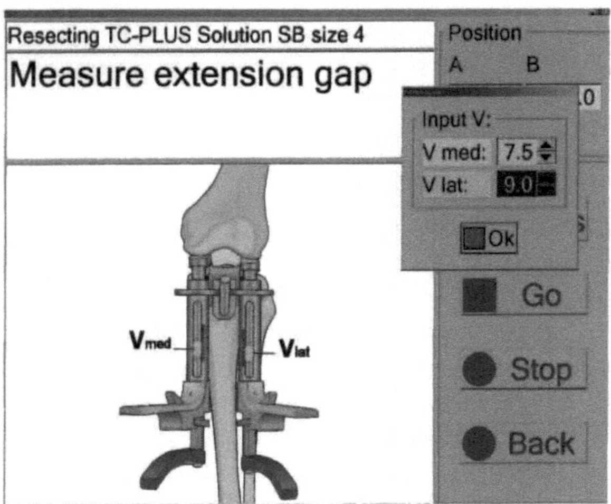

Fig. 39-6. After entering the distance: »Variable medial and Variable lateral« the robot moves the cutting block to the calculated position for the distal cut. This results in rectangular flexion and extension gaps of equal tension and equal size

template into the pre-calculated position and the distal cut can be performed.

The end result is an equally tensioned, rectangular flexion and extension gap together with perfect implant fit.

Clinical Data and Precision Measurement

In order to answer the question of how accurately the centre of the femoral head and the centre of the ankle joint can be determined with the Galileo navigation system, a specially designed intraoperative measuring device was set up [3] (Fig. 39-7). Analysis of the results gives the deviation of the calculated mechanical axis from the centre of the femoral head/centre of the ankle joint in mm. The deviation in angular degrees can be determined by comparing with the known femoral and tibial lengths obtained from navigated measurements. The measurement error of this device is 0.5° (max. 1.3, min. 0°) [11].

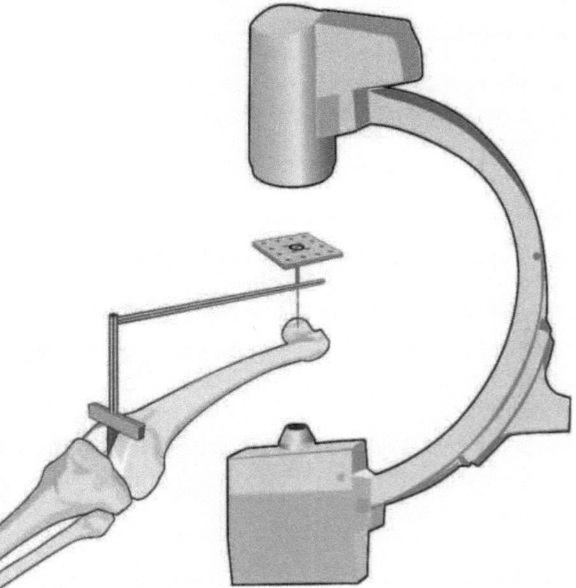

Fig. 39-7. According to the method, an extra-medullary alignment rod is mounted of the robot and positioned over the center of the knee joint. The proximal end of the rod over the hip joint is fitted with a marked plate. This plate has set into it a central metal ring for parallax-free projection and spheres in the form of a coordinate grid to correct for image distortion. An identical alignment on the tibial alignment guide is set up on the ankle joint. By using an image converter, it is thus possible to achieve parallax-free projection. The distortion effects can be corrected by mathematical methods

In order to assess the effects of this new instrumental technique on intraoperative and perioperative results, a comparison with conventional OP techniques was also carried out.

For this purpose basic information relating to 50 patients operated using the Galileo navigation system (TC-SB, Plus Endoprothetik AG) was compared with that of 50 patients operated using conventional techniques (LCS, DePuy Inc.).

Additionally, operation time for the first 100 navigated patients is shown against that for 100 conventionally implanted patients.

Results

Precision in measurement refers to the femoral and tibial mechanical axis in the frontal plane.

For 69 consecutive implantations, an average deviation of the femoral mechanical axis of 7.5 mm (max.: 25 mm, min.: 0 mm) was measured. In angular degrees this is a deviation of an average of 1° (max.: 3.5°, min.: 0°) from the ideal line.

Values at the upper ankle joint in 37 patients show an average deviation of 7.8 mm (max.: 18, min.: 0), corresponding to an average value in angular degrees of 1.2° (max.: 2.9°, min.: 0°). For the clinically more relevant determination of the centre of the femoral head and its axial deviation, a deviation of <1° was measured in 68.3% of patients and a maximum measurement error of 3.6° in 99.9% of all patients (■ Fig. 39-8).

The analysis of blood loss and blood requirements, length of hospitalization, range of motion (ROM) on dis-

■ Table 39-1

	Galileo	Conventional
Intraoperative blood loss [ml]	417	423
Required blood reserves [units]	1.3	1.4
Hemoglobin drop preoperative to the 10th postoperative day [mg/dl]	3.2	3.0
Median hospitalization postoperative [days]	15	15
ROM/extension deficit on discharge	91°/2°	89°/3°
Local/systemic complications	6/2	9/0

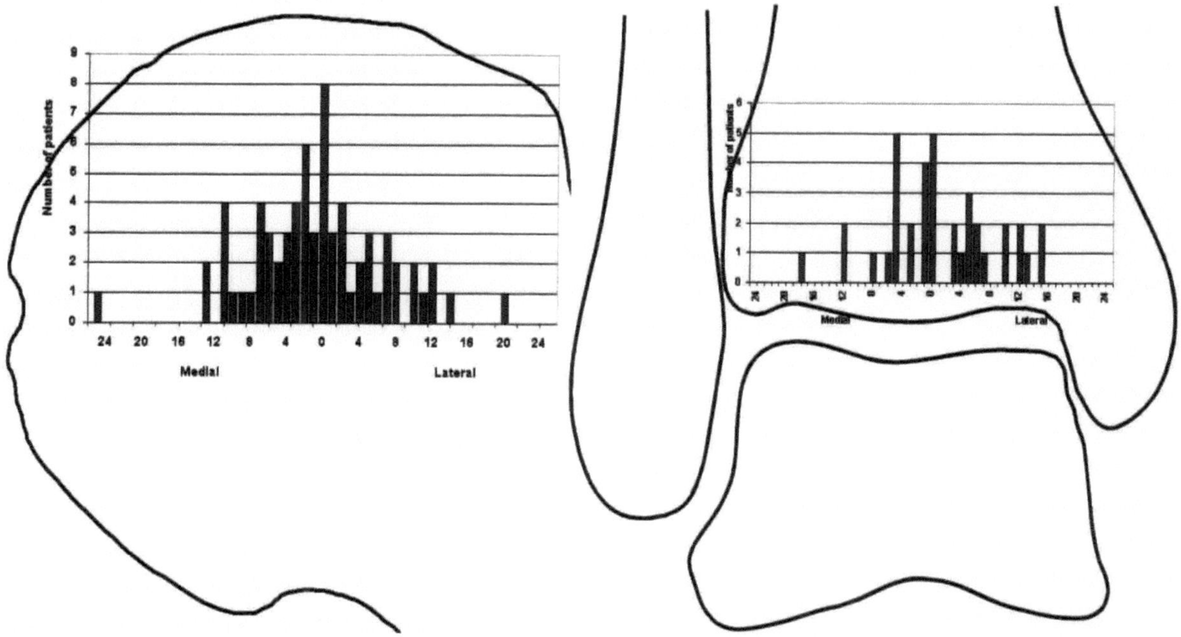

■ **Fig. 39-8.** The diagrams of the intraoperative measurement show the achieved accuracy in the determination of the femoral and tibial mechanical axes in the frontal plane. One can observe the Gauss-like distribution around the centre of the femoral head and the ankle joint

charge and complications does not show any significant differences between the two groups (■ Table 39-1). Comparing the length of operation time for navigated implants against conventional prostheses shows a difference of 36 min (137 vs. 99). However, account should be taken for the time incurred with the navigated system for the learning curve, development time, X-rays of the axes, as well as inquiries from interested visitors. A senior surgeon not involved with the development required an average time of 105 min (difference = + 6 min) for 17 operations.

There were thus no indications that modifying the implantation technique and the prolonged OP time affected the hospitalization phase.

Summary

The Galileo system is a practical, modern knee navigation system. The only preoperative examination required is a conventional radiograph. Expensive preoperative CT examination and planning steps are not required. By using an integrated autoclavable mini-robot in the system it is possible to achieve both highly precise bone resection of the femur and also ligament balancing. Ligament balancing is mainly achieved by it being possible to position the cutting guide in 0.5 mm steps in both cranial-caudal and ventral-dorsal direction. If a ligament tensioner is also integrated into the system, perfect balancing of the flexion and extension gaps can be achieved with correct axial alignment even with significant axial mal-alignments and pathologically deformed ligaments. Very high and reproducible accuracy is achieved when reconstructing the mechanical axis without any need to fix a marker pin to compensate for movements of the pelvis.

References

1. Anouchi YS, Whiteside LA, Kaiser AD, Milliano MT (1993) The effects of axial rotational alignment of the femoral component on knee stability and patellar tracking in total knee arthroplasty demonstrated specimen. Clin Orthop 287: 177
2. Berger RA, Rubash HE, Seel MJ, Thompson WH, Crossett LS (1993) Determining the rotational alignment of the femoral component in total knee arthroplasty using the epicondylar axis. Clin Orthop 286: 40–47
3. Broers H, Hemken H, Luhmann T, Ritschl P (2002) Photogrammetric calibration of a C-arm X-ray system as a verification tool for orthopaedic navigation systems. ISPRS Journal of Photogrammetry & Remote Sensing 56: 338–346
4. Berger RA, Crossett LS, Jacobs JJ, Rubash HE (1998) Malrotation causing patellofemoral complications after total knee arthroplasty. Clin Orthop 356: 144–153
5. Eckhoff DG, Metzger RG, Vandewalle MV (1995) Malrotation associated with implant alignment technique in total knee arthroplasty. Clin Orthop 321: 28–31
6. Farris PM, Ritter MA, Keating EM (1988) Sagittal plane positioning of the femoral component in total knee arthroplasty. J Arthroplasty 3: 355–358
7. Insall J, Easley M (2001) Surgical techniques and instrumentation in total knee arthroplasty. In: Insall J, Scott N (eds) Surgery of the knee, vol 2, 3rd edn. Churchill Livingstone, Philadelphia, pp 1553–1620
8. Jeffery RS, Morris RW, Denham RA (1991) Coronal alignment after total knee replacement. J Bone Joint Surg Br 73: 709–714
9. Milner CE, Soames RW (1998) A comparison of four in vivo methods of measuring tibial torsion. J Anat 193: 139–144
10. Olcot CW, Scott RD (1999) The Ranawat Award. Femoral component rotaing during total knee arthroplasty. Clin Orthop 367: 39–42
11. Ritschl P, Zettl R, Fuiko R (2002) Precision measurement of the navigated, reconstructed mechanical axis on implanting a total knee prosthesis. Description of method and results. Poster 2nd annual meeting of the International Society for Computer assisted Orthopaedic Surgery (CAOS), June 19–22, 2002, Santa Fe, USA
12. Ritter MA, Faris PM, Keating EM, Medino JB (1994) Postoperative alignment of total knee replacement. Its effect on survival. Clin Orthop 299: 153–156
13. Stiehl JB, Abbott BD (1995) Morphology of the transepicondylar axis and its application in primary and revision total knee arthroplasty. J Arthoplasty 10: 785–789
14. Whiteside LA, Arima J (1995) The anteroposterior axis for femoral rotational alignment in valgus total knee arthroplasty. Clin Orthop 321: 168–172
15. Yoshioka Y, Siu DW, Scudamore RA, Cooke TD (1989) Tibial anatomy and functional axes. J Orthop Res 7: 132–137

40 Clinical Experiences with the Surgetics System in TKA

U. Böhling, J. Scholz, R. Nassutt, H. Grundei

Introduction

Navigation has developed to an inherent part of orthopaedic surgery. Navigation technology seems to void the same fate compared with robotics as demonstrated in numerous successful practical experiences and scientific reports [4, 5, 7, 9]. In addition, navigation does not try to replace surgeons skills, but enhances intraoperative accuracy by delivering geometric data, thus keeping surgical control in the hand of the surgeon. Navigation tools differ considerably from conventional instruments such as capture blades and resection blocks because of its opto- and magnetic-electronics. However, one should keep in mind that classical tool still represent mechanical navigational instruments.

Electronic navigation has evolved rapidly in the past three years, such that one begins anticipating further fields of applications. This perspective increases the imminent conflict of technical possibilities and practical necessities. Close teamwork of surgeon and engineers is required for future software updates and to avoid a drift from serious technology into gadgets, a development recently observed with robotics. Operating room logistics such as sterile conditions, limited space, minimally invasive techniques, and time issues are challenging factors for navigation. These requirements may collide with implantation of an arthroplasty [2, 7].

Current political discussion and decreasing resources for health insurances are a further disadvantage for electronic equipment. An optimal cost-benefit equation is required for successful development of navigation in orthopaedics. Electronic navigation improves the reliability of reproduction, quality of prosthetic implantation, and digital documentation of the surgery. However, relatively increased capital investment has to be addressed. We, therefore, look for a future-oriented navigation concept and standard with a view to improving economics, ergonomics, practicality, and ease of use.

Navigation in the Operating Room

Navigation in the OR is considered to solve identical problems as noted in the fields of navy navigation, air traffic control, and automotive industry: assistance of detecting previously defined positions. Medical navigation consist of a computer, tracking system, monitor, and hand or foot switches. The tracking system includes stereo infrared cameras capable of identifying diodes in the operating field (◘ Fig. 40-1, *right*). Position and relation of instruments and bone landmarks can be identified during surgery. Digital information is transferred into graphical images with the help of customized software and implemented data from CT scans, fluoroscopy, MRI, and ultrasonography [7, 8, 11]. The surgeon is guided via visual information on the monitor in order to overlap pre- and intraoperative positions. The main advantage of navigation includes exact calculation and visualization of intraoperative geometries, which, so far, were not accessible for the surgeon. Best example is the mechanical axis of the leg, Mikulicz line, running from the femoral head center to the middle of the ankle joint. Preoperative and postoperative predictability of this line is often estimated utilizing conventional tools, but accuracy significantly improves function and long term outcome of total knee arthroplasty [1, 2, 4, 5, 10, 12]. Navigation allows for continuous control of numeric and graphic data during surgery. Today's orthopaedic navigation includes joint arthroplasty, pedicle screws intra-medullary nailing, and osteotomies [7, 8]. Further fields of application are neurosurgery, dental surgery and ENT.

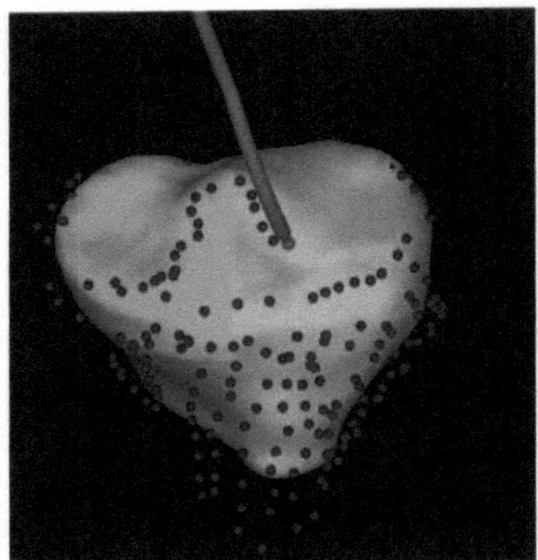

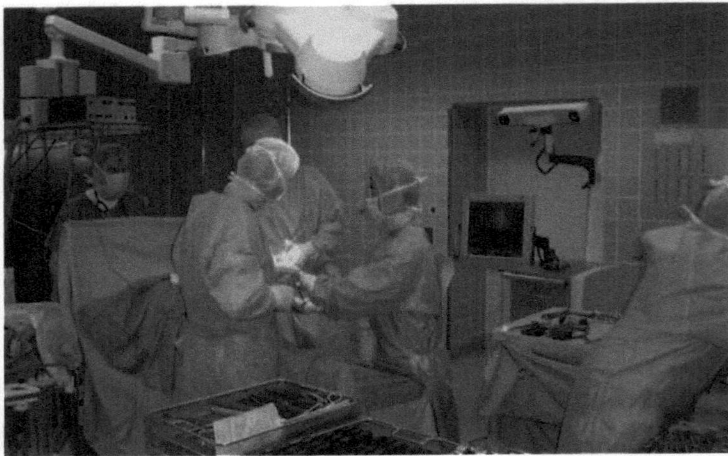

■ **Fig. 40-1.** Screen design during bone morphing procedure *(left)*. There is no information overflow, everything can be seen from the distance. The position of the Surgetics station is outside the operation field *(right)*

40

Navigation of Total Knee Arthroplasty

Standard instrumentation is based upon intra-medullary alignment allowing for precise preoperatively planned bone resections. So far resection guide were set utilizing bone pins and resection gauges. For navigation of the ESKA Knee system/Type RP (a mobile-bearing knee), this principle was transferred into the navigation system, except resection block setting is defined by navigation instead of intra-medullary rods. Six pins in total are required for all femoral and tibial cuts.

According to medical regulations both navigation tools and conventional instruments must be present at all times during surgery in order to allow for instant switching to manual methods, however, this has rarely been the case. This navigation requires one additional set of instruments with rigid bodies, fixing material, bone pins, and two listed tools that provide a smooth work-flow: quick drill clamp that takes all required drills and pins, which can be easily attached and detached without chuck key. Secondly, a ligament balancing pliers that is clamped into flexion and extension gaps, thus delivering visible data of ligament tension (see Figs. 40-3 and 40-4). The pliers has a link that adapts according to the local forces within the knee joint, this creates a non-quadrilateral space capable of measuring physiologic tension without enforcing symmetric gaps. The navigation system computes the relative position of performed resection planes delivering valuable information of individual ligament tension

Fixation of rigid bodies on instruments and bones are required for navigation. In order to avoid cable required for active light emitting diodes and possible damage, all reference markers are equipped with reflectors. Four rigid bodies are required: femur (F), tibia (T), pointer (P), and universal pin guide (G) (■ Fig. 40-2, *right*). There is no marker necessary on the pelvis or the foot. Alteration of rigid bodies is not necessary during surgery. All rigid bodies are equipped with snapped-on reflectors, which have a flat disc in comparison to usually spherical shapes. The advantage of a flat disc includes simplified intraoperative cleaning and reduced costs in a single used set of 20 reflectors.

Operative Procedure

The used Surgetics navigation is straight forward providing the surgeon with all information required without gimmicks and consists of four steps:

Installing the Equipment

Installation includes mounting of two patient's rigid bodies and camera positioning. Both steps are guided on the screen by illustrations and text messages.

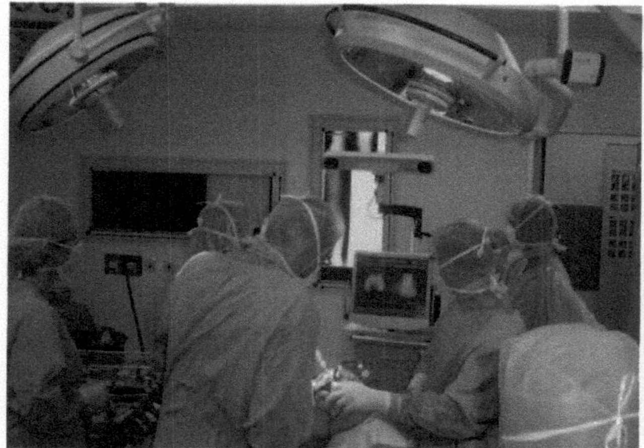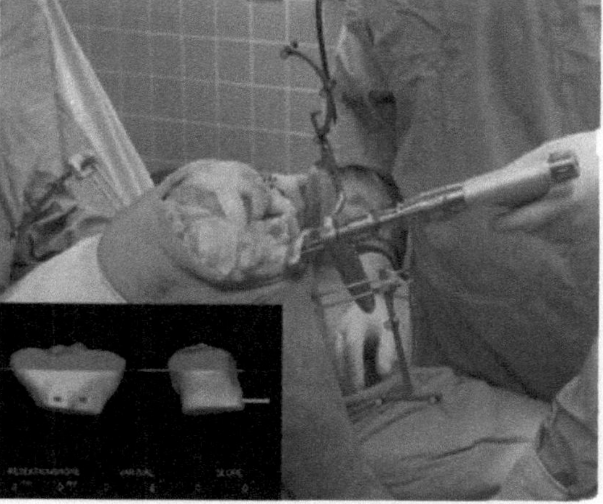

Fig. 40-2. Typical navigation arrangement in the OR *(left)*. The surgeon places the universal guide onto the bone surface and sets the pin *(right)*. With the drilling machine in one hand and the guide in the other the tools are well balanced and easy to place correctly into the »green area«

Feeding of Data

All anatomical data collection is performed online without need of preoperatively collected images or information. This includes anatomical landmarks on tibia and femur, which are identified with a pointer or kinematic motion of a joint. With the new bone morphing procedure the surgeon creates a three-dimensional model of femur and tibia by digitizing the bone surface with the pointer tip.

Planning

On basis of the calculated anatomy, the system suggests both size and position of the implants considering ideal alignment, minimal bone resections, external femoral component rotation and slight flexion. If desired, the surgeon can alter or adapt all parameters. The result of this procedure determines all navigational parameters at the same time.

Navigation

During navigation the position of the universal guide tool is guided by graphic and numeric information on the monitor (see Fig. 40-2). After positioning a pair of pins the resection blocks are attached and the resection is per-

formed. Three pin pairs are navigated for tibial, horizontal femoral and four remaining femoral resection planes.

The surgeon can evaluate ligament tension in both extension and flexion after tibial resection. In doing so graphical and numerical information of the mechanical axis and paralleled resection planes are provided on the monitor (**Fig. 40-3**). Finally the patient's and prosthetic parameters are added via the touch screen. A navigation report (readable by most PC systems) includes all patient's parameters and is copied onto a CD-ROM. This allows a reconstruction of the operation if desired.

Handling Comfort

The monitors play an important role as a link between surgeon and navigation system and can be compared with arthroscopical techniques. However, the orthopaedic surgeon has the ability to easily switch between navigation monitor view and site. The Surgetics monitors are equipped with a touch screen surface allowing finger tip handling of active screen windows. In general, the monitor needs a sterile cover when entering the operating field, which reduces the visual quality. The Surgetics system is designed for a distance of 2 to 3 meters and is placed outside the sterile field. Size, contrast, and geometric distorsion are optimized due to TFT technology, thus avoiding quick tiring and confusion of the surgeon. A straight

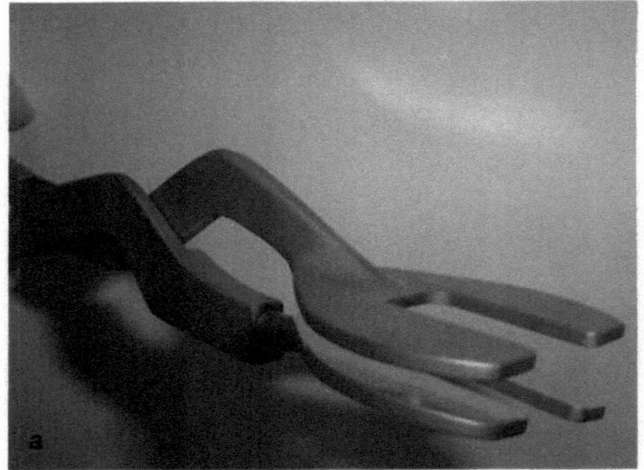

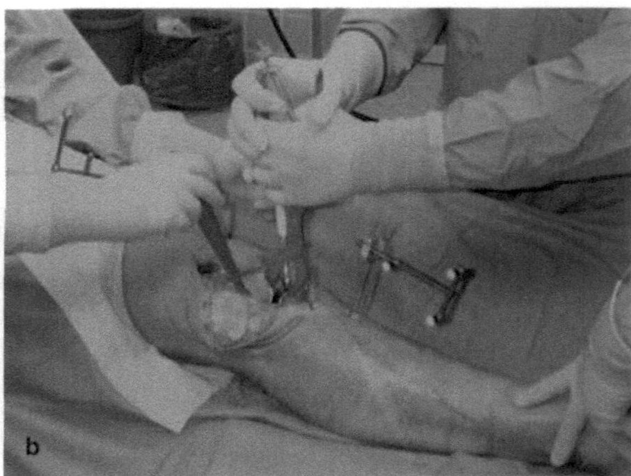

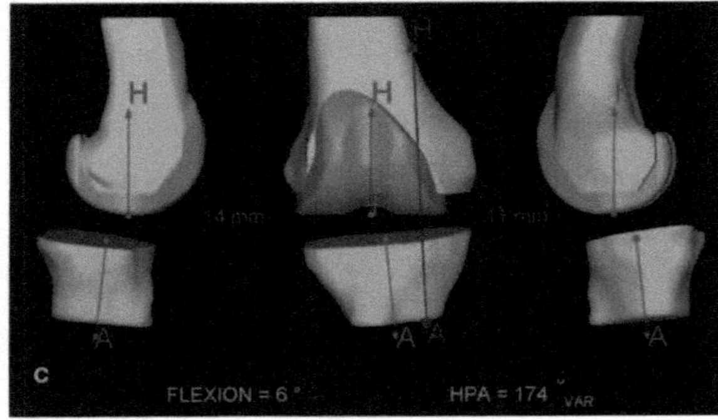

Fig. 40-3a-c. Due to an additional hinge joint the balancing pliers allow to put tension on the knee ligaments without forcing it into parallel position (**a**). The pliers are inserted in extended (**b**) or flexed position and the medial/lateral ligament condition is displayed on the screen (**c**)

forward graphic user interface is supported by short text messages and guides the surgeon through software settings, patients demographics, prosthetic selection, and navigation of bone resections. The manual is basically included on the screen. During TKA implantation the screen can be left alone without touching it due to foot switches or manual handling by non-scrubbed personnel.

Discussion

Future success and continued existence of navigation technology depend on acceptance and compatibility within the OR. Little to no changes of routine follow-up will cause a positive attitude to this technology. Education of staff and easy to handle additional steps should cause little disturbances. Economics is another important factor. Independent of clinical setup (type of health insurance, orthopaedics, or trauma), increased operating time influences capacity and cost effectiveness. Navigation

should have no negative implication. This leads to five postulations for successful navigation: navigation must be quick, universal, easy to handle, economic, thus providing increased quality. The latest generation Surgetics navigation system fulfills these requirements as demonstrated in practical OR experiences.

Navigation seriously revolutionizes operating methods in orthopaedic surgery. And we believe that not only in Europe navigation will establish very quickly in many clinics as a standard technology. Due to additional information the surgeon can enhance his or her effectiveness and skills. The quality and consistency of surgical results is significantly improved, also in our hospital. In addition Navigation reduces invasiveness and allows to work on highly deformed bone structures without loosing any precision. Bone loss is reduced to a minimum (**Fig. 40-4**).

The described Surgetics concept demonstrates adaptation of routine surgery and navigation without decreasing its benefit. Quite the contrary, improvement of

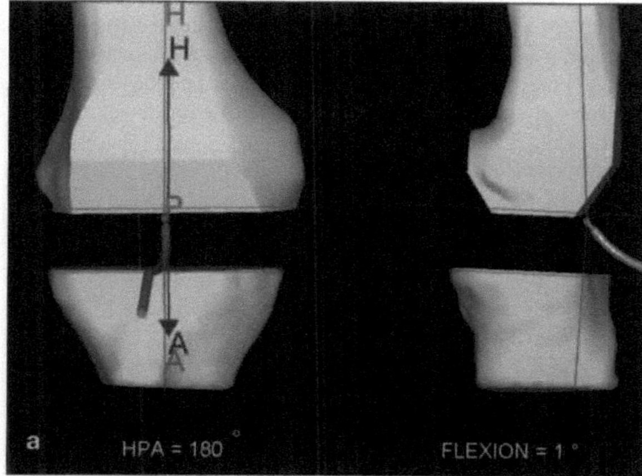

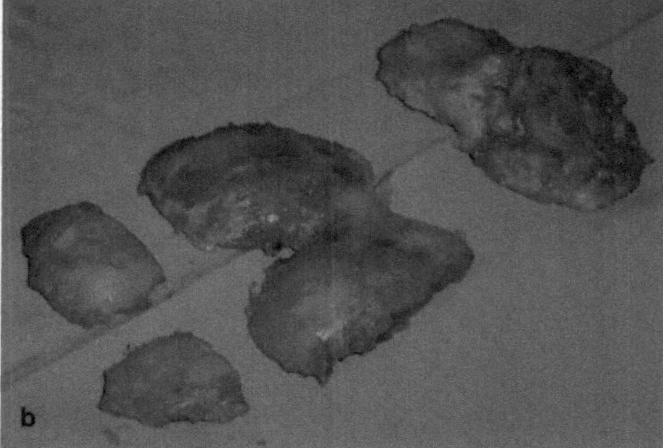

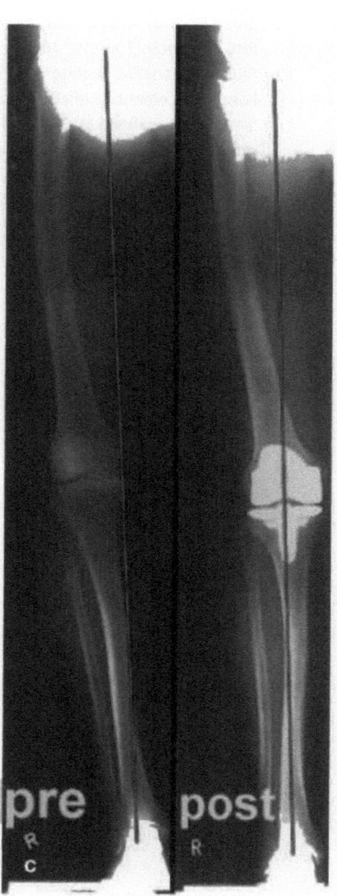

■ **Fig. 40-4a-c.** After resections have been performed the actual situation including the orientation of the leg axis is displayed (**a**). The resected bone is minimized due to planning the smallest implant height (**b**). Pre- and postoperative X-rays prove the perfect geometric result (**c**)

user-friendly handling and reduction to a convenient amount of information the surgical team can profit from the assistance of navigation without loosing focus. The Surgetics system is future-oriented, is open for further data acquisition via hospital networks and encourages future applications for the user. The Surgetics system including the presented application is clinically proven and will be transferred to hip surgery focusing on as minimal and vital information as possible needed by the surgeon. This improves the quality and expenditure-benefit relation of navigation.

References

1. Bargren JH, Blaha JD, Freeman MA (1983) Alignment in total knee arthroplasty. Correlated biomechanical and clinical observations. Clin Orthop 173:178–183

2. Cartellieri M, Kremser J, Vorbeck F (2001) Comparison of different 3D navigation systems by a clinical »user«. Eur Arch Otorhinolaryngol 258: 38–41

3. Insall JN, Binazzi R, Soudry M (1985) Total knee arthroplasty. Clin Orthop 192:13–22

4. Jenny JY, Boeri C (2001) Navigated implantation of total knee endoprostheses–a comparative study with conventional instrumentation. Z Orthop Ihre Grenzgeb 139:117–119

5. Konermann W, Saur MA (2003) Postoperatives Alignment von konventionell und navigiert implantierten Knietotalendoprothesen. In: Konermann W, Haaker R (eds) Navigation und Robotic in der Gelenk- und Wirbelsäulenchirurgie. Springer, Berlin Heidelberg New York Tokyo

6. Krugluger J, Steinwenter A, Knahr K 81998) Uncemented Miller-Galante total knee replacement. The influence of alignment on clinical and radiological outcome in a 5 to 8-year follow-up. Int Orthop 22:230–233

7. Lavallee S, Bainville E, Bricault I (2000) An overview of computer-integrated surgery and therapy. Crit Rev Diagn Imaging 41:157–236

8. Merloz P, Tonetti J, Cinquin P (1998) Computer-assisted surgery: automated screw placement in the vertebral pedicle. Chirurgie 123: 482–490

9. Miehlke RK, Clemens U, Jens JH (2001) Navigation in knee endoprosthesis implantation–preliminary experiences and prospective com-

parative study with conventional implantation technique. Z Orthop Ihre Grenzgeb 139: 109–116

10. Ritter MA, Faris PM, Keating EM (1994) Postoperative alignment of total knee replacement. Its effect on survival. Clin Orthop 299: 153–156

11. Simon DA, Lavallee S (1998) Medical imaging and registration in computer assisted surgery. Clin Orthop 354: 17–27

12. Smith JL, Tullos HS, Davidson JP (1989) Alignment of total knee arthroplasty. J Arthroplasty 4 [Suppl]: S55–61

13. Stindel E, Briard JL, Merloz P et al. (2002) Bone morphing: 3D morphological data for total knee arthroplasty. Comput Aided Surg 7: 156–168

14. Wasielewski RC, Galante JO, Leighty RM et al. (1994) Wear patterns on retrieved polyethylene tibial inserts and their relationship to technical considerations during total knee arthroplasty. Clin Orthop 299: 31–43

41 Navigation in TKA with the *Navitrack* System

T. Mattes, W. Puhl

Introduction

Navigation systems are gaining popularity in total knee arthroplasty (TKA). These systems should improve the exactness of implant positioning [5]. A reduction of aseptic loosening and better functional results are expected [3, 4, 10].

Based on the established CT-based application of the Navitrack system (Fa. Centerpulse, Winterthur, Switzerland; Orthosoft Inc., Montreal, Canada) for pedicle instrumentation of the lumbar and thoracic spine, instruments and software were developed for a CT-based Navitrack application for use in TKA. The 3D CT data allow a virtual planning and well-controlled surgery. On the other hand the procedure of CT-based navigation is expensive and complex related to time-consuming preoperative data management. Clinical experience has demonstrated that this complex system is necessary only in special indications, e.g. severe posttraumatic or congenital deformities. Therefore a CT-free application for routine cases was integrated in the Navitrack platform. We have used the CT-based application since January 2000, the CT-free since January 2002 for Implantation of the Natural Knee II (Fa. Centerpulse, Winterthur, Switzerland), since October 2002 additional form implantation of the Innex (Fa. Centerpulse, Winterthur, Switzerland) endoprostheses.

System Components

System components of the Navitrack system include a UNIX workstation (O2 Workstation, Fa. Silicon Graphics, Mountain View/USA), a high-resolution monitor, and special surgical instruments with passive optolectronic or electromagnetic markers. The computer realization of surgical tools and anatomic objects follows the principle of dynamic referencing (tracking). A special quality of the Navitrack system is the possibility of choice between an optoelectronic tracking system (Polaris, Fa. Northern Digital Inc., Waterloo/Canada) – or a magnetic tracking system (Motion Star, Fa. Ascension Corp., Burlington, USA) (magnetic only CT-based). To operate the system from the sterile area, a footswitch and a draped remote control is used.

Virtual Model

The principle difference between the applications is the origin of the virtual model, which is used for navigated cutting guide positioning. While in the CT-based version, as the name tells, the model is reconstructed from preoperative CT scan, In the CT-free application all data are collected intraoperatively using kinematic analysis or digitizing points on the patient. The positioning of the cutting guides and bone resection is the same in both applications, using the same adapted surgical instruments.

CT-Based Application

Besides the roentgenograms (a.p., sagittal and full-length standing roentgenograms) used for indication, a CT scan of the whole leg – from the femoral head to the upper level of the talus – is performed in spiral technique (Somatom 4Plus, Fa. Siemens, Erlangen, Germany). Following parameters are used for CT scan – slice thickness 3 mm in the femoral head (spacing 4.5 mm/increment 5 mm), 2 mm in the knee area (spacing 2 mm/increment 2 mm) and 3 mm in the ankle joint (spacing 3 mm/increment 4 mm). Within the femoral and tibial shaft, the slice thickness is 100 mm (spacing 20 mm/increment 40 mm).

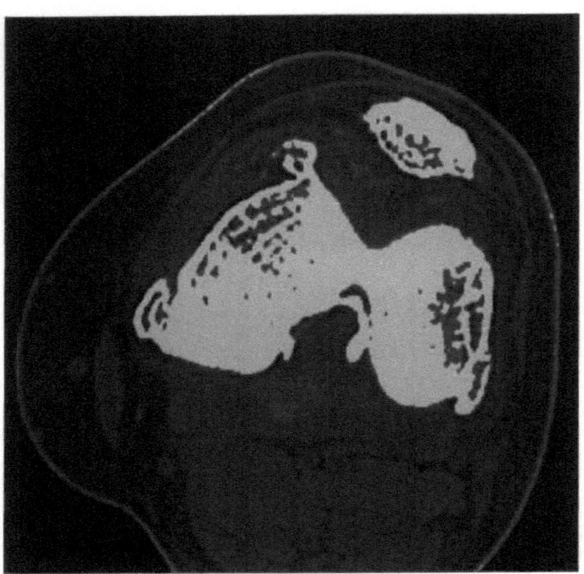

◼ Fig. 41-1. CT data preparation – segmentation CT slide epicondylar region

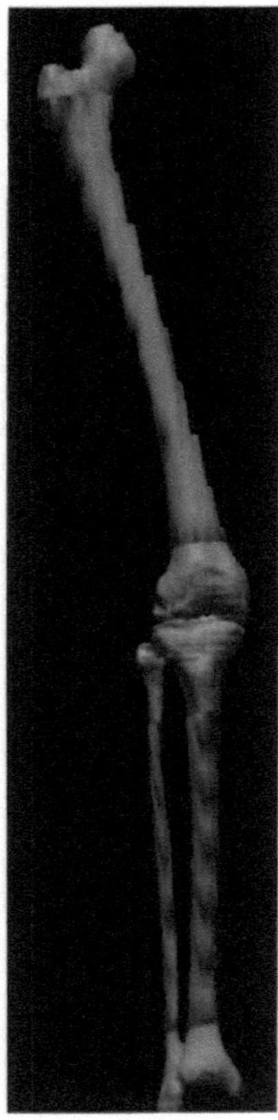

◼ Fig. 41-2. Reconstructed virtual 3D surface model CT-based application

The data from the CT scan are transferred in the workstation as DICOM files using CD-Rom, MOD or direct network transfer. The preparation of the CT data is done in the planning station (O2 Workstation) in 4 steps.

First a semiautomatic segmentation is done by separating bone structure by grayscale thresholding – manual segmentation in some slides, especially in the joint line is necessary (◼ Fig. 41-1). Changes of normal anatomy, like big osteophytes, bone defects or artifacts in the CT scan make this step time-consuming. The segmentation always leads to a compromise between real bone structure and segmented bone structure. Therefore, in our opinion the surgeon should do the CT preparation to know the difference between real and segmented data. If this is not possible at least the surgeon must be informed about the changes and manipulation of the data.

Using the segmented data the software calculates a 3D model by automatic rendering of a 3D volume model (voxels; ◼ Fig. 41.2). In our experience the quality of the 3D model and also the time needed for segmentation correlates with the quality of the original CT data. Therefore, a compromise must be found between the contrast of the images and the radiation energy.

In the 3D model 5, better 7 landmarks must be defined for each bone/femur and tibia/fibula; ◼ Fig. 41-3). These landmarks (matching points) are probed during intra-operative registration on the patients bone surface.

The last step of the preoperative procedure is the definition of the leg axis and planning of implant positions and size. Additional lines and axis, like the »Whitesideline« or the epicondylar axis can be drawn as 3D lines in the model.

During the described clinical trial the planning module of the software is in a beta phase and not available in routine used systems.

Intraoperative Axis Definition CT-free Application

Apart from the roentgenograms for indication, the CT-free application needs no further preoperative image data. All relevant data for generating an axis model and implant sizing are collected intraoperatively.

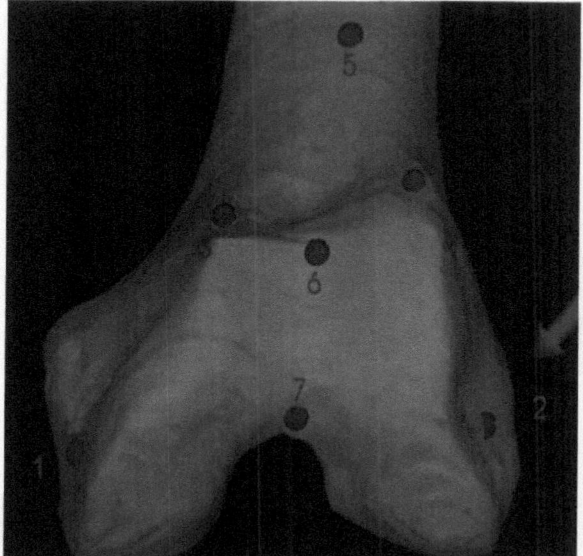

Fig. 41-3. Monitor view femoral registration points (matching points)

Therefore, it is possible to focus on very few points in special areas, depending on surgery technique and 3D imagination of the surgeon, e.g. for the natural knee the anterior femoral cortex to prevent anterior notching, the posterior condyles and a few points on the highest and lowest level of the tibial joint line. For better visualization the size and color of the mosaic points are variable.

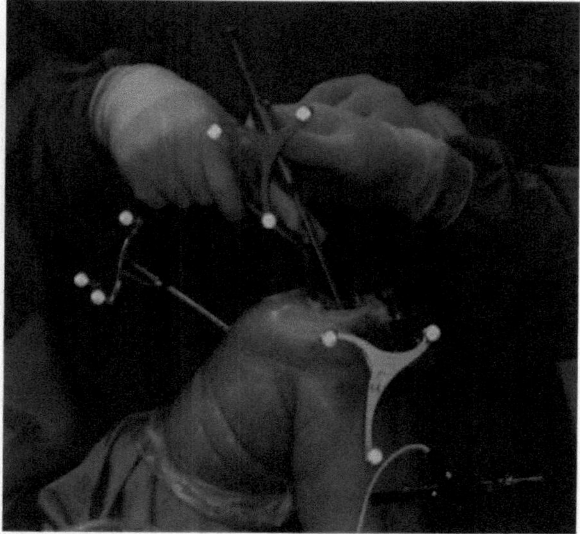

Fig. 41-4. Intraoperative situs probing for mosaic model tibial joint line

The hip center results out of kinematic analysis, the knee center and ankle center and also axis definition for femoral rotation are determined digitizing landmarks on the tibia, fibula and femur. The axis points in the knee are mainly comparable with the entrance points of intra-medullary rods in conventional technique. The middle of the ankle joint is calculated by digitizing the malleoli transcutaneously. For tibial rotation alignment, the medial third of the tibial tuberosity and tibial insertion of the PCL are digitized. For the femoral rotation of the natural knee we probe the posterior condyles, the epicondylar line or »Whitesideline«, which is similiar for the Innex knee. After complete probing, the axis model is shown on the system monitor.

With a special instrument, the mosaic pointer, surface points in the knee joint are digitized (**Fig. 41-4). These mosaic points (white points in **Fig. 41-5) give a virtual image of the patient's anatomy, exactly related to the pre-operatively determined axis.

By digitizing infinite surface points, theoretically a nearly 1:1 image of the real anatomy is possible. In contrast to the CT model, the mosaic model does not accurately determine the bone surface as in some regions, the carti-lage surface is probed. However, these models are mainly necessary for implant sizing and intraoperative validation.

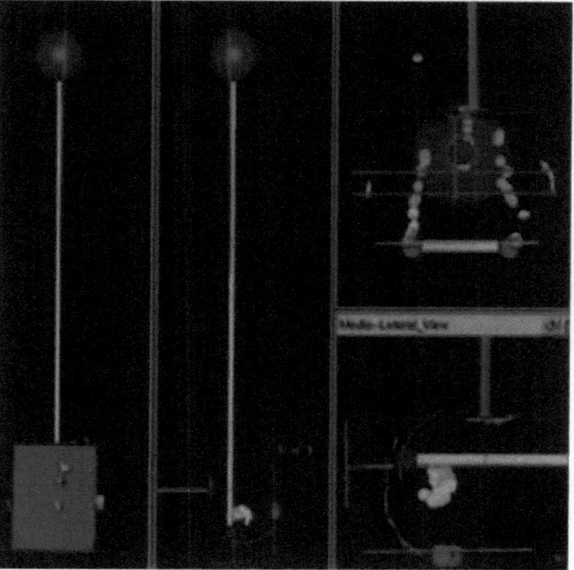

Fig. 41-5. Monitor view CT-free application – femoral alignment and sizing

A validation point, for control of the system, is digitized on the medial tibial tuberosity and the medical femoral epocondyle. The bone is there marked with the electro coagulation. By probing these points with the pointer at any point of surgery the conformity of the virtual model and the real anatomy can be checked. Problems with loosening of registration, e.g. because of movement of the rigid bodies (see below) can be detected.

OP Technique

We use the same surgery technique for navigated and conventional TKA.

Additional steps are fixation of a dynamic reference base (DRB), so-called »rigid bodies«, one on the femur and one on the tibia. The femoral DRB is attached on the bone with a bicortical screw within the normal approach, the fixation of the tibial DRB needs an additional small incision in the middle of the tibia. Using the optoelectronic tracking system, the position of the DRBs must be chosen in the line of sight of the camera and also in adequate distance from the joint line, preventing an interference with the markers from the instruments. On the tibial side, one must be also considered that the DRB is far enough below from the impactor and the tibial stem. We use a tourniquet and an anterior approach. A prolongation of the surgery caused by the calibration can be avoided by doing the tool calibration (pointer, mosaic pointer, universal positioning block – UPB) by the first assistant while the surgeon does the initial exposure. The pointer and the mosaic pointer are calibrated with an automatic calibration tool. The UPB is calibrated by probing drillholes on its surface.

A validation of the calibration must be done, and if the internal calculation of the accuracy is poor, a recalibration is necessary. A visual validation – pointer vs. UPB – is recommend checking the result on the system monitor. For CT-based navigation, bone registration is necessary. Therefore, the 5 (or 7) surface points (matching points), determined on the virtual model (see Fig. 41-3), must be probed with the pointer. For CT-free, the kinematic and probing of the landmarks and generating of the mosaic model must be done.

After successful registration a validation based on the clinical aspect is mandatory. It is easy to perform probing

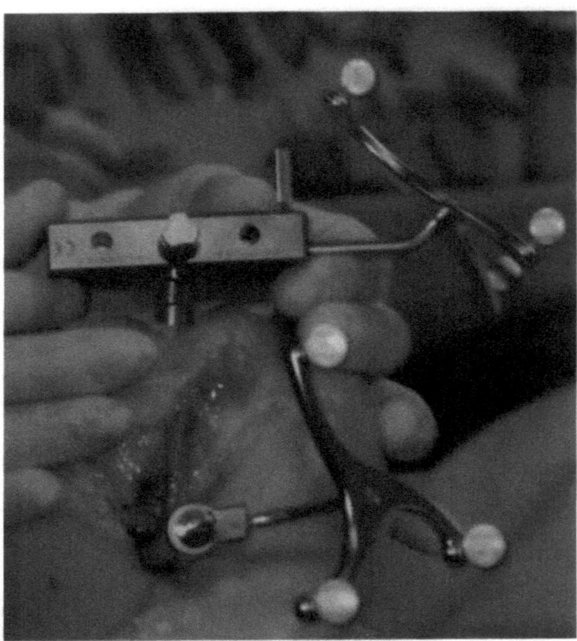

◘ Fig. 41-6. Femoral alignment with UPB fixed on polyaxial screw (monitor view see Figs. 41.5 and 41.7)

points on the joint line, the epicondyles or the tibial tubercle and check the position of the pointer in the anatomy with that shown on the system monitor. If validation is good navigated positioning can start. Depending on the preferred surgery technique (tibia first or femur first) a polyaxial screw is fixed on the proximal tibia or in the distal femur first. Soft tissue balancing may be done before making cuts and in some cases is mandatory. The following steps show the technique for the natural knee II. Using other implants, the sequence of the steps and the monitor views may differ according to the philosophy of the system.

Attaching the UPB on the polyaxial screw (◘ Fig. 41-6) a three-dimensional positioning of the virtual cuts based on the axis-/mosaic model or 3D bone model is possible. Additionally, the system gives numeric information for the ankle of the mechanical axis, posterior slope and component rotation.

The determination of the femoral implant size results in the lateral view portrayal of the posterior condylar cuts (◘ Fig. 41-7, see also Fig. 41-5) The pointer can be used for validation of the correct anterior level.

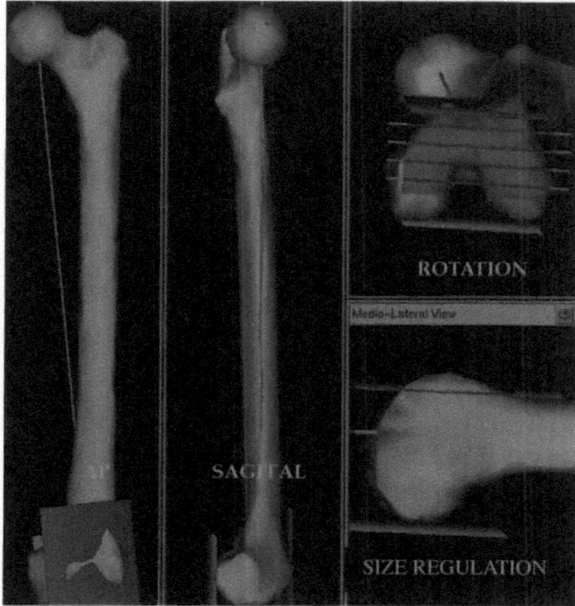

◘ Fig. 41-7. Monitor view CT-based application – femoral alignment and sizing

The conventional cutting guide for the posterior condylar resection is attached, the resection level for a standard resection will be adjusted, and the UPB will be removed allowing the bone resection to be done using the oscillating saw. Bringing up the UPB on the resection plane allows a validation and if necessary (e.g. deviation of the saw in sclerotic bone) a correction can be done. As mentioned before every final cut, a probing of the validation point makes sense to validate the registration and determine possible errors, like movement of the DRBs. If the distal cut and validation gives no error the femoral rotational alignment and final sizing is done with the UPB on the distal cut, respecting the level of the anterior cortex. In the correct position again, two pins are fixed over the UPB. Then the UPB can be removed and the conventional drill guide can be attached to the pins and the femoral holes can be drilled. Over the holes the conventional cutting guide for the a.p., posterior and oblique cuts brought in and bone resection again is done with the oscillating saw. NK II specific grooving is done conventionally with the chisel.

In the CT-free application all important angles are shown in the monitor, in the CT-based application the angles are only given in the prototype of the planning module. On the tibial site the alignment is based on the a.p.- and sagittal axis. The posterior slope depends on the implant and the patient's »natural slope«. The resection level can be adjusted in millimeter steps screwing down the UPB. The positioning again is done by attaching the UPB on the polyaxial screw. In the final position pins are brought in over the UPB. Afterwards the UPB and the polyaxial screw must be removed and the conventional tibial cutting guide is attached to the pins. Bone resection is done with the oscillating saw. For validation and controlled correction of cutting errors, the same steps as shown in the femur are possible.

Total limb alignment based on the performed cuts, and can be controlled with the UPB in the gap for the CT-based version. In the CT-free application the angles are calculated from the dynamic system and in real time. The trial implants are then applied. A navigated supported soft tissue balancing is now possible using the deviation angles under varus and valgus stress. Also a range of motion analysis and documentation is possible. For the Innex there is the possibility to navigate only the bone cuts, but one also may use a special software version with preliminary integration of soft tissue balancing. After this conventional sizing and tibia preparation (drilling and impacting) must be done.

The preparation of the patella is conventional. Final implantation is done with cement in all cases. After hardening of the cement a final control is be done with the navigation system and the data of final axis, maximal extension and flexion are stored for documentation.

Clinical Trial

Material und Method

Patients

In a first clinical trial with the CT-based application, we performed 31 surgeries (12 male, 19 female) in 2000. From March 2002 to October 2002 we performed 23 surgeries (9 male, 14 female) with the CT-free version. The indication for TKA was in all cases primary or posttraumatic osteoarthritis.

The mean patient age at time of surgery was in the CT-based group 69,8 (49–81); in the CT-free 67 (54–86). The mean body-mass index was 28,8 kg/m^2 in CT based group; 29,7 in the CT-free.

Surgery time, time for preoperative data treatment (CT-based), preoperative leg axis, post-operative leg axis and complications has been recorded. Angles measured has been done according to the knee society evaluation system [2]. In the CT-based group the measurements are related to the anatomical axis AP and sagittal in short roentgenograms of the knee, in the CT-free group on full-length standing roentgenograms a.p. For the CT-based group the alignment score [7] has been calculated. Maximum points, means perfect component position, result in a score of 100. A precise implant position in the CT-based surgeries was not possible in this first clinical trial, because there was no implementation of the preoperative planning module or an intraoperative angle measurement in the system.

Results

In both clinical trials the system was safe and reliable. The intraoperative handling was problem-free for the computer-experienced surgeon and other OR staff after instruction. The preoperative time in the CT-based group and surgery time in both application could be reduced substantially. The mean surgery time was in the CT-based trial 108 min (min. 85 min – max. 130 min), in the CT-free 107 min (min. 85 min – max. 154 min). A learning curve was realized in both applications. Time for preoperative data reconstruction could be reduced from initial 180 min to about 45 min per case. Problems still exists in patients where there are implants in the scanned regions (e.g. THR or TKA of opposite side) leading artifacts in the CT data. A qualitative sufficient segmentation and 3-D model was even possible in these cases.

The mean alignment score in the CT-based group was 80 (SD 11.2). Worst individual position was with 18 points in mean (SD 5.24) for femoral component alignment a.p. (maximum possible 25).

In the CT-free group, deviation from the ideal mechanical axis was in mean 1.39° (SD 1.01°). The maximum deviation was 3.5° of varus.

Three patients had superficial wound healing problems while two patients required manipulation. One patient had a cardiac arrhythmia while three patients required treatment for urinary tract infection with antibiotics.

Discussion

In a first clinical trial of the Navitrack system we could show that computer-navigated component positioning in TKA is possible with this system either based on preoperative CT data or based on intraoperative analysis of leg axis and geometry.

For both applications the results are preliminary, as they are not out of a controlled, prospective randomized study. In addition, the CT-based version lacked preoperative planning and an intraoperative measurement tool. For CT-free, the results are promising, even if some of them are out of the alpha testing of the system and all of them are within the learning curve of the system. There where no minor problems in the CT-free surgeries from the beginning of the trial. Experiences out of the CT-based application from the surgeon and the engineer led to a faster developing process and an elaborated software from the beginning of this project.

A learning curve must be respected for both procedures, as seen by other groups using navigation systems [5]. In our experience the learning curve is easier in the CT-free application. The reason is the deletion of the more complex procedure for the CT based, especially the preoperative CT data preparation. Although in these steps, a tremendous learning curve could be seen, the main challenge for evolution for the CT-based navigation would be simpler and faster CT data segmentation and a better planning tool. We still require 30 to 40 min for preoperative planning.

Intraoperative creation of the axis and mosaic in CT-free navigation is fast and easy to perform. We found that after a few surgeries the tendency was to reduce the mosaic points to a minimum. Mosaic points are utilized only to get a more 3D imagination of the anatomy, and too many points may be more confusing.

Based on the experiences and the long process of developing the CT-based version, we introduced a new concept for development and training of the CT-free version. Both surgeons and engineers participated in cadaver studies to understand specific needs of the system. Inexperienced surgeons must participate in the training before venturing into the operating room.

In the majority of CT-based cases a good post-operative limb alignment was achieved. The alignment index [7] is comparable to results from conventional surgeries. The main effort in clinical trial of the CT-based software was the feasibility and accuracy of segmentation and registration. Reasons for minor aberration are the missing planning tool and intraoperative angle measurement in the Navitrack software for CT-based TKA. Another deficiency seems to be the femoral registration. In contrast to the tibial registration (tibial-proximal tibia and ankle joint) the allocation of the points is closer in the femur in relation to the femur length. A combination of CT-based surface matching combined with kinematic determination of hip center may improve this problem in future.

For the complex and time-consuming CT-based navigation, we are unable to confirm the accuracy of the system. Essential studies to demonstrate this must be done after release of the planning- and measuring software, which is in development at the moment.

However, even with the existing software there is the tendency to benefit in severe posttraumatic or congenital deformities especially from CT-based navigation. We found the preoperative 3D model to be helpful as we are able to measure and define limb axis, limb torsion and rotational deviations or location and expansion of bone defects to plan exact implant positioning and size. With bone defects, this information can be invaluable to select bone transplants or wedges in the reconstruction. In these special cases the higher expense (technical, time and money) seems to be justifiable.

A clear definition of indications for CT-based (hereafter also MRI based?) TKA navigation must be determined from the experiences in centers with complex cases.

For »standard cases« with normal or only less axis deviation or bone defects the benefit of 3D preoperative planning seems to be marginal. Conventional 2D planning gives enough information for implant choice. The goal of CT-free navigation in these cases is a more precise positioning of cutting guides than can be done with conventional intra- or extra-medullary rods [8, 9].

Already with the alpha 1 software version for CT-free TKA navigation we could show that a precise implant positioning is possible with the Navitrack system with low expense.

The easy for registering the intraoperative mosaic model enables an adaptation of the system to different surgical techniques. Probing existing TKAs with the mosaic technique for sure will be helpful in TKA replacements after implementation of special fixation devices and instruments in the system. Because of image artifacts CT-based navigation is impossible with this indication.

For further analysis and development in the alpha phase of the CT-free software, detailed documentation (intraoperative fluoroscopy control, video documentation, screenshot documentation) was done. The analysis detected several reasons for minor deviation of ideal position. There may be problems intrinsic to the surgical technique or conventional instrumentation utilized. Additional problems may arise from bone cuts made on dense sclerotic bone or from areas where the bone is too soft. The implant companies must manufacture and adapt the instruments to the high standard of precision of the navigation system. Manufacturing tolerances for the instrument must decrease.

The ability of the Navitrack system to use different tracking systems is not as important in TKA. None the less, an advantage of the magnetic system is that the DRBs and instruments can be positioned without respect of visibility of the camera and the instrument dimension can be reduced. A disadvantage, however, is the ability of an ferromagnetic object to interfere with the tracking system. The principle advantage of magnetic tracking may be realized with minimally invasive surgery.

Further analyses are necessary for kinematic determination of axis points, like the hip center, to pinpoint indications and contraindications (e.g. dysplastic hips with deformity of femoral head) for CT(image)-free navigation.

A main factor for good results in TKA, beside the correct alignment, are well-balanced soft tissues. Further biomechanical studies and software and hardware developments therefore are still in progress. Other software changes are necessary for online documentation.

It must be pointed out that information obtained from either robotics or navigation are significantly more accurate than that obtained from a standard postoperative X-ray. Furthermore, the three-dimensional data available after total knee arthroplasty will be more comprehensive. We believe a future interest will be to use these tools to determine the etiology and diagnosis of implant failures and loosening.

Conclusion

The Navitrack system enables an experienced knee surgeon reliable navigated TKA with or without preoperative image data (CT scan). The modular concept of the system, concerning the tracking system and the different applications allows the surgeon the ability to chose the CT-free navigation for standard cases or CT-based navigation in severe deformities of the lower extremity depending on the indication or required surgical technique. Particular the CT-free Navitrack application seems to be more advantageous than conventional alignment techniques with rods.

A new generation of instruments, which meet the high precision standard of navigation will improve the results in TKA. and other indications for navigated surgeries such as THR, spine surgery and osteotomies.

To justify the expense of navigation, in time of reduced budgets in health care systems, of course the benefit of both applications, like for all new techniques, must be demonstrated in prospective randomized studies. For the CT-free application of the Navitrack system a prospective, randomized multicenter study is still in progress to examine the effect of navigation on functional and long-term outcome in TKA.

From the view of a clinical user and adviser of a developing system I hope for an evolution of the navigation systems to expand beyond the primary applications currently used in total hip and total knee arthroplasty. This approach may be particularly useful in situations where elaborate three-dimensional determination is need such as pelvic osteotomies or dorsal cervical spine instrumentation.

References

1. Amiot LP, Lang K, Putzier M, Zippel H, Labelle H (2000) Comparative results between conventional and computer-assisted pedicle screw installation in the thoracic, lumbar, and sacral spine. Spine 25:606–614
2. Ewald FC (1989) The Knee Society total knee arthroplasty roentgenographic evaluation and scoring system. Clin Orthop 248:9–12
3. Gill GS, Mills DM (1991) Long-term follow-up evaluation of 1000 consecutive cemented total knee arthroplasties. Clin Orthop 273:66–76
4. Jeffery RS, Morris RW, Denham RA (1991) Coronal alignment after total knee replacement. J Bone Joint Surg Br 73:709–714
5. Kiefer H, Langenmeyer D, Schmerwitz U (2001) Computerunterstütze Navigation in der Knieendorprothetik. Europ J Trauma E [Suppl 1]: S128–123
6. Krackow KA, Bayers-Thering M, Phillips MJ, Bayers-Thering M, Mihalko WM (1999) A new technique for determining proper mechanical axis alignment during total knee arthroplasty: progress toward computer-assisted TKA. Orthopedics 22:698–702
7. Lotke PA, Ecker ML (1977) Influence of positioning of prosthesis in total knee replacement. J Bone Joint Surg Am 59:77–79
8. Teter KE, Bregman D, Colwell CW Jr (1995) Accuracy of intramedullary versus extramedullary tibial alignment cutting systems in total knee arthroplasty. Clin Orthop 321:106–110
9. Teter KE, Bregman D, Colwell CW Jr (1995) The efficacy of intramedullary femoral alignment in total knee replacement. Clin Orthop 321:117–121
10. Windsor RE, Scuderi GR, Moran MC, Insall JN (1989) Mechanisms of failure of the femoral and tibial components in total knee arthroplasty. Clin Orthop 248:15–19; discussion 19–20

42 Clinical Experience with the CT-Based *VectorVision* System

M. Wiese, K. Schmidt, R. E. Willburger

Introduction

Since the very beginning of total knee arthroplasty for osteoarthritis and rheumatoid arthritis the number of procedures performed worldwide has continuously increased in the last decades. The component design has changed from hinged to non-constrained implants with the advantage of more preserving bone resections and ligament stability. The femoral component in particular changed from a single radius to more anatomical radii for conforming the femoral shape and appreciation of the patellar groove. Modern TKA kinematics rely on both active and passive soft tissue kinematics and provide increased bone mass for revisions.

Clinical long-term outcome depends on a variety of factors, particularly on implant positioning and soft tissue balancing [17]. Rand and Coventry [13] reported a correlation between implant alignment and survivorship. Polyethylene wear is decreased in cases with optimal component alignment and soft tissue balancing [9, 12, 14–16].

In order to reproduce optimal implant positioning newer instrument sets have evolved such as intra- and extra-medullary alignment rods and resection blocks. Preoperative planning is usually determined on non-standardized plain radiographs in two planes. This technique includes its known potential errors with regards to anatomical landmarks and the mechanical axis. Deviation may result especially in deformed knee joints with flexion deficit. When using the PFC Sigma conventional TKA instrumentation (Johnson & Johnson, Warsaw, USA) a deviation of up to 4 degrees was observed in about 8% of the cases [14, 15].

The potential errors of preoperative planning on 2D images could be considerably reduce utilizing 3D images from CT scans with the VectorVision system. This concept has proven to be successful in spine surgery, ACL reconstruction, and total hip arthroplasty [2, 10, 12].

CT-Based Brain-LAB Navigation System

Equipment

The VectorVision navigation system (Brain-LAB, Germany) works passively via an optical camera tracing in a three-dimensional space. Three markers are required in order to precisely identify the location of the instrument (see Fig. 42-5a,b). The markers have a range of 120 degrees allowing weight sparring design without the need for cable connection or batteries. The navigation system includes both hardware and software plus camera and a sterile touch screen reducing the amount of extra instruments (◘ Fig. 42-1), it is, furthermore, modular and open allowing multiple applications for knee, hip and spine surgery for different implants.

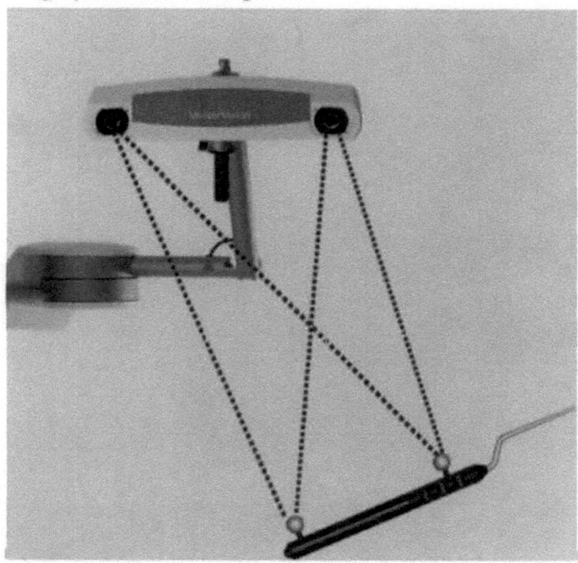

◘ **Fig. 42-1.** Computer navigation system with camera, and pointer and a reference marker

Preoperative Planning

The current version requires a preoperative hip, ankle CT with 2 to 4 mm cuts and a knee CT scan with 1 to 2 mm cuts for planning and execution of the TKA procedure. Acquired data are transmitted via intranet or portable storage media. Preoperative planning can be performed on external PCs or on the navigation system itself. All digital CT are primarily reconstructed to a 3D model. Mechanical leg axis and anatomical landmarks are calculated suggesting bone cuts and implant sizes. The surgeon can alter the angle of view as well as component size from a library. One may also virtually implant femoral and tibial components (Fig. 42-2).

Femoral component rotation is defined by either the transepicondylar axis or both posterior condyles (Fig. 42-2). Intra-medullary alignment rods are included in the virtual system. For tibial component positioning the malleolar axis and the posterior plateau are optional references. Completed data are stored on the navigation system or transferred via a portable storage medium. A print-out of all patients' data is helpful for file documentation (Fig. 42-2).

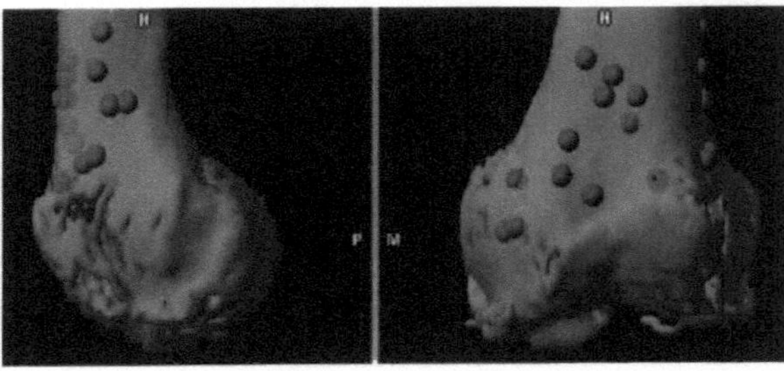

Fig. 42-3. Example of femoral surface matching. *Red spots* indicate a perfect surface, *blue spots* indicate withdrawn surface points

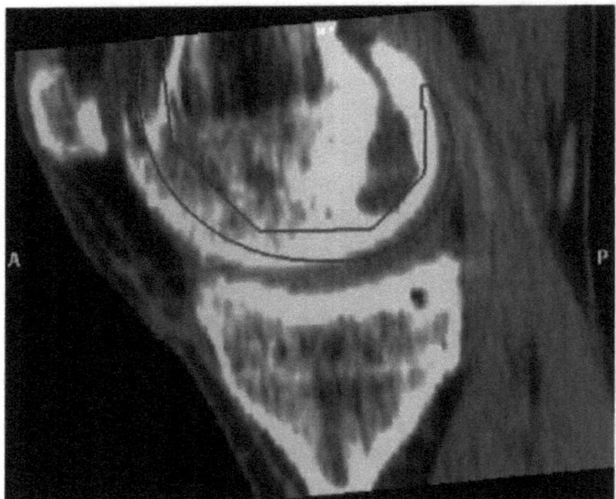

Fig. 42-4. Planning view of the position of the protheses in single layers

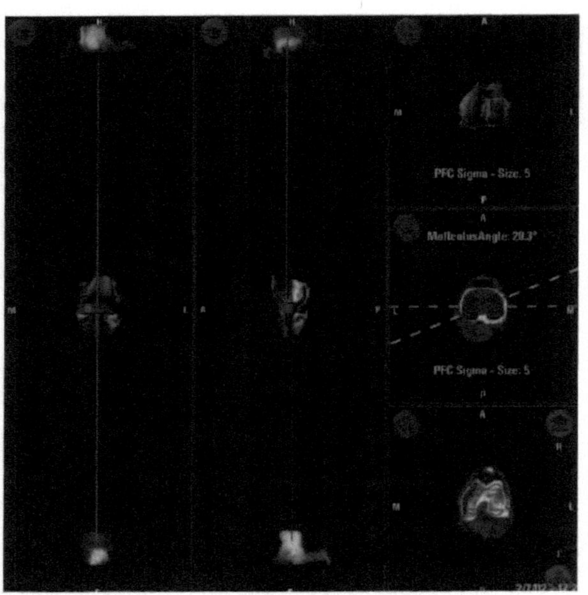

Fig. 42-2. Planning of the mechanical axis using a virtual radiograph

Computer Navigation in TKA: Surgical Technique

The navigation tower is positioned distal to the feet on the side of the surgeon and the touch screen, which is held by a moveable arm, close to the knee joint. Routine approach of the knee until 90 degrees of flexion are achieved. A three-pointed reference marker is screwed into the femur 2 cm proximal and medial to the patellar groove (Fig. 42-5a). The hip center is calculated using a pivoting algorithm by slowly rotating the femur in the view window of the cameras. CT data of the knee are registered pointing at anatomical landmarks (paired point matching) or pointing at over 20 different location at the bone surface (surface matching; see Fig. 42-3). Finally the referencing is verified with the pointer touching at various bone sur-

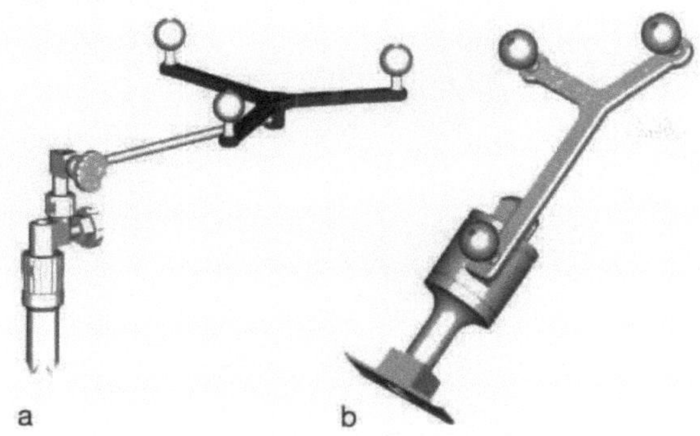

a   b

Fig. 42-5a,b. Additional instruments for resection block alignment. **a** Minimally invasive reference marker, **b** adapter for knee resection blocks

faces comparing these structures with the image on the screen.

The femoral cutting block can be positioned using intra-medullary rods or free hand with pin track navigation, when one attaches reference diodes onto the cutting guide (**Fig. 42-5b**). The reference marker fits also onto the four-in-one femoral cutting block, which allows free-hand navigation as well. All resection planes can be double-checked with the pointer. The tibial resection follows the same principles as on the femoral side, requiring one referencing screw (see **Fig. 42-6**). Extra-medullary instruments are used for final positioning of the resection block. Tibial rotational alignment is calculated as well. After preparation of the specific implant pegs and trial component, the final implants can be cemented.

The current software version (1.1) does not include soft tissue tensioning, however, prototype instruments are already in use on special cadaver knees (Thiel solution)

mimicking near to normal forces and will hopefully be implemented in the near future.

The precision of paired point matching or surface matching was compared with the fiducial CT marker technique and showed no significant difference compared to the literature. However, component alignment was more precise, when compared to conventional instruments.

References

1. Bargren JH., Blaha JD, Freeman MAR (1983) Alignment in total knee arthroplasty: Correlated biomechanical and clinical observations. Clin Orthop 173: 178–183
2. Bernsmann K, Langlotz U, Ansari B, Wiese M (2000) Computerassistiert navigierte Pfannenplazierung in der Hüftendoprothetik – Anwendungs-studie im klinischen Routinealltag. Z Orthop 138: 515–521
3. Clayton ML, Thompson RT, Mack RP (1986) Correlation of alignment deformities during total knee arthroplasties staged soft tissue releases. Clin Orthop 202: 117–124
4. Hoffman AA, Bachus KN, Wyatt RWB (1991) Effect of tibial cut on subsidence following total knee arthroplasty. Clin Orthop 269: 63–69
5. Hood RW, Vanni M, Insall JN (1981) The correction of knee alignment in 225 consecutive total condylar knee replacements. Clin Orthop 160: 94–105
6. Hungerford DS, Kenna RV (1983) Preliminary experiences with total knee prosthesis with porous coated used without cement. Clin Orthop 176: 95–107
7. Hvid I, Nielsen S (1984) Total condylar knee arthroplasty: Prosthetic component positioning and radiolucent lines. Acta Orthop Scand 55: 160–165
8. Insall JN, Binazzi R, Soundry M, Mestriner LA (1985) Total knee arthroplasty. Clin Orthop 192: 13–22
9. Jeffery RS, Morris RW, Denham RA (1991) Coronal alignment after total knee replacement. J Bone Joint Surg Br 73: 709–714
10. Laine T, Schlenzka D, Mäkitalo K, Tallroth K, Nolte L-P, Visarius H (1997) Improved accuracy of pedicle screw insertion with computer assisted surgery – A prospective clinical trial of 30 patients. Spine 22: 1254–1258
11. Miehlke RK, Clemens U, Jens J-H, Kershally S (2001) Navigation in der Knieendoprothetik – vorläufige klinische Erfahrungen und prospektiv vergleichende Studie gegenüber konventioneller Implantationstechnik. Z Orthop 139: 109–116
12. Nolte L-P, Zamorano L, Visarius H, Berlemann U, Langlotz F, Arm E, Schwarzenbach O (1995) Clinical evaluation of a system for precision enhancement in spine surgery. Clin Biomech 10: 293–303
13. Rand JA, Coventry MB (1988) Ten-year evaluation of geometric total knee arthroplasty. Clin Orthop 232: 168–173
14. Teter K, Bregman D, Colwell CW (1995) Accuracy of intramedullary versus extramedullary tibial alignment cutting systems in total knee arthroplasty. Clin Orthop 321: 106–110
15. Teter K, Bregman D, Colwell CW (1995) The efficacy of intramedullary femoral alignment in total knee replacement. Clin Orthop 321: 117–121
16 Wasiliewski RC, Galante JO, Leighty R, Natarajan RN, Rosneberg AG (1994) Wear patterns on retrieved polyethylene inserts and thier relationship to technical considerations during total knee arthroplasty. Clin Orthop 299: 31–43
17. Windsor RE, Scuderi GR, Moran MC, Insall JN (1989) mechanisms of failure of the femoral and tibial components in total knee arthroplasty. Clin Orthop 248: 15–20

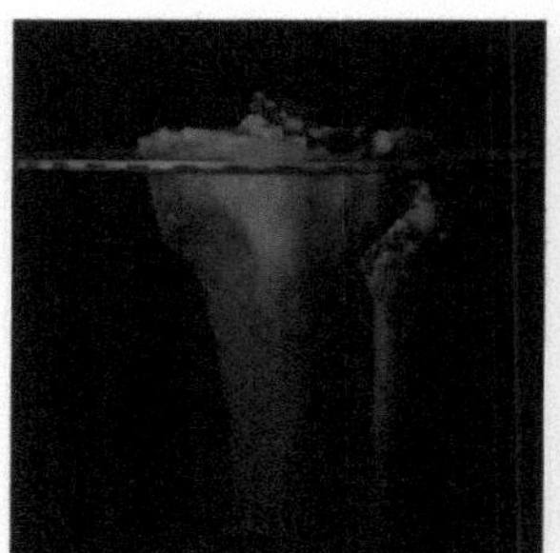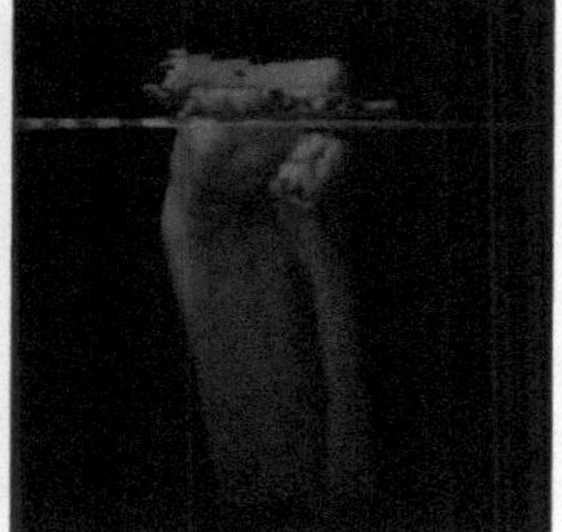

Fig. 42-6. Positioning of tibial resection block. *Yellow* plane indicating calculated plane, *blue* indicating actual plane

43 CT-Based and CT-Free Navigation with the BrainLAB *VectorVision* System in Total Knee Arthroplasty

L. Perlick, H. Bäthis, C. Lüring, M. Tingart, J. Grifka

Introduction

Accurate alignment of knee implants is essential for the success of total knee replacement. Although mechanical alignment guides have been designed to improve alignment accuracy, there are several fundamental limitations of this technology [2]. Petersen and Engh [8] reported radiological results of 50 primary knee arthroplasties. 26% (13/50) failed to achieve a satisfactory post-operative limb alignment (±3°). In several studies the rotational alignment of the femoral component has shown to be crucial for patellofemoral mechanics and balancing of flexion and extension gaps, and a significant correlation was found between patient outcome and prosthesis alignment [1].

Navigation systems are supposed to guarantee a higher precision of implant positioning. The application of navigation in primary total knee arthroplasty (TKA) started in 1998 [9]. During the last years several systems for image-guided surgery in TKA have become available.

Since August 2001 we have performed 85 CT-based navigated TKAs in our department, working with the CT-based version of BrainLAB's VectorVision. In February 2002 we started using a prototype of the CT-free module of this navigation system, within a development cooperation of our department with BrainLAB and DePuy, Germany. As a part of this cooperation, different software versions have been evaluated and the clinical usability has been improved in a clinical study supervised by the local ethics committee. Furthermore, a navigation procedure for determining a ligament based axial rotation of the femoral component was developed. Until November 2002 more than 70 TKAs have been implanted using this CT-free module.

Technical Aspects

The VectorVision compact system is very compact, due to the integration of the camera and computer in one unit. This allows using the system under conditions with limited space like in most operation rooms.

It is an optical system which detects the reflecting marker spheres by an infrared camera. The software is controlled by touch screen so that foot switches or additional cables are not necessary.

CT-Based Module

CT scans of the leg (femoral head, knee, ankle) are performed according to a standard protocol the day before operation. Then an automatic pre-planning can be performed, based on 3D surface images or the original CT scans. This planning allows a precise orientation of the prosthetic components, representing an optimal alignment to the mechanical limb axis. As default settings, the surgeon can either use the epicondylar axis for rotational adjustment of the femoral component or the posterior condylar axis. The whole planning procedure can be performed in about 20 min.

After planning, data are transferred from the planning station to the navigation system either via network or ZIP disc. However, so far, planning and navigation are based on bone landmarks, and no additional tools for evaluating ligament tension and long leg axis are integrated.

At the beginning of the operation, a reference frame is attached to the distal femur or the proximal tibia, respectively, instead of intra-medullary femoral reaming using a bicortical pin. This is followed by a surface matching process, where the surgeon has to digitize up to 20 points of free choice on the bone surface of both, the femur and tibia. Next, the conventional cutting blocks of the knee system are orientated in real time visualization, using the navigation system, for the distal femur and 4-in-1 cutting block.

A similar procedure is performed for the proximal resection of the tibia and the orientation of the tibial tray. After resection, the planes can be checked by a verification function.

CT-Free Module

In contrast to the CT-based module, the CT-free version does not require any preoperative image sets or planning time. With this technique, reference arrays with passive marker spheres are rigidly attached to both, the femoral and the tibial bone (◘ Fig. 43-1). At the beginning of the surgical procedure landmarks are needed for navigation. Information about the bone surface is given to the system by sliding a pointer above the tibial plateau and the femoral condyles using a fast and user-friendly algorithm. Then, the system creates an adapted bone model of the specific patient's anatomy and offers the surgeon an automatic planning of the implants. This default planning can be modified depending on surgeon's preferences regarding component size and orientation. To avoid ventral femoral notching a special routine for controlling the ventral femoral plane has been integrated in the software (◘ Fig. 43-2).

Before any cuts are performed, the surgeon has the opportunity to examine and document the leg axis and to test the ligament tension when applying varus and valgus stress.

The system provides different opportunities for rotational orientation of the femoral component to achieve a perfectly balanced extension and flexion gap. The femur component can be orientated according to the posterior condyles, to the transepicondylary axis or based on the ligament tension (gap technique).

In our opinion, this ligament-balanced technique is preferable for different reasons. Previous studies (e.g. Olcott et. al [7]) indicate that a 3° external rotation of the femoral component according to posterior condylar line only creates a rectangular flexion gap in about 70%. The

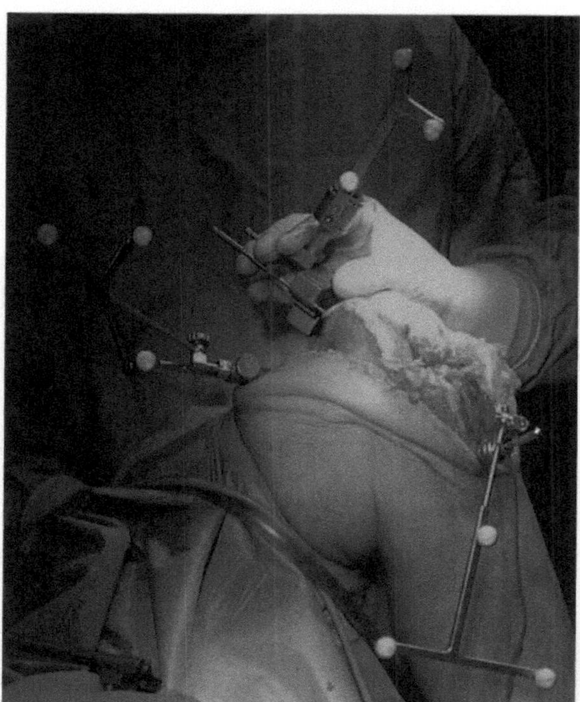

◘ **Fig. 43-1.** Reference arrays with passive marker spheres are rigidly attached to the femur and tibia. A reference tool is attached to the conventional distal femur cutting block

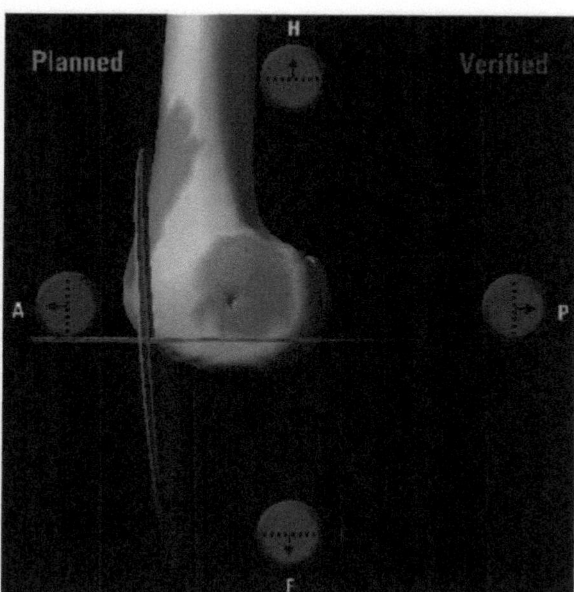

◘ **Fig. 43-2.** Before performing the ventral femur cut the ventral femur plane is checked to avoid notching of the ventral cortex in a flexed femur

transepicondylar axis most consistently creates a balanced flexion gap. On the other hand, Jerosch et al. [4] demonstrated a poor reproducibility in defining the transepicondylary axis, even for experienced surgeons with a deviation of up to 23°.

One possible solution for this problem could be the orientation of the femoral component based on the collateral ligament tension in flexion by using spreader tools or spacer blocks, as successfully performed in the conventional LCS technique.

According to Katz et al. [5] flexion gap tensioning may offer superior reliability, because of its independence of obscured or distorted bone landmarks.

Using the navigation-based ligament-balanced technique, the proximal tibia and the distal femur cuts are performed as primary steps. Similar to the CT-based system, the conventional cutting blocks are positioned to the defined cutting planes using the navigation system. After bone resection, the achieved planes are checked and documented by a verification function. Then, a ligament balancing is performed using a spreader tool, to achieve a rectangular extension gap (□ Fig. 43-3). Gap size and deviation of the leg axis are displayed by the navigation system.

After creating a rectangular extension gap, the knee is moved to a 90° flexion position. Again, the spreader tool is inserted between the tibia and the posterior femoral condyles. The navigation system stores this position and recommends the optimal femoral-component orientation to achieve a balanced, rectangular flexion gap. If there are any deviations between the flexion and extension gap, resizing of the femoral component or a modification of the distal femur cut can be performed. The expected values for the extension and flexion gap are notified. Then, the anterior and posterior femoral cuts are prepared by placing the conventional 4-in-1 cutting block.

After insertion of the trial implants it is possible to check the range of motion, the achieved leg axis and joint stability applying stress examination. Every parameter can be documented intraoperatively. Afterwards adjustment of the tibia tray can be performed either by using the navigation system similar to the CT-based software (□ Fig. 43-4) or by dynamic self-adjustment of the trial component.

Materials and Methods

The CT-based system has been evaluated in a prospective study, which started in September 2001. In this study, 40 prostheses were implanted using the navigation system, while another 40 prostheses were implanted in the conventional technique.

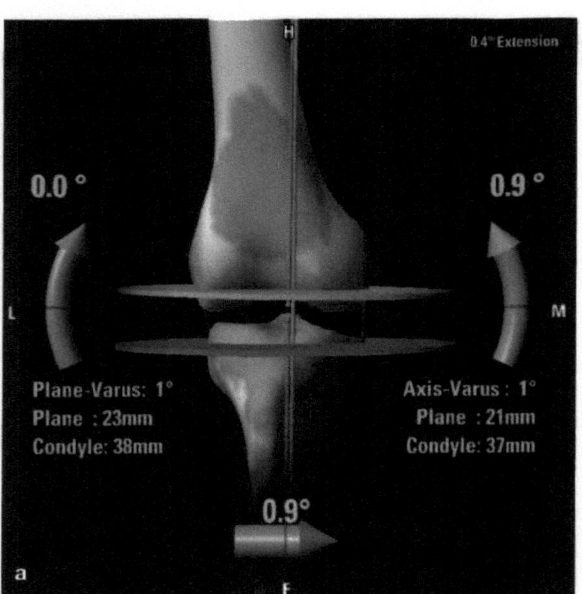

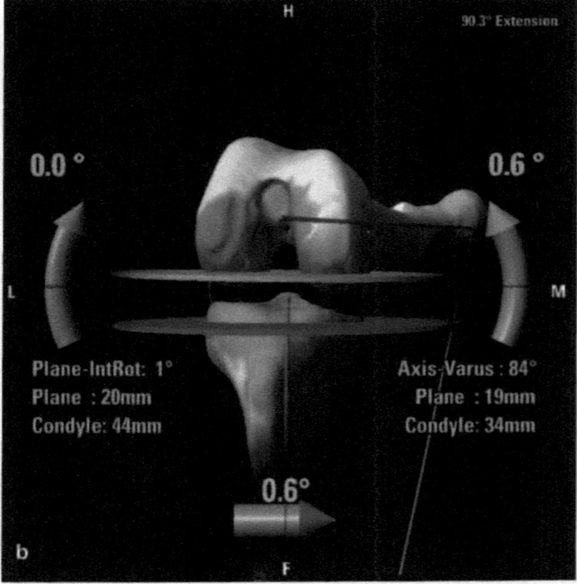

□ **Fig. 43-3a,b.** The (achieved) extension gap and the expected flexion gap are displayed during the surgical procedure

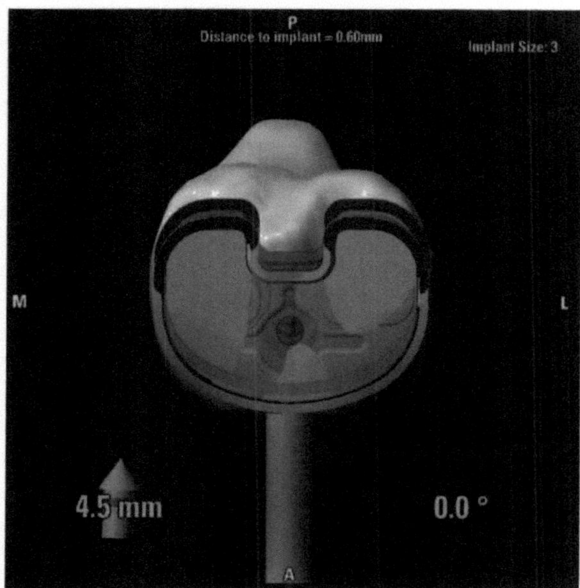

■ Fig. 43-4. The system offers the opportunity of placing and sizing (better: measuring) the tibial tray

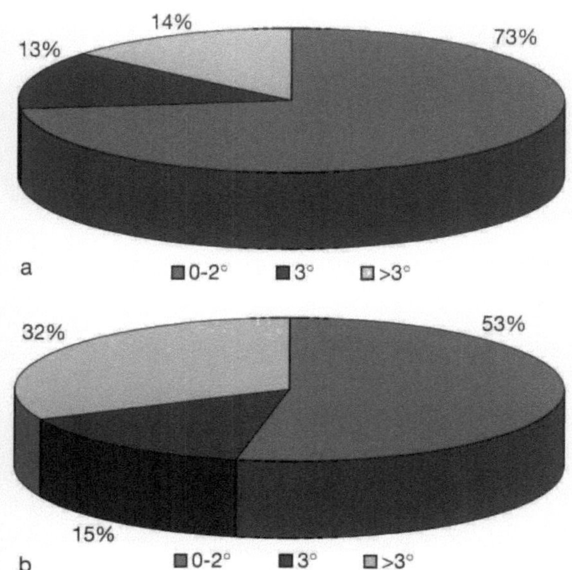

■ Fig. 43-5a,b. 88% of patients in the CT-based group (*n*=40) showed a good postoperative long leg axis (deviation: ±3°) compared to 68% of patients in the control group (*n*=40)

In a second prospective study, which started in April 2002, the CT-free navigation system (VectorVision Knee, Brain-LAB, Munich, Germany) was used. 40 total knee arthroplasties (PFC Sigma, DePuy Inc., Warsaw) were performed with the CT-free system, and a control group of 40 patients was operated on in a conventional technique. No significant differences in age, BMI and deviation of the leg axis existed between the two groups. Data were analyzed with respect to axial alignment, determined on post-operative standardized long leg weight bearing radiographs.

Results

CT-Based Module

In the navigation group a significantly better mechanical limb axis (±2°) was obtained in 73% of patients than in the control group (53%). Further, 88% of patients had an angle within ±3° in the study group, compared with 68% in the control group ($p<0.05$; ■ Fig. 43-5). An axis deviation of >4° was seen in 2 patients in the study group (maximum: 5°), and in 6 patients in the control group (maximum: 10°; $p<0.05$). The average time for surgery was

increased by 14 min in the navigation group compared to conventional technique.

CT-Free Module

The time of surgery increased by a mean of 16 min. There were no adverse effects resulting from the use of the navigation system. All operations performed with the navigation system could be completed.

In the navigated group, 96% of the patients showed post-operative mechanical limb axis of ±3°, and 78% of ±2°, respectively.

In the control group, 76% of the patients had an angle of ±3° and 56% of patients one of ±2°, respectively (■ Fig. 43-6).

Using the ligament-balanced navigation tool for femoral component rotation, a balanced flexion and extension gap with a maximum angulation of less than 4° under varus/valgus stress was achieved in all patients of the navigation group. Referring to the posterior condylar line, the mean external rotation of the femoral component was 3,9° (standard deviation: 3,3°, range 1° internal rotation – 10° external rotation).

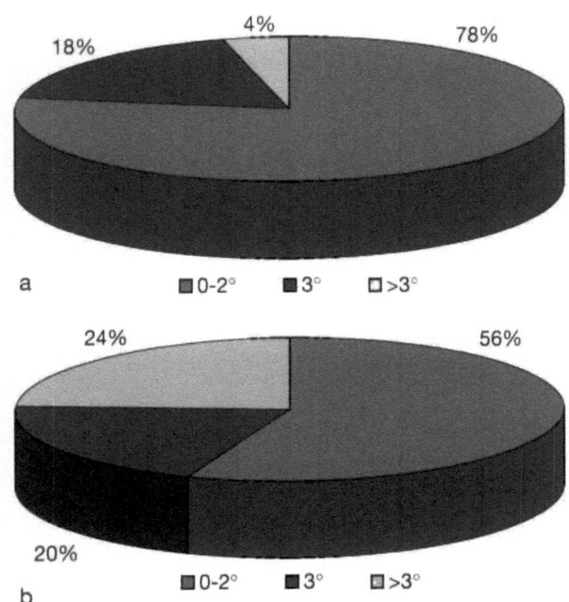

Fig. 43-6a,b. When using a CT-less system, 96% of patients in the CT-less group (*n*=40) had a good postoperative result (deviation of the long leg axis: ±3°) compared to 76% of patients in the control group (*n*=40)

Discussion

Both software versions (CT-based and CT-free) of the VectorVision navigation system show an easy and user-friendly handling in clinical routine.

The VectorVision system in general uses passive reflecting marker spheres for instruments and reference arrays. From our experience, these passive marker spheres guarantee a good visualization during the whole surgical procedure regardless of the leg position. This might be an advantage compared with active (LED-based) reference arrays.

The VectorVision system is a wireless system, which ensures a higher acceptance by the operation room stuff, since problems regarding cable breakage and sterility are minimized. Minor problems inherited in every optical navigation system such as contamination of marker spheres with blood can be easily solved by simple intra-operative cleaning.

Additional operating time is needed when using navigation systems in total knee arthroplasty. However, as a result of our prospective studies, mean duration of the surgical procedure is only prolonged by 16 min after an initial learning curve. This additional time seems tolerable in clinical routine. In the future, the time needed, might be further reduced by improvement of the navigation workflow and development of navigation-specific instruments.

The CT-free VectorVision system offers the orthopaedic surgeon important information regarding axis alignment, range of motion and ligament tension. Further, it can be easily adjusted to the surgeon-specific preferences concerning the method of femoral rotational alignment and level of bone resection. The ligament tension module shows a high functionality in clinical routine, particularly, if used in combination with a spreader system.

In contrast, the CT-based software, so far, does not offer any tool for determination of ligament tension, since the femoral and tibial navigation can not be performed simultaneously. To date, this is a limitation of the CT-based version compared with the CT-free software. However, in the future, also the CT-based software will contain this functionality.

In our series both the CT-based and CT-free navigation system showed a significantly improved restoration of the post-operative mechanical axis. These results are in agreement with the data reported by others. Miehlke et al. [6] reported only 6.7% unacceptable results (>4°) after computer-assisted total knee arthroplasty. In another study performed by Jenny and Boeri in 2001 [3] 33 of 40 patients had a mechanical leg axis of ±3°.

Different reasons might be relevant for deviation of the mechanical leg axis even if using a navigation system. An explanation might be that most systems are used in combination with conventional implantation instruments. For example, placing the pins to fix the 4-in-1 cutting bloc can result in an axis deviation up to 1.5°. Therefore, the manufacturers are working on the development of new and more precise instruments.

Another reason for variations of the leg axis is a possible deviation of the saw blade in dense bone stock. However, an important advantage of navigation systems is that some of the errors discussed before can be verified and corrected intraoperatively. Other factors are variations in cementing the prosthetic components as well as inaccuracies in determining the leg axis on post-operative weight bearing long leg radiographs.

However, it also has to be discussed that some factors for a deviation of the leg axis might be immanent to the navigation system.

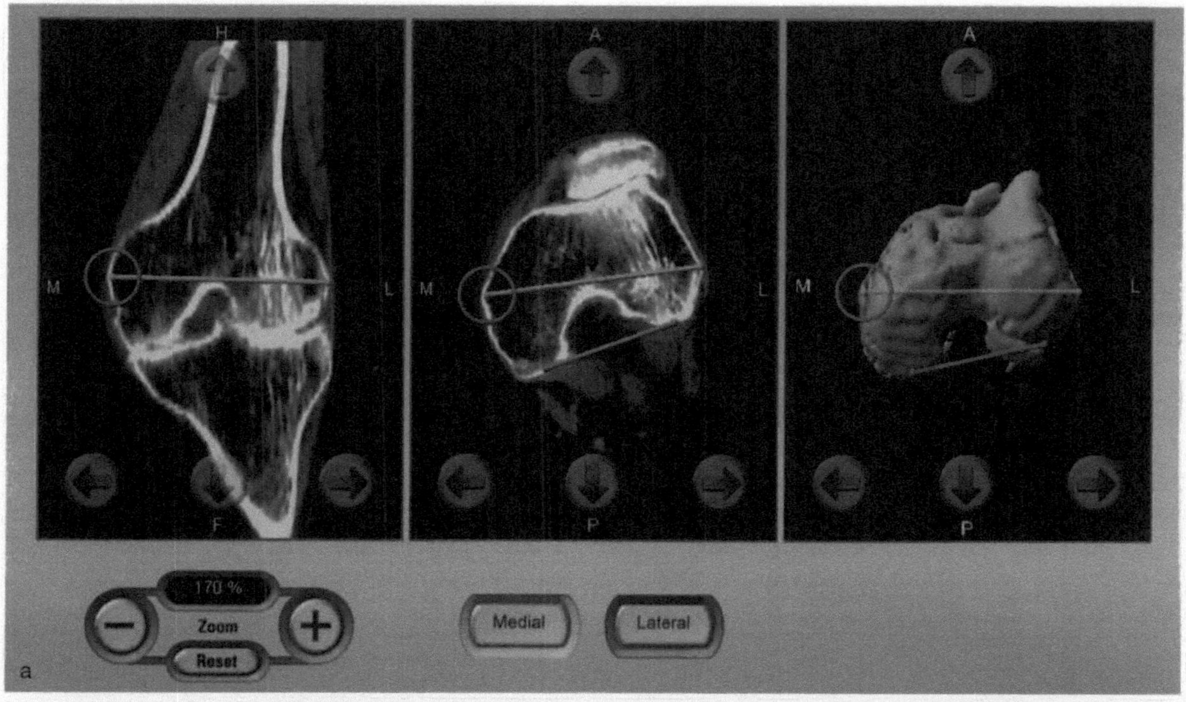

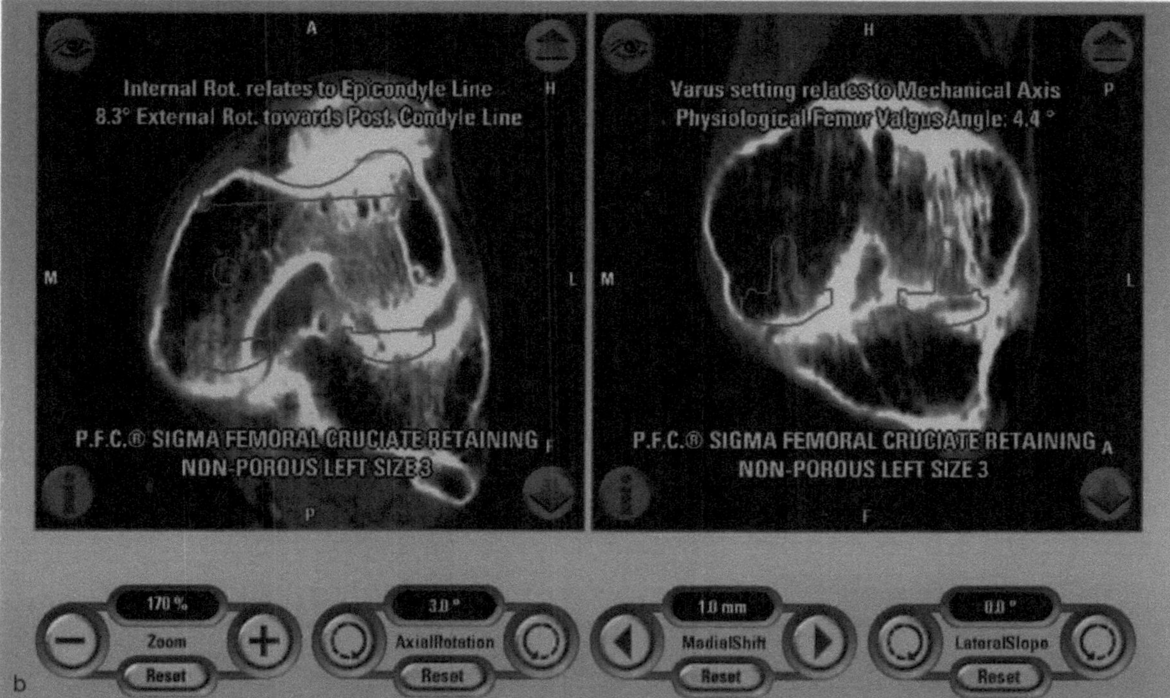

Fig. 43-7a,b. The CT-based system offers the opportunity of preoperative planning which is useful in cases with severe bone loss. In this case of a 34 year old patient with rheumatoid arthritis, using the posterior condylar axis as orientation would have led to insufficient component placement. Furthermore the surgeon can get information, if bony or metal augmentation is necessary

In all image-based systems (e.g. CT-based), the accuracy of navigation depends on the quality of CT-data and the intraoperative acquisition of reference points, which are necessary to correlate the image set to the patients real anatomy. On the other side, the accuracy of the CT-free system depends on the quality of the acquired landmarks and surface points at the beginning of the surgical procedure.

Comparing the CT-based and the CT-free system the main advantages of the CT-free system are information about the achieved leg axis and ligament tension. For most surgeons the required preoperative CT-scans are a costly and time consuming disadvantage of the CT-based navigation. In contrast, in special cases these CT scans and the opportunity of preoperative planning might be helpful.

The CT-free system allows performing revision arthroplasties. So far, this is not possible with the CT-based system due to artefacts from the implants.

As mentioned before, the CT-free VectorVision system offers the surgeon detailed data regarding leg axis, implant positioning and ligament tension. However, this raises new questions regarding the optimal ligament tension and how long term results are influenced by this. Future studies might answer these questions. Nevertheless, navigation systems give the opportunity of detailed data acquisition and result documentation.

Conclusion

The CT-based navigation system offers the opportunity of preoperative planning and correct intraoperative navigation of cutting blocks. Particularly, in situations with femoral or tibial bone defects (◨ Fig. 43-7) this planning might be helpful; however, additional costs and time due to the CT-scanning and pre-planning have to be discussed.

Our first results using the CT-based and CT-free VectorVision navigation system show, that limb alignment is significantly improved compared with the conventional technique. The ligament balancing tool is useful in achieving a balanced flexion and extension gap. Alignment, range of motion and ligament situation as well as each step of bone resection can be verified and documented during surgery.

References

1. Anouchi YS, Whiteside LA, Kaiser AD, Milliano MT (1993) The effects of axial rotational alignment of the femoral component on knee stability and patellar tracking in total knee arthroplasty demonstrated on autopsy specimens. Clin Orthop 287: 170–177
2. Delp SL, Stulberg SD, Davies B, Picard F, Leitner F (1998) Computer assisted knee replacement. Clin Orthop 354: 49–56
3. Jenny JY, Boeri C (2001) Navigiert implantierte Knietotalendoprothesen – Eine Vergleichsstudie zum konventionellen Instrumentarium. Z Orthop Ihre Grenzgeb 139: 117–119
4. Jerosch J, Peuker E, Philipps B, Filler T (2002) Interindividual reproducibility in perioperative rotational alignment of femoral components in knee prosthetic surgery using the transepicondylar axis. Knee Surg Sports Traumatol Arthrosc 10: 194–197
5. Katz MA, Beck TD, Silber JS, Lotke PA (2001) Determining femoral rotational alignment in total knee arthroplasty. J Arthroplasty 16: 301–305
6. Miehlke RK, Clemens U, Jens JH, Kershally S (2001) Navigation in der Knieendoprothetik – vorläufige klinische Erfahrungen und prospektiv vergleichende Studie gegenüber konventioneller Implantationstechnik. Z Orthop Ihre Grenzgeb 139: 109–116
7. Olcott CW, Scott RD (1999) Femoral component rotation during total knee arthroplasty. Clin Orthop 367: 39–42
8. Petersen TL, Engh GA (1988) Radiographic assessment of knee alignment after total knee arthroplasty. J Arthroplasty 3: 67–72
9. Saragaglia D, Picard F, Chaussard C, Montbarbon E, Leitner F, Cinquin P (2001) Computer-assisted knee arthroplasty: comparison with a conventional procedure. Results of 50 cases in a prospective randomized study. Rev Chir Orthop Reparatrice Appar Mot 87: 18–28

44 Extra-Medullary Computer-Assisted Total Knee Replacement: Towards Lesser Invasive Surgery

R.L. Wixson

Introduction

Modern total knee replacement has emerged as one of the most successful and reproducible surgical procedures performed today [26, 41]. Much of this success has been due to the advances made with improved instrumentation with an understanding of the importance of restoring normal alignment of the mechanical axis of the knee [1, 12, 13, 15, 22, 29, 36, 46]. However, even with modern intra-medullary alignment systems there is still variability in the overall results achieved. There is further continued concern about fat embolization with intra-medullary techniques. Computer-assisted extra-medullary techniques offer the opportunity for improved accuracy and reproducibility while avoiding instrumenting the intra-medullary canal. As total knee replacement continues to evolve with minimally invasive surgery, the incorporation of computer-assisted techniques has the potential to allow the surgeon to continue to place the knee components accurately with less trauma to the patient.

Rationale for Extra-Medullary Approach

Mal-alignment, perhaps greater than 3°, has been shown to cause higher incidences of loosening in long term studies [7, 8, 15, 20, 38, 39, 43, 46, 47]. To achieve normal alignment, most modern knee instrument systems rely on the insertion of a femoral intra-medullary guide set at a predetermined angle or measured from long-standing radiographs. On the tibial side, most knee instrument systems are designed to cut the proximal tibial at 0° to the long axis of the tibia through the use of either intra-medullary guides or an extra-medullary guide aligned with the estimated center of the ankle.

There are a number of limitations inherent in the use of intra-medullary alignment guides. One of these is that not all patients have normal intra-medullary canals that are suitable, due to deformity or a history of trauma. ◻ Figures 44-1a and 44-1b demonstrate the long standing radiographs of a patient before and after total knee

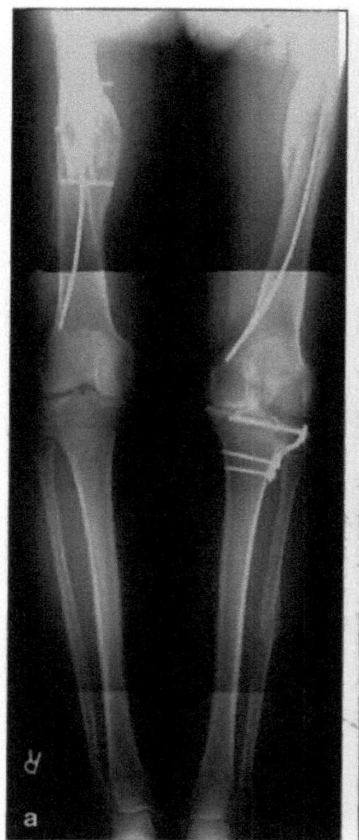
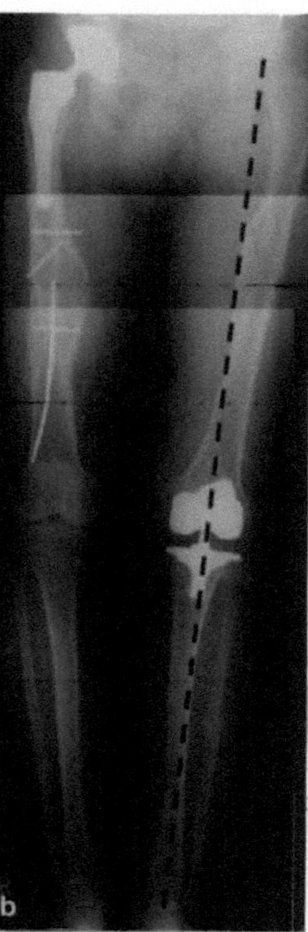

◻ **Fig. 44-1a, b.** Pre-operative and post-operative long standing radiographs of a patient with both femoral and tibial deformity not suitable for intra-medullary instrumentation. Restoration of neutral alignment in a total knee replacement using an extra-medullary computer-assisted technique

replacement using a computer-assisted approach to restore normal alignment in the face of both femoral and tibial mal-alignment with internal fixation devices. This patient would have been difficult to manage with conventional IM technique.

In addition, there is normal variation in the anatomy of both the femur and the tibia. Based on long standing radiographs of normal human volunteers without arthritis, Oswald et al. [31] compared the mechanical axis to the anatomic axis. For the mechanical axis a line was drawn from the center of the femoral head to the center of the knee and across the bottom of the femoral condyles. The mean valgus angle was 5.4° with a standard deviation of ±1.5° and a range of 2.0°–7.5°. On the tibial side, a line was drawn from the center of the tibial plateaus to the center of the talar dome and across the tibial plateaus. This had a mean varus angulation of 1.7° with a standard deviation of ±1.3° and a range of –0.5°–3.0°.

When intra-medullary alignment systems are used, long standing radiographs are frequently used to determine the accuracy that was achieved during surgery. While the mean restoration of alignment was very close to the mechanical axis, there was also a range of values in most studies. This has been attributed to both variations in the long bone anatomy, the effect of varying widths of the intra-medullary canal and variations from the X-ray technique [21]. A variety of studies that summarize these results are shown in ■ Table 44-1.

McGrory [24] compared a prospective series of patients with intra-medullary femoral guides and an extra-medullary tibial technique. The alignment in one group of patients was based on long-standing preoperative radiographs and averaged 6.2°. This was compared to a group where the distal femoral alignment was arbitrarily

set at 5°. He found no difference between the groups based on the percentage where the mechanical axis fell in the central one-third. This was 86% (95% C.I., 75%–93%) for patients with long leg preoperative radiographs and 92% (95% C.I., 80%–97%) for patients with short films only preoperatively. Similarly, there was no difference in the distance in millimeters from the center of the knee to the mechanical axis with both groups being in slight varus. The mean was 1.5 ± 8.4 mm for patients with and 1.9 ± 8.5 mm for patients without long leg radiographs. He concluded that in uncomplicated total knees, there was not a benefit to using long-standing radiographs for preoperative planning. Essentially, the variation in results achievable with the intra-medullary measurements overcame and benefits of preoperative planning.

Using conventional intra-medullary instruments for thirty-five total knees, Stulberg [44] used a computer-assisted knee navigation system to measure the preoperative and postoperative alignment, stability, and range of motion of the knee. Using a femoral rod set at 5° of valgus and cutting the tibia at 0° in the coronal plane resulted in coronal plane alignment of 2.6° varus with a range of 3.7° varus to 1.5° valgus. When long-standing radiographs were used to evaluate the patients postoperatively, there was also a significant discrepancy between the readings from the knee navigation system and the X-rays that averaged 3.5° with a range of 0° to 8°.

In addition to concerns about the accuracy of intra-medullary instrumentation, the introduction of rods into the canal has been shown to increase the intra-medullary pressure and produce embolization of fat particles into the circulation. In the extreme situation, this has resulted in the classic fat emboli syndrome with Gurd's [11] triad of petechiae, respiratory symptoms with chest radiographic changes and neurologic symptoms and even death [3, 6, 27]. Fahmy et al. [9] demonstrated the need to decompress the femoral canal by over drilling the femoral entrance hole in order to avoid high intra-medullary pressures and embolization.

With modern intra-medullary alignment methods, multiple studies have shown the persistence of echogenic material with transesophageal ultrasound when the tourniquet is released [2, 18, 32, 33]. In a prospective study of the use of regional heparinization to control embolization, Giachino [10] found no impact of heparinization but all of the total knee patients had embolic material detected

■ **Table 44-1.** Accuracy of intra-medullary instrumentation

Author	Goal	Achieved [%]
McGrory (2002) [24]	Central 1/3 (±4°)	89
Mahaluxmivala (2001) [23]	4°–10° valgus	75
Peterson (1988) [34]	4°–10° valgus	74
Reed (1997) [37]	Tibial IM	85
	Tibial EM	65
Teter (1995) [45]	Fem 2°–10° valgus	91
	Tibia ±4°	93
Jeffery (1991) [15]	Central 1/3	68

by transesophageal echocardiography in the right atrium after the tourniquet was released.

Postoperative mental status changes and confusion are common following total knee replacement. In a study of 262 patients with total knee replacements, Williams-Russo [48] found acute mental status changes in 41% with long-term changes in 5%. There is concern that some total joint patients may experience sub-clinical embolization with potential cognitive impairment [5,19], although to a lesser degree than that described for coronary artery bypass surgery patients [4,17].

Morawa [28] used transesophageal echocardiography to compare a group of total knee patients operated on with an intra-medullary technique to a group operated on with a mechanical extra-medullary knee alignment system. He reported substantial reductions in the level and duration of embolic events for the extra-medullary group as compared to the patients where conventional intra-medullary instrumentation was used. However, the extra-medullary group did show evidence of emboli with the implication that even without intra-medullary activities, other manipulations of the bone with the saw cuts, trial reductions and cementing may still be producing some emboli.

The development of techniques and equipment for computer-assisted total knee surgery allows accurate implant positioning without instrumentation of the intra-medullary canal [16,25,30,40,42,44]. Concerns about the accuracy of manual intra-medullary instrumentation and the possibility of fat embolism led to an interest in using computer-assisted navigation with an extra-medullary technique for routine total knee replacement

Surgical Technique

The Styrker Leibinger Knee Navigation system used in this series uses an imageless approach that does not require preoperative computer-assisted CT images. Patients undergo routine preoperative planning and assessment for total knee replacement with conventional X-rays. Long-standing films are not required unless there is a suspected significant long bone deformity.

The equipment used is based on trackers with infrared light emitting diodes (LED) that are attached to the skeleton with rigid fixation. These are active, in that they produce the signal rather than reflect a signal from another source.

In addition, they are battery powered and do not require external wires for power or communication. Each tracker has multiple LEDs that emits a series of unique infrared light flashes which are detected by three cameras in a localizer mounted on a movable arm several meters from the operating field. The received signals from each LED to each camera are processed by the knee navigation software to establish the location of each tracker in a three-dimensional coordinate system. In this series, threaded pins to attach the trackers are rigidly fixed to the anterior iliac crest, distal femur and proximal tibia. Once the trackers are in place, an anatomic survey is done with another instrument, the pointer, with LEDs on its handle and a metal tip at a precise distance from each LED. By touching various anatomic points on the knee, each of the bony landmarks has a known position in the coordinate system created by the computer. The information collected is converted into graphical images and data displays for the surgeon to visualize on a computer screen attached to the system on another movable arm. The accuracy of the instruments is to 0.1 mm and 0.1° which far exceeds the surgeon's ability to plan and execute the bone cuts themselves [35].

Once the knee has been exposed through a standard midline incision, the pins for the tracking devices are placed. In the series reported here, an iliac pin was placed percutaneously through a stab wound three centimeters behind the anterior superior iliac spine. A second pin was placed bicortically from anterior to posterior on the lateral side of the distal femur several centimeters above where the anterior flange of the femoral component would be placed. A third bicortical pin was placed through separate 1.5 cm incision over the anterior tibial crest. The location of the pins is shown in Figs. 44.2 to 44.4.

In the anatomic survey, the center of the femoral head was found first by placing trackers on the iliac crest pin and distal femur. The leg was then moved around in a cone shaped area creating a large sphere with the femoral tracker and the computer algorithm locating the center of the sphere which is also the center of the femoral head. With future software developments, it is anticipated that the iliac pin will not be needed to establish the location of the femoral head center. The remaining anatomic points surveyed are listed below. From these points the long axes of the bones, sagittal, coronal and transverse planes, joint line position, limb alignment and range of motion are assessed and the information stored.

Anatomic Survey

- Hip
  - Center of femoral head
- Distal Femur
  - Medial epicondyle (sulcus)
  - Lateral epicondyle
  - Mapping of distal medial condyle
  - Mapping of distal lateral condyle
  - Center of distal femur
  - Line of trochlear groove
- Proximal Tibia
  - Center of proximal tibia
  - Mappping surface of medial condyle
  - Mapping surface of lateral condyle
  - Neutral tibial anterior-posterior axis
- Ankle
  - Tip of medial malleolus
  - Tip of lateral malleolus
  - Center of ankle

Using this system with an extra-medullary approach has been described by Sikorsky et al. [42]. Either the femur or tibia can be approached first depending on the patient's anatomy and soft tissue exposure. For all of the cuts, the sequences is to

- place the cutting block and adjust it to the correct position;
- pin it in place;
- record the cutting jig position;
- execute the cut;
- verify the accuracy of the cut and adjust as indicated.

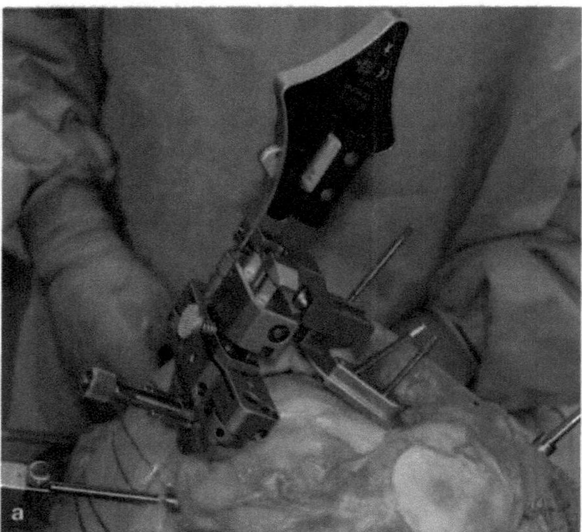

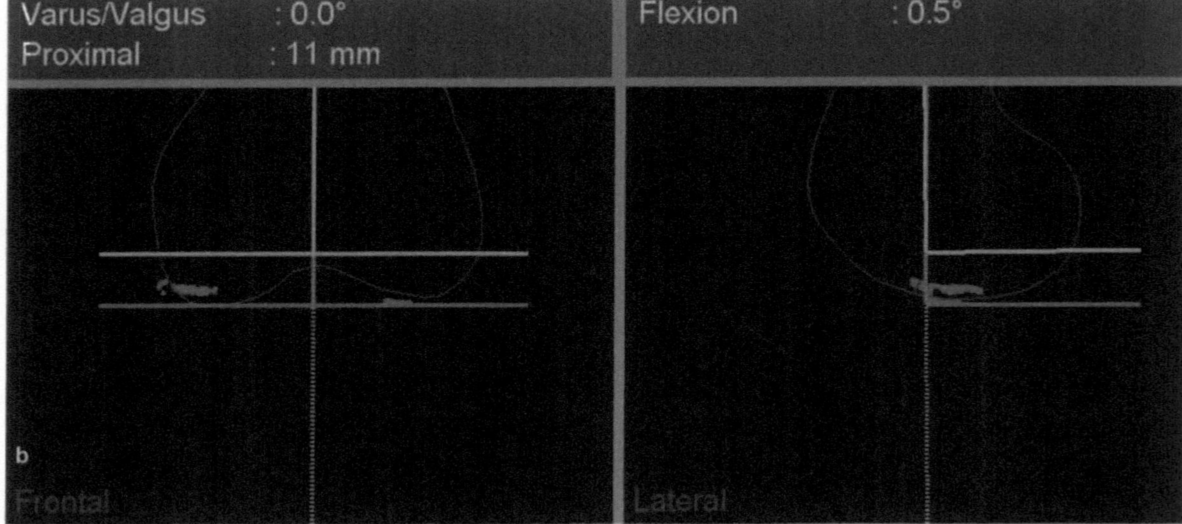

■ Fig. 44-2a,b. Distal femoral pivotal resection guide in place with the LED tracker attached to the distal femur with a fixation pin and another attached to the resection guide. The image on the computer display indicates the orientation of the planned cut in two planes as well as the depth of cut. Once the desired position is achieved with the adjusting screws on the device, the guide is pinned in place, the adjustment component and tracker removed and the cut can be made

For the femoral distal cut, our initial approach was similar to that described by Sikorsky [42] where a standard distal cutting block with an attached tracker was positioned freehand and pinned in place when the computer screen indicated that the block was at 0° varus-valgus; 0° to 1° flexion; and 10 mm resection from the most distal aspect of the femur. The current technique uses the same principle but uses a femoral pivotal resection cutting guide that can be attached to the distal femur and moved in all three planes to the desired position with adjusting screws at which point it is pinned in **place**. The use of this device is illustrated in ◘ Fig. 44-2a with the graphic display in ◘ Fig. 44-2b. Once the cut has been made, the accuracy is verified by placing a flat plate attached to the tracker on the bone cut surface.

Neutral femoral rotation is based on the anatomic survey with an average of the line perpendicular to the epicondylar axis and a line through the trochlear groove. By placing a tracker on the femoral rotation guide, the rotation can be adjusted to conform to the neutral femoral rotation at 0°. The same device is used to size the femur and make the distal femoral drill holes which the femoral cutting block will be placed in for the remaining condylar and chamfer cuts.

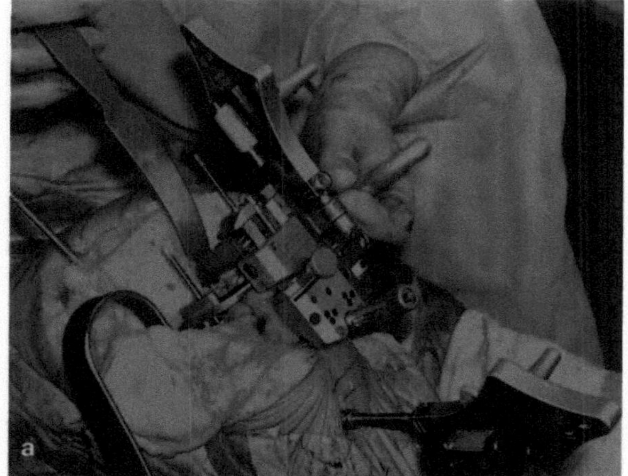

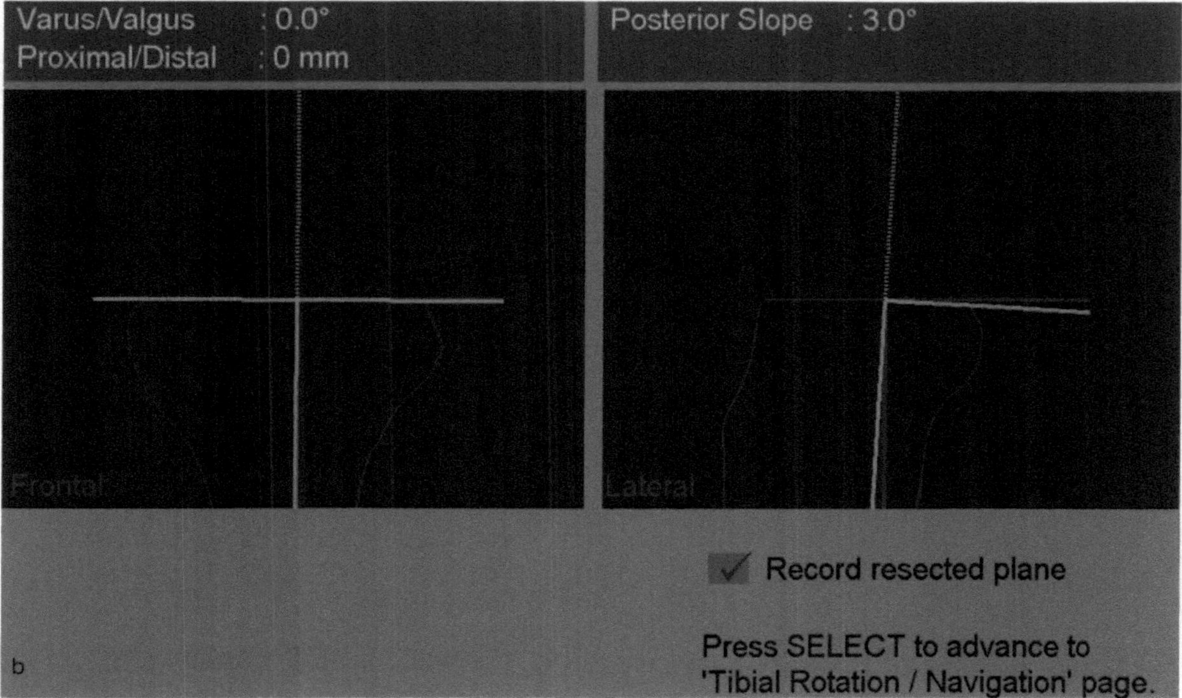

◘ **Fig. 44-3a,b.** Proximal tibial pivotal resection guide in place with the LED tracker attached to a tibial fixation pin and another one attached to the top of the resection guide. Once the desired position is achieved with the adjustment screws, the guide can be pinned in place and the cut made after removal of the tracker and adjustment component. The computer display shows the verification of the final cut achieved with this method

The desired proximal tibial cut is 0° to the long axis of the tibia in the coronal plane with some amount of posterior flexion in the sagittal plane depending on the individual patient anatomy. A tibial pivotal resection guide is seen in ◘ Fig. 44-3a and b that allows the jig to be moved to the desired position by using adjusting screws to bring the cut level to 0° varus-valgus, the desired amount of flexion, and the depth of bone resection needed. An alternative approach would be to use a Uniball guide that attaches to the tracker pin and allows the cutting block to be moved to the proper position and pinned in place. Once the cut has been made, the cut surface is verified for accuracy. Based on the neutral anterior-posterior tibial axis, the trial tibial jig is also positioned in 0° of rotation for placement of the peg holes and slots for this component.

Having completed the essential bone cuts, the trial components are put in place and the knee put through a range of motion with assessment of ligament tension and overall limb alignment. These results are displayed on a separate screen for intraoperative assessment both graphically and in tabular form. Appropriate ligament releases, changes in component position and thickness of the tibial insert can then be made to achieve complete extension with neutral alignment through the range of motion and appropriate ligament stability. Once the definitive components are put in place and the knee is completed, an outcome assessment is performed that shows the same information. An example is shown in ◘ Fig. 44-4a and b where neutral alignment at 0° was achieved throughout the range of motion.

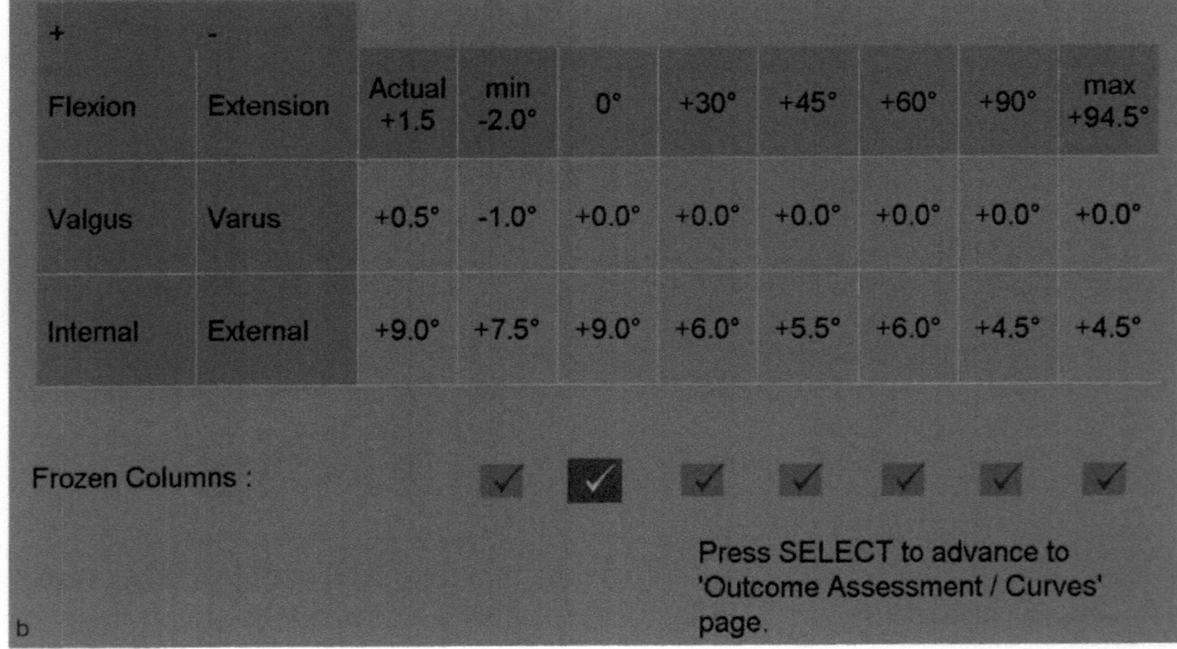

+	−	Actual	min	0°	+30°	+45°	+60°	+90°	max
Flexion	Extension	+1.5	-2.0°	0°	+30°	+45°	+60°	+90°	+94.5°
Valgus	Varus	+0.5°	-1.0°	+0.0°	+0.0°	+0.0°	+0.0°	+0.0°	+0.0°
Internal	External	+9.0°	+7.5°	+9.0°	+6.0°	+5.5°	+6.0°	+4.5°	+4.5°

◘ **Fig. 44-4a,b.** Total knee in place with the proximal tibial and distal femoral LED trackers. The computer display is the final outcome assessment that shows the alignment throughout the range of motion

Results with Extra-Medullary Computer-Assisted Technique

This approach was used in sixty-six consecutive patients with osteoarthritis of the knee. There were 67% female and 33% male patients with a mean age of seventy-three (range 56–91). Based on intraoperative computer assessment prior to making the bone cuts, 67% of the patients had varus deformity with a mean of 6.4° (± 3.3°) while 33% had valgus deformity with a mean of 7.4° (± 4.2°).

Once the initial assessment was completed, each bone cut was made as described above. We then adjusted the cuts as needed, selected the appropriate size of the components to be inserted, performed ligament releases if they were required to balance the knee and cemented the components into place. Following placement of the real tibial insert, the final outcome assessment was performed. The results of this series are in Table ◻ 44-2. The distribution of the final tibial-femoral alignment from the computer output is in Fig. ◻ 44-5.

◻ **Table 44-2.** Output of computer-assisted extra-medullary technique

Measurement [degrees]	Mean	Std Dev	Range]
Femoral varus-valgus	0.0	0.3	–1.0–1.0
Femoral extension	1.1	1.3	–3.0–4.5
Femoral rotation	0.1	0.3	–1.0–0.5
Tibial varus-valgus	0.0	0.2	–0.5–0.5
Tibial rotation	–0.1	0.3	–1.0–0.5
Femoral tibial alignment	0.0	0.7	–1.5–1.5

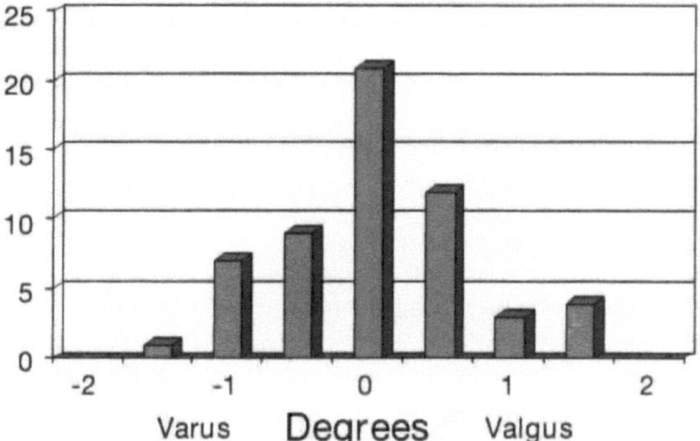

◻ **Fig. 44-5.** Distribution of the number of cases for each half degree of femoral-tibial alignment around the neutral, zero degree mechanical axis of the femoral head, knee and ankle

These measurements reflect the reproducibility of the extra-medullary technique using a computer assisted surgery. Long standing radiographs will provide information on the accuracy of the system but are limited by the variation in technique and position with the radiographs [21]. The definitive answer on the accuracy of computer techniques with manual methods may require more sophisticated analysis techniques that recreate the three dimensional relationships of the lower extremity with CT scans (computed axial tomography scans) [14,49].

Summary

Modern total knee replacement has evolved into a reproducible operation that provides significant pain relief and restoration of normal function to arthritic patients. The success of the surgery involves the use of total knee designs and appropriate materials that have been developed over the last several decades. Computer-assisted extra-medullary knee alignment system for total knee replacement allows the surgeon to make the same decisions and sequence of bone cuts during the performance of the surgery as with conventional techniques relying on mechanical guides. While the outcome of the surgery is dependent on the surgeon's choice of anatomic landmarks in both systems, the computer-assisted approach provides a high level of accuracy and is more independent of variations in patient's anatomy. The surgery can also be done without violation of the intra-medullary canal. The series of patients described here demonstrates that this approach is a reproducible and reliable method of achieving appropriate alignment in total knee arthroplasty. In the future, this method should also be applicable for surgical approaches with less invasive methods and surgical incisions.

References

1. Bargren JH, Blaha JD, Freeman MAR (1983) Alignment in total knee arthroplasty: Correlated biomechanical and clinical observations. Clin Orthop 173: 178–183
2. Berman AT, Parmet JL, Harding SF et al. (1998) Emboli observed with the use of transesophageal echocardiography immediately after tourniquet release during total knee arthroplasty with cement. J Bone Joint Surg 88A: 389
3. Caillouette JT, Anzel SH (1990) Fat embolism syndrome following the intramedullary alignment guide in total knee arthroplasty. Clin Orthop 251: 198–199

4. Clark RE, Brillman J, Davis DA et al. (1995) Microemboli during coronary artery bypass grafting: Genesis and effect on outcome. J Thorac Cardiovasc Surg 109: 249–258

5. Colonna DM, Stump DA, Kilgus DJ et al. (1999) Total hip arthroplasty produces intraoperative brain embolization and neuropsychologic dysfunction up to 6 weeks postoperatively. Anesthesiology A79: 91

6. Dorr LD, Merkel C, Mellman MF et al. (1989) Fat emboli in bilateral total knee arthroplasty. Clin Orthop 248: 112–118; discussion 118–119

7. Dorr LD, Boiardo RA (1997) Technical considerations in total knee arthroplasty. Clin Orthop 205: 5–11

8. Ecker ML, Lotke PA, Windsor RE et al. (1987) Long-term results after total condylar knee arthroplasty: Significance of radiolucent lines. Clin Orthop 216: 151–158

9. Fahmy NR, Chandler HP, Danylchuk K et al. (1990) Blood gas and circulatory changes during total knee replacement: The role of the intramedullary alignment rod. J Bone Joint Surg 72A: 19–26

10. Giachino AA, Rody K, Turek MA et al. (2001) Systemic fat and thrombus embolization in patients undergoing total knee arthroplasty with regional heparinization. J Arthroplasty 16: 288–292

11. Gurd AD (1970) Fat embolism: an aid to diagnosis. J Bone Joint Surg 52B: 732–737

12. Hood RW, Vanni M, Insall JN (1981) The correction of knee alignment in 225 consecutive total condylar knee replacements. Clin Orthop 160: 94–105

13. Insall JN, Binazzi R, Soudry M et al. (1985) Total knee arthroplasty. Clin Orthop 192: 13–22

14. Jazrawi LM, Birdzell L, Kummer FJ et al. (2000) The accuracy of computed tomography for determining femoral and tibial total knee arthroplasty component rotation. J Arthroplasty 15: 761–766

15. Jeffery RS, Morris RW, Denham RA (1991) Coronal alignment after total knee replacement. J Bone Joint Surg 73B: 709–714

16. Jenny JY, Boeri C (2001) Computer-assisted implantation of a total knee arthroplasty: a case-controlled study in comparison with classical instrumentation. Revue de Chirurgie Orthopedique et Reparatrice del Appareil Moteur 87: 645–652

17. Kilo J, Czerny M, Gorlitzer M et al. (2001) Cardiopulmonary bypass affects cognitive brain function after coronary artery bypass grafting. Ann Thoracic Surg 72: 1926–1932

18. Klein AL, Stewart WC, Delos M et al. (1990) Visualization of acute pulmonary emboli by transesophageal echocardiography. J Am Soc Echocardiogr 3: 412

19. Koessler MJ, Pitto RP (2002) Fat embolism and cerebral function in total hip arthroplasty. Intern Orthop 26: 259–262

20. Laskin RS (1990) Total condylar knee replacement in patients who have rheumatoid arthritis: A ten-year follow-up study. J Bone Joint Surg 72A: 529–535

21. Lonner JH, Laird MT, Stuchin SA (1996) Effect of rotation and knee flexion on radiographic alignment in total knee arthroplasties. Clin Orthop 331: 102–106

22. Lotke PA, Ecker ML (1977) Influence of positioning of prosthesis in total knee replacement. J Bone Joint Surg 59A: 77–79

23. Mahaluxmivala J, Bankes MJK, Nicolai P et al. (2001) The effect of surgeon experience on component positioning in 673 press fit condylar posterior cruciate-sacrificing total knee arthroplasties. J Arthroplasty 16: 635–640

24. McGrory JE, Trousdale RT, Pagnano MW et al. (2002) Preoperative hip to ankle radiographs in total knee arthroplasty. Clin Orthop 404: 196–202

25. Miehlke RK, Clemens U, Jens JH et al. (2001) Navigation in knee endoprosthesis implantation: preliminary clinical experiences and prospective comparative study with conventional implantation technique. Z Orthop Ihre Grenzgeb 139: 109–116

26. Mont MA, Booth RE Jr, Laskin RS et al. (2003) The spectrum of prosthesis design for primary total knee arthroplasty. Instructional Course Lectures 52: 397–407

27. Monto RR, Garcia J, Callaghan JJ (1990) Fatal fat embolism following total condylar knee arthroplasty. J Arthroplasty 5: 291–299

28. Morawa LG, Manley MT, Edidin AA et al. (1991) Transesophageal echocardiographic monitored events during total knee arthroplasty. Clin Orthop 331: 192

29. Moreland JR (1988) Mechanics of failure of total knee arthroplasty. Clin Orthop 226: 49–64

30. Nizard R (2002) Computer assisted surgery for total knee arthroplasty. Acta Orthop Belg 68: 215–230

31. Oswald MH, Jakob RP, Schneider E et al. (1993) Radiological analysis of normal axial alignment of femur and tibia in view of total knee arthroplasty. J Arthroplasty 8: 419–426

32. Parmet JL, Berman AT, Horrow JC et al. (1993) Thromboembolism coincident with tourniquet deflation during total knee arthroplasty. Lancet 341: 1057–1058

33. Parmet JL, Horrow JC, Singer R et al. (1994) Echogenic emboli upon tourniquet release during total knee arthroplasty: pulmonary hemodynamic changes and embolic composition. Anesth Analg 9: 940–945

34. Petersen TL, Engh GA (1988) Radiographic assessment of knee alignment after total knee arthroplasty. J Arthroplasty 3: 67–72

35. Plaskos C, Hodgson AJ, Inkpen K et al. (2002) Bone cutting errors in total knee arthroplasty. J Arthroplasty 17: 698–705

36. Ranawat CS, Boachie-Adjei O (1988) Survivorship analysis and results of total condylar knee arthroplasty. Clin Orthop 226: 6–13

37. Reed SC, Gollish J (1997) The accuracy of femoral intramedullary guides in total knee arthroplasty. J Arthroplasty 12: 677–682

38. Ritter MA, Faris PM, Keating EM et al. (1994) Postoperative alignment of total knee replacement: Its effect on survival. Clin Orthop 299: 153–156

39. Ritter MA, Herbst SA, Keating EM et al. (1994) Radiolucency at the bone-cement interface in total knee replacement: The effects of bone-surfacing preparation and cement technique. J Bone Joint Surg 76A: 60–65

40. Saragaglia D, Picard F, Chaussard C et al. (2001) Computer-assisted knee arthroplasty: comparison with a conventional procedure: Results of 50 cases in a prospective randomized study. Rev Chir Orthop Reparatrice Appar Mot 87: 18–28

41. Scuderi GR, Scott WN, Tchejeyan GH (2001) The Insall legacy in total knee arthroplasty. Clin Orthop 392: 3–14

42. Sikorski JM, Chauhan S (2003) Computer-assisted orthopaedic surgery: Do we need CAOS? J Bone Joint Surg 85B: 319–323

43. Stern SH, Insall JN (1992) Posterior stabilized prosthesis: Results after follow-up of nine to twelve years. J Bone Joint Surg 74A: 980–986

44. Stulberg SD, Loan P, Sarin V (2002) Computer-assisted navigation in total knee replacement: results of an initial experience in thirty-five patients. J Bone Joint Surg 84A [Suppl 2]: 90–98

45. Teter KE, Bregman D, Colwell CW Jr (1995) Accuracy of intramedullary versus extramedullary tibial alignment cutting systems in total knee arthroplasty. Clin Orthop 321: 106–110

46. Tew M, Waugh W (1985) Tibiofemoral alignment and the results of knee replacement. J Bone Joint Surg 67B: 551–556

47. Wasielewski RC, Galante JO, Leighty R et al. (1994) Wear patterns on retrieved polyethylene tibial inserts and their relationship to technical considerations during total knee arthroplasty. Clin Orthop 299: 31–43

48. Williams-Russo P, Sharrock NE, Mattis S et al. (1995) Cognitive effects after epidural vs. general anesthesia in older adults. JAMA 274: 44–50

49. Yoshino N, Takai S, Ohtsuki Y et al. (2001) Computed tomography measurement of the surgical and clinical transepicondylar axis of the distal femur in osteoarthritic knees. J Arthroplasty 16: 493–497

45 Knee Endoprosthesis Navigation with the *Stryker System*

M. Sparmann, B. Wolke

Strategic Considerations

Cooperation with industrial navigation developers should be made dependent upon whether these companies are prepared to fulfill medical demands on navigation surgery:

- Navigation systems should not only be regarded as aids for positioning endoprostheses (electronic spirit levels), but should also provide for intraoperative kinematic analysis. Particularly in the case of frictional joints such as the shoulder or knee, the analysis of intraoperative kinematics is of far-reaching importance for postoperative function. A reduction of the navigational measurements solely to an alignment of the prosthesis at the same time means a reduction of quality management to the postoperative X-ray image.
- The development of navigation systems should be organized in such a way that the systems are available to the user as open systems, i.e. the user must be free to choose the design of prosthesis during the operation. A reduction of the software to individual products – possibly those of the developing company – leads to a restriction of the physician's freedom of action and thus to a disadvantage for the patient. Open systems not only make it possible to freely choose the implant design, but also to check the kinematic qualities of different endoprostheses, to use kinematic navigation systems in prosthesis development and, above all, to determine mal-positioning of the in-situ prosthesis and its abnormal kinematics in revision cases.
- The development of navigation systems should take into account the economic situation of the health-care institutions. Real-time navigation must be demanded that does not lead to an increase in the costs of individual treatment due to additive imaging diagnostics and manpower, but also a navigation that appropriately exceeds the normal operation times.
- The development of modern navigation systems should include the possibility of allowing interactive processes between the senders and the central hardware. This will make it possible to rapidly build up modules for further joint regions and to change software in quick development steps, in order to make it even more user-friendly. This will minimize the secondary costs, and interactive processes between the LED and the central computer system will thus enable industrial development work that will rapidly encompass the different regions of the body.

Development Steps

The Stryker-Leibinger navigation system has been jointly developed in our department since the autumn of 1999, initially in cadaver experiments, and since March 2000 in a pilot project. Over this period and up to today, the navigation has been repeatedly modified and the software repeatedly coordinated, in order to translate the understanding of the generated data more clearly for the operating team. Further development of the tools for implantation also represented a major development step, especially the development of thin fixation pins for closing the soft-tissue coat at any time. The system is now available in a wireless design. Navigation of the section blocks without additional intra-medullary anchorage is possible; further development steps are envisaged in the use of mini-robots that will perform the osseous sections in the future.

Description of the System

The Stryker knee navigation system is a module for analysis of the leg axes, the alignment of the resection surfaces and thus of the prosthesis components, as well as the kinematics of the knee. The system is a so-called image-less navigation system, i.e. a preoperative three-dimensional reconstruction of the knee based on CT scans is not necessary. Two hardware platforms are available: a laptop and a workstation version. Both platforms are for mobile application and, in addition to the computer, include an infrared camera system, a flat screen and all entry aids. The working area of the system comprises a spherical space with a diameter of 1 m. The system should be set up around 1.5 m from the area of surgery. Communication between the navigation instruments and the camera is wireless via active, light emitting diodes (LEDs). The process is controlled by the operator himself using a specially developed pointer. Foot pedals and similar aids are not necessary. This means that the method does not require people who are familiar with computer systems. No additional persons are necessary in the operating theatre.

To begin with, the first tracker is fixed in place via a small incision in the iliac crest. A further fixation pin is attached to the distal femur and to the proximal tibia within the surgical incision. For this purpose, special rotationally stable fixation pins were developed, which are available both as monocortical and as bicortical. Particular importance was attached to a slim form of the pins in order to avoid soft-tissue compression and to be able to follow joint kinematics both with an opened and a closed joint capsule. After entry of the individual patient data, the system set-up and initialization of the pointer and trackers takes place. The anatomical landmarks are then defined and the center of the femoral head is ascertained by determination of rotation. The epicondylar axis, the Whiteside line, the femur and the tibial center, the malleolae and the center of the ankle are also determined via single-point digitalization. Defects in the femoral condyles and on the tibial plateau are recorded by means of surface digitalization, in order to exactly define the level of resection and to prevent displacement of the joint line.

The actual pathological situation is calculated from the data and the deformities present preoperatively are shown. The calculation is made using mathematical algorithms. From the relative distances between the individual landmarks during different movements, such as varus/valgus, rotational stress or a.p. shifting, a calculation of the kinematic curve is made.

Navigation of the individual resection blocks is done in part with specially developed instruments or using universal gauges. The advantage of this is not only that the Stryker prosthesis families are supported, but also that the system can be used with other prosthesis types (■ Figs. 45-1 to 45-4).

The navigation system analyzes the original pathology, not only in relation to the axis, but also in relation to the kinematics at the initial measurement. intraoperatively, the bone sections can be measured in all freedoms of movement, the surfaces of the bone can be examined after the bone has been prepared, and the intraoperative kinematics after bone resection and soft-tissue balancing are visualized, along with the result after insertion of the original prosthesis and closure of the capsule.

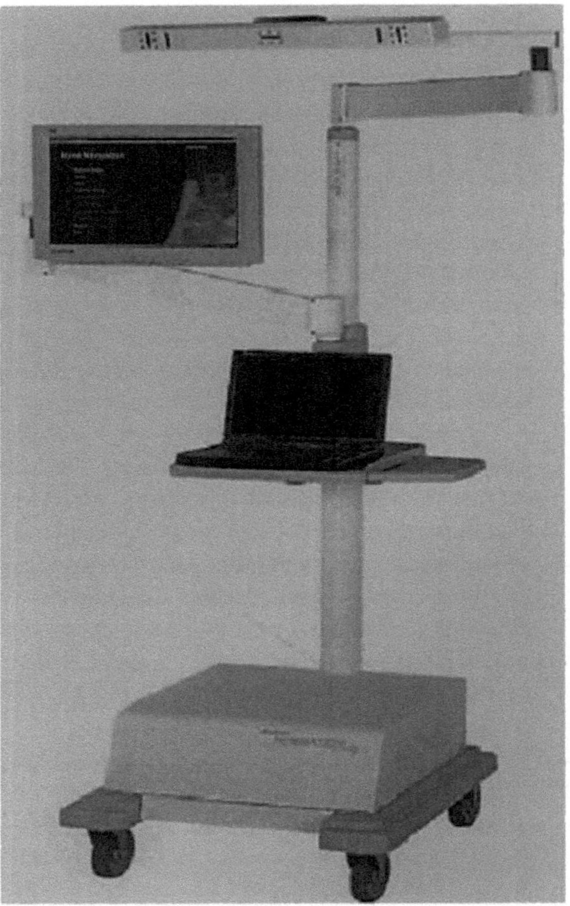

■ Fig. 45-1. Hardware of the Stryker-Leibinger navigation system (three infrared cameras, localizer, laptop and monitor)

In the period from March 2000 to February 2002, a total of 400 knee endoprostheses were implanted under navigation. In order to examine the quality of navigation surgery in knee arthroplasty, a prospective randomized study was conducted from 1 Nov. 2000 to 26 Nov. 2000. Since we were not in a position to conduct a study on this system in our role as its developers, a completely external evaluation was performed. The project was handed over to the German Rheumatism Research Centre, Department of Epidemiology (Prof. Dr. Zink), analysis of the post-operative X-rays was done by an independent radiology institute. A total of 240 patients were included in the study, so that both 120 patients with and 120 patients without navigation underwent surgery. The results showed

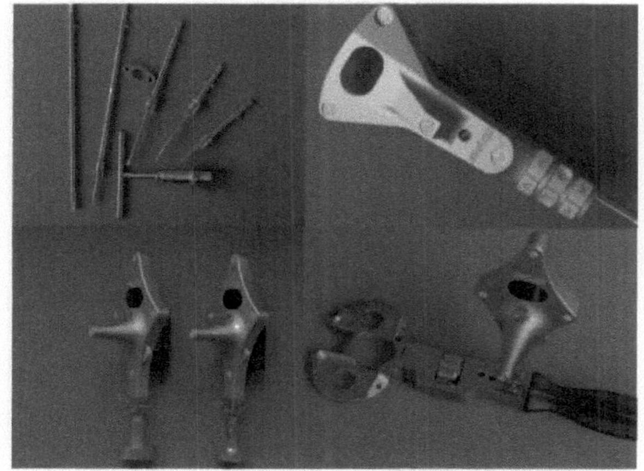

■ **Fig. 45-2.** Pins, LEDs, handle all for rotational alignment on the two beer, pointer

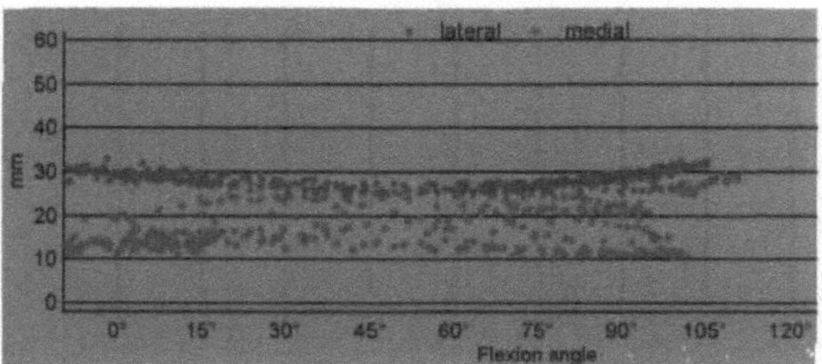

■ **Fig. 45-4.** Kinematic curve for a medial instability. The medial and the lateral joint cavity are displayed separately. In the event of multiple movements and varus/valgus stress, the amplitude of the curve decides stability. This image shows a broadening of the red curve, corresponding to a pronounced medial instability secondary to medial ligament insufficiency

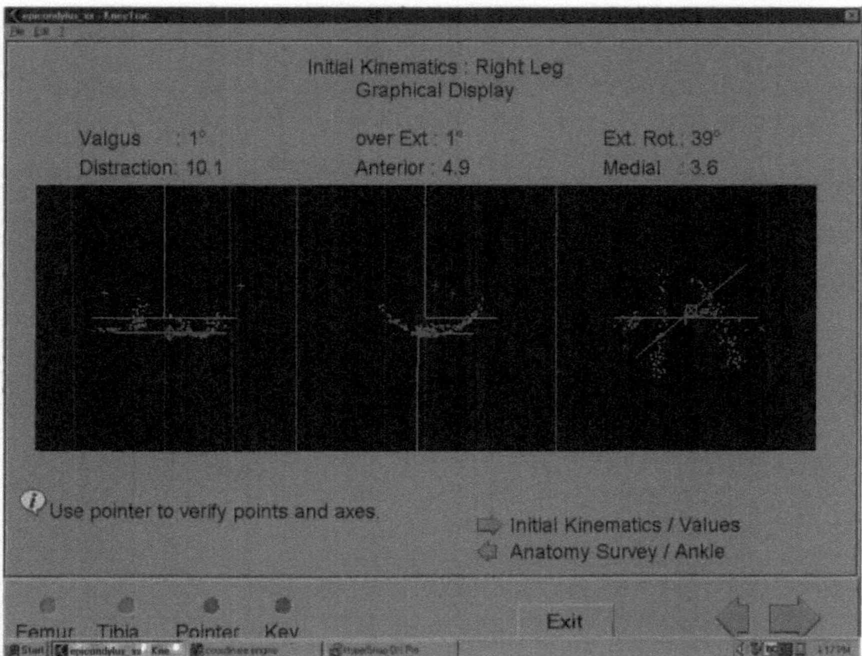

■ **Fig. 45-3.** Primary graphic presentation of the leg axis for varus/valgus, flexion/extension and rotation

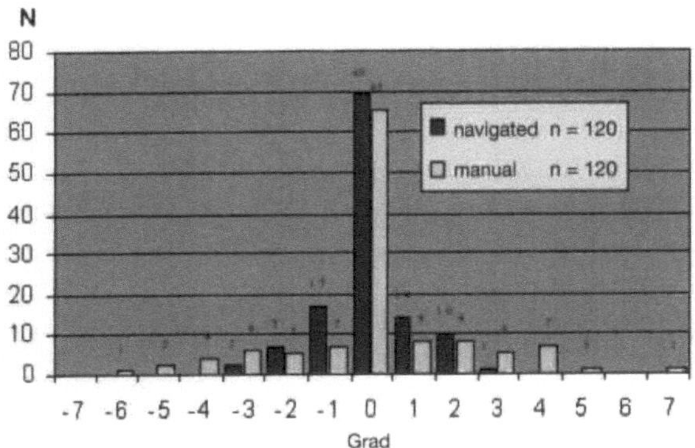

◘ Fig. 45-5. Biomechanical axis of the entire leg. Mechanical axis and prosthesis implant 90° on the mechanical axis (corresponding to 0), the major deviations are only detectable in the manually implanted group

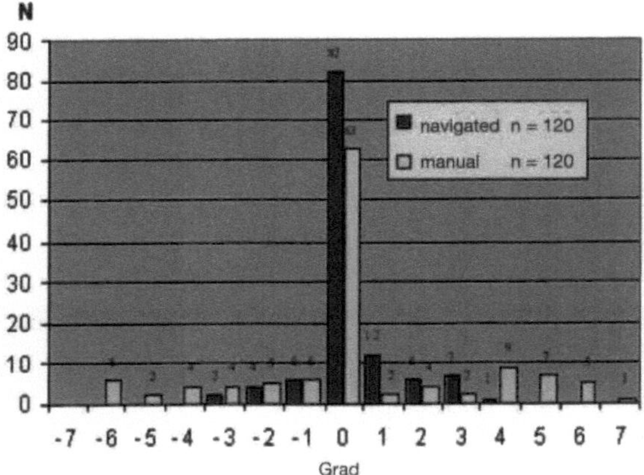

◘ Fig. 45-6. Femoral axis sagittal. In the manual group, considerable deviations result, the 0-degree position is only achieved in individual cases, because the antetorsion of the femoral neck is not optically detected and thus the position of the femoral head cannot be analyzed via the anatomical femoral axis

that there is a highly significant difference between the two groups (Chi-squared test: up to $p<0.0001$), although both groups were operated on by only two surgeons who had both performed more than 1500 primary implantation is. This clearly proves that even experienced surgeons can markedly improve the quality of positioning by using a navigation system. The analysis of the functional results has not yet been completed (◘ Fig. 45-5 and 45-6).

Revision Surgery

Since the Stryker-Leibinger navigation system is an open navigation system, all early revisions of mal-implanted prostheses can also be performed. This dissatisfied patient group is generally composed of patients from surrounding hospitals, which means that a large number of very different implants have to be revised in such revision operations. This navigation system helps to determine the mal-positioning of the implants and the pathological kinematics. The procedure is the same as for primary implantations, the surface measurements of the femur and tibia are taken on the implants. If the implants are successfully removed without loss of bone, the osteotomy can also be examined (◘ Fig. 45-7).

In a total of more than 20 implants, there was a relative mal-rotation of the femoral component. In Germany, it is normal to measure along the condylar line and an external rotation of 3° is preset in the implantation tools, which means that the actual degree of external rotation is often overlooked, since the external rotation is often more

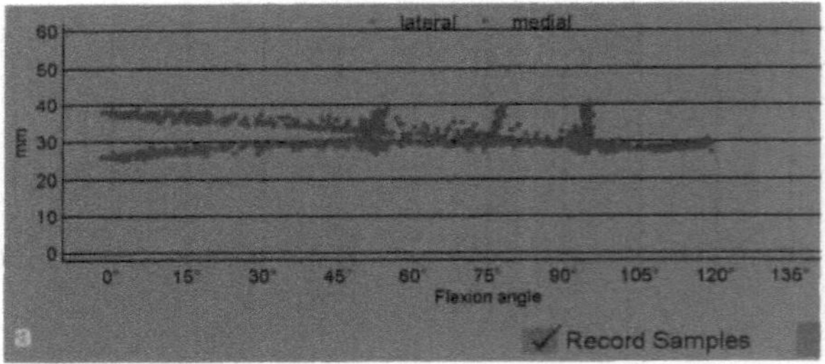

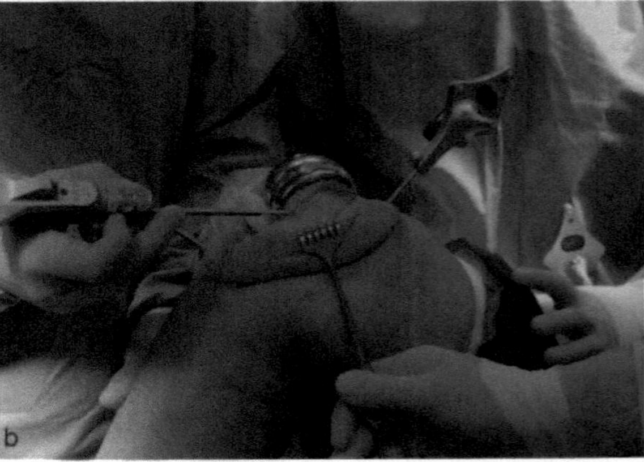

◘ Fig. 45-7a,b. Revision surgery: LED on implant with simultaneous kinematic curve. It can be determined to what extent mal-positioning of the primary implant occurred

than 6°. If, in such cases, the prosthesis is implanted in 3° external rotation, there is a relative internal mal-rotation. This can be very clearly demonstrated on kinematic curves, since increased internal rotation of the femur in flexion results in increasing compression on the medial side and increasing instability on the lateral side (see Fig. 45.4). This mal-positioning then generally leads to a marked restriction in movement or to a feeling of instability, thus necessitating a revision operation. Analysis of the pathologically stressed polyethylene is now possible in biomechanical laboratories with exact angle data.

Future Challenges

Analysis of the intraoperative kinematic data is basically dependent upon the quality of the mathematical algorithms. These were markedly improved over the period of development, so that even incorrectly entered landmarks can be largely eliminated. Serious errors in anatomical localization lead to clearly pathological kinematic curves, so that the surgeon can check the entered anatomical points with the kinematic curve at the beginning of the operation and, if necessary, make a new primary setting. Nevertheless, rotational errors are possible in the case of minor fluctuations of up to 2°. Here, the uptake of additional landmarks and the adjustment of the landmarks among each other is a challenge for the future.

Rotational analysis of the tibia poses a special problem, since few landmarks are available for calculating the rotation. This problem can lead to erroneous rotation data being produced. In such cases, the kinematic curve again shows a markedly pathological change, so that the surgeon is warned of erroneous rotation analysis. However, no navigation systems are capable of determining exact rotational alignment using landmarks at present.

Summary

The Stryker-Leibinger navigation system basically fulfills the demands now formulated by the German Society for Orthopaedics and Orthopaedic Surgery, since it is an open system, a system that analyzes alignment and kinematics, and a system that, in a prospective external study, enabled a clearly significantly better positioning of the implant than with conventional methods. The results of the study show that the improvement in positioning is highly significant, not only in the sum of the mechanical axis, but also in the individual section levels. This navigation system thus represents a considerable improvement for the patient, while helping in the development of new implants, in the entire field of revision surgery and in examining existing implants and their intraoperative kinematics.

References

1. Aglietti P, Buzzi R (1988) Posterior stabilized total condylar knee replacement. Three to eight year follow-up of 85 knees. J Bone Joint Surg 70B : 211–216
2. Aglietti P, Buzzi R, Gaudenzi A (1988) Patellofemoral functional results and complications with the posterior stabilized total condylar knee prosthesis. J Arthroplasty 3: 17–25
3. Delp SL, Stulberg SD, Davies B, Picard F, Leitner F (1998) Computer Assisted Knee Replacement. Clin Orthop Rel Res 354: 49–56
4. Figgi HE, Goldberg VM, Heiple KG, Moller HS, Gordon NH (1986) The influence of tibial-patellofemoral location on function of the knee in patients with posterior stabilized condylar knee prosthesis. J Bone Joint Surg 68A: 1035–1040
5. Jenny JY, Boeri C (2001) Navigiert implantierte Knietotalendoprothesen – Eine Vergleichsstudie zum konventionellen Instrumentarium. Orthopopaede 139: 117–119
6. Krackow KA, Serpe L, Philips MJ, Bayers-Thering M, Mihalko WM (1999) A new technique for determining proper mechanical axis alignment during total knee arthroplasty: Progress toward computer assisted TKA. Orthopedics 22: 698–702
7. Merkow RL, Soudry M, Insall JN (1985) Patella dislocation following total knee replacement. J Bone Joint Surg 67A: 1321–1327
8. Miehlke RK, Clemens U, Jens J-H, Kershally S (2001) Navigation in der Knieendoprothetik – vorläufige klinische Erfahrungen und prospektiv vergleichende Studie gegenüber konventioneller Implantationstechnik. Z Orthop 139: 109–116
9. Oswald MH, Jakob RP, Schneider E, Hoogeworud H (1993) Radiological analysis of normal axial alignment of femur and tibia in view of total knee arthroplasty. J Arthroplasty 8: 419–426
10. Picard F, Digioia AM, Jaramaz B et al. (2000) Computerassistierte Navigationssysteme in der Wiederherstellungschirurgie der Hüft- und Kniegelenke. Orthopädische Praxis 36: 771–778
11. Stern SH, Insall JN (1992) Posterior stabilized prosthesis: Results after follow-up of 9–12 years. J Bone Joint Surg 74A: 980–986
12. Vince KG, Insall JN, Kelly MA (1989) The total condylar prosthesis: 10 to 12 year results of a cemented knee replacement. J Bone Joint Surg 71B: 793–797
13. Wasielewski RC, Galante JO, Leighty R, Natarajan RN, Rosenberg AG (1994) Wear patterns on retrieved polyethylene tibial inserts and their relationship to technical considerations during total knee arthroplasty. Clin Orthop 299: 31–43

46 Capabilities and Limits of Kinematically Based Navigation Systems in Total Knee Arthroplasty

C. Stukenborg-Colsman, C. Hurschler, S. Ostermeier, K. Knabe, H. Windhagen, F. Gossé

Introduction

Soft-tissue balancing and geometrically correct positioning with respect to the bony axes both play an equally important role during prosthesis implantation in total knee arthroplasty. The possible presence of ligamentous instabilities, and the thereby resulting incorrect loading of the prosthesis increase the risk of polyethylene wear and early loosening of the prosthesis.

Even for the experienced surgeon, it is a technical challenge to achieve optimal component alignment while still taking soft tissue balancing into consideration. Conventional instruments in use today utilize intra- and extra-medullar mechanical alignment aids in order to achieve correct alignment. The alignment aids are often of only limited accuracy since their alignment is determined more by eye than based on objective landmarks. Furthermore, positioning of the cutting blocks is often not possible in a continuous manner, but restricted to predetermined adjustment increments. Since mechanical orientation aids must be constructed for an »average« standard leg, limited adaptation to individual variations can be achieved.

Computer-Aided Knee Prosthesis Implantation

First experiences with robot-assisted implantation have been made. However, these systems are, not least because of their high acquisition costs, only being used in a small number of centers. First accounts suggest that correct leg axis alignment was achieved using this procedure. It was further shown that active robotic surgical systems could produce more precise bone resection surfaces than was possible with conventional saw blades. The amount of effort involved, however, is much higher in comparison to manual navigation systems due to the required preoperative planning and computed tomographic (CT) imaging. Furthermore, the possibility of intraoperatively changing preoperative planning is not possible in these systems. Soft tissue balancing is also not taken into consideration.

The manual navigation system is most commonly found in service today. The first manual navigation system was the OrthoPilot system, which was presented in 1999 by the Aesculap company (Aesculap AG & CO. KG, Tuttlingen, Germany). Today, multiple additional systems can be found on the market. Most of the presently available systems function according to the principle of »Surgeon-Defined Anatomy« since the data necessary to carry out and plan the operation are obtained intraoperatively from anatomical landmarks: Preoperative CT image data and their intraoperative display are thus not necessary.

Knee Track Navigation System

The Knee Track navigation system, which has been in service in our clinic since 2001, was developed by the Stryker/Leibinger company (Stryker Leibinger GmbH & Co KG, Freiburg, Germany). This system is of the so-called »open« type with which, in principal, any knee prosthesis may be navigation-implanted. The dynamic reference base, with light emitting diode equipped surgical instruments and implant-guides, sends infrared light impulses which are captured by an infra-red camera. The infrared camera is in turn interfaced with a personal computer (PC) which is capable of processing three-dimensional images in real-time. The intraoperatively attained patient-landmark information is linked to the current position of the instruments by the PC. In order to correct for intra-operatively occurring relative motions of the bone and instruments, it is necessary to continuously acquire the relative motion of the instruments with respect to bone. It is thus necessary to establish a dynamic basis of reference on the operated bones (femur and tibia). The entire system is controlled by the operating surgeon by means of a sterile LED pointer device (☐ Fig. 46-1).

The navigated total knee arthroplasty is performed with the Knee Track system according to the following steps:

1. Attachment of the reference pins on the anterior iliac spine, the distal femur, and the proximal tibia.
2. Measurement of the anatomic landmarks, and determination of the centers of the hip and ankle joints.
3. Measurement of knee joint kinematics.
4. Navigation of the saw guides and completion of the saw cuts.
5. Insertion of the trial prosthesis components.
6. Measurement of intraoperative knee joint kinematics.
7. Performance of soft-tissue balancing.
8. Check knee joint kinematics.
9. Implantation of prosthesis components.
10. Check post-operative knee kinematics.
11. Documentation.

Navigation systems for knee arthroplasty are currently being implemented with great enthusiasm. Whether or not the use of these systems leads to longer survivability of knee prosthesis can at this point in time still not be answered. Nonetheless, based on already attained experience, it is possible to answer the question whether the Knee Track system in particular addresses known problems occurring during knee prosthesis implantation.

Preoperative Planning

preoperative analysis of alignment, the possible occurrence of bony defects, and the degree of soft tissue contraction are relevant. It is difficult to avoid inaccuracies in measurements from roentgenographs such as the anterior-posterior overview under load bearing, the medial-lateral view of the knee joint, and the patella tangential view, even when the pictures are of a high quality. Morland et al. defined the radiologic exact position of the center of the hip, knee and ankle joints [4]. Nonetheless, the neck-shaft-angle (CCD-angle) is changed by projection effects in the roentgenograph, which leads to a tendency to underestimate the angle between the anatomic femoral axis and the mechanical axis (Mikulic line or load bearing axis) of the leg.

Three dimensional alignment can only be partially estimated, even after careful planning, because possible transverse plane mal-rotations of the distal femur and the tibia cannot be reliably recognized in standard roentgenographs.

Preoperative planning in free-hand systems is also based on conventional roentgenographs since capture of the necessary data for planning and execution of the operation first occurs intraoperatively after measurement of the anatomic landmarks. The use of an active navigation system (i.e a surgical robot) requires the acquisition

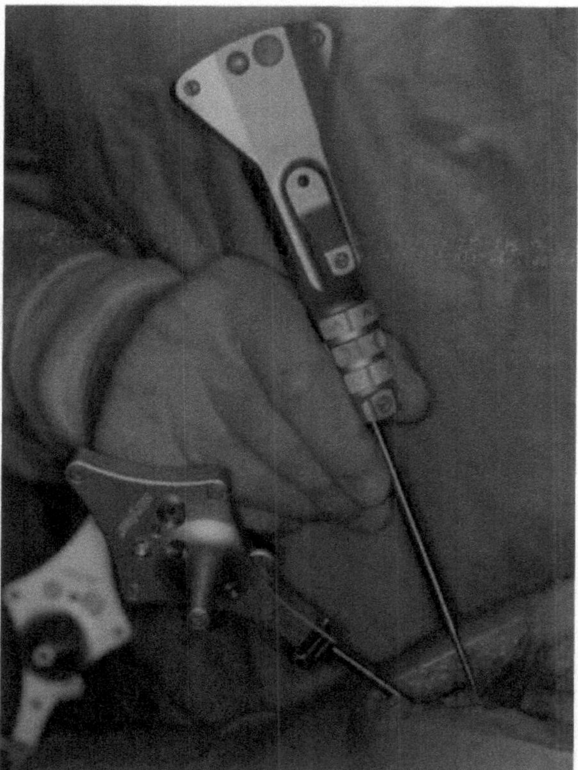

☐ **Fig. 46-1.** Knee track pointer

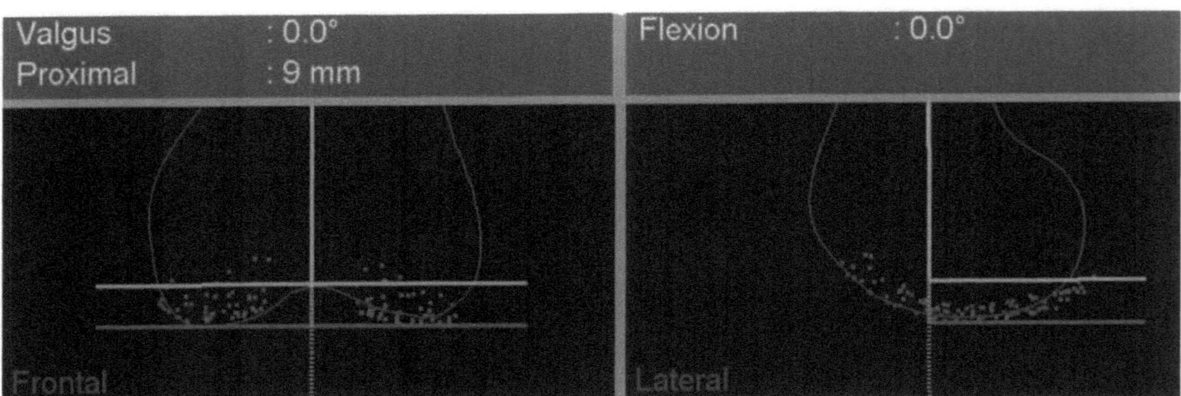

Fig. 46-2. Alignment of the femoral cutting guide

of a planning CT image of the to be operated extremity. Computed tomography or fluoroscopy based navigation systems are nonetheless also already undergoing clinical trials (Brainlab, Heimstetten, Germany; Medivision, Oberdorf, Switzerland).

Preparation of the Femur

Alignment of the femur component in the frontal plane (varus-valgus orientation) and sagittal plane (slope) already occurs through the placement of the distal femoral saw cut. The goal is to achieve 90° alignment of the femur component in both planes relative to the load-bearing axis of the femur. The width of the extension gap is influenced by the superior-inferior orientation of the resection. Conventionally, this sagittal resection is usually guided through the insertion of an intra-medullar alignment rod which follows the axis of the femoral shaft. The height of the resection is aligned on the further distally reaching femoral condyle, while the resection itself is then made with a valgus angle of from 5° to 7° relative to the intra-medullar axis.

Alignment along the femoral axis can, however, be problematic in the presence of large anatomic deviations, as for example often seen during post-traumatic deformities of the femur. The use of thicker guide rods improves the accuracy of the alignment, but also increases the risk of fat embolism. The entrance opening of the guide rod, which is conventionally located from preoperative roentgenograms and the intraoperative situation presents an additional problem.

The insertion of the guide rod is no longer necessary when using the Knee Track system. The cutting block for this important first cut is aligned according to the kinematic and mathematical computation of the mechanical axis of the leg by the navigation system (**Fig. 46-2**). The distal femur is finally prepared by further cuts with support of the Knee Track system which controls transverse plane rotation since this rotation has a large effect on the later function of the prosthesis. Insufficient external or even internal rotation of the femoral component can lead to lateralization or subluxation of the patella caused by over tensioning of the lateral retinaculum. Mal-rotation of the femoral component relative to the tibial component can lead to increased pressure or shear loading and increased polyethylene wear. A mal-rotation of the femoral component can not least lead to varus or valgus instability.

The following alignment tools were used during programming of the Knee Track software to allow for correctly aligned implantation of the femoral component.

- Orientation on the posterior condyle tangent and external rotation of 3°.
- Alignment parallel to the »Whiteside-Line«.
- Alignment parallel to the transepicondylar axis.
- Creation of a symmetrical flexion gap.

Preparation of the Tibia

Navigation-aided alignment of the tibial plateu follows in the frontal and sagittal planes. The frontal plane saw cut is aligned at a right angle to the loading axis. Intra- and extra-medullar guide tools are available to perform this alignment using conventional instruments. During extra-medullary alignment, the center of the ankle joint is visually determined and the instrument is connected to the center of the tibial plateau by the surgeon. The use of an intra-medullar guide dependent on the presence of a suitable anatomic shape of the tibia. During use of the Knee Track system, the previously defined landmarks are again used as an aid for alignment of the saw guide in the frontal and sagittal planes.

The alignment of the tibial saw cut in the sagittal direction can be adjusted according to anatomic variations so that either a dorsally falling slope or a right angle to the loading axis is achieved (◘ Fig. 46-3). The depth of the resection of the tibial cut is determined by conventional means with help of a depth gauge when utilizing the Knee Track system. The size of the implanted component as well as the navigated orientation of the tibial component in the transverse direction (rotation) are determined after completion of the tibial bone resection. The determination of well-defined anatomic landmarks is even more difficult in the tibia than in the femur. The following suggestions for rotational orientation of the tibial base plate can be found in the literature:

- Medial third of the tibial tuberosity.
- Posterior tangential to the tibial head.
- Transverse to the tibial head axis.

- Second midfoot vector.
- »Free« rotational »self« positioning.

The carrying out of the tibial saw cut is thus not influenced by the use of a navigation system.

Soft Tissue Balancing

The goal of soft-tissue balancing is a uniform flexion- and extension joint gap and therefore there are identical pressure conditions between the lateral and medial components of the prosthesis in flexion and extension. Conventional instruments, such as the Balancer (Stryker/Howmedica/Osteonics, Duisburg, Germany) for example, today offer orientation and measurement aids to achieve this goal. Through the use of the Knee Track system, the surgeon has access to a dynamic representation of the joint gap, both in graphical and tabular form, during the entire range of motion both with the trial components as well as after implantation of the final components (◘ Figs. 46-4 and 46-5). This representation permits subtle intraoperative soft-tissue balancing, and furthermore delivers an objective representation of this important operative step in the operating protocol. The operative technique actually used for soft tissue balancing does not depend on a

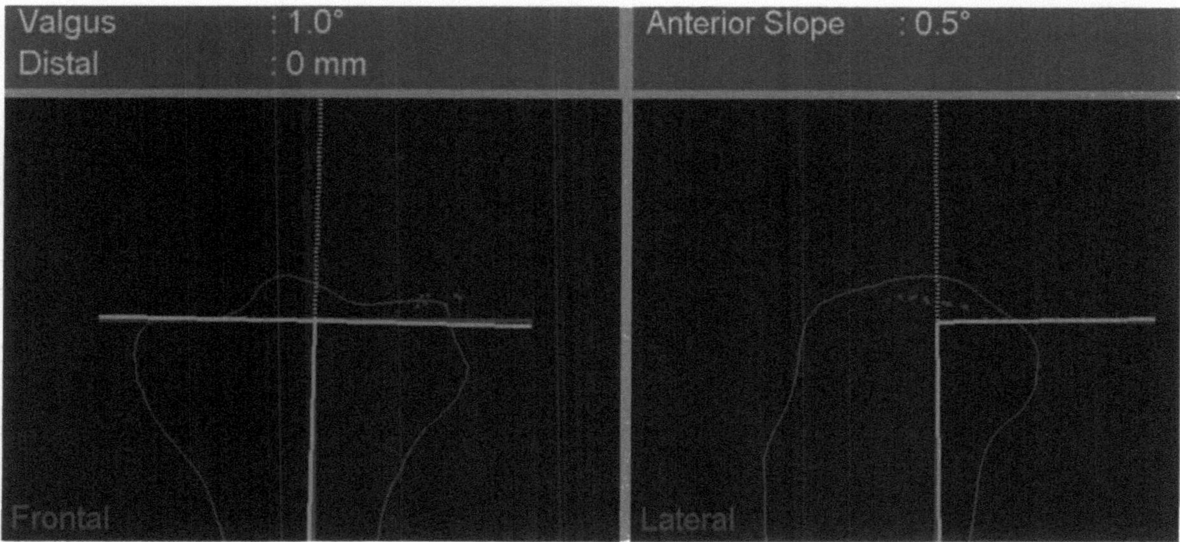

◘ **Fig. 46-3.** Alignment of the tibial cutting guide

+ Flexion	− Extension	Actual -2.0	min -5.0°	0°	+30°	+45°	+60°	+90°	max +90.5°
Valgus	Varus	-0.5°	-4.0°	-3.0°	-5.5°	-4.5°	-6.0°	-4.0°	-3.5°
Internal	External	-6.5°	-23.0°	-18.0°	-17.0°	-21.5°	-18.5°	-8.5°	-7.0°
Frozen Columns :		✓	✓	✓	✓	✓	✓	✓

Fig. 46-4. Table of kinematic parameters

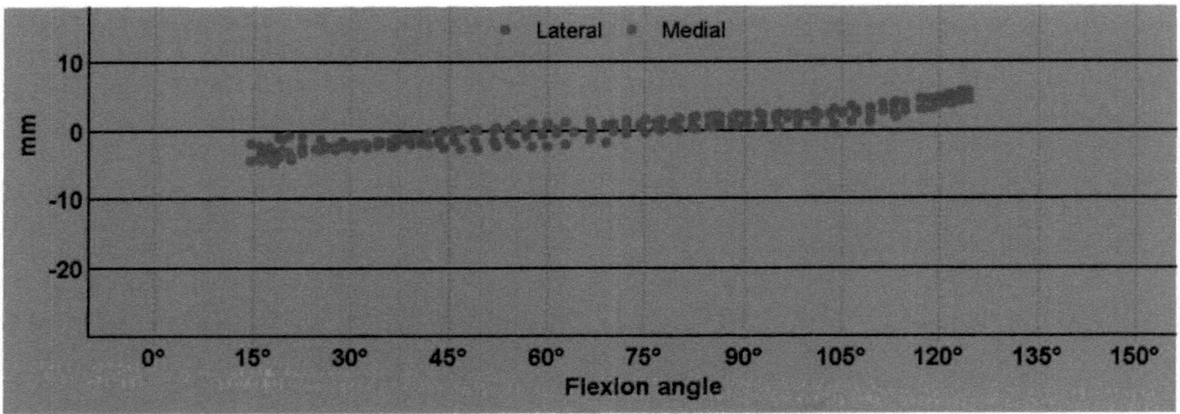

Fig. 46-5. Graphical representation of kinematics

navigation system and will thus not be discussed. The ability to dynamically check soft tissue balancing both before and after implantation of the knee prosthesis is a unique feature of the Knee Track system.

Summary

Navigation systems represent a promising broadening of the operative possibilities in knee arthroplasty. Besides the few systems that offer preoperative planning aids, most systems in use depend on the ability to clearly measure and define anatomical landmarks intraoperatively. The mechanical loading axis is one orientation aid which can be established correctly by means of a kinematic analysis in conjunction with defined bony landmarks. The location of other orientation points used in most systems, such as the epicondyler line of the femur, and the joint line, can be problematic, especially after partial destruction of the condyler joint surfaces as well as the rotation of the tibial component.

Furthermore, until now there exists a lack of consensus regarding how a prosthesis should be optimally aligned relative to the anatomic landmarks. It therefore still remains to be shown whether or not navigation aided cutting guides and prosthesis alignment can provide real benefits in knee arthroplasty long term results despite the presence of these background imprecisions and uncertainties. Besides meeting geometric criteria, modern navigation systems must also be in the position to intraoperatively support the particularly important soft tissue balancing as well as its documentation. The ability to objectively document all operative steps will be of particular interest in joint arthroplasty in view of the ever increasing demands on quality control.

References

1. Clarke HD, Scott WN (2001) Knee: axial instability. Orthop Clin North Am 32:627–637
2. Delp SL, Stulberg SD, Davies B, Picard F, Leitner F (1998) Computer assisted knee replacement. Clin Orthop 354:49–56
3. Gebhard F, Arand M, Fleiter T et al. (2001) Computer assisted surgery, 2001 development and prospects. Results of a congress at Reisenburg Castle, 23–4 November 2000. Orthopäde 30:666–671
4. Kohn D, Rupp S (2000) Knieendoprothetik – Operationstechnische Aspekte. Orthopäde 29:697–707
5. Laskin RS (1995) Flexion space configuration in total knee arthroplasty. J Arthroplasty 10:657–660

47 Fluoroscopy-Based Navigation in Genesis II Total Knee Arthroplasty with the *Medtronic »Viking« System*

F.-W. Hagena, M. Kettrukat, R.M. Christ, M. Hackbart

Introduction

Mal-alignment reduces the survival of total knee replacements. The imbalance of the soft-tissue results in instability of the replaced knee joint. This leads to functional deficits and increased wear.

Computer-assisted technology has been introduced into orthopaedic surgery based on the knowledge that it can improve the precision of surgical procedures. Computerized three-dimensional imaging has been the prerequisite to adapt these techniques. In total knee replacement an optimized alignment to the mechanical axes of the lower limb in comparison to the traditional instrumentation is required. The additional aim is to achieve a correct soft-tissue balancing.

Computer-assisted surgical procedures are based on CT-scan analysis and kinematic evaluation of the anatomy of the lower limb. The acquisition of fluoroscopic imaging for navigation has been described in traumatological procedures [3] Fluoroscopic navigation with the Medtronic system has been widely used in spine surgery [2].

The advantages are a minimum of radiation exposure and the exact and reproducible fixation of pedicle screws. Fluoroscopic-assisted navigation offers a high level of precision and surgical safety [3].

These advantages of minimal radiation and of reproducible accuracy are adapted for the development of a stable software and new instruments for fluoroscopic-assisted navigation in total knee arthroplasty.

The goal is to plan preoperatively and to adjust intraoperatively to the individual anatomy, and to navigate the surgical tools and cutting guides to reduce the human errors. After evaluation of medical images (CT, MRI, fluoroscopy) and correlation to anatomical landmarks, determined by sensors mounted on surgical instruments the physician can be guided during performance [2,3]. At any time the surgeon is able to simulate and to control the precision of each single step of the procedure. This technology leads to a new approach to documenting the individual procedure and performing follow-up studies in the future.

Requirements

Data related to the individual patient's anatomy are required for computer-assisted surgery. Function of the extremity is a prerequisite for the kinematic acquisition of these data. In case of an ankylosis of the adjacent joints (i.e. the hip or ankle joints) the necessary mobility can not be expected. The ankylosing osteoarthritis of the knee also may be an exclusion for kinematic evaluation of the extremity.

For the CT-based navigation preoperative imaging and evaluation has to be performed. This technique needs very sophisticly logistic planning. Even more the radiation exposition for the patients is critical in the routine of total knee replacement. Additionally, the amount of costs have to be considered in relation to the achieved improvement of accuracy on a regular base.

Navigation is »only« a supplementary instrument for the implantation of the knee arthroplasty. For optimal use a learning curve is necessary. Failures may be expected if navigation is only used in »special« cases. Navigation integrated in the routine surgical procedure has to follow these principles: availability, reproducibility, cost-effectiveness and safety. To correspond with these criteria the effort and the costs have to correlate with efficacy. The equipment has to be appropriate to the integration into the routine. Under these postulations the CT-based navigation is at least controversial for the routine of total knee arthroplasty.

In fluoroscopy-assisted navigation of TKA the individual lower limb is evaluated radiographically including all joints: the hip, the knee and the ankle joint. After acquisition of these images in two planes the mechanical axis of the limb is calculated in 3 dimensions.

The availability of these data is not restricted in any way. This information is stored and is available for controls and quality management. The time for fluoroscopic investigation and image acquisition is 8 min and less than 1 min of fluoroscopic radiation.

The surgeon estimates the individual quality of the images and is able to include this information into the further decisive steps of the surgical procedure. The additional time of data acquisition in the operation theatre does not increase the overall time considerably.

Having registered the axes of the limb the surgeon outlines the anatomic landmarks of the femoral condyles and of the tibia plateau with a mobile diode which is mounted to a probe. After complete data evaluation a 3D model of the extremity is calculated. The discrimination of the data is of less than 2 mm and smaller than 2° within the acceptable limits.

Surgical Procedure

The patient is in supine position. A tourniquet is put on the thigh. It may be inflated at any time during the procedure.

A pre-patellar longitudinal skin incision is carried out. To mount the femoral navigation frame this incision is proximally extended about 4 cm longer. Mediopatellar opening of the joint. Proximal and distal of the joint line the navigation frames are mounted to transosseous fixed pins.

Two fluoroscopic images are taken of the joints: the femoral head in 45° angle and in a.p. and lateral view of the knee and ankle joint. The center of the femoral head is identified on the monitor. After registration of the mechanical axes the intra-articular landmarks of the femoral condyles and of the proximal tibia are determined with a free diode. The mechanical femoral axis is defined by the relation of the intercondylar center, the epicondylar axis and the »Whiteside line« at the distal femur to the center of the femoral head. The tibial axis is determined by the a.p. alignment perpendicular to the center of the tibial head and to the center of the distal tibia. The rotational alignment is depending on the midtransversal axis at the

tibial head diverging 10° of the posterior corticalis axis and at the center of the joint surface of the distal tibia.

The resection guides are registered and the osteotomies of the joint surfaces are performed with the navigated instruments. During each step it is possible to adjust the cutting guides within the limits of less than 2 degrees of deviation to the navigated axes.

At any time an intraoperative clinical control and revision is possible. The program and the controls have to be coordinated.

The system offers of the alignment of the trial implants. Dynamic testing during continuous motion and at 0°, 30° and 90° flexion enables the test of the soft tissue balancing. All these tests are documented automatically.

Experience with Fluoroscopic Navigation

Experimental data of fluoroscopic navigation had been presented after cadaver surgery [1]. After further clinical testing the technology of fluoroscopic-assisted navigation had been introduced for clinical studies. At each stage of development a very sophisticated documentation of all data had been collected. The documentation of each step of the surgical procedure is an excellent contribution to quality control and quality improvement. This is a very important advantage of navigation.

During the phase of development of fluoroscopic-assisted navigation an integration of the system into the routine program was not possible. The testing of new instruments has been time consuming. With up to 4 total knee replacements the same day it is not possible to use the navigation system at each procedure because there has been only one set of instruments for navigation available. After some experience and the development of adequate equipment, we are now able to state that the application of the system is now stable, safe and reproducible.

Results

We had the opportunity to start with the clinical application of the fluoroscopic navigation »Viking« in our clinic in May 2001. Out of a total of 240 TKA within the last year, we were able to use the fluoroscopic-assisted navigation system in 50 of the Genesis II TKA. During the early phase of this study we were not able to increase the frequency of application considerably. It is our goal to use the navigation system in each case to achieve optimal results for all patients.

To evaluate the accuracy of the new fluoroscopic navigation system all these patients are introduced into a prospective study design in comparison to traditional implantation techniques. The results of this study is not yet available.

Alignment

The advantage of this system is a control of accuracy at any time of the procedure and it allows an online documentation. Surgical time is slightly increased by the acquisition of the fluoroscopic images (◘ Fig. 47-1). We have to admit that it is still a more time-consuming procedure in comparison to the traditional instrumentation with alignment rods.

We check the alignment of the resection planes regularly during the surgical procedure. The real presentation

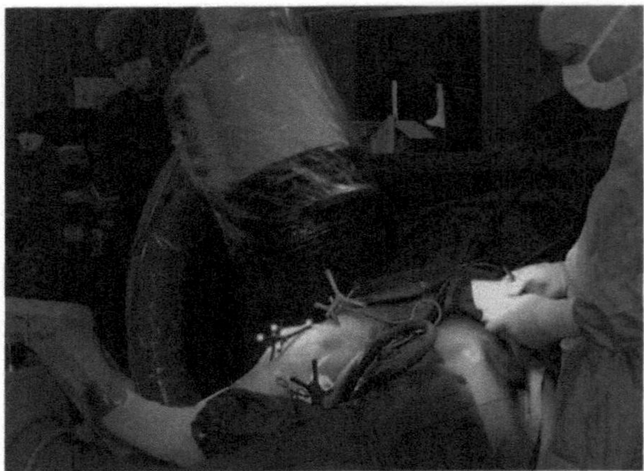

◘ **Fig. 47-1.** Acquisition of the center of the femoral head with mounted navigation frames at the knee

of the fluoroscopic images on the touch-screen facilitates the imagination of the surgeon during the procedure. A virtual line representing the anatomical structures and the position of the limb may have a negative influence on the surgeons' compliance. The intraoperative control shows a very high accuracy of less than 2° degrees deviation (◘ Fig. 47-2).

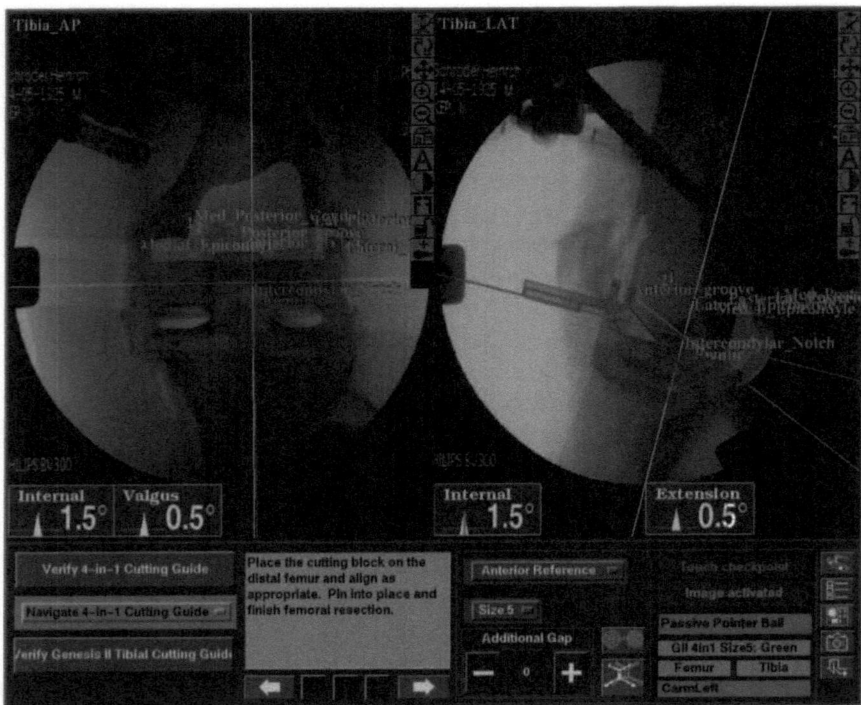

◘ **Fig. 47-2.** The real fluoroscopic image of the knee in combination with the virtual image of the implant on the screen and the results after resection

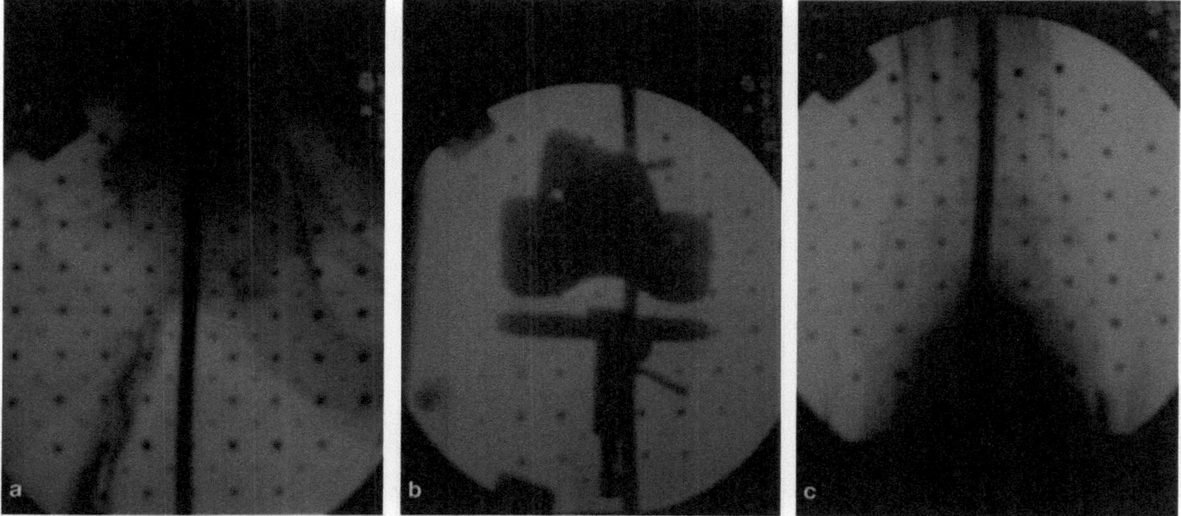

Fig. 47-3a-c. Intraoperative fluoroscopic control after insertion of the trial-implants with the alignment rod. **a** Center of the femoral head, **b** the knee, **c** center of the ankle

It is essential that there are no contraindications for the application of the fluoroscopic-assisted navigation. In contrast, kinematic-based navigation may be limited in case of ankylosing disease of the hip and of the knee which is going to be operated.

Control of the Results Intraoperatively

It is possible to control the results of alignment. The control studies did not show any failure that was related to the navigation system. Even in cases of very severe deformities of the femur or of the tibia (i.e. posttraumatic deformities) the intraoperative control with alignment rods did confirm the exact alignment and the correct implantation of the arthroplasty (◘ Fig. 47-3).

Testing of Soft-Tissue Balancing

Fluoroscopic-assisted navigation with the »Viking« system (Medtronic) offers a great advantage after implantation of the trial implants. It is now possible to check the soft-tissue balancing dynamically and in various degrees of flexion. The tests are documented in neutral 0° and in 90° of flexion. The tests are performed for the following parameters:

- a.p. translation (anterior drawer sign),
- varus- and valgus stress,
- rotational stability.

After these dynamic tests it is still possible to improve soft-tissue balancing by adequate procedures. It is interesting to note that using the »Viking« navigation system we can see that there is hardly any correction of the resection necessary because of the accuracy of implantation of the TKA.

The mean values show excellent results. The tests before the closure of the capsule cause an increased laxity at 90° flexion. The rotating platform of the Genesis II TKA provides a high degree of rotational capacity (◘ Fig. 47-4). After finishing the knee replacement the manual controls did not give any sign of pathologic laxities (◘ Table 47-1).

Limitations of Alignment

The improvements of the designs of knee arthroplasties include the development of better instrumentation techniques to achieve a reproducible alignment to the mechanical axis of the lower limb.

There are still some controversial publications in terms of the navigation-guided instruments. Some of the critical cuts and positions of the implants are depending on the visual analysis by the surgeon.

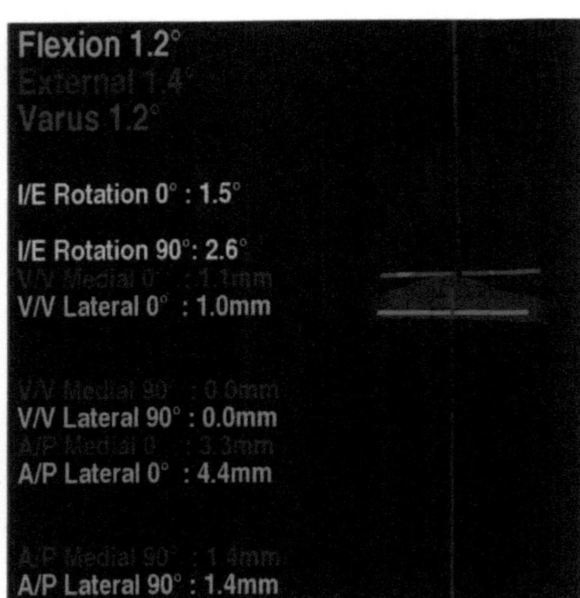

Fig. 47-4. Visualization and documentation of the soft-tissue balancing at 0° and 90° of flexion

Table 47-1. Fluoroscopic-assisted navigation: Genesis II/rotating platform (n=50)

Level of evaluation	Results (median)	Standard deviations
V/V lateral 0°	2,3 mm	0,1 – 5,8 mm
V/V lateral 90°	2,9 mm	–2,7 – 14,3 mm
a.p. lateral 0°	1,9 mm	–5,4 – 6 mm
a.p. lateral 90°	2,9 mm	–8,0 – 6,4 mm
I/E rotation 0°	3,6°	0 – 7,0°
I/E rotation 90°	9°	2,0 – 16,9°

V/V Varus/Valgus, *a.p.* Translation, *I/E* internal/external rotation.

Variables for alignment in TKA

- Intercondylar femoral center
- Transepicondylar axis of the femur
- Rotation of the tibia
- Center of the distal tibia
- Position of the patella implant

It is well accepted that it is not possible to define the epicondyles as a point at the distal femur. Using the fluoroscopic-assisted navigation system it is possible to exactly define the center of the femoral head and of the distal tibial joint surface. But still it is difficult to accurately describe the rotation of the tibia.

Time of Surgical Procedures

A continuous reduction of the total time of the surgical procedures have been registered for the fluoroscopic-assisted navigation during the experience of more than 12 months. With a total time of 90 min cut to finish of surgery a reasonable time has been achieved. This is not only true for the senior author but also for 3 senior surgeons at our hospital. This could be demonstrated during various visits of other colleagues. We are now going to include the online documentation of the timing into our software program.

The testing of soft-tissue balancing is a new part of the surgical procedure which justifies additional time. The graph demonstrates the »learning curve« during the first applications of the navigation system (**Fig. 47-5**). The black line »trial alignment« of this graph shows the time of laxity tests that are about 10 minutes unchanged. It is expected that this time will be reduced in the future also.

Additional Efforts for Navigation

Navigation in total knee arthroplasty is in a stage of development. At the phase of application it is not only time-consuming. During the first 20 navigated TKA one more

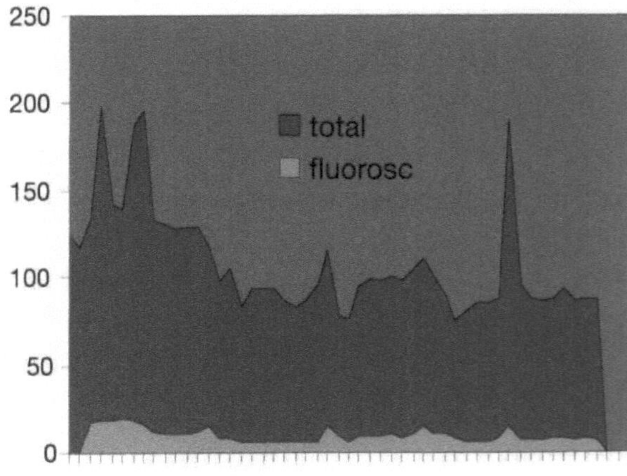

Fig. 47-5. Additional time for navigation

nurse has been needed to adjust the camera during the navigation. The use of fluoroscopic investigation and registration took more time during the first cases than it was necessary later. The exact positioning and the stable fixation of the navigation frames has been established after our experience. The development of special instruments for navigated total knee arthroplasty will help to reduce the time of surgery even more.

Discussion

Various systems to navigate the total knee arthroplasties are already available. Kinematic-based navigation shows the advantage that it is applied independently of any imaging. The disadvantage seems to be the limitation in case of severe joint contracture and ankylosis of the knee and of the adjacent hip joint. Also patients with greater masses of soft tissues surrounding the knee are excluded of this method. The results do not confirm a higher degree of reproducibility. As limiting factors for kinematic based-navigation

- the variability of the surgeons,
- the value of surface registrations and
- movements of the navigation frames

had been identified as problems [4].

The CT-based navigation may give the highest degree of accuracy. The fact that this method is depending on CT scan preoperatively is restricting its application. This technology is not available in all hospitals and it needs more time and more radiation exposure for the image acquisition and it is very expensive in the routine.

Fluoroscopic navigation seems to give the best solution. It offers a very high degree of accuracy and the best way of reproducibility. The reduction of radiation using the fluoroscopy is an advantage for the surgeon [5]. At any time the update of the imaging is available. It is less time-consuming than the CT-based navigation. The online imaging on the screen offers an excellent compliance for the surgeon. The time for surgery used for documentation and laxity tests seems in good relation to the improved quality.

Prospective studies are planned to verify the significance of this system.

References

1. Carson C, Lyons C, Salehi A (2002) Accuracy validation of an image guided surgical system for total knee arthroplasty. Orthopedic Research Society, 48th Annual Meeting, Dallas, Abstract
2. Foley KT, Simon DA, Rampersaud YR (2000) Virtual fluoroscopy. Oper Tech Orthop 10:77–81
3. Hofstetter R, Slomczykowski M, Sati M, Nolte L-P (1999) Fluoroscopy as an imaging means for computer-assisted surgical navigation. Computer Aided Surg 4:65–79
4. Stulberg D, Loan P, Sarin V (2001) Computer-assisted total knee replacement surgery: an analysis of an initial experience with Orthopilot system. Computer Aided Surg 6:124
5. Suhm N, Jacob Al, Nolte L-P, Regazzoni P, Messmer P (2000) Surgical Navigation based on fluoroscopy – clinical application for computer-assisted distal locking of intramedullary implants. Computer Aided Surgery 5:391–400

48 CT-Based Planning and Individual Template Navigation in TKA

F. Portheine, J.A.K. Ohnsorge, E. Schkommodau, K. Radermacher

Introduction

Among the various modalities of alloarthroplasty of the knee joint the total endoprosthesis is the most often executed intervention in the world. Severe arthrosis and axial deformities up to 30° varus or valgus can thereby be equalized. Today's high quality standard of surgical treatment requires anatomically correct orientation and fitting of the implant aiming at optimal biomechanical functionality. Thus, the single components must be taken into account as well as functional changings of tension in the surrounding soft tissue.

Besides the individual wear and tear of the prosthesis depending on a more or less active patient its durability is influenced to a great extent by the accuracy of its implantation. There is a common consensus about inexact alignment and negligent placement causing early failure of artificial knee joints several authors [1–3, 7, 12] and little later Insall et al. [4] report on axial deviation of hardly more than 3°, or the Maquet line passing by the medial third of the prosthesis in the a.p. view, respectively, being the most frequent reason. These findings are remarkable, as conventional TKA often leads to unfavorable results despite conscientious planning and responsible performance of the operation. ◘ Table 48-1 reviews postoperative data published in literature concerning the articular alignment after conventional and computer-assisted implantation.

Jeffrey et al. [5] and Tew et al. [16] assessed persisting axial deficiency in approximately one third of all conventionally operated cases all affecting the longevity of the implant. In the same context Stern et al. [15] reported on various cases of extreme deviation.

Various computer-assisted planning systems and navigation tools have been developed lately to realize a higher degree of surgical accuracy regarding geometric conformity between preoperative concept and postoperative outcome. Relative improvement of results e.g. by the use of the OrthoPilot system as also shown in Table 48.1 go

◘ **Table 48-1.** Postoperative results for total knee arthroplasty

Author	Deviation				Cases	Type of intervention
		Area		Absolut		
	Angle	Percent	Varus	Valgus		
Jeffery et al. [5]	>3°	32			115	Conventional
Tew et al. [16]	>5°	34			428	Conventional
Tew et al. [16]	>9°	7			428	Conventional
Stern et al. [15]			6°	16°	289	Conventional
Kiefer et al. [6]	>2°	55	8°	8°	50	Conventional
Kiefer et al. [6]	>2°	25	8°	10°	100	OrthoPilot
Saragaglia et al. [13]	>3°	25			25	Conventional
Saragaglia et al. [13]	>3°	16			25	CATKA/OrthoPilot
Miehlke et al. [9]	>2°	38,3	7°	4°	60	OrthoPilot
Miehlke et al. [9]	>2°	43,3	6°	8°	30	Conventional
Miehlke et al. [9]	>2°	36,6	4°	7°	30	OrthoPilot

together with an important intraoperative expenditure of time and manpower for technical execution. Attempts of a so-called »soft-tissue balancing« turned out to be insufficient so far. Therefore, research at the IBMT (Institute of Biomedical Technologies, Aachen, Germany) and at the Orthopaedic department of the University of Aachen focused on the development of a system for preoperative planning based on CT scans that allows a realistic simulation of functional extension of the collateral ligaments of the knee according to differing position and size of the implant that likewise can deliberately be adapted to the individual requirements. For optimal transposition of the planning result to the anatomy the approved individual templates [11] are an especially suited tool for its intraoperative use is technically simple and can be performed both quickly and with high accuracy. Triple pelvic osteotomy and pedicle screw implantation have successfully been carried out with the help of individual templates in the past. Scientific findings from clinical evaluation studies have led to decisive improvements of the new CAOS system (computer-assisted orthopaedic surgery). With the module for knee arthroplasty it has been supplied with an application offering geometric accuracy and ergonomic proceeding.

Problems of Conventional TKA

Instrumentation sets and conventional assisting tools for correct total knee replacement depend on the producers standardizations and are universally employed to all patients. The individual anatomy or particular biomechanical details can only partly be considered in the standardized procedures. The intraoperative definition and control of the mechanical axes is decisive for the successful completion of the operation but sometimes also difficult. Due to the vast covering with blankets of the patient rested in an abnormal position on the operation table – sometimes in combination with important deformities of the long bones – incorrect determination of osseous landmarks and correlation with extra-medullary adjustment devices are quite likely.

The plane of the femoral reference osteotomy, which has to be oriented relative to the mechanical axes of the femur, cannot be defined exactly just by using the intra-medullary rod, as this only permits detection of the anatomical axis. Cutting is usually performed according

to measurements in two-dimensional radiographs quantifying the discrepancy of both axes. Moreover, numerous studies showed that differing radii of femoral curvature are responsible for incoherency of the anatomical axis with the one suggested by the intra-medullary rod [8] and that just by inconstant choice of the point of insertion variations up to 8.3° are possible [10].

The conventional planning is limited regarding the size of the implant as well as regarding the assumption of the postoperative range of motion and the over-all functionality of the artificial joint, as the latter is strongly dependant on all factors debated above. As a tribute to the solution of this complex problem a singular approach was made up.

CT-Based Operation Planning System

The preoperative planning software used for soft-tissue management and implant selection is based on DISOS (Desktop Image Processing System for Orthopaedic Surgery) that is applied clinically since several years together with individual templates for the above mentioned applications. The system is easy to handle, the menu can be controlled intuitively by the medical staff without the need of extensive instruction. This uncomplicated applicability was achieved by integration of medical knowledge and skills focusing algorithms on the specific task, leaving to the operator the responsibility for just a few decisions. With DISOS-TKA the surgeon himself disposes of a number of auxiliary devices and functionalities that before were only available to specialized engineers on CAD systems (computer-aided design). The software guides the user through a series of planning steps, provides him with additional information if requested and helps verifying the plausibility of the interactive process. That is composed of four consecutive sequences:
- individual biomechanical analysis,
- selection of implants and planning of osteotomies,
- functional analysis and soft-tissue balancing,
- fabrication of individual templates.

Individual Biomechanical Analysis

Quantification of axial deformities requires the exact definition of the mechanical axes of the femur and the tibia. Image-based measuring is possible by means of CT-generated topographic scout-views or in a 3D model after reconstruction out of CT slices. Especially the reduction of radiation exposure and costs favor the use of two scout views that offer the complete aspect of the extremity in orthogonal planes like classic radiographs do, which makes the comparison to postoperative X-ray control much easier. Schkommodau et al. [14] proved that data can be transferred from one modality to the other if coordination follows equal parameters. As it gives a more realistic impression, measurements are set to be done by landmark identification within the topographic overview, all preserving the possibility of doing so in the 3D model (◘ Fig. 48-1, left).

The conventional depiction of the femoral and tibial mechanical axes is based on the punctual determination of the center of the femoral head and of the intercondylar notch as well as of the center of the intercondylar eminence and that of the ankle joint. The method is limited to 2D information, unlike the new planning system that allows 3D depiction by assembling calculations from a.p. and lateral plane taking into account the position of the joint and the leg itself. The degree of rotational deviation from the neutral position of the leg for instance can easily be detected in a single CT slice by virtual connection of the epicondyles (◘ Fig. 48-1, right). These deviations can be mathematically neutralized in order to avoid misjudgement of the 2D X-ray projection as a varus or a valgus deformity.

Selection of Implants and Planning of Osteotomies

Exact planning and execution of the osteotomies are essential for perfect fitting and correct position of the prosthesis. They can be classified subsequent to their function as a reference to the planning and as a profile cutter to the implant. The **reference osteotomy** is dependent on the individual biomechanical analysis and is supposed to guarantee ideal function and alignment according to the result of the preoperative planning procedure.

Whereas the mutual relations of the **clear-cutting osteotomies** are directly defined by the design of the elected implant (◘ Fig. 48-2), their orientation depends on the reference osteotomy. Once that cut is made, a multi-cutting block usually procures reliable profiling all-in-one. As a matter of course the main interest of computer-assisted total knee arthroplasty applies to precise planning and performance of the reference osteotomies as decisive factors to a favorable out-come.

Aiming at a so-called **classic alignment**, the specific reference osteotomies would be planned and executed rectangular to the previously defined mechanical axes. Usually preoperative deformities up to 30° of deviation can be equalized this way. However, in cases of extreme deformity, for example where a complete compensation is not desirable, the system leaves all options to the planning surgeon. In cases of a recommended anatomic alignment the relative inclination of the resection plane can be

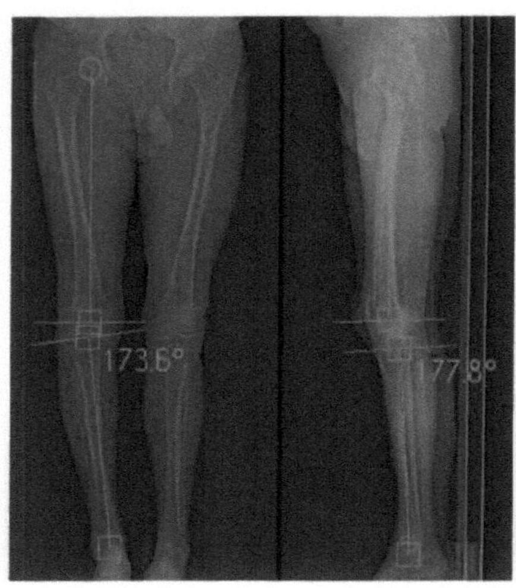
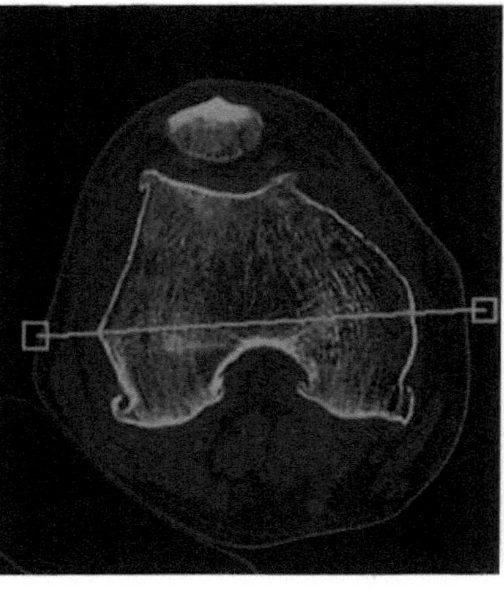

◘ **Fig. 48-1.** Measurement of the anatomical and mechanical axis

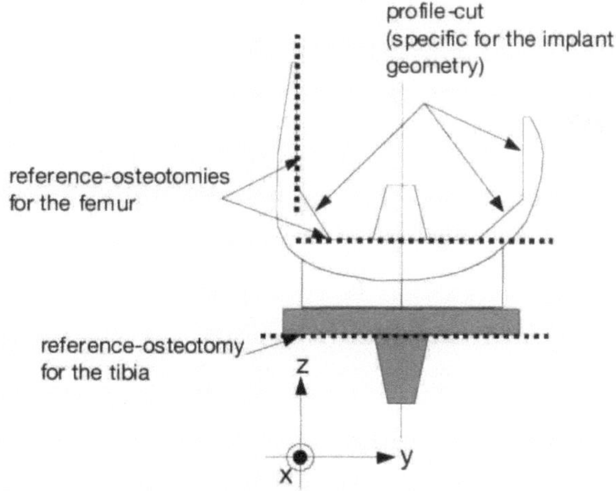

Fig. 48-2. Classification of the osteotomies for TKA

realized to the corresponding degree. Another option refers to a slope that is sometimes required from the manufacturing side as the design of the implant is founded on such a basic ventro-dorsal inclination. By implementation of the specific CAD data of the implants in question such specific standards are automatically represented in the setting of DISOS-TKA so that the planning of the reference osteotomy always follows individual conditions.

After the orientation of the plane being definitely accomplished its position along the mechanical axis still stays adjustable by tuning one single degree of freedom (**□** Fig. 48-3). This proceeding is necessary to enable soft-tissue balancing and is analogous for the tibial and the femoral side. For simultaneous quality control of bone, the corresponding sectional view is reconstructed out of

3D CT data to ensure a sufficient osseous support to the prosthesis (see Fig. 48-3).

Virtual simulation assists on selecting the perfect fitting implants out of a broad variety of different designs and sizes. The specific geometric data of the preferred products can deliberately be added to the software according individual needs.

Functional Analysis and Soft-Tissue Balancing

Not only can the implant itself be simulated in company with the 3D anatomy model but also physiological joint motion and consecutive alteration of length of the collateral ligaments. This is realized by the use of a volumetric elastic model called »**mass-spring-model**« of each ligament consisting of around 10,000 elements of defined physical properties. As CT imaging does not allow automatic segmentation of the ligamentous insertions these are defined over a stereometric approach based on statistical models and demographic data. In combination with the segmented surface of the bone the elastic deformation of the ligaments during flexion-extension and differing degrees of rotation can be simulated (**□** Fig. 48-4). By means of an integrated analysis algorithm the most favorable position of the implants in terms of biomechanical functionality can be determined. Hence the suitability of the designated implant and its position can be tested and adjusted. The necessity and the extent of intra-operative soft-tissue release can be estimated preoperatively. The risk of postoperative dysfunction with inconstant tension of the soft tissue and incongruity of the ar-

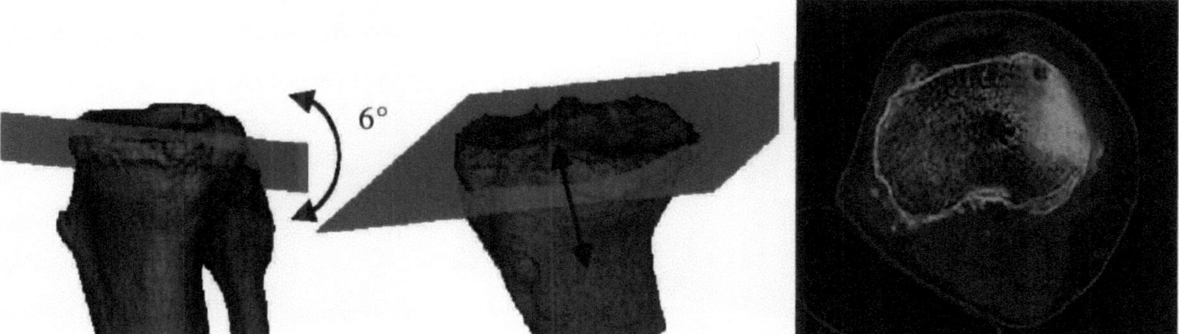

Fig. 48-3. Determination of the tibia reference osteotomy with grey-cut control view (showing the quality of bone)

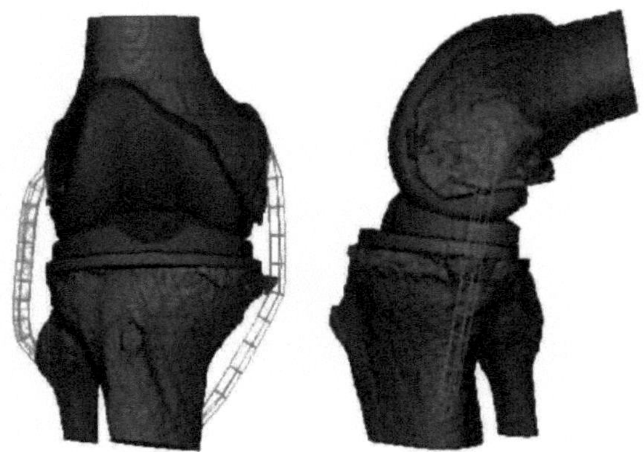

Fig. 48-4. Simulation of the changing length of the ligaments during motion enables the surgeon to define optimal position and suitable size of the femoral and tibial components

tificial articular surfaces should thus be diminished. Consequent failure due to excessive wear and early loosening for instance might decrease as well on the long term.

Definition of Individual Templates

When the planning is completed the results must be transferred to the patient. Inaccurate proceeding for this purpose endangers all improvement gained by the previous planning process. In this context, any form of navigation comes into question, but particularly the individual template [11] bears the possibility of direct reference to the 3D model that the planning is based upon.

The technique relies on the exact reproduction of the bone surface as a negative print. The individual pattern is copied from the virtual reality by computer-controlled milling into a blank block of polycarbonate. This template is to be firmly connected to the cutting block of the given implant (**Fig. 48-5**). Intra-operatively set on the knee, it only fits to a distinct area and thereby defines clearly the position of the cutting block which can be pin-fixed as usual. The mechanical junction of both is standardized (see Fig. 48.5, center). As all geometric data of the instruments, the template and the anatomy assemble in the same planning software, an unequivocal relation can be established between one and the other. This indicates that the defined reference osteotomy corresponds via the steering slot of the cutting block to a characteristic profile of the template.

The synchronized projection of a virtual model of the template attached to the cutting block during the planning process permits permanent control of the intraoperative feasibility (see Fig. 48.5, left). If the template virtually comes to be situated in a region which would be difficult to expose in reality, the surgeon may displace it along the formerly planned reference osteotomy towards a more appropriate area. This is a very important feature because undisturbed contact of the individual template with the corresponding bone is elementary for successful computer-assistance in this case (see Fig. 48-5, right).

The fabrication of the template takes 15–20 min, depending on the diversity of the contact profile. The blank block can always be shaped according to special demands,

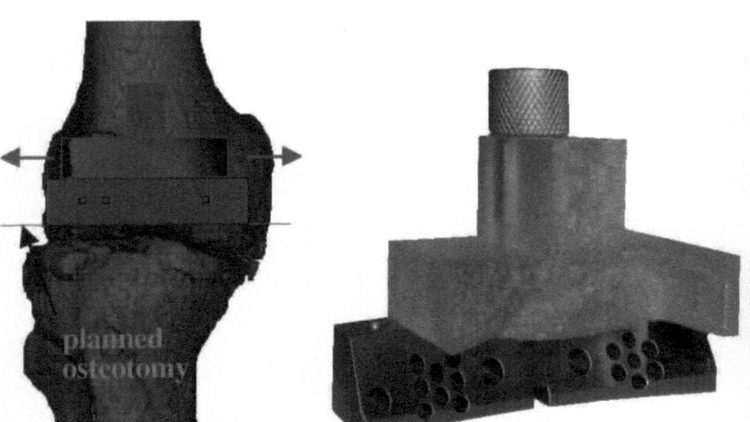

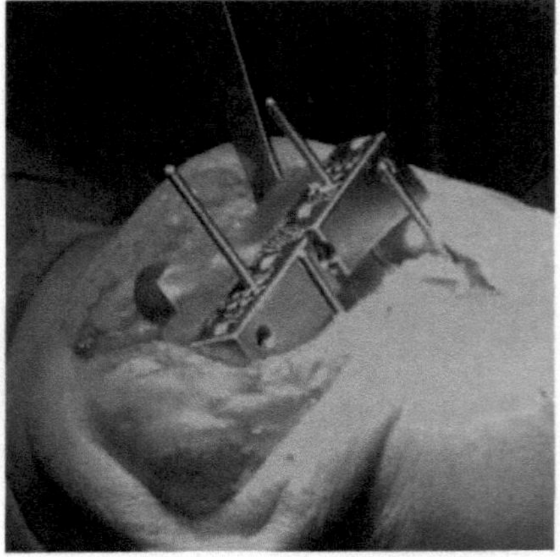

Fig. 48-5. Virtual model and real sample of the individual template attached to the cutting block for femoral reference osteotomy (*right:* intra-operative pin-fixation of the template)

whilst the costs as well as those for the milling machine are moderate, compared to other high-priced CAOS alternatives. The plastic material weighs light and is apt to be sterilized by autoclave joining the other instruments. The intraoperative workflow is hardly prolonged, for the template almost automatically slides into the single correct position. The mounted cutting block can immediately be fixed with two pins and does not need to be scrupulously balanced as known from the conventional routine. Right afterwards the template can be removed and the operation just follows the classic course.

The procedure is equal to the femoral as to the tibial application on principle. But as the tibial side usually offers less room for instrumentation it is preferable not to mount the cutting block to the template from the beginning. Instead the template ought to be fixed with pins through preformed holes. With the template removed, the remaining pins guide the cutting block to the planned position when slipped over.

Clinical Results

Up to now, ten total knee replacements have been executed using the new DISOS-TKA planning system in combination with the presented individual template method. Stable positioning of the template on the bone was easily realized without need of extension of the surgical approach. Unlike other CAS systems, this technique requires no additional technical devices intraoperatively and the operating routine is barely disturbed if at all. As a benefit of the simple and precise template placement by usage of the cutting block the time-consuming and often even inaccurate application of intra- and extra-medullary guiding tools has become completely dispensable. Despite a learning-curve that inevitably entails delay, the total operating time was not prolonged compared to the conventional procedure. The actual average time ranged at 70 min from the opening incision to the closing suture. The postoperative radiological control was affected again as a CT scout view of the entire leg, as it had been originally done to be used for the planning. This made the computer-assisted control easier and more reliable, although digital X-ray showed to work as well. The evaluation of the follow-up cases showed an optimal alignment with a maximum deviation of 3°. Alone the unavoidable

radiation exposure due to the preoperative CT and the time spent on oppose the encouraging results. Especially for cases of severe dysplastic deformity and important axial deviation the new planning and navigation tool assures the opportunity of subtle implant accommodation and accurate incorporation.

Conclusion

The studies shows, that by the use of DISOS-TKA a lot of information could be supplied to the surgeon preoperatively, that otherwise would only be accessible after terminated osteotomies. Above all the integration of functional soft-tissue modeling offers the unique opening to estimate resulting conditions of the ligaments and to modify the planning of the implantation for best biomechanical function. Such design should be represented in planning systems for other applications accordingly. Except for minimal-invasive surgery, the planning results can consistently be transported by individual templates with high accuracy. The introduced new approach represents a simple and economic alternative for elective operations that allow preoperative planning.

References

1. Decking R (2001) Computernavigation in der Knieendoprothetik. 26. Kolloquium Computerunterstützte Chirurgie in der Unfallchirurgie und Orthopädie, Baden-Württemberg, pp 22–25
2. Feng EL, Stuhlberg SD, Wixon RL (1994) Progressive subluxation and polyethylene wear in total knee replacements with flat articular surfaces. Clin Orthop Rel Res 299: 60–71
3. Goodfellow JW, O'Connor JJ (1986) Clinical results of the Oxford knee. Clini Orthop Rel Res 205: 21–24
4. Insall JN, Binzzir R, Soudry M, Mestriner LA (1985) Total knee arthroplasty. Clin Orthop Rel Res 192: 13–22
5. Jeffery RS, Morris RW, Denham RA (1991) Coronal alignment after total knee replacement. J Bone Joint Surg 73-B: 709–714
6. Kiefer H, Langemeyer D, Schmerwitz U (2001) Computergestützte Navigation in der Knieendoprothetik. Urban & Vogel, München, S 128–132
7. Laskin RS (1990) Total condylar knee replacement in patients who have rheumatoid arthritis. A ten year follow-up study. J Bone Joint Surg 72-A: 529–535
8. Mai S, Lörke C, Soebert W (2000) Implantation von Knieendoprothesen mit dem neuen Operationsroboter-System CASPAR. Orthopädische Praxis 36: 792–800

9. Miehlke RK, Clemens U, Jens JH, Kershally S (2001) Navigation in der Knieendoprothetik – vorläufige klinische Erfahrungen und prospektiv vergleichende Studie gegenüber konventioneller Implantationstechnik, Z Orthop 139: 109–116

10. Nuño-Siebrecht N, Tanzer M, Bobyn JD (2000) Potential errors in axial alignment using intramedullary instrumentation for total knee arthroplasty. J Arthroplasty 15: 228–230

11. Radermacher K, Portheine F, Anton M, Zimolong A, Kaspers G, Rau G, Staudte H-W (1998) Computer assisted orthopaedic surgery with image-based individual templates. Clin Orthop Rel Res 354: 28–38

12. Ritter M, Merbst WA, Keating EM, Faris PM (1992) Radiolucency at the bone-cement interface in total knee replacement. J Bone Joint Surg 74-A: 980–986

13. Saragaglia D, Picard F, Chaussard C, Montbarbon E, Leitner F, Cinquin P (2001) Computer assisted total knee arthroplasty: Comparison with a conventional procedure. Results of a 50 cases prospective randomized study. Proceedings of the International Society for Computer Assisted Orthopaedic Surgery, p 130

14. Schkommodau E, Portheine F, Radermacher K (2001) Geometric co-relation between topogram-tomogram for computer assisted surgical planning of total knee replacement. Proceedings of the International Society for Computer Assisted Orthopaedic Surgery, p 115

15. Stern H, Insall JN (1992) Posterior stabilized prosthesis. J Bone Joint Surg (Am) 74-A: 980–986

16. Tew M, Waugh W (1985) Tibiofemoral alignment and the results of knee replacement. J Bone Joint Surg 67-B: 551–556

III B Unicompartmental Knee Arthroplasty

49 Implantation of Unicondylar Prosthesis Using the *OrthoPilot* System

One Way Towards a Minimally Invasive Operation

J.-Y. Jenny, C. Boeri

Introduction

The unicompartmental knee endoprosthesis (UKP) remains the subject of controversial discussion. Although no one denies that the functional results are better than those for total knee prostheses (TKP) [6], and possibly also than those for valgus corrective osteotomy [9], the long-term results of these implants are still often regarded as unsatisfactory. However, certain authors have reported remarkable results which stand comparison with the best results from total prosthesis implantations [2]. These specially selected series of very experienced centers are confirmed by the results of the Swedish Knee Arthroplasty Register [7], which finds only a minimal difference in the survivor rates after ten years: 88% for the TKPs, 84% for the UKPs. One must try to discover the causes for failure of certain UKA implantations, rather than condemning the principle as such.

The quality of implantation of a UKP is a recognized prognostic factor determining the long-term result. The traditional implantation instrumentation allows an acceptable level of reproducibility, but with a error rate that cannot be ignored [4]. These errors can be held responsible for certain implantation failures, especially those involving premature wear.

Computer-assisted implantation makes it possible to improve the technical quality of TKP implantation [8]. One can thus suppose that, after suitable technical adaptation, the same systems will make the same progress possible in UKP implantation, too. Most current computer-assisted navigation systems require preoperative CT scanning or even advance implantation of metallic landmarks. The OrthoPilot system is used exclusively intra-operatively, and could therefore demonstrate a better cost benefit ratio.

Validating the OrthoPilot System in TKA Implantation

Reproducibility of Intra-Operative Data Recording

Twenty prostheses were used in a study on the variability of the intra-operative determination of the mechanical knee axes between two users, as well as the variability of various measurements made by the same user. The data on the mechanical axes of the operated leg was recorded following the manufacturer's recommendations. Three kinematic registrations were performed on the same patient without altering the position of the anatomical points required by the system: two registrations were made by the main surgeon and one by the second surgeon.

The following angles were measured by the system:
- the frontal femorotibial angle in maximum extension,
- the lateral femorotibial angle in maximum extension,
- the frontal femorotibial angle in 90° flexion,
- the frontal femorotibial angle in extension from 0° under manually induced load with maximum valgus und varus,

- the frontal femorotibial angle in 90° flexion under manually induced load with maximum valgus und varus.

The variability of the two registration processes carried out by the same surgeon and that between two surgeons was determined using Wilcoxon's T test for dependent samples and Spearman's calculation of correlation coefficients.

- The intrapersonal variability of the measurements in measuring the frontal and lateral femorotibial angle in extension was in all cases less than or equal to 1°.
- The intrapersonal variability for all the other measurements was always less than or equal to 2°.
- The interpersonal variability between the two observers in measuring the frontal and lateral femorotibial angles in extension was in 19 cases less than or equal to 1°, in one case 2°.
- The interpersonal variability in measuring the angles with no load was always less than or equal to 2°.
- The interpersonal variability in measuring the angles under load was in 5 cases more than 2°.

There was no significant difference between the intrapersonal and the interpersonal observer analysis.

From this study one can conclude that the variability of the intra-operative registration of the frontal and lateral mechanical axes of the operated leg is reproducibly. The uncertainty linked to this reproducibility lies in the magnitude of the error connected to the measuring process itself. The greater variability in measurements under load can be explained through the failure to calibrate the force used to produce the varus and valgus manoeuvres.

Validity of Intra-Operative Data Recording

The design team of this method carried out a prospective, comparative, randomized study in order to validate the system used [8]. The differences observed were in favor of the computer-assisted implantation in respect of both the absolute angle values and their distribution, but did not reach the level of significance.

We have conducted a radiographic investigation into the quality of implantation of a total knee endoprosthesis (Search, Aesculap, Chaumont) in 100 patients with primary gonarthrosis [5]. 50 patients (Group A) were operated on using the OrthoPilot computer-assisted navigation system. 50 patients (Group B) were taken from a series of 400 patients operated on for the same indication and with the same prosthesis, after pair matching with Group A in respect of age (in intervals of 5 years), sex, frontal mechanical femorotibial angle preoperatively (in intervals of 5° around the theoretical ideal value of 180°) and severity of the degenerative lesions, which were classified according to Ahlbäck [1]. Where there were several pair matching possibilities the measurements analyzed were determined by drawing lots from a table of random numbers.

The quality of the TKA implantation was examined on frontal and lateral whole leg X-rays on monopodal support with maximum extension. The images were analyzed using a technique derived from the recommendations of the Knee Society [3].

The specification for implantation of the prosthesis used was, according to the concept and wishes of the authors, as follows:

- frontal mechanical femorotibial angle 177°–183°,
- frontal orientation of the femoral component 88°–92°,
- sagittal orientation of the femoral component 88°–92,
- frontal orientation of the tibial component 88°–92°,
- sagittal orientation of the tibial component 88°–92°.

Global implantation of the prosthesis was regarded as optimal in 33 patients from group A and 15 patients from group B ($p<0.001$). The frontal mechanical femorotibial angle was 180°±2° in group A and 180°±3° in group B ($p=0.43$); it was regarded as optimal in 47 patients from group A and 39 patients from group B ($p<0.05$). The frontal orientation of the femoral component was 90°±1° in group A and 90° ± 2° in group B ($p=0.71$); it was regarded as optimal in 48 patients from group A and 42 patients from group B ($p=0.05$). The sagittal orientation of the femoral component was 89°±2° in group A and 88°±3° in group B ($p=078$); it was regarded as optimal in 38 patients from group A and 32 patients from group B ($p<0.05$). The frontal orientation of the tibial component was 90°±1° in group A and 89°±2° in group B ($p=0.03$); it was regarded as optimal in 48 patients from group A and 40 patients from group B ($p<0.05$). The sagittal orientation of the tibial component was 90°±1° in group A and 90°±3° in group B ($p=0.90$); it was regarded as optimal in

47 patients from group A and 33 patients from group B ($p<$0.001).

The navigation system used permitted a significant improvement in the quality of implantation of the TKA in the frontal and sagittal planes. The effect of this improvement on the long term result of this prosthesis still has to be investigated, and the measurement of ligamentary stability in the frontal plane could contribute further interesting elements.

Using the OrthoPilot System in the Implantation of Unicompartmental Knee Endoprostheses (UKP)

The authors have to date implanted 60 UKPs with the help of the OrthoPilot computer system.

Operating Technique

The system is based on an intra-operative, kinematic analysis of movements of the pelvis, femur, tibia and foot. It consists of a central unit with a PC, monitor and infrared camera (Polaris, Northern Digital, Toronto, Canada; 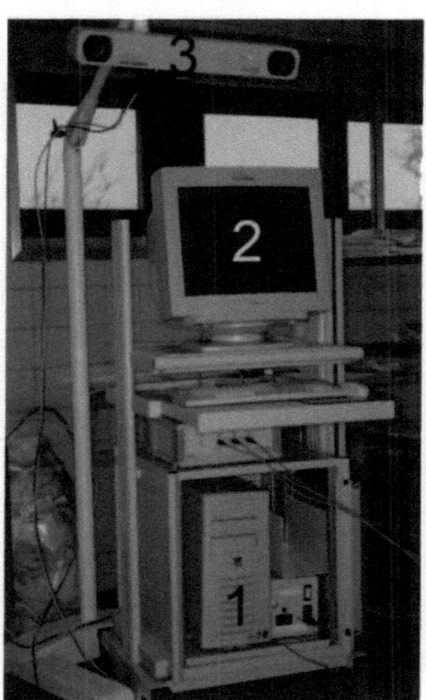 Fig. 49-1). Four infrared transmitters are placed onto the anterior superior iliac spine, the distal femur, the proximal

tibia and the back of the foot. The relative movement of two adjacent infrared transmitters makes it possible, purely through intra-operative kinematic analysis, to determine the joint centers of the hip, knee and ankle (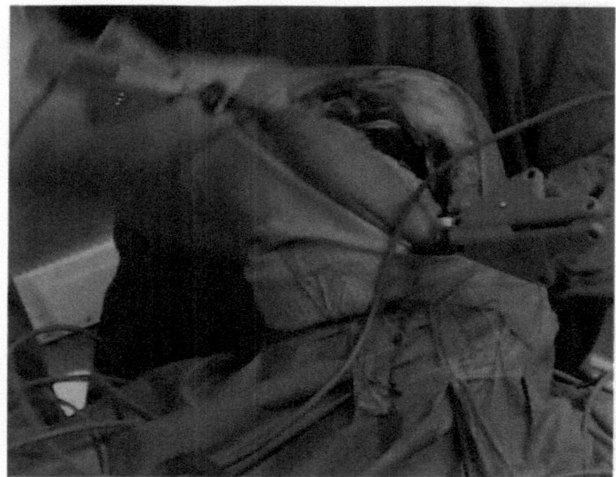 Fig. 49-2) and thereby to define the frontal and sagittal mechanical axes of the femur and tibia. Palpation of the dorsal points of both femoral condyles (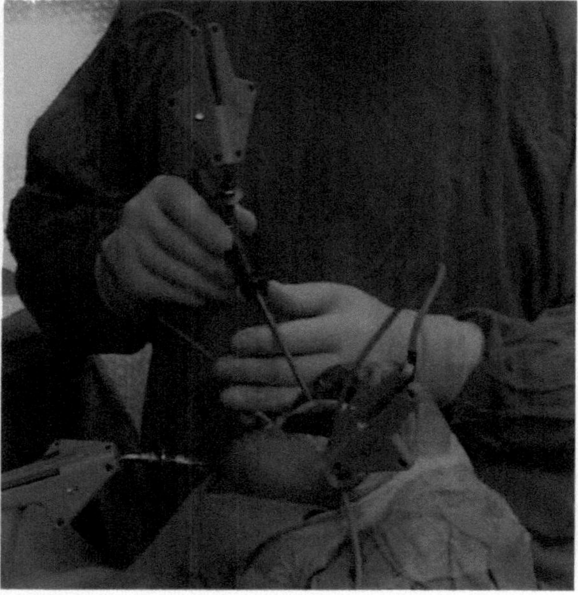 Fig. 49-3), combined with the joint center of the hip, makes it possible to define the frontal reference plane, to which the sagittal

Fig. 49-2. Determination of the joint center of the knee

Fig. 49-1 The Ortho Pilot system: PC (1), monitor (2) and infrared camera (3)

Fig. 49-3. Palpation of the anatomical points

49

plane stands at right angles. Palpation of the deepest tibial point of both tibia plateau and the distal femoral point of both femoral condyles completes the collection of reference data for the resection height. The mechanical frontal and lateral femorotibial angles can subsequently be measured (Fig. 49-4). An infrared transmitter fixed onto the cutting blocks of the tibial (Fig. 49-5) and then the femoral resection (Fig. 49-8) permits very precise orientation of these resections in the three spatial planes, using micrometer screws. As soon as the optimal position has been achieved in the three planes (frontal and sagittal orientation and resection height; Figs. 49-6 and 49-9),

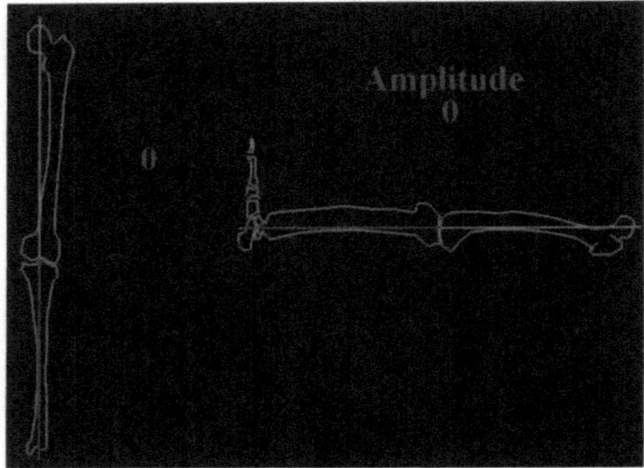

Fig. 49-4. Control screen: femorotibial frontal and sagittal mechanical axes

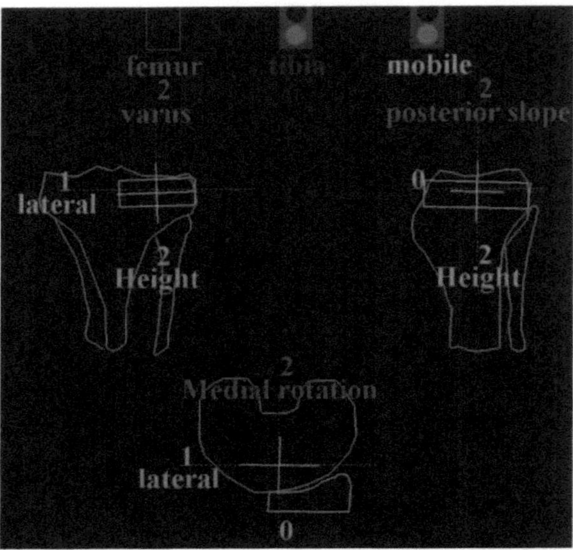

Fig. 49-6. Control screen: orientation of the tibial cutting block

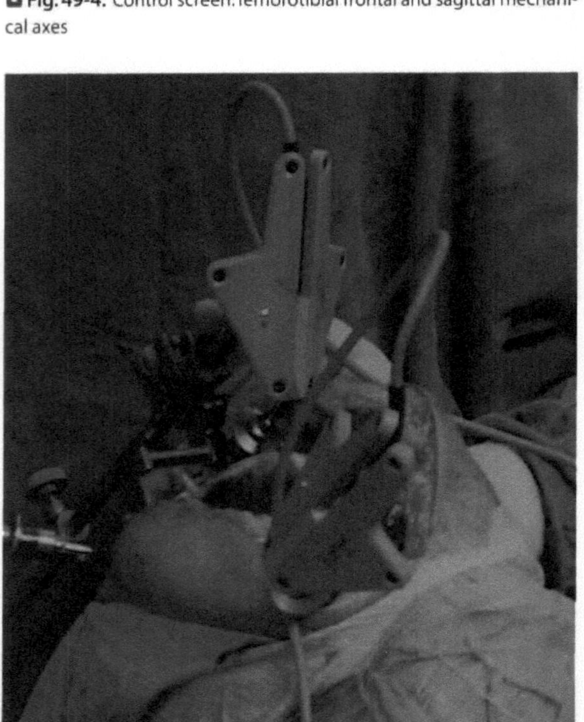

Fig. 49-5. Fixing the tibial cutting block equiped with an infrared transmitter

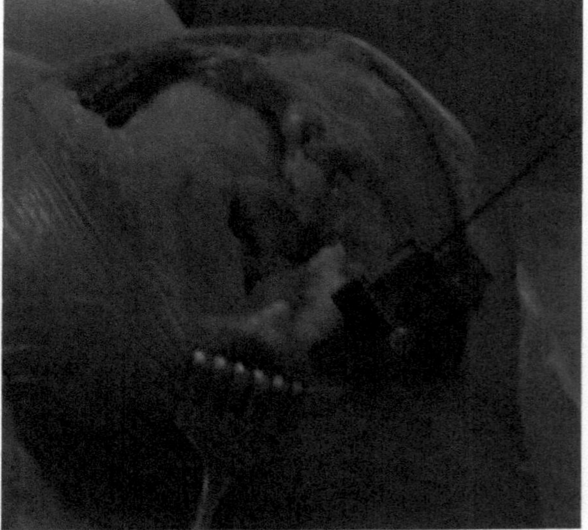

Fig. 49-7. Proximal tibia resection

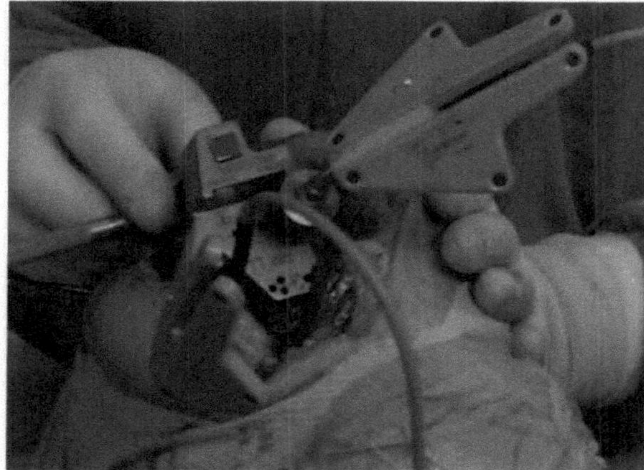

Fig. 49-8. Fixing the femoral cutting block equiped with an infrared transmitter

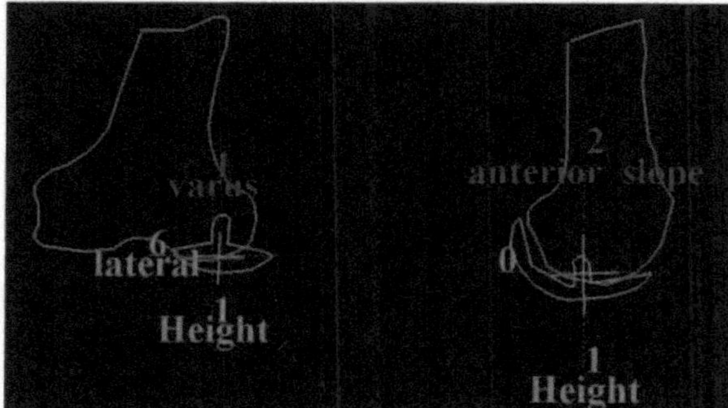

Fig. 49-9. Control screen: orientation of the femoral cutting block

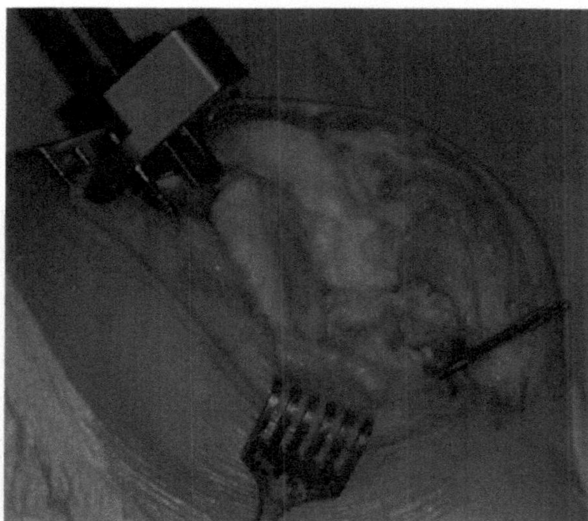

Fig. 49-10. Distal femur resection

the cutting blocks are fixed onto the respective bones. The bone resections are then performed in the classical technique using an oscillatory saw (■ Figs. 49-7 and 49-10). After implantation of the trial prosthesis the system can be used to display the axial correction which has been achieved in the frontal and sagittal plane.

Validation Study

The group of the first 30 cases (group A) was used for radiographic comparison of the quality of implantation, using frontal and lateral axis X-rays, with a control group of 30 unicompartmental prostheses implanted with conventional instrumentation using intra-medullary femoral orientation (group B). All patients were operated on for primary medial gonarthrosis by the same surgeon using the same implant (Search prosthesis, Aesculap). The control group was selected from a series of 250 consecutive cases, after pair matching with the group under investigation with respect to age, sex, severity of arthrotic lesion [1] and frontal mechanical femorotibial angle.

The quality of the UKP implantation was examined on frontal and lateral whole leg X-rays on monopodal support with maximum extension. The images were analyzed using a technique derived from the recommendations of the Knee Society [3]. The frontal X-ray was used to establish the mechanical femoral axis (line connecting the center of the femoral head with the center of the knee), the mechanical tibial axis (line connecting the center of the tibia with the center of the ankle), the axis of the femoral component (line parallel to the medial margin of the posterior segment of the prosthesis) and the axis of the tibial component (axis of symmetry of the prosthesis stem). The following angles were measured:

- frontal mechanical femorotibial angle (angle measured on the medial side between the mechanical axes of the femur and tibia),
- frontal orientation of the femoral component (angle measured on the medial and distal side between the mechanical axis of the femur and the axis of the femoral component),
- frontal orientation of the tibial component (angle measured on the medial and distal side between the mechanical axis of the tibia and the axis of the tibial component).

The lateral X-ray was used to establish the femoral axis (axis of the last ten centimeters of the femoral diaphysis), the tibial axis (line connecting the center of the tibial plateau with the center of the tibial pilon), the axis of the femoral component (axis of symmetry of the prosthesis stem) and the axis of the tibial component (axis of symmetry of the prosthesis contact stud). The following angles were measured:

- the sagittal orientation of the femoral component (angle measured on the proximal and posterior side between the femoral axis and the axis of the femoral component),
- the sagittal orientation of the tibial component (angle measured on the distal and posterior side between the tibial axis and the axis of the tibial component),
- the vertical height of the joint space (vertical distance between the tangent at the inferior margin of the femoral component and its parallel tangent on the upper margin of the fibula, both perpendicular to the tibial axis).

The objectives in implanting the prosthesis used, in accordance with the concept and wishes of the authors, were as follows:

- frontal mechanic femorotibial angle 175°–180°,
- frontal orientation of femoral component 88°–92°,
- sagittal orientation of femoral component 88°–92°,
- frontal orientation of tibial component von 88°–92°,
- sagittal orientation of tibial component 86°–90°,
- vertical height of reconstructed joint space with a margin of ±2 mm compared with the preoperative height.

All measurements were taken by one of the surgeons (JYJ), who was not aware of the implantation technique used (navigated or conventional) in the measuring procedure. The angles were measured with a protractor.

The angle results for each criterion were regarded as optimal if the angle measured was within the desired interval, and as not optimal if this was not the case. The number of optimal criteria was calculated for each patient and the patient's implant was regarded as optimal if all the criteria were fulfilled, and as not optimal if this was not the case.

The frontal mechanical femorotibial angle was within the required limits in 26 patients from group A and in 20 patients from group B. The frontal orientation of the femoral component was within the required limits in 27 patients from group A and in 19 patients from group B ($p<0.02$). The frontal orientation of the tibial component was within the required limits in 26 patients from Group A and in 19 patients from group B ($p<0.05$). The sagittal orientation of the femoral component was within the required limits in 27 patients from group A and in 19 patients from group B ($p<0.02$). The sagittal orientation of the tibial component was within the required limits in 28 patients from group A and in 21 from group B ($p<0.02$). The preoperative height of the joint space was reconstructed with a margin of 2 mm in 30 patients from group A and in 24 patients from group B ($p<0.05$). 18 patients from group A and 4 patients from group B had an optimal implantation with regard to all the criteria investigated ($p<0.001$). There were no system related complications.

Discussion

According to the criteria selected for this study, the quality of implantation of a UKP with the OrthoPilot navigation system was significantly better than that of the prostheses implanted using a conventional manual technique. The technique and the program used also allow reproducible frontal and lateral measurement of the mechanical axes of the femur and tibia.

Choosing this navigation technique does involve certain disadvantages. The first software version required a screw to be inserted temporarily into the pelvic crest, which needed an additional surgical incision, but this never gave rise to any complications. In the current software versions of the program this screw is no longer required. The requirement for temporary implantation of a femoral and tibial screw is less disturbing, as it is done using the normal surgical incision. As with each new procedure, the technique requires a learning period, which can be estimated as around ten implantations. It also involves a longer operation time, at present around 20 min on average. Finally, the system also takes up some room in the operating theater, but not more than an arthroscopy tower.

On the other hand, a navigation technique which does not require CT has numerous advantages. Even if the essential point is naturally the improvement in quality of the implantation, proven beyond doubt by this study, the absence of any imaging (including CT) in addition to classical X-ray diagnosis must be named as an advantage over those techniques based on preoperative imaging. The conventional operating technique is only slightly modified and it is possible to return to the conventional technique at any time without any difficulty whatsoever. The system is not directive, but always leaves the surgeon free to choose whether to follow the instructions given or not. Above all, it is an ingenious measuring system, that intraoperatively provides more reliable data than the best surgeon's eye. Furthermore, it is very moderate from the cost point of view, particularly because it does not require any specific consumables.

Conclusion

Computer-assisted instrumentation works more reliably and more reproducibly than conventional instrumentation for the implantation of a unicompartmental knee endoprosthesis. The long-term results of these type of implanted prostheses could be improved. The systematic use of preoperative imaging procedures (including CT) or even the preoperative implantation of metallic landmarks is not necessary. The OrthoPilot navigation system used appears to offer the best cost benefit ratio.

Special instruments for the navigated implantation technique are currently being developed. With the conventional instrumentation previously available, the surgical approach is relatively large, since relevant anatomical reference points have to been found. The navigation system allows these reference points to be established through kinematic analysis without additional skin incisions. Thus a minimally invasive approach (6 cm skin incision) can be used in future without having to give up the high level of precision (■ Fig. 49-11). This could make the postoperative rehabilitation phase shorter and simpler.

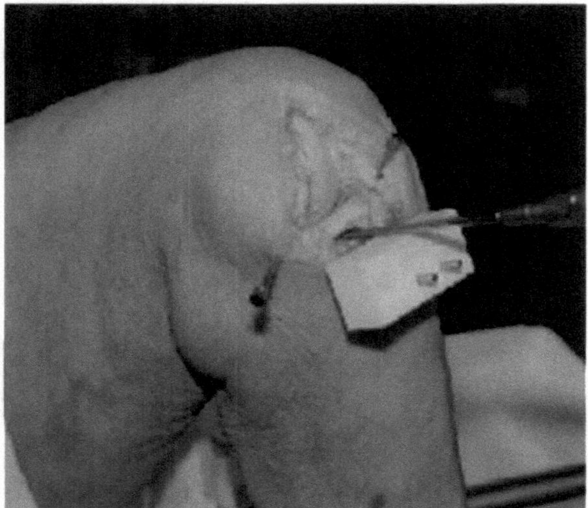

■ **Fig. 49-11.** Minimally invasive surgery (cadaver study)

References

1. Ahlbäck S (1968) Osteoarthrosis of the knee. A radiographic investigation. Acta Radiol Diagn 277 [Suppl]: 7–72
2. Ansari S, Newman JH, Ackroyd CE (1997) St. Georg sledge for medial compartment knee replacement. 461 arthroplasties followed for 4 (1–17) years. Acta Orthop Scand 68: 430–434
3. Ewald FC (1988) The Knee Society total knee arthroplasty roentgenographic evaluation and scoring system. Clin Orthop 248: 9–12
4. Hernigou P, Deschamps G (1996) Prothèse unicompartimentales du genou. Rev Chir Orthop 87 [Suppl 1]: 23–60
5. Jenny JY, Boeri C (2001) Implantation d'une prothèse totale de genou assistée par ordinateur: étude comparative cas-témoin avec une instrumentation traditionnelle. Rev Chir Orthop 87: 645–652
6. Newman JH, Ackroyd CE, Shah NA (1998) Unicompartmental or total knee replacement. Five-year results of a prospective, randomised trial of 102 osteoarthritic knees with unicompartmental arthritis. J Bone Joint Surg 80-B: 862–865
7. Robertsson O, Borgquist L, Knutson K, Lewold S, Lidgren L (1999) Use of unicompartmental instead of tricompartmental prostheses for unicompartmental arthrosis in the knee is a cost-effective alternative. 15,437 primary tricompartmental prostheses were compared with 10,624 primary medial or lateral unicompartmental prostheses. Acta Orthop Scand 70: 170–175
8. Saragaglia D, Picard F, Chaussard C, Montbarbon E, Leitner F, Cinquin P (2001) Mise en place des prothèses totales du genou assistée par ordinateur: comparaison avec la technique conventionnelle. Rev Chir Orthop 87: 18–28
9. Weale AE, Newman JH (1994) Unicompartmental arthroplasty and high tibial osteotomy for osteoarthrosis of the knee. A comparative study with a 12- to 17-year follow-up period. Clin Orthop 302: 134–137

III C Robotics: Total Knee Arthroplasty

50 Clinical Results with the Robot-Assisted »CASPAR« System and the »Search-Evolution Prosthesis«

S. Mai, C. Lörke, W. Siebert

Introduction

The number of Total Knee Arthroplasty (TKA) operations per annum is increasing. This is possibly due to the increasing life expectancy of the older population and their demand for painless mobility. The high life expectancy of people with implants also calls for long-term durability which is to be achieved by an improvement of the implantation techniques.

The complex anatomy and mechanics of the knee joint place high demands on the preoperative surgical planning and the implantation strategy. The endoprosthesis position achieved with traditional manual techniques, supported by the development of intra- and extra-medullary guides as well as saw templates, is not always satisfactory, even when performed by experienced surgeons [3, 9]. Just the choice of the insertion point of the femoral intra-medullary rod can cause deviations of the mechanical axis of up to 8.3° [6]. There are several additional influencing factors like femur flexion, thickness and length of the rod.

The leg's mechanical axis has a special significance for the knee's implant alignment as the prosthesis is to be implanted perpendicularly to the axis in order to enable a balanced stress of the components and bones. If the alignment is not correct, early loosening can be expected. Deviations outside the optimal range of 3° in a follow-up study over a period of 8 years [3] show a higher revision rate of 24%, in contrast to 3% associated with optimal implantation. Literature reports deviations of more than 3° in 32% of 115 patients [3], of more than 5° in 34% of 428 reexamined patients, with 7% of these cases displaying a deviation of more than 9° [8]. The range of the measured deviations was between 6° varus and 16° valgus in the frontal plane, and, in the sagittal plane, between –3° and

+40° flexion for the femur, and between 84° to 95° for the tibia [1]. In our patients, the postoperative leg axes of 31% of the cases are outside the optimal range, with a dispersion of up to 7°.

In order to achieve a stress-balanced implantation and corresponding longer longevity (of the implant), different passive, semi-active and active systems are in development. The aim is to improve the preoperative planning, as well as the implantation technique, so that the implant can be inserted in an exact, standardized and reproducible manner, achieving consistent mechanical axis, rotation, slope and ligament tension in all three planes. Furthermore, the patella is to run central in its articulation. Since March 2000, our clinic has been performing TKA (total knee arthroplasty) with assistance from the CASPAR-system (U.R.S. Ortho Rastatt/Germany).

Surgical Technique

Placement of Fiducial Markers

For the intraoperative orientation of the robot (registration), each bone to be operated on has to be marked with screws (fiducial markers) before the patient undergoes a CT scan for preoperative planning. A femoral and a tibial pin are needed in each case. Both pins have different, self-tapping, bone screws, suitable for the respective bone structure. The pins are placed into the femur by an anterior approach and into the tibia via an anteromedial approach. The stab incisions are positioned in such a way that they can later be incorporated into the primary surgical incision. To maintain the pins stable in the required position, they are placed bicortically. The skin is closed over the pins so that the main procedure can be performed on the same or on the following day.

CT-Scan-Based Pre-Operative Planning

Following the placement of the fiducial markers, a helical CT of the whole leg is taken. Particular attention is paid to the areas of the femoral head, the knee with the markers, and the ankle joint. For detection of possible motion artefacts, a calibration rod is fixed to the leg. As we insert the pins in spinal anesthesia, and subsequently take the CT, the quality of all scans has always been good. The CT data are transferred to the planning station. First of all, the position of the pins and the quality of the CT are checked.

On the 3D scans, which are presented in all three planes at the same time, the anatomical landmarks of the femur and tibia have to be marked. By scrolling through the scans, one can obtain an exact orientation. The mechanical axis in the frontal, sagittal and transversal planes is set. The epicondylar line, also known as »Insall line«, is determined, and the epicondylar twist (angle between epicondylar line and dorsal condylar line) [5] is calculated. The torsion of the tibia (angle between dorsal part of the tibial plateau and the malleolar line of the ankle joint) and its relation to the femur are calculated as well.

After that, the implant is selected and placed virtually (◘ Fig. 50-1).

A further important advantage of the system is that one can scroll through the CT scans in all three planes in order to prove and optimize the exact position of the implant components in all areas. One can immediately notice how a change affects other planes and the mechanical axis. An unintended »notching« can always be avoided. There is an option to plan the joint line and the dorsal

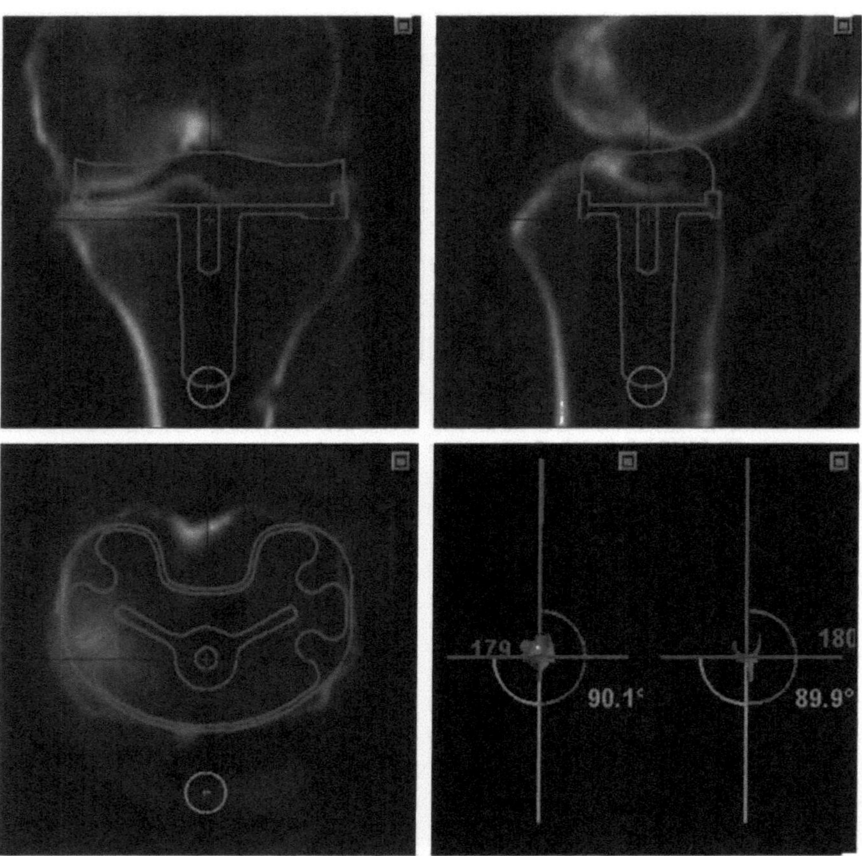

◘ **Fig. 50-1.** 3D planning of the position of the tibial component with indication of the planned mechanical axis

slope in an anatomical or classical way, to influence the slope and translation, as well as to set the components' external rotation in order to ensure a central patellar tracking. After selecting the height of the inlay, the software informs the user about changes in the extension and flexion gaps with possible effect on the ligament tension. This is an indication that a release might be needed and the implant position might need to be reconsidered. Since the indications regarding the soft-tissue tension are only relative, the definite decisions on the thickness of the inlay and on soft-tissue balancing are made by the surgeon intraoperatively, in the traditional way.

Finally, the milling areas are determined to ensure an accurate, time-saving milling procedure without risk of hurting the soft-tissue. As a last step, the system prints an overview of the final plan, and the data are stored on a PC card and transferred to the robot control unit in the OR.

Robot-Assisted Surgery

The patient is positioned in the same way as in a conventional TKA implantation. A conventional median incision with parapatellar medial approach to the knee joint is used. The knee joint is secured by a transfemoral and transtibial self-cutting screw with a specially designed frame (fixateur externe). On the holding device, there are fixtures for hooks and levers (◘ Fig. 50-2).

In exceptional cases with a very extensor mechanism, a quadriceps snip might be necessary in order to keep the patella unstressed aside. The fixation frame is firmly connected to the robot.

The total procedure is surveyed by a Polaris infrared camera system (NDI, Waterloo, Canada) so that the milling procedure can be stopped immediately in case of inacceptable movement. The reflecting »rigid bodies« are firmly attached to the Schanz screw of the bone that is being worked on and to the link to the robot.

To register the position of the bone to the robot, the corresponding CT cross (fiducial marker) is prolonged with a registration cross which is then registered semi-automatically by the robot (see Fig. 50-2). The result of the measurement is compared with the CT data. In accordance with these data, the milling on the femur and tibia can be performed (◘ Fig. 50-3).

Two different milling heads with internal water-cooling and a splash guard are used for the milling procedure which takes approximately 20 min. After the fixation frame is removed, the soft tissues are balanced. The selection of the polyethylene inlay, the insertion of the implants, and the wound closure are performed in the classical technique.

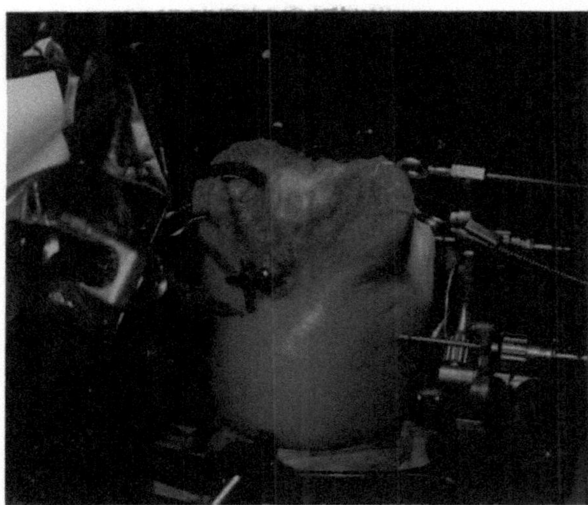

◘ **Fig. 50-2.** Fixateur externe with hooks and levers. Referenciation at the CT-cross elongation

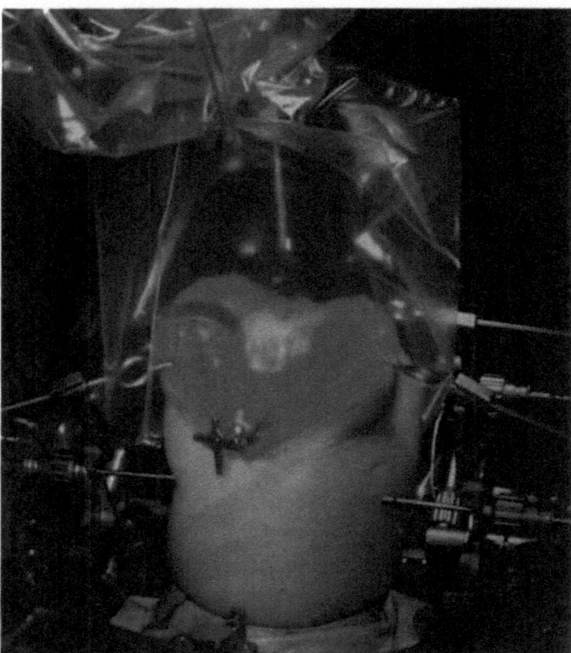

◘ **Fig. 50-3.** Milling of the femur under a splash-guard

Material and Methods

The development of the clinical procedure of TKA using the CASPAR (computer-assisted surgery planning and robotics) robot took place in our clinic [4, 8]. The system is based on a Stäubli industrial robot with 6 joints, which gives it a range of movement similar to human arms. The system was first experimented and standardized on artificial bones and then on human bones. In March 2000, a successful first operation was performed. In the course of a clinical study, supervised by an ethics committee, we performed 70 TKA with the assistance of the robot. We exclusively used the implant LC Search Evolution of the company Aesculap (Tuttlingen) (◘ Fig. 50-4).

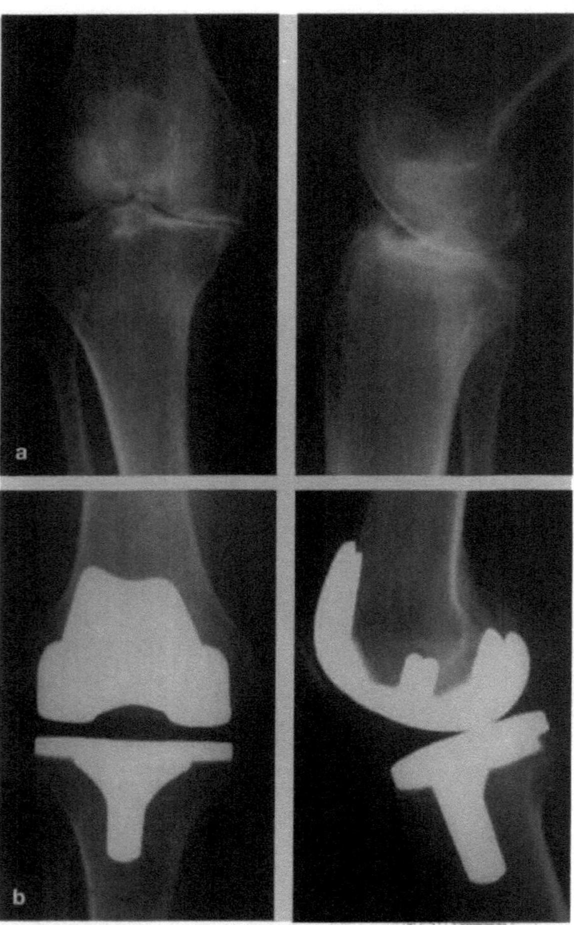

◘ **Fig. 50-4a, b. a** Preoperative medially emphasized gonarthrosis. **b** Surface replacement by prosthesis Search Evolution Aesculap milled with the CASPAR-system

One female patient, with bilateral severe pain due to arthrosis, received a simultaneous, bilateral TKA with considerable success. The mean age of the patients (48 women, 21 men) was 66 years (46–87 years). All patients were enlisted in a prospective study and re-examined after 3, 6 and 12 months. The indication for the operation was primary arthrosis. Patients with diseases weakening the bones (e.g. rheuma, osteoporosis), with immune deficiencies, neurologic basic diseases, reduced general condition or reduced willingness to cooperate were excluded from the study.

The aim of the study was to prove the reproducible precision and reliability of the CASPAR system and to recognize possible complications associated with the system. To check this, standing long-leg anteroposterior roentgenograms were taken of all patients and the mechanical axis of the leg was measured by one person. The postoperative value of the mechanical axis was compared to the nominal value aspired to in the planning. The Knee Society Score (KKS) [2] and the score of the Hospital for Special Surgery (HSS) [7] were used for clinical judgement.

For the measurements of the mechanical axes, 52 patients (40 women, 12 men) served as a control group. For the KSS, the control group consisted of 176 patients with idiopathic gonarthrosis, who received a comparable implant of the Nex-Gen knee system (Zimmer Inc., Warsaw. IN, USA), in the same period, with the manual technique.

Results

General Observations

The operating time for the first 70 robotic cases averaged 135 min (80–220). The delay is mainly due to the set-up and fastening of the fixation frame. Current operating times are about 2 hours.

In the postoperative days, there were no essential differences in comparison with the patients operated with the manual technique. At first, in the early postoperative phase, there seemed to be lower soft-tissue swelling and a better flexibility in the robotic group compared to the patients operated with the traditional technique. In the robotic group no nerve damage appeared, in contrast to the control group with 2 peroneus lesions, which have completely resolved within a year. At discharge, the patients reached full extension and a flexion of at least 90°.

Complications

Neither intra- nor postoperative complications have been noted which could be related to the use of the robot.

In one intraoperative case there was a mechanical problem at the elongation cross causing a slight mis-milling of the femur, which was corrected manually. Once a tibial pin got loose due to osteoporosis and the operation was finished manually.

Post-operatively, one cutaneous necrosis on a patient with adipositas permagna, and three superficial skin infections at the pin sites have been noted, which rapidly healed under conservative treatment. One had to be revised. Those were exclusively patients with a special incision for the pin placement. At the site of the Schanz screws there was no complaint in any of the cases. One patient suffered a late infection of the knee, half a year after the operation, which was cured without consequences by one arthroscopic irrigation and by a course of antibiotics. A deep vein thrombosis was noted in two cases.

Function Score

Between the compared groups, there were no considerable differences as expected (◨ Fig. 50-5).

The »Knee Society Score« is divided into a »knee score« and a »function score«. Preoperatively, and after one year, the total score of the manual group was 48/159 points, whilst the robotic group scored 91/166 points. Since restrictions due to other existing diseases are involved in the score, full score (200) has not been achieved.

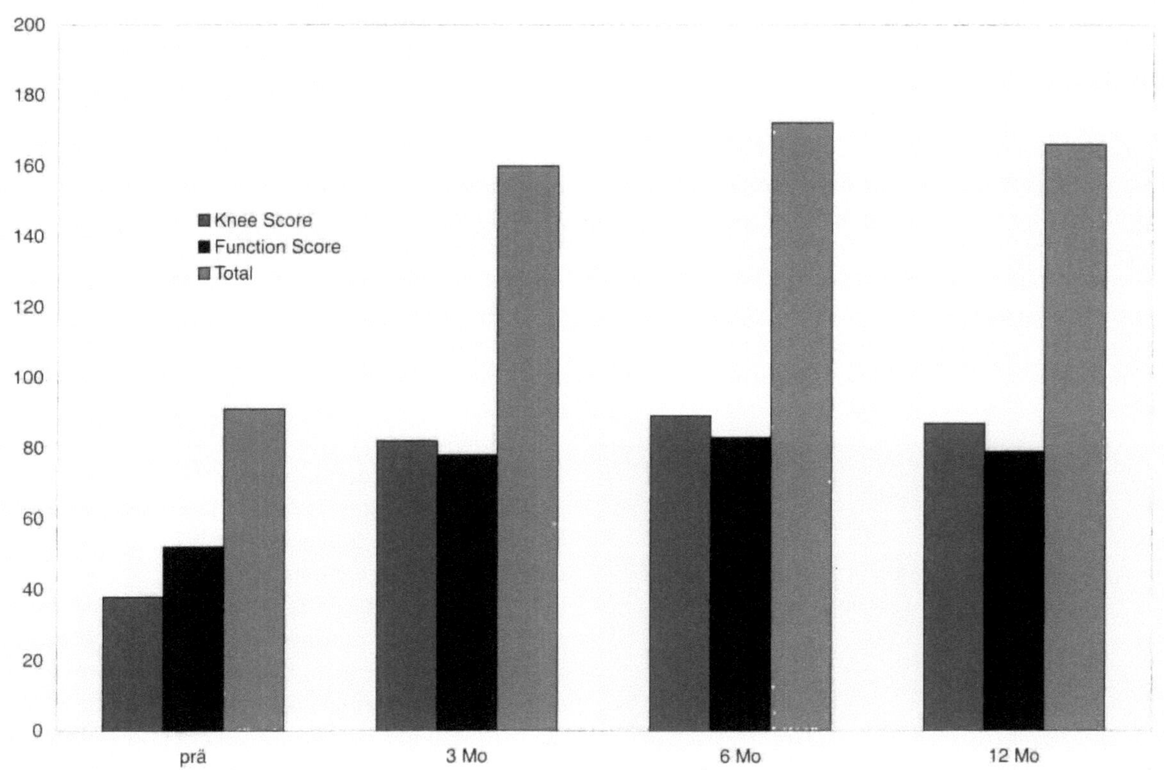

◨ Fig. 50-5a. Knee Society Score for the robotic group.

50

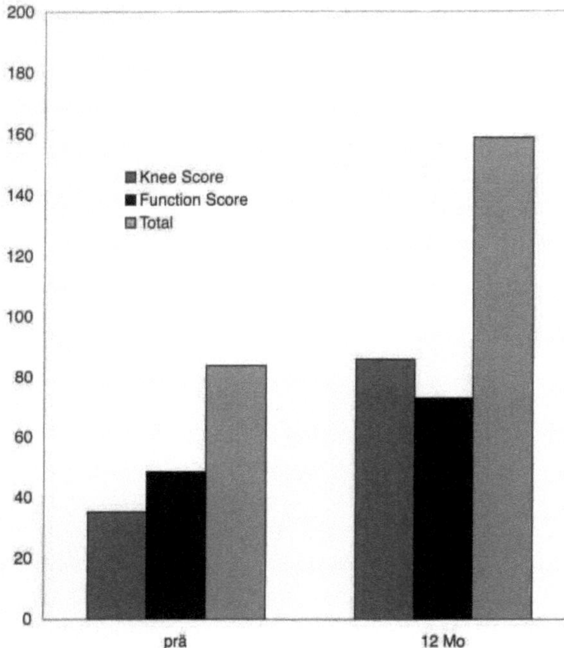

Fig. 50-5b. Knee Society Score for the manual group

Mechanical Leg Axis

A fundamental sign of quality in TKA is the achieved mechanical axis of the leg, i.e. the tibiofemoral angle, as this mainly reflects the precision of the method. Standing long-leg roentgenograms have been measured. Usually, an angle of 0° is desired. In one case of a female patient in the robotic group with a varus deformation of 20°, an angle of 3.7° varus was planned to avoid too much resection and to maintain sufficient ligament tension. The

comparison of the planned aim with the postoperatively achieved mechanical axis showed an overall mean difference of only 0.8° (0° to 3°) in the robotic group and of 2.6° (0° to 7°) in the manual comparison group (■ Table 50-1). The difference between the plan and the achievement in the robotic group is significant ($p<0.0001$).

Conclusions and Prospects

The robot system CASPAR stands out for high precision and safety so that very good results can be achieved, especially regarding the position of the implant. An essential part is the preoperative planning, in which one can plan the surgery with respect to all axes, angles, rotations and tilts. The exact position of the implant, and its effects on the mechanical axis, can be defined in all planes, without haste. In contrast to that, even with high clinical experience and visual estimation, manually one can only plan approximately by means of roentgenograms with inexact enlargement factor and distortions.

A further special feature is that this exact planning is used intraoperatively and executed reliably and very precisely. One prerequisite is that the technique is performed in a correct way and a second demand is that the reference screws do not move during the whole procedure. Intra- and extra-medullary guides containing a certain inaccuracy [6] and which could trigger complications like fat embolism are not necessary. It is not possible to change the plan during the operation but, because of the sufficient preoperative planning with the help of a CT, we have not seen a reason to do this so far. In case of emergency problems, one can revert to the manual implantation at any time.

The milling track is defined exactly preoperatively. For that reason, a good support of the endoprosthesis is guaranteed and injuries of soft tissues, kept aside with help of the fixation frame, are avoided. The loss of bone can be restricted to a minimum and the bone block with the attachment of the posterior cruciate ligament can be maintained. When cutting the dorsal femur condyles, small bone pieces remain, with which cysts of weak bone might be filled. Instruments specified for implantation of the prosthesis are not necessary. The cutting planes are absolutely flat so that the implants fit perfectly – independently of the operator's skill. Cementless implants are

Table 50-1. Evaluation of the mechanical axis in the robot-assisted and manual group. Clinical results with the robot-assisted »CASPAR« system and the »Search-Evolution Prosthesis«

Femorotibial angle	CASPAR (70 patients)	Manual comparison group (52 patients)
0–2°	97,2%	69%
3°	2,8%	–
>3°	–	31%
Standard deviation	1°	2,2°
Median deviation, planned/achieved axis	0,8°	2,6°

expected to have a good ingrowth conduct. In further discussion, the sort of surface coating, hydroxylapatite or porous coated, will surely become the focus of attention. This precision of the cutting planes cannot be achieved in either manual or navigated procedures, despite sawing guides, as the saw blades themselves are not rigid and are deviated by sclerosed bone. Even the soft tissues, like tendons, ligaments, nerves and vessels, can be affected in case of manual sawing.

A disadvantage is the use of reference screws which require a small operation beforehand. To avoid this, a pinless technique is in development, which of course has to achieve a similar precision. A further disadvantage is the additional physical exposure to radiation due to the necessary CT, which could already be reduced by the development of spiral CTs. However, the high precision of the planning and execution can only be achieved with CTs. In future developments, other imaging techniques, which are also steadily improving and extending, such as sonography, MRI, Iso-C 3D image converter, will surely offer interesting alternatives.

An aim of the application of robots is to shorten the operation time. Unfortunately, the set-up of the system requires a lot of time, so, in case of primary TKA, the operation will be prolonged, even with a well-coordinated team. One has to pay attention to the ipsilateral hip which has to allow a flexion of 50°. Intensive work is done to facilitate the setting up and to avoid the need for a rigid fixation. Technical possibilities of a simpler and faster registration are not yet exhausted.

A problem still unsolved is the precise soft-tissue balancing which is of considerable importance to the result and the knee joint's stability. The CASPAR system only gives hints. Navigation systems also need further development in this area. A combination of different techniques could perhaps lead to success. As new methods are being developed analyzing the virtual mobility and dynamic function of the knee under stress further new findings will influence our ideas about the knee joint, which has a very complex anatomy and mechanics.

To sum up, it can be said that robotics, which is in the initial stage of a promising development, enables a new approach to TKA. It offers the possibility of accurate and careful 3D planning, executed in a reliable and reproducible way, with high accuracy. It could be proved that an essential quality criteria, i.e. the biomechanical integration of the implant in the load line of the body, is achieved with high significance. This precision at present is achieved by additional expenditure and high costs. Long-term studies will show if these advantages will pay off for the patients in future.

Constantly new knowledge is achieved by means of new techniques of examination, planning and implantation regarding the knee function and TKA. It will highly influence and improve techniques of joint replacement, the design of endoprostheses as well as the kind of the applied materials in the next few years. High intelligent high technologies do not represent a competition but each has particular advantages that can complement each other. Only by means of combination of these advantages, the highest degree of accuracy of fitting and position as well as biocompatibility can be achieved.

References

1. Insall JN, Binzzir R, Soudry M, Mestriner LA (1985) Total knee arthroplasty. Clin Orthop 192: 13–22
2. Insall JN, Dorr LD, Scott R, Scott WN (1989) Rationale of the knee society clinical rating system. Clin Orthop 248: 13–14
3. Jeffery RS, Morris RW, Denham RA (1991) Coronal alignment after total knee replacement. J Bone Joint Surg 73B: 709–714
4. Mai S, Lörke C, Siebert W (2000) Implantation von Knieendoprothesen mit dem neuen Operationsroboter-System CASPAR. Orthopädische Praxis 12: 792–800
5. Malzer U, Schuler P (1998) Die Komponentenausrichtung beim Oberflächenersatz des Kniegelenkes. Orthopädische Praxis 3: 141–146
6. Nuño-Siebrecht N, Tanzer M, Bobyn JK (2000) Potential errors in axial alignment using intramedullary instrumentation for total knee arthroplasty. J Arthroplasty 15: 228–230
7. Ranawat CS, Adjei OB (1988) Survivorship analysis and results of total condylar knee arthroplasty. Clin Orthop 323: 168–173
8. Siebert W, Mai S, Kober R, Heeckt P F (2002) The Knee: technique and first clinical results of robot-assisted total knee replacement. Knee 9: 173–180
9. Tew M, Waugh W (1985) Tibiofemoral alignment and the results of knee replacement. J Bone Joint Surg 67B: 551–556

51 Clinical Experiences with *ROBODOC* and the *Duracon* Total Knee

M. Börner, U. Wiesel, W. Ditzen

Objectives

A surgical robot (ROBODOC) is used for total knee replacement (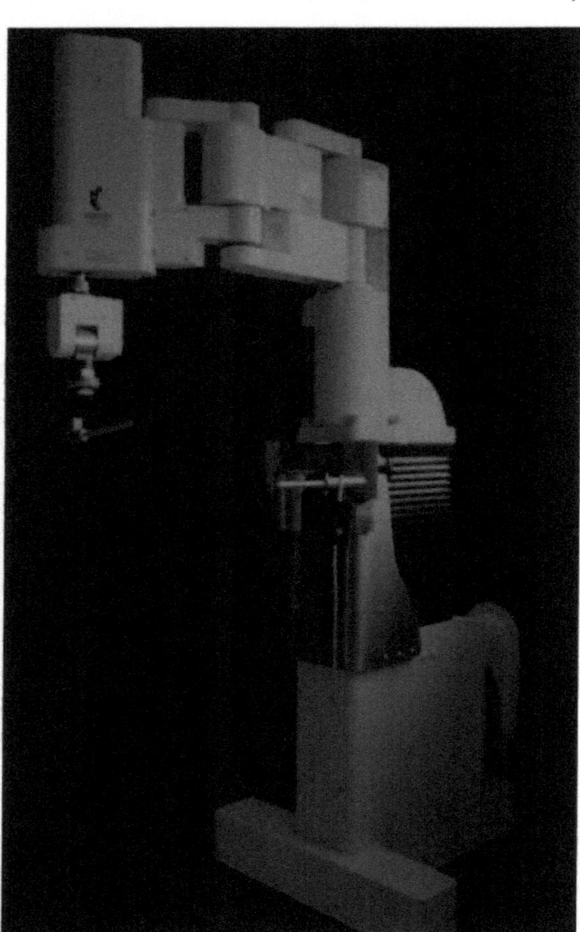 Fig. 51-1). The system has been used as clinical routine for total hip replacement at the Trauma Clinic of Trade Associations (BGU) Frankfurt, Germany since 1994. Since March 2000 it has also been used for total knee arthroplasty.

This article is intended to give an overview of the system and the first clinical experiences.

Background

The results in conventional TKA have so far been very dependent on the surgeon's experience and routine. The most common mistakes are varus and valgus mal-positionings as well as mal-rotations of the implant causing mal-alignment of the anatomical axis postoperatively. These mistakes often lead to untimely loosening of the implant.

Materials and Methods

The system enables to do a 3D preoperative planning of the correct axes and rotation as well as the correct implant size. The intraoperative execution is performed by the robot according to the preoperative planning.

The ROBODOC system consists of the three components:
- the preoperative planning workstation (Orthodoc),
- the surgical robot,
- the control unit which receives all the preoperative planning data and controls the robot's actions.

Presently four titanium pins need to be implanted preoperatively, two in the distal femur and two in the proximal tibia. These pins serve as »landmarks« for the following steps. After pin implantation a CT scan of the femoral head, the distal femur, the proximal tibia and the ankle including all four pins is obtained (Fig. 51-2). An aluminium

Fig. 51-1. ROBODOC cutting block (Fa. ISS, Davis, California, USA)

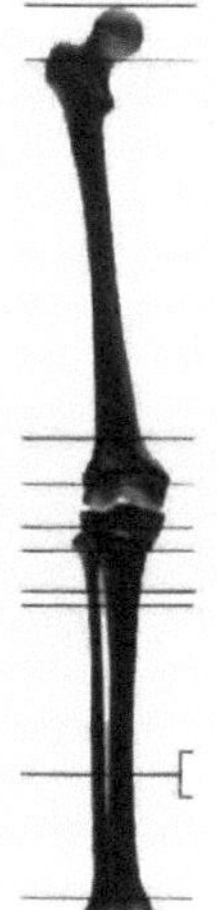

□ Fig. 51-2. Region of interest in the CT scan of the whole leg

rod is attached to the patients leg to detect motion during the CT scan.

The data is transferred to Orthodoc using an optical disc (MOD) or a network.

Orthodoc shows a 3D view of the bone in the following aspects:

- a.p. level,
- lateral level as well as
- the cross-section (□ Fig. 51-3).

Moving the bone in one view automatically moves the other views as well.

The first step is to find the four pins on the CT-scan and to check their position. Then the femoral (FMA) and tibial (TMA) mechanical axes are created using four markers: The femoral head, the center of the femoral condyles, the center of the tibial plateau and the center of the ankle. The femoral and tibial component are planned independently, then the FMA and the TMA are put together. To plan the femoral component, the axis and rotation of the bone are aligned, the right implant size is selected and the implant is positioned. The rotation is found by using the epicondylar line. For the tibial component the rotation is set using the tibial tuberosity and the notch. The implant is selected and positioned according to those landmarks. Finally the tibial line is selected (□ Fig. 51-4).

When the planning is finished a synthetic X-ray can be generated to virtually see the postoperative result. The X-ray shows the post-operative anatomic axis of the lower extremity. This way possible mistakes in planning can be corrected. The data is stored on a CD-ROM. Those data are loaded into the control unit of ROBODOC.

The patient's leg is positioned in a specially designed leg holder (□ Fig. 51-5). The knee should be flexed to about 70° to 80°. Draping is done in the conventional manner

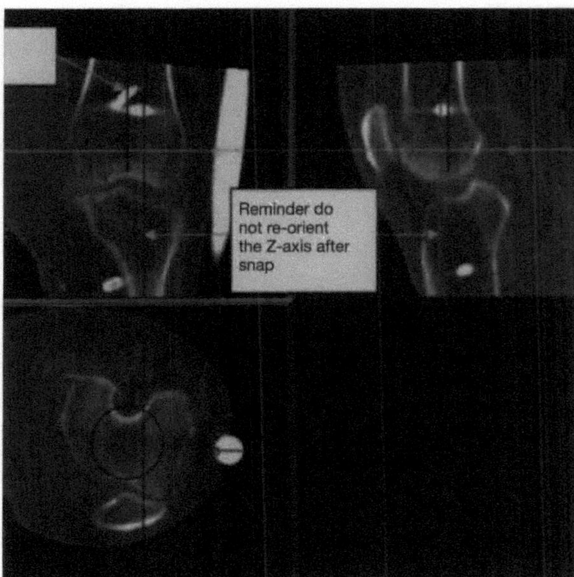

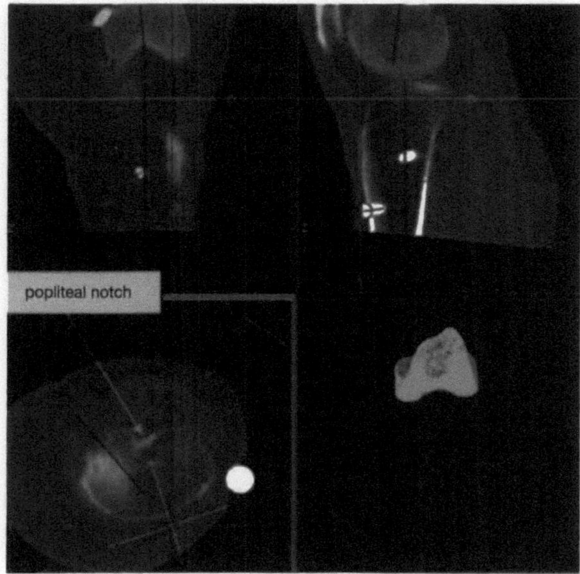

□ Fig. 51-3. Orthodoc, 3D view of the bone

and the normal approach is used for surgery. The knee is exposed and the 4 pins are identified. A Steinmann pin is implanted in the femur and the tibia. The two pins are connected with the Hoffmann II fixator system and the joint is distracted.

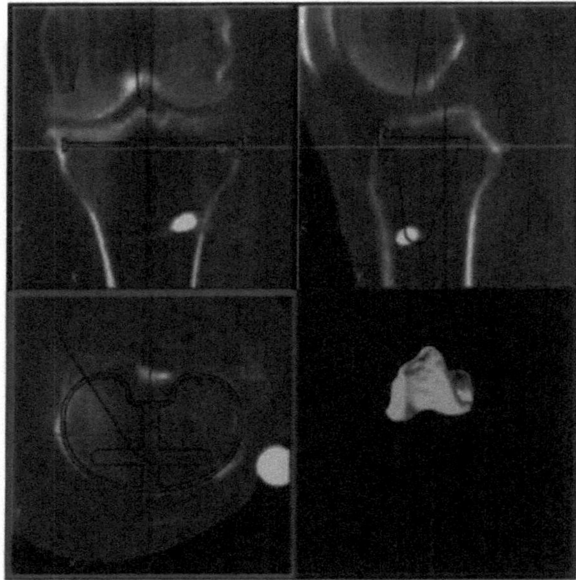

□ Fig. 51-4. Preoperative planning of the femoral and tibial component

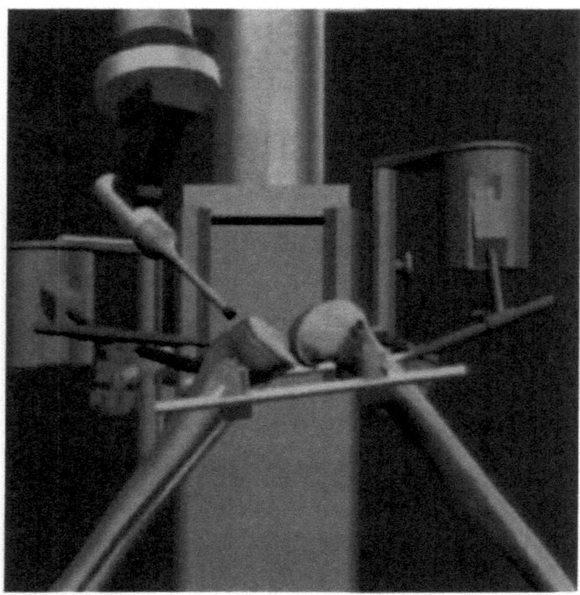

□ Fig. 51-5. Fixing of a model joint in the leg holder

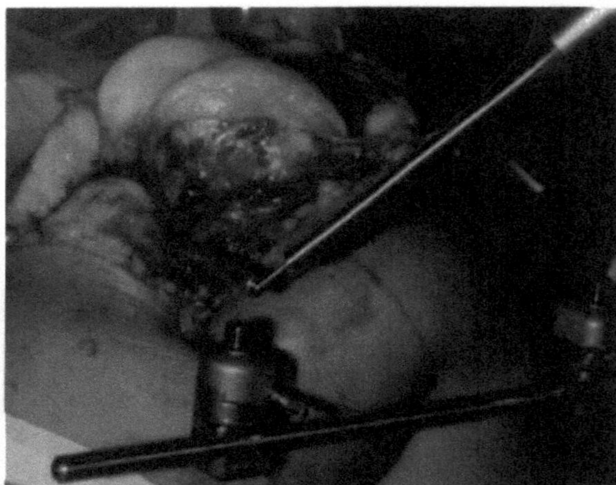

□ Fig. 51-6. intraoperative scanning of the pins after fixing the knee joint

The robot is moved to the OR-table and femur and tibia are connected to the robot. The registration algorithm is started, the robot registers the four pins and their angles. The data is matched with the CT-data. After successful registration the cutter and the irrigation system are installed (□ Fig. 51-6). First the femoral part is cut by the robot (□ Fig. 51-7), then the tibial part and the tibial emminentia (□ Fig. 51-8).

Should bone motion occur during the cutting process this is registered by two bone motion monitors (femur and tibia) and the robot is stopped immediately. The pins then need to be re-registered.

After the cutting is finished the robot is moved away from the OR-table, the four pins are removed and the planned components are implanted by the surgeon manually (□ Figs. 51-9 to 51-11).

Soft-tissue-balancing so far is done the conventional way. The exposure is closed by the surgeon.

Results

In the first 100 patients 76 cases were done cementless, in 16 cases the tibial component was cemented and in 8 cases both components had to be cemented due to poor bone quality.

The preoperative axis was neutral in 2 cases, 28 patients had a valgus deviation and 70 patients had a varus deviation. The postoperative axes are shown in □ Tables 51-1 and 51-2. In no case we found a postoperative varus mal-

Table 51-1. TKA using ROBODOC (*n*=100)

Post-operative anatomical axis			
Optimal	99	47	(0°)
Sub-optimal	1	38	(1°)
Inefficient	–	3	(3°)
Varus: None			

Table 51-2. Knee Society Score (KSS); ROBODOC KTEP (*n* =100)

KSS day 0	111 (49–156)
KSS 3 months	147 (83–174)
KSS 6 months	161 (74–185)
KSS 12 months	176 (111–200)

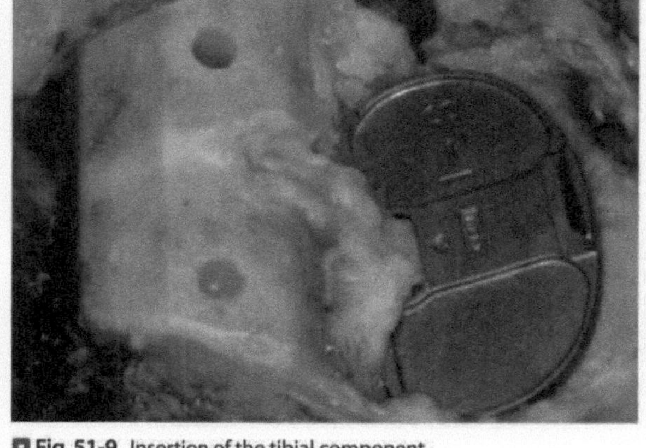

Fig. 51-9. Insertion of the tibial component

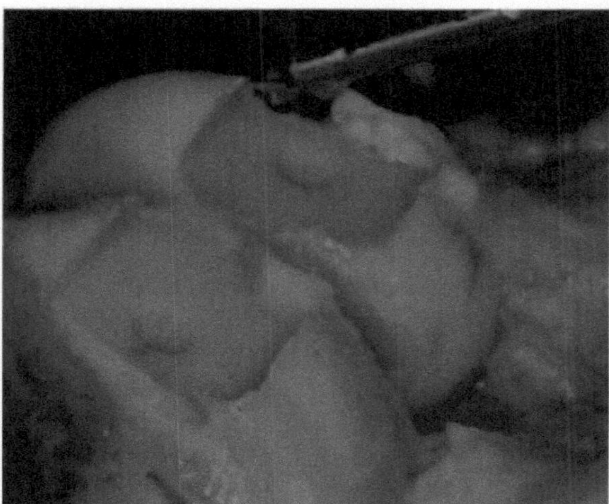

Fig. 51-7. Cutting of the femur

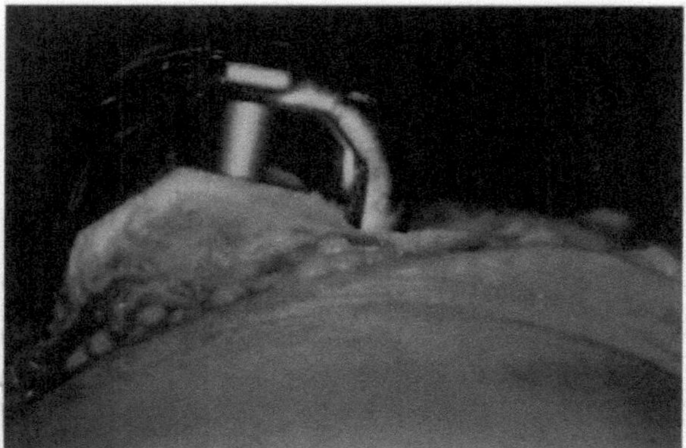

Fig. 51-10. Insertion of the femoral component

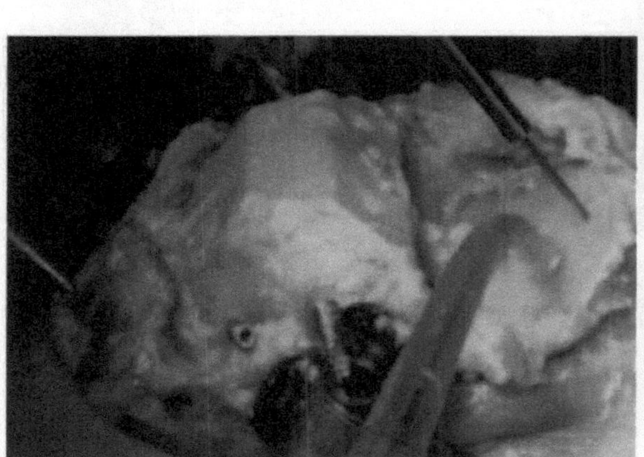

Fig. 51-8. Cutting of the tibia

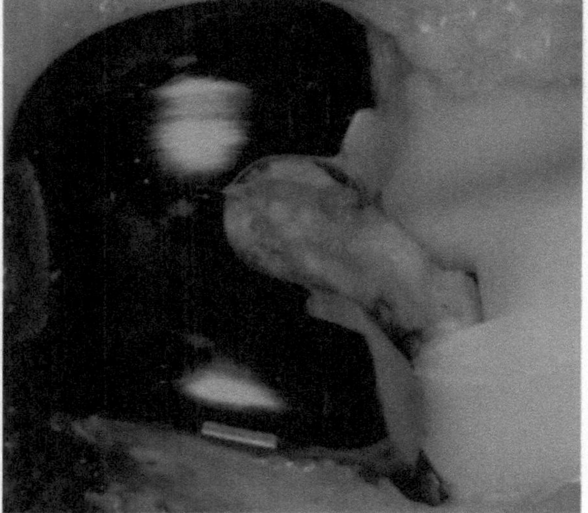

Fig. 51-11. Final placement of the inlay

positioning. The optimal implant size was planned and implanted in all cases. Within the first 100 surgeries the robot could not be used in 5 cases (1 pin problem, 1 positioning problem and 3 hardware problems). Those patients received conventional TKA and are not included in the above patients.

We found an obvious learning curve. The first surgery that was performed March 27th, 2000, took 130 min, meanwhile the average OR-time is 90–100 min. By January 2002 500 patients had been operated on successfully using the ROBODOC system.

inary results show that this goal can be achieved using the system and that the outcome is very consistent.

The present disadvantages of the system are soft-tissue management including ligament balancing, the rigid fixation and the use of pins (markers). These disadvantages will be resolved in the near future by integrating a special navigation system (ROBONAV) into the ROBODOC-system.

By January 2002 500 patients had been operated on successfully using the ROBODOC system at BGU Frankfurt. The pinless system is in a very advanced stage and clinical trials are presently performed at BGU Frankfurt.

Conclusion

The system permits an optimal 3D preoperative planning of the correct axis, rotation and implant size. The intraoperative cutting is entirely executed by the surgical robot according to the preoperative planning. Due to the exact cut surfaces the cementless technique can be used in the majority of cases. The patients are permitted full weight bearing immediately postoperatively.

No conventional instruments are necessary for the procedure. The OR-time is slightly increased compared to the conventional method. The surgeon has immediate control of the system and the surgery can always be finished manually. Correct alignment and rotation are the known preconditions for durability in TKA. Our prelim-

References

1. Börner M, Wiesel U (1999) Einsatz computerunterstützter Verfahren in der Unfallchirurgie. Trauma Berufskrankh 1: 85–90
2. Hungerford DS, Krackow KA, Kenna RV (1984) Total knee arthroplasty: A comprehensive approach. Williams & Wilkins, Baltimore London
3. Krackow KA (1990): The technique of total knee arthroplasty. Mosby, St. Louis Baltimore Philadelphia Toronto
4. Paul HA, Bargar WL et al. (1992) Development of a surgical robot for cementless total hip arthroplasty. Clin Orthop Rel Res 285: 57 – 66
5. Wiesel U, Lahmer A, Tenbusch M, Boerner M (2001) Total knee replacement using the ROBODOC system. CAS 2: 116
6. Wiesel U, Boerner M (2001) First experiences using a surgical robot for total knee replacement. Proc. CAOS/USA, July 6th – 8th, 2001 Pittsburgh, USA, pp 143–146

IV Navigation and Robotics: Anterior Cruciate Ligament (ACL) Reconstruction

52 Fundamentals in ACL Reconstruction: »The American View«

V. Musahl, F.H. Fu

Introduction

In ACL reconstruction procedures, the position of femoral and tibial tunnels is known to significantly affect the clinical outcome. Despite this knowledge however, great variability exists in tunnel placement among surgeons and the rate of misplaced tunnels in ACL reconstruction surgery has been reported between 10–40% [13, 16]. The result of misplacement of tunnels as well as a number of other reasons is revision ACL reconstruction [9]. Surgeons frequently use preoperative radiographs during surgery to assist with tunnel placement, however no direct links exist to the intraoperative situation. Computer-assisted surgery (CAS) is now assumed to help improve precision in ACL reconstruction and to provide this link. This manuscript will review fundamentals of ACL reconstruction and briefly discuss the different available CAS systems.

Background for ACL Reconstruction

The »perfect« ACL replacement graft should be free of any associated donor site morbidity, should reproduce the insertion site anatomy and biomechanics, should have complete biological incorporation, and should resume neuromuscular control. Unfortunately, such a »perfect« graft does not exist to date. Historically, bone-patella tendon-bone (B-PT-B) grafts have been used since the late 1970s and hamstring tendon grafts have been used since the late 1980s. Quadriceps tendon grafts, synthetic graft materials, as well as allografts can also be used for reconstruction of the ACL. A recent survey on a global panel consisting of 14 expert surgeons from all five continents revealed equal use of B-PT-B and hamstring grafts, whereby two thirds of the surgeons used multiple grafts in their practice [10].

An evaluation of different grafts and their advantages and disadvantages reveals a consistent size and shape for the B-PT-B graft, bone-to-bone healing in the tunnels, as well as consistent fixation. However, harvesting the graft can be complicated by intraoperative patella fracture and postoperative donor site morbidity. Hamstring tendons provide higher stiffness and show no interference with the extensor mechanism while harvested. Hamstring tendons have the disadvantage of tendon-to-bone healing and inconsistency with various fixation systems. Allograft materials can be used from the patella tendon, Achilles tendon, or tibialis anterior tendon. The advantages of allografts are better cosmesis, no donor site morbidity, and less postoperative pain. However, allografts show a prolonged healing response, decreased tensile strength, and have the risk of disease transmission. As difficult as the graft selection process might seem, clinical outcome has not been proven significantly better in one or the other technique [5].

Surgical Technique

After harvesting of the graft and performing a systematic diagnostic arthroscopy, the intraarticular notch will be prepared for graft placement in a one-incision technique. Notch preparation involves removal of residual ACL tissue from the lateral femoral condyle and the ACL stump at the tibia. Care must be taken not to injure the posterior cruciate ligament (PCL) during this preparation. A minimal notch plasty is then performed in cases of a narrow notch to provide an impingement-free placement of the ACL graft. After placement of the tunnels and testing for

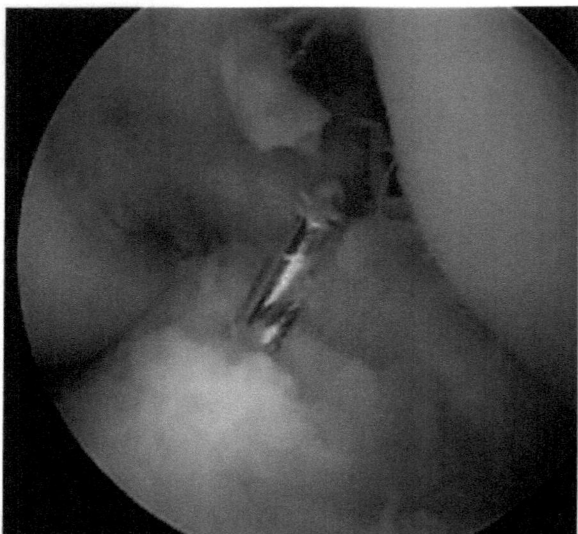

Fig. 52-1. Guide wire insertion into the tibial ACL footprint, arthroscopic view

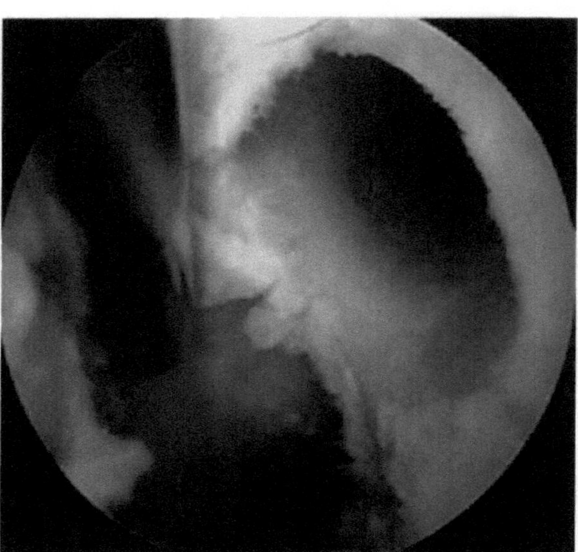

Fig. 52-2. Drill hole position in the femoral ACL footprint, arthroscopic view

impingement utilizing a tunnel dilator, a more extensive notch plasty can be performed if impingement is present.

The placement of the tibial tunnel should be in the posterior half of the anterior-posterior diameter and the center of the medial-lateral diameter of the ACL footprint (**Fig. 52-1**). This position minimizes the risk of anterior graft impingement and allows for creation of the femoral tunnel in an endoscopic fashion. Landmarks that are helpful in anatomical positioning of the tibial tunnel include the anterior horn of the lateral meniscus, the tibial spines, the anterior border of the PCL, and the intercondylar roof. A tibial tunnel aimer is then inserted through the anteromedial portal and used to insert a guide wire into the ACL footprint from outside-to-in. The angle of the tibial tunnel aimer from the horizontal plane can be adjusted from 30 to 60° and matched with the length of the graft construct. The guide wire should enter the tibia medial from the midline to provide for a femoral position that needs to be on the lateral femoral condyle. The tibial tunnel is then created with a cannulated reamer of the appropriate diameter.

For creation of the femoral tunnel, it is crucial to identify the posterior cortical margin of the lateral femoral condyle and to probe the over-the-top position. Care must be taken to avoid anterior femoral tunnel placement by mistaking the »resident's ridge« for the over-the-top position. In order to place the femoral tunnel into an anatomical position, a posterior position just anterior to the over-the-top position is recommended (**Fig. 52-2**). Usually, 7 mm-offset guides are used to achieve this. In the other dimension, the o'clock position is the most widely used method. The roof of the notch thereby serves as the 12:00 o'clock reference position and is also called Blumensaat's line as viewed in a lateral roentgenogram. A 10:30 to 11:00 o'clock position for a right knee (and a corresponding 1:00 to 1:30 o'clock for a left knee) is used as the tunnel entrance position. With the knee flexed at 90°, the femoral tunnel is drilled in a trans-tibial fashion with an endoscopic reamer after placement of a guide wire retrograde trough the tibial tunnel into the center of the selected tunnel location. The length of the femoral tunnel should be the length of the femoral portion of the graft construct. Special considerations are thereby additional length needed for »flipping« of an endobutton or adjusting the length in case of a tibial graft-tunnel mismatch. The final step in preparation of the femoral tunnel is to penetrate the anterolateral femoral cortex to provide for passage of the graft.

The graft preparation is completed at the back table in the meantime and should include a mark with a sterile marking pen. This mark is for visualization during arthroscopic graft insertion and is at the bone tendon junction for the femoral tunnel (B-PT-B) or indicates the femoral tunnel length plus 8 mm if an endobutton is to be used (hamstring tendon). The graft is then inserted from the tibia using the Beath pin and no. 5 Ethibond sutures. For a B-PT-B graft, the construct will be pulled into the femoral tunnel until the femoral bone block is flush with the articular margin. The femoral bone block will be fixed with a metal interference screw. Final fixation of the graft will be accomplished with the knee close to full extension, a manually applied posterior drawer, and tension on the graft. Tibial fixation can then also be achieved with a metal interference screw.

For a hamstring tendon graft, the construct will be pulled into the femoral tunnel until the mark for the femoral tendon portion is flush with the articular margin. Fixation can then be achieved with a bio-absorbable interference screw. If an endobutton is used, the graft needs to be pulled an additional 8 mm into the femoral tunnel in order to rotate the endobutton. Another option for fixation are cross-pins that are inserted from outside-to-in. Tibial fixation can be accomplished with a screw and washer, staple, cross-pins, or bio-absorbable interference screws. A flexion-extension test should be performed to assure impingement-free range of motion as well as a Lachman test to assure successful fixation of the ACL replacement graft.

Complications and Pitfalls

The arthroscopically assisted one-incision technique of ACL reconstruction differs in several ways from the traditional two-incision technique. Therefore, several pitfalls can be encountered that require the surgeon to have alternatives available. As previously mentioned, the preparation of the over-the-top position is critical, as a failure to do so can result in anterior placement of the femoral socket and failure of the ACL reconstruction. If the femoral socket is placed too posterior, on the other hand, the back wall can be perforated, resulting in a femoral socket »blowout«. In this case, one must be prepared to obtain fixation through other means, e.g. over-the-top fixation. Similarly, if significant osteoporosis or poor fixation with an interference screw is encountered, different

fixation techniques should be available. The no. 5 Ethibond sutures from the femoral bone block can be tied to a suture post that is placed in the lateral femoral cortex or an endobutton can be used.

In case of a graft tunnel mismatch in a B-PT-B graft, the surgeon must have different technical options available. The femoral bone block can either remain flush with the articular margin and will be fixed with a metal interference screw, while the tibial bone block will be fixed outside the tunnel with a screw and washer or a staple. Or the femoral bone block will be pushed further up into the femoral tunnel to provide for the tibial bone block to be flush with the tibial cortex. In this case, the femoral bone block can be fixed with a bio-absorbable interference screw and the tibial bone block can be fixed with a metal interference screw or a bio-absorbable interference screw.

Basic Principles of Computer-Assisted Surgery

Prior to the utilization of CAS in the orthopaedic operating room, surgeons commonly used guides and imaging techniques to achieve greater precision of their surgical technique. The femoral quadrant method that was proposed by Bernard and Hertel is a technique that can be utilized intraoperatively to determine the anatomical femoral tunnel position using K-wires and fluoroscopy [3] (Fig. 52-3). Many others have introduced similar techniques with the common goal of achieving greater precision.

CAS is now assumed to facilitate ACL reconstruction in many ways, one of which is to increase precision. Two types of CAS systems have been developed: passive and active systems. Passive systems generally perform no action and provide the surgeon with additional information prior to and during the surgical procedure. Passive navigation systems can be subdivided into three general categories, CT- and MRI-based systems, fluoroscopy-based systems that allow real time imaging during surgery, and non-image based systems that obtain data from kinematics or anatomical landmarks [18]. Active systems have the ability of performing certain surgical steps autonomously and to carry out repetitive motions tirelessly (e.g. drill holes in ACL reconstruction). These systems consist of two main components, a planning station and a control unit with a robot.

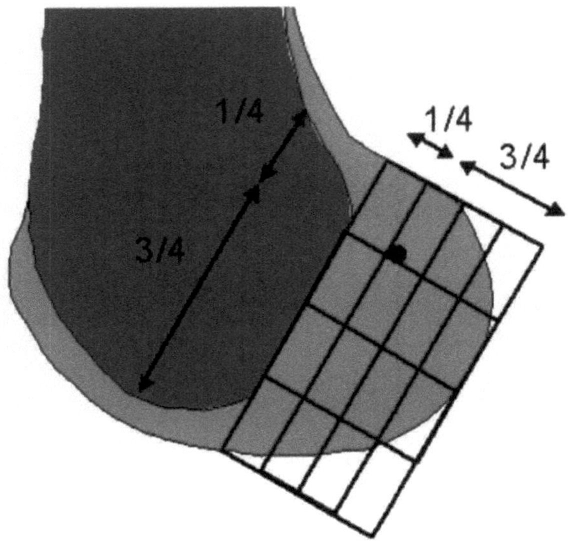

Fig. 52-3. Schematic of a femur, lateral view, femoral quadrant method [3]. The ACL footprint is approximately 1/4 of the distance from Blumensaat's line and 1/4 of the distance from the posterior margin of the femoral condyle

While CAS may allow surgeons to be more precise and enduring, precision and accuracy need to be separately defined. Precision is defined as the degree of agreement between repeated results whereas accuracy is defined as the maximum amount by which a result differs from a true value [1]. Therefore, CAS can only be as precise as the surgeon who plans it, which is especially important in ACL reconstruction, since a universal agreement on the »correct« tunnel position does not exist. Medical imaging, such as magnetic resonance and computed tomography has also experienced many developments in the past years. Yet, preoperative images are presented to the surgeon as a series of two-dimensional scans or radiographs.

Passive Navigation and Active Robotic Systems

Surgical navigation or passive CAS systems include several necessary steps:
1. preoperative planning;
2. intraoperative registration to relate preoperative imaging with the patient's anatomy and position on the operating table;
3. tracking to confirm at all times the position of bony structures and tools (guides, drills, etc) and their movement during surgery.

intraoperative registration or data points-collection can be accomplished with direct or percutaneous probes [8] from fluoroscopic radiographic images [12], or using ultrasonic probes [14]. Two major tracking systems, optical and electromagnetic, are presently available. All systems require attachment of tracking devices to bones and tools. Optical tracking devices sense the position using optical cameras and infrared light emitting diodes or optical reflective markers.

The accuracy of traditional arthroscopic ACL reconstruction and a passive CAS system (KneeNavACL) was compared on 20 identical knee models [17]. This study demonstrated that the passive CAS system could be more accurate than the traditional arthroscopic technique when utilizing 3D data from the CAS system. However, when using planar radiographs as the basis for comparison of accuracy, no statistical difference was noticed, because of poor correlation with the 3-D data. This study critically reviews the lack of accuracy when using 2D images.

Active CAS systems have the ability of performing certain surgical steps autonomously. Digital data for the planning station of active CAS systems are acquired utilizing CT scans of the injured knee. The planning station then displays anterior-posterior, lateral, and cross-sectional images of the knee, allowing the identification of all necessary anatomical landmarks and calculation of 3D orientation of the placement of the ACL graft. On completion of the plan, the data is transferred to the control unit, which can then guide the robot. During surgery, femur and tibia are rigidly attached to the robot, using custom made clamps and pins. Subsequently, a registration process is performed to orient the robot in space. A high-speed drill attached to the robot arm then reams the tunnels. The surgeon supervises the reaming, holding a sterile remote control in his hand with the possibility of interrupting the process at any point in time. A separate bone motion detector is attached to the femur/tibia and monitors relevant motion between the bone and the robot, stopping the reaming process if excessive bone motion occurs.

The precision of tunnel placement during ACL reconstruction was compared between a robotic system

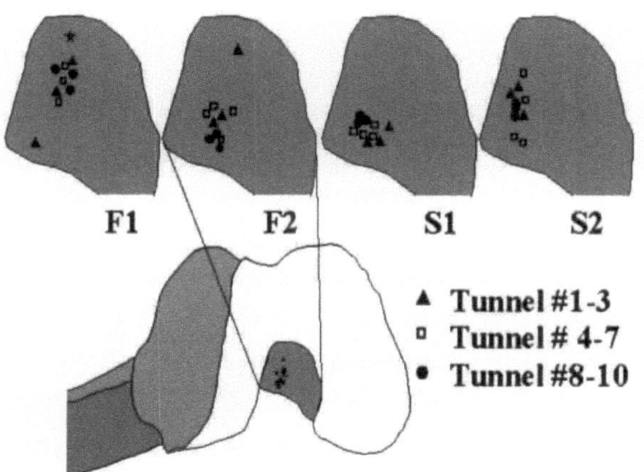

Fig. 52-4. Schematic of femur. Learning curve of femoral tunnel placement (10 tunnels) by four surgeons (Fellows: F1, F2; Surgeons: S1, S2) (with permission from Burkart et al [4])

(CASPAR, U.R.S. ortho, Rastatt, Germany) and traditional arthroscopic techniques using Sawbones. In 10 consecutively drilled tunnels, a learning curve for three (surgical fellows F1, F2, and expert surgeon S2) out of four tested surgeons was shown, as compared to the robot, respectively (**Fig. 52-4**). However, no significant difference in tibial graft tunnel placement between traditional surgeons and the active robot system could be shown. For the femoral tunnel, the robotic technique seemed to be advantageous over the surgeons [4].

In an attempt to assess accuracy of the CASPAR system, a human cadaver trial was conducted. A preoperative tunnel, planned by the surgeon at the surgical planning station and an actual drilled tunnel (autonomously by the robot) revealed a mean difference of <2 mm in tunnel vector, and <1.50 in tunnel angle. Measurements were taken at the intraarticular tunnel points, demonstrating that both consistency in tunnel placement and orientation of the tunnel with respect to the joint line are provided by the active robot system. The results of that study proved the testing hypothesis that the active CAS system is highly accurate [15]. For clarification however, it needs to be stated that improved accuracy of the system does not necessarily mean improvement of ACL surgery.

In summary, advantageous for passive navigation systems is the surgeon-assistance by providing feedback on surgical tool position and surface anatomy in real time. Current literature reveals significant reduction of variability for example in graft tunnel placement for ACL reconstruction when using these systems [6, 12, 20]. Advantageous for active robotic systems, is the tirelessness and ability to carry out a preoperative plan reproducibly. However, for both systems, the registration process bears the risk for imprecise matching of the pre- and intraoperative anatomy and is subject of current research studies. Another problem is the deformation of tools that are being used for drilling into bones. This deformation is known to reduce accuracy of surgical procedures. The disadvantages of active robotic surgery are preoperative placement of fiducials to register the patient's anatomy, reduction in operating room workspace, and difficulties with patient motionless fixation.

Future of ACL Reconstruction

Both active and passive CAS systems are currently subject of basic science and clinical investigations and are being established in the orthopaedic operating room. Specifically, it has been shown that rates of inappropriate tunnel placement are lower when using these systems [6, 11, 12, 19]. Active robot systems however, leave the surgeon with no possibility of intervention, once the preoperative plan is established and the procedure is ongoing. Furthermore, the rigid fixation and preoperative insertion of fiducial markers add morbidity. It is however proven, that both active and passive CAS systems are precise [2, 4, 7].

Although initial results, mainly from clinical experience in Europe, are positive, problems like acceptance by surgeons, high costs, performance validation, and safety issues need to be addressed. At present, CAS can be used to work more precisely inside the musculoskeletal system. For active CAS, robotic technology allows for bones to be machined or drilled during procedures according to the surgeon's specifications. The question, however, remains if more precise surgery can improve clinical outcome.

As described in the introduction section, accuracy can only be achieved if the true value is known. For example in ACL reconstruction, surgeons are still debating whether to place the tunnels for soft tissue fixation of the graft into the geometrical center of the ACL footprint or elsewhere. Unless surgeons will agree to a single point of »correct« tunnel placement on a global consensus, CAS will only be able to accurately carry out a preoperative plan. CAS will therefore not be able to replace surgeons and will only be able to be as accurate as the surgeon who plans the procedure.

For sports medicine applications, navigation systems are currently the »hot topic«. Integration of arthroscopic and 3D images as well as virtual kinematics thereby enables the surgeon to better and more consistently assess graft placement. In the future, arthroscopy, computer navigation, and surgical robotics will be integrated. Virtual kinematics and 3D images can then increase precision in surgical techniques and hopefully the outcome of orthopedic surgery.

References

1. Beckwith T, Buck N, Marangoni R (1993) Treatment of uncertainties. Mechanical Measurements, Fifth Edition, Addison-Wesley
2. Bernard M (2000) Robot-assisted tunnel placement in ACL-surgery. 9th ESSKA Meeting, London
3. Bernard M, Hertel P, Hornung H, Cierpinski T (1997) Femoral insertion of the ACL. Radiographic quadrant method. Amer J Knee Surg 10: 14–21; discussion 21–22
4. Burkart A, Debski R, Rudy T, Musahl V, McMahon P, Fu F, Woo SLY (2002) A comparison of precision for ACL tunnel placement using traditional and robotic technique. Comput Aided Surg 6: 270–278
5. Corry IS, Webb JM, Clingeleffer AJ, Pinczewski LA (1999) Arthroscopic reconstruction of the anterior cruciate ligament. A comparison of patellar tendon autograft and four-strand hamstring tendon autograft. Am J Sports Med 27: 444–454
6. Dessene V, Lavallee S, Julliard R, Orti R, Martelli S, Cinquin P (1995) Computer-assisted knee anterior cruciate ligament reconstruction: first clinical tests. J Image Guid Surg I: 59–64
7. DiGioia AM 3rd, Jaramaz B, Colgan BD (1998) Computer assisted orthopaedic surgery. Image guided and robotic assistive technologies. Clin Orthop 354: 8–16
8. DiGioia AM, Jaramaz B, Blackwell M et al. (1998) The Otto Aufranc Award. Image guided navigation system to measure intraoperatively acetabular implant alignment. Clin Orthop 355: 8–22
9. Eriksson E (1997) How good are the results of ACL reconstruction? Knee Surg Sports Traumatol Arthroscopy 5: 137
10. Harner CD, Fu F, Irrgang JJ, Vogrin TM (2001)) Anterior and posterior cruciate ligament reconstruction in the new millennium: a global perspective. Knee Surg Sports Traumatol Arthroscopy 9: 330–336
11. Julliard R, Lavallee S, Dessenne V (1998) Computer assisted reconstruction of the anterior cruciate ligament. Clin Orthop Rel Res 354: 57–64
12. Klos TV, Habets RJ, Banks AZ, Banks SA, Devilee RJ, Cook FF (1998) Computer assistance in arthroscopic anterior cruciate ligament reconstruction. Clin Orthop Rel Res 354: 65–69
13. Kohn D, Busche T, Carls J (1998) Drill hole position in endoscopic anterior cruciate ligament reconstruction. Results of an advanced arthroscopy course. Knee Surg Sports Traumatol Arthroscopy 6 [Suppl 1]: S13–15
14. Kowal J, Amstutz CA, Nolte LP (2001) On B-mode ultrasound based registration for computer assisted orthopaedic surgery. in computer assisted orthopaedic surgery – CAOS/USA. Pittsburgh, PA
15. Musahl V, Burkart A, Debski R, VanSyoc A, Fu FH, Woo SL-Y (2002) Accuracy of ACL-Tunnel Placement with an active robot system – CASPAR: A cadaveric study. Arthroscopy 18: 968–973
16. Musahl V, Cierpinski T, Hornung H, Hertel P (1999) Sekundäre vordere Kreuzbandplastik nach primärer Naht und Kreuzbandplastik. 63. Jahrestagung der DGU, November 1999, Berlin, Germany
17. Picard F, Moody JE, DiGioia AM et al. (2001) Knee Nav-ACL computer assisted measurement reliability. Comput Aided Surg 6: 6
18. Picard F, Moody JE, Jaramaz B, DiGioia AM, Nikou C, Labarca RC (2001) A classification proposal for computer assisted knee systems. CAOS International, Davos, Switzerland
19. Sati M, Bourquin Y, Staeubli H, Nolte LP (2000) Considering anatomic and functional factors in ACL reconstruction: new technology. 4th CAOS USA meeting, Pittsburgh, PA, USA, pp 121–123
20. Sati M, de Guise JA, Drouin G (1997) Computer assisted knee surgery: diagnostics and planning of knee surgery. Comput Aided Surg 2: 108–123

53 Fundamentals in ACL Reconstruction: »The European View«

S. Rupp, D. Kohn

Introduction

Tears of the anterior cruciate ligament are common injuries. Today the incidence is 1 injury per 1000 people per year [102]. It occurs typically during sports due to a external rotation valgus movement of the flexed weight bearing knee e.g. during skiing or football. An overextension mechanism is also possible.

This article reviews the current treatment options.

Anatomy and Function

The anterior cruciate ligament (ACL) runs in an anterior direction from the femur to the tibia. From the femur the ACL originates from the lateral condyle on the posterior aspect of the medial surface (◘ Fig. 53-1). The average length is 31 mm [77]. The ACL fans out in the distal part of the ligament resulting in a larger tibial attachment. The tibial attachment is located at the anterocentral region of the tibial plateau between the tibial eminences, medial to the insertion of the anterior horn of the lateral meniscus.

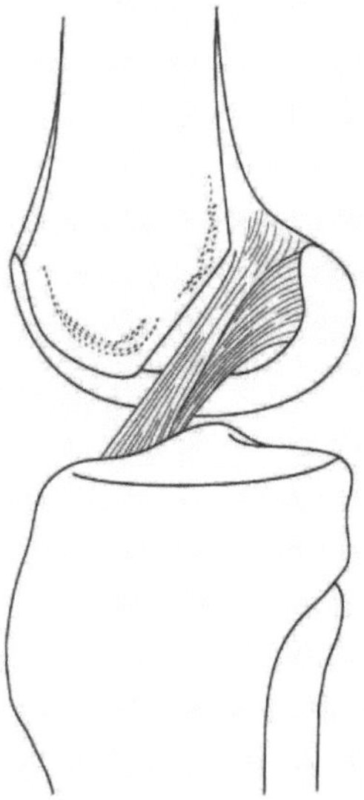

◘ **Fig. 53-1.** Anatomy of the ACL

It is suggested that the ACL has two complementary roles: proprioceptive function and mechanical restraint.

The role as a load carrying structure has been defined extensively. The ACL resists forces that cause the tibia to translate anteriorly relative to the femur. In addition, the ACL provides a restraint to internal rotation of the tibia, varus and valgus angulation, and hyperextension of the knee. In concert with the posterior cruciate ligament the bony geometry the ACL controls the extension flexion kinematics of the knee.

The ACL deficiency leads to an increased tibial translation in anterior direction laxity of the joint. In many knee joints the increased laxity results in an overuse of secondary restraints as the posterior horn of the medial meniscus and the posterior oblique ligament. In the long run ACL deficiency may result in damage to the articular cartilage and osteoarthritis.

The role as a proprioceptive element is not outlined as clearly as the mechanical role. The proprioceptive function has to be quantified further.

Therapy

Treatment Options

The treatment of ACL deficiency should be individualized. The decision should be based on the degree of instability, the age of the patient and the activity level.

Non-operative treatment may be an issue for people without giving way. The activity level should be low. The focus of non-operative treatment is on the strengthening of the knee stabilizing muscles (hamstrings are agonists of the ACL) and on the improvement of coordination. However, it can be expected that the complex kinematics is not controlled on a physiologic level. In the long run lesions of the menisci and the hyaline cartilage may occur.

In the case of higher activity levels (high risk pivoting sports) or giving ways during activities of daily living ACL reconstruction is recommended.

There are two main goals:

1. Prevention of giving way and restoration of gross stability.
2. Prevention of osteoarthritis due to instability.

Principles of ACL Reconstruction

Today the torn ACL is commonly replaced with an autologuos tendon graft that is fixed in femoral and tibial tunnels.

The replacement is commonly done arthroscopically. Surgery via miniarthrotomy is possible.

The success of ACL reconstruction depends on several key factors:

- graft selection,
- graft placement,
- graft fixation,
- rehabilitation.

Graft Selection

Autografts and allografts are the two graft options. The use of allografts has the risk of infection with HIV or hepatitis. The sterilization and storage compromises the mechanical and biological quality of the tissue. Commonly autografts are used.

Two grafts are widely used [21]:

- The mid third of the patellar tendon with bone plugs from the patella and the tibia (bone – patella tendon – bone graft).
- The semitendinosus graft (quadrupled) or the semitendinosus/gracilis graft (doubled)

Other graft options are:

- quadriceps tendon [35, 101],
- plantaris-longus tendon (eight strands) [42].

There is a scientific debate about the pros and cons with respect to the different graft options. To our opinion there is no ideal graft.

In the clinical setting the graft selection should be based on several factors:

- mechanical properties of the graft fixation construct,
  - tendon,
  - fixation
- biology of healing of the graft,
- donor site morbidity.

Mechanical Properties of the Graft Fixation Construct

The basic question is: How much load the graft sees during rehabilitation? Morrison estimated the resulting forces during activities of daily living using a mathematical model base of reaction forces measured under the foot. The resulting forces should range from 27 N (stair-climbing) to 445 N (going downhill) [70]. Noyes and Grood suggested that the ACL should be loaded up to 1/5 of its maximum strength during activities of daily living. They estimated that the resulting forces range from 200 to 400 N [74]. From direct measurements of the resulting forces it is known that a graft which is pretensioned with 40 N in 30 degrees of flexion is loaded up to 125 in full extension. If the knee is fully extended against gravity using quadriceps pull the load increases up to 250 N [92].

The strength of the graft and the strength of the graft fixation to the bone should be assessed independently.

The strength of the BPTB-graft ranges from 1700 to 2900 N [15, 25, 31, 32, 75, 84, 106]. The semitendinosus tendon or the gracilis tendon has a maximum strength of 1200 N [75]. In theory, a four strand graft would tear at 4000 N [40] under the condition that all strands are equally loaded. However, this is not realistic in vivo.

The maximum strength of the graft tissue is superior to the resulting graft forces during rehabilitation.

The graft fixation is the weak link during the first weeks after surgery. Interference screw fixation of the BPTB-graft is a widely used procedure. It achieves a very stiff (ca. 4000 N/mm) [3] fixation with a high initial pull-out force (400–900 N in younger patients) [18, 49, 62, 65, 80, 89, 91, 104]. In the case of a divergence between the screw and the bone plug of more than 15° to 30° the initial stability decreases [54, 66, 82].

Some surgeons use a press-fit fixation of the BPTB-graft without any implant [16, 17, 43]. At the moment a valid biomechanical evaluation of this technique is lacking.

Several techniques of fixation are available for the hamstring graft. The tendon graft fixation can be achieved with techniques that secure the graft near the tibial and the femoral cortices using an endobutton or suture plate on the femoral side and a post screw or a suture disc on the tibial side (◘ Fig. 53-2a). This construct fixes the graft distant to the joint line and may allow for increased graft tunnel motion [44] which may result in a bone tunnel enlargement [24, 51] and may compromise the graft-tunnel healing. With respect to the mechanic behavior of the graft a stiffer construct seems desirable. This can be achieved using a transfixation (◘ Fig. 53-2c) or an interference fixation (◘ Fig. 53-2b). The interference fixation may fail during submaximum loading due to graft slippage [3]. Up to now none of these fixation techniques has proven to be superior.

Biologic Properties

Bone plug-patellar tendon-bone plug grafts in a bone tunnel are incorporated after 8 weeks. However, in most cases the graft is too long resulting in a position of the bone plug distant from the joint line. Tendon graft incorporation has been shown to occur in an indirect manner. Sharpey fibers connect the tunnel wall and the graft [69, 85, 108]. To promote healing it is important that the graft fits snugly within the osseous tunnel.

Donor Site Morbidity

The harvesting of an autologous graft may be associated with donor site symptoms. Especially the use of the central third of the patellar tendon is reported to have a high rate of donor site morbidity as

- muscle weakness,
- anterior knee pain,
- shortening of the patellar tendon,
- pain with kneeling.

Muscle Weakness. The harvest of the central third of the patella tendon is associated with a weakness of the extensor mechanism. Six months after surgery the quadri-

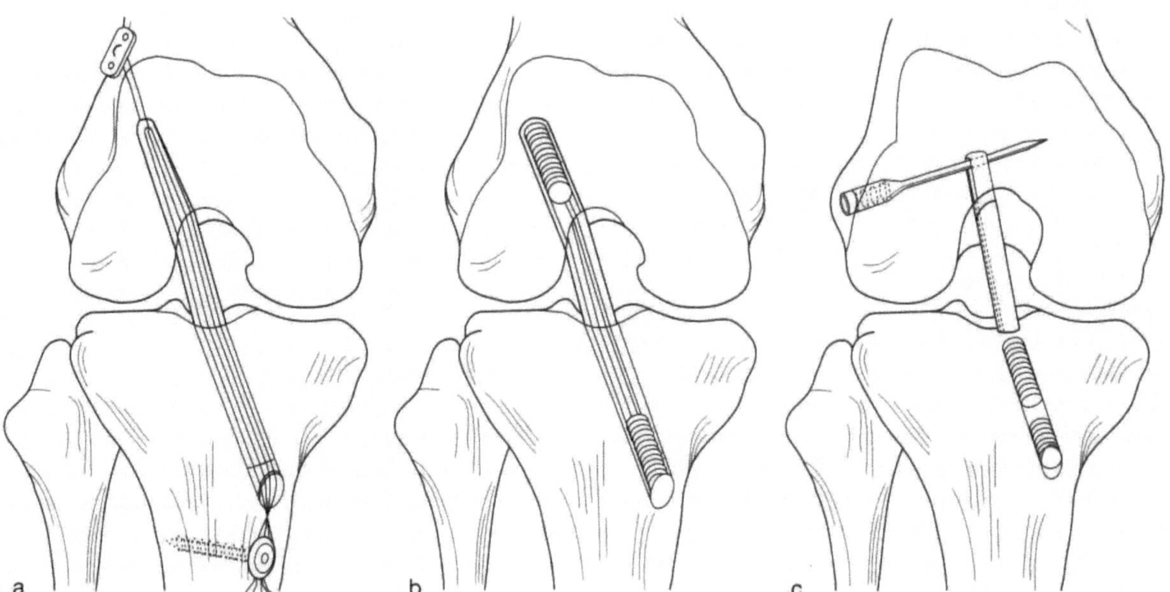

◘ Fig. 53-2a–c. Fixation of a semitendinosus gracilis graft. **a** Suture plate and post screw. **b** Interference screw. **c** Cross pin on the femoral side and interference screw on the tibial side

ceps strength his 70% during isokinetic testing [22, 59]. However, in a prospective study, Carter et al. [22] failed to demonstrate a significant difference between BPTB-grafts and hamstring grafts with respect to muscle strength.

Keays et al. [60] found 6 months after the use of a hamstring graft a 12% reduction of the strength of the quadriceps muscle and a 12% reduction of the strength of the hamstrings. Similar reductions are seen after the use of allografts [67]. The graft harvest seems to be only one out of several factors responsible for the reduction of strength.

Anterior Knee Pain. Anterior knee pain was reported in up to 35% of patients 3 to 6 years after ACL reconstruction using the BPTB graft. However in most cases the pain level was very low [71]. In only 10% of the patients the pain interfered with their sports activities.

Jarvela et al. [53] found 7 years after ACL-reconstruction with a BPTB graft a moderate arthritis of the femoropatellar joint in 12% and severe arthritis in 1% of the patients.

Despite these data anterior knee pain is not due exclusively to the harvest of the central third of the patellar tendon. It seems reasonable to suppose that the pathogenesis is based upon several independent factors.

This conclusion is based on several facts: Even after the use of allografts retropatellar crepitation was found [76]. Harvesting the graft from the opposite knee Rubinstein et al. [88] did not find any anterior knee pain.

After the use of hamstring grafts anterior knee pain was reported in up to 23% of the patients [4,56,95]. Spicer et al. [100] found relevant anterior knee pain during sports activities in 7% of the patients with a hamstring graft. Eriksson et al. [28] compared in a prospective randomized study 80 patients with a BPTB graft and 73 patients with a 4 strand semitendinosus gracilis graft. The minimum follow-up was 24 months. There was no difference between the 2 groups with regard to the patellofemoral pain score according to Werner [105].

Feller et al. [30] compared in a prospective randomized study 31 patients with a BPTB graft and 34 patients with a hamstring graft. After 4 months 81% of the patients with a BPTB graft and 70% of the patients with a hamstring graft complained about anterior knee pain. The difference was not significant.

Besides the graft harvest other factors as the initial trauma with resulting chondral lesions, secondary changes as fibrosis of the Hoffa fat pad and unphysiologic joint kinematics may be responsible for the anterior knee pain.

There is a relevant percentage of patients (up to 57%) after having undergone ACL replacement with a BPTB graft who complain about patellar pain due to kneeling [27, 57, 71]. Even if there are reports about pain with kneeling after ACL replacement with hamstring grafts [100] most surgeons agree that the hamstring graft should be used in patients working in kneeling position.

Shortening of the Patellar Ligament. A shortening of the patellar ligament has been reported after harvesting of the mid third of the patellar ligament. However, this phenomenon is seen only in a minority of cases [96] In a study based on sonographic length measurement 75% of the patients had none or only a minimal shortening of the tendon. In only 6% of the cases a shortening of 7–9 mm was found [71].

»The Ideal Graft«

The BPTB graft has been the gold standard over years. The scientific data base is better for the BPTB graft than for other potential grafts. With regard to clinical outcome and donor site morbidity BPTB grafts and hamstring grafts seem to be equivalent. Each graft has advantages and disadvantages.

However, there are distinct situations in which the hamstring graft may be preferable.

In children with open physes a hamstring graft with extracortical fixation should be used. The application of a bone block or a screw across the open physes would cause a premature closure and a consecutive axe deviation of the leg. Patients which work often in kneeling position may be disabled after the use of a BPTB graft. On the other hand bone to bone healing has been shown to be more predictable and faster than soft tissue to bone healing. Interference screw fixation of the bone plug to the tunnel has proven to be considerably strong. Therefore, the BPTB graft may be advantageous in high demand athletes which need an accelerated rehabilitation and early return to sports.

Advantages and Disadvantages of Different Grafts

BPTB graft

- Advantages
  - High maximum strength of the tendon
  - High initial stability of fixation (interference screws)
  - Bone to bone healing
  - Broad scientific basis
- Disadvantages
  - Anterior knee pain with kneeling
  - Graft geometry (rectangular cross section, graft sometimes to long to fix it on joint level)
  - Extensor mechanism weakness

Hamstring graft

- Advantages
  - High maximum strength of the tendon
  - Small incision for graft harvest (cosmesis)
  - Geometry (four strands, round cross section)
  - No anterior knee pain with kneeling
- Disadvantages
  - Fixation of the graft
  - Tendon to bone healing
  - Weakness of knee flexion and internal rotation

It is reasonable that a surgeon is experienced in several techniques to design graft selection and fixation individually adapted to the special needs of each patient.

Graft Position

Graft positioning is crucial. However, there still is some controversy about the optimal position.

Strain of 4% to 20% of the resting length causes irreversible structural lesions of collagen tissue [2, 68, 83]. The intraarticular length of a graft is about 31 mm [77]. The maximum strain should be less than 1,2 to 6,2 mm. Therefore, the distance between the femoral and tibial tunnel should be constant during the full range of motion. This would mean »isometric«.

The position of the femoral tunnel strongly determines the forces seen by the graft during a flexion extension movement. Zavras et al. analyzed 13 so-called isometric

points given in several papers [109]. Some points were located outside of the femoral footprint of the ACL. The points proposed by Friederich, Hefzy and Sidles [33, 34, 41, 99] were associated with the smallest change of the femorotibial distance [109].

The best tunnel position seems to be at the cranial circumference of the ACL footprint at the posterolateral edge of the intercondylar roof (Blumensaat's line in the X-ray; ◘ Fig. 53-3).

The most common error in ACL surgery is a too anterior position of the femoral tunnel. This position is unisometric and results in an inappropriate strain pattern [72]. Flexion of the knee causes unphysiologic strain and the graft may stretch out (◘ Fig. 53-4). In extended knee position the graft is loose.

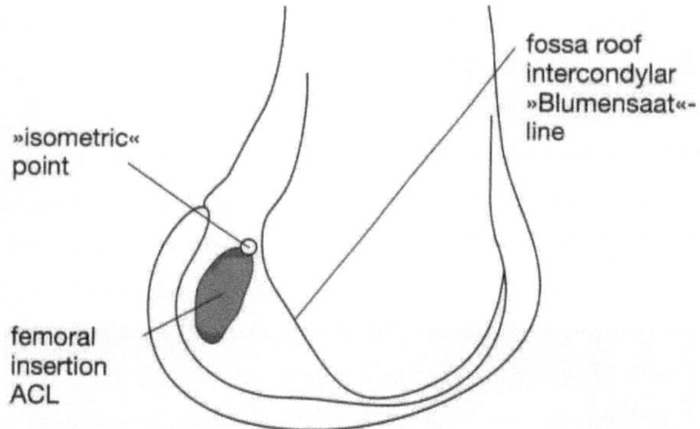

◘ Fig. 53-3. »Isometric« position

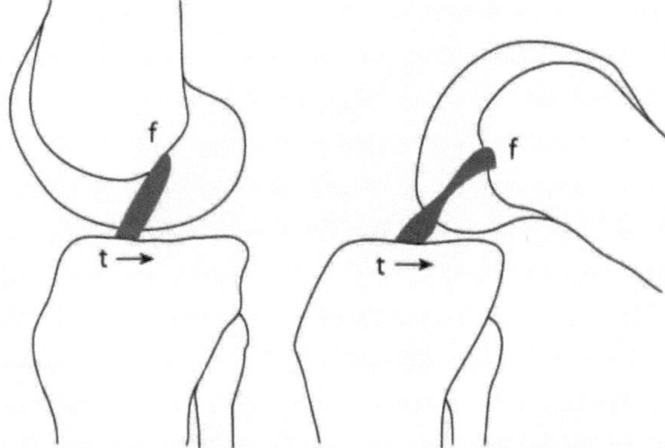

◘ Fig. 53-4. Anterior malposition of the femoral tunnel. t tibial graft attachment site; f femoral graft attachment site. Flexion of the knee leads to a significant increase of the distance t – f. In this situation the knee flexion may be blocked or the graft stretches out with knee laxity

In order to identify the ideal position it is mandatory to expose the posteriolateral edge of the intercondylar roof (Fig. 53-5). An aiming device can be used to position a guide wire for the definite tunnel reamer in a defined distance from the edge of the roof (Fig. 53-6). This ensures a posterior tunnel wall of 1–2 mm. In the frontal plane the tunnel should be positioned between the 10 and 11 o'clock position for the right knee and between the 1 and 2 o'clock position for the left knee.

The tibial tunnel defines the relation between the graft and the roof of the intercondylar notch (Blumensaat's line) in knee extension [8, 45, 46, 47, 73, 107]. The tunnel position should be far enough posterior so that the extension of the anterior tunnel wall lies behind the roof of the intercondylar notch in knee extension. This position avoids that the notch impinges on the graft during knee extension (so-called »notch-impingement«), which would cause an extension lag and a attrition of the graft. [45, 46] (Fig. 53-7). The center of the tunnel should intersect with the tibia at about 43% of the a.p. diameter [8]. How-

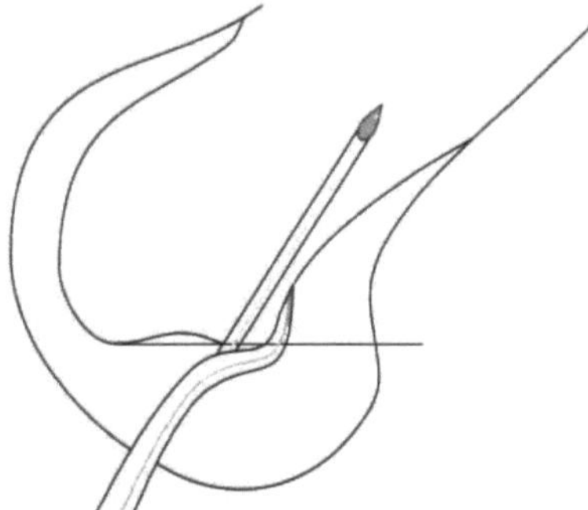

Fig. 53-5. Use of the aiming device during positioning of the femoral tunnel

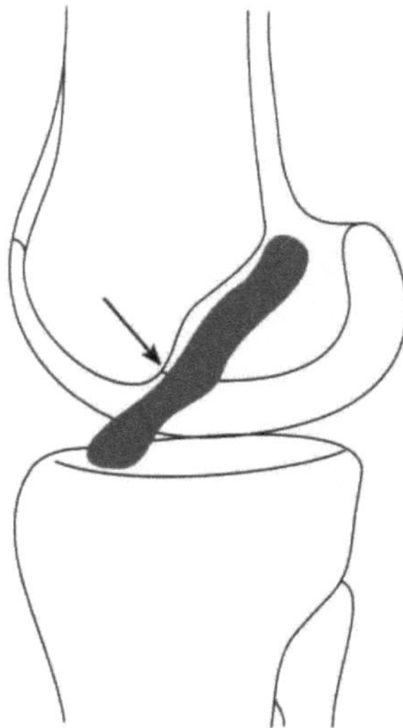

Fig. 53-7. »Notchimpingement«. The tibial tunnel lies too far anterior. During knee extension the intercondylar roof impinges on the graft (arrow). This situation results in extension lag and graft lesion

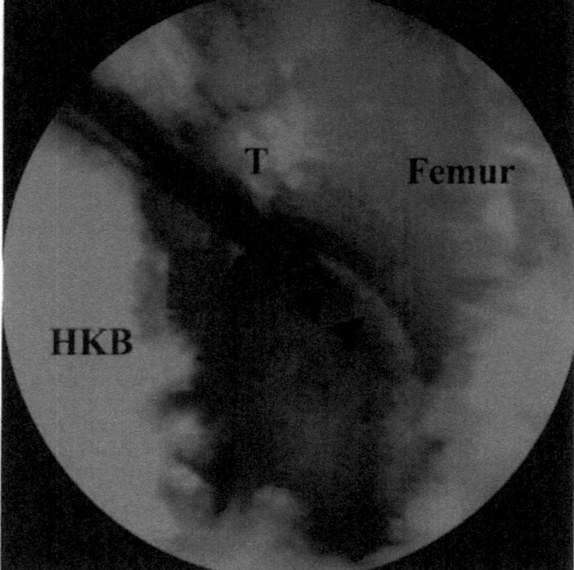

Fig. 53-6. ACL reconstruction. The posterolateral edge of the intercondylar roof is exposed. The position is verified with a probe (T). HKB posterior cruciate ligament

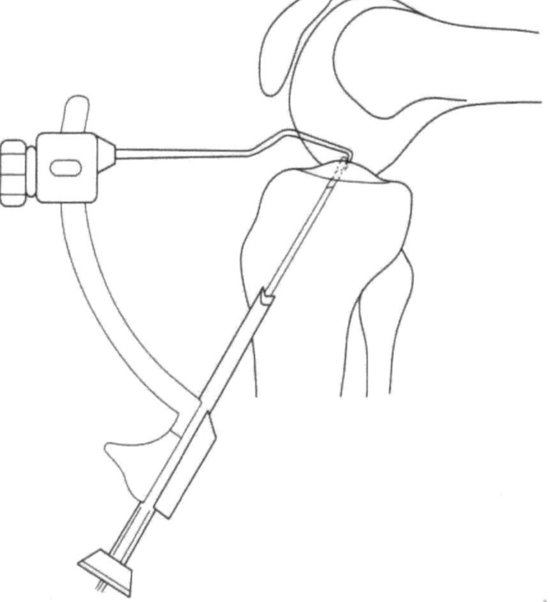

Fig. 53-8. Use of an drill guide for the positioning of the tibial tunnel

ever, there are great variations of the inclination of the roof of the intercondylar notch in relation to the long axis of the femur. The angle ranges from 26° to 46°. Knees with a steep roof (small angle) which can be hyperextended are problematic (»unforgiving notch«) [45, 46]. The tibial tunnel has to be drilled in a more posterior position [46].

The tibial tunnel is placed using a drill guide (◻ Fig. 53-8). Anatomic landmarks are the stump of the ACL, the medial tibial spine, the anterior horn of the lateral meniscus and the PCL. Some drill guides use the PCL as reference. The center of the tunnel is 7 mm from the PCL with the knee at 90 degrees. However, all these landmarks are highly variable. Especially a fixed distance to the PCL seems not to be appropriate in alls knees. To validate the planned tunnel position the K-wire can be controlled fluoroscopically.

Special Considerations in Children

The type of ACL injuries in the skeletally immature patient, either tibial spine avulsion or mid-substance tear, depends on the load conditions and the maturity of the knee. Avulsion fractures predominate in children and under lower loads whereas mid-substance tears predominate in adolescents in conditions of larger loads.

Non-displaced or minimally displaces fractures of the tibial spine are treated in a long-leg cast for 6 to 8 weeks. Hinged or displaced fractures are reduced under arthroscopic control and fixed.

Mid-substance tears in skeletally immature patients receive increasing attention. Poor results have been reported after non-operative treatment in the presence of instability and unlimited activity. Surgical reconstruction should be preferred [6,29]. There is some debate whether the reconstruction should be transphysal or physeal sparing. Transphysal drilling has a potential risk of inducing growth abnormalities. This risk seems to be low when using a hamstring graft which fills the bone tunnels snug fit and is fixed extraarticularly using an endobutton and a suture disc.

Rehabilitation

Rehabilitation following ACL reconstruction must take into account the initial graft strength, the fixation method and the ligament healing process.

During the first 6 to 8 weeks after surgery the graft fixation is the weak link. The graft is avascular in this period. However, the collagen fibers remain grossly intact. The intrinsic strength of the graft tissue remains high under the condition of avascularity [93]. Based on animal experiments [7, 10, 13, 19, 20, 23, 37] and on biopsy studies in humans [1, 87] one can suggest that revascularisation weakens the graft which reaches its definite strength during a remodeling process between 12 and 24 months after the ACL reconstruction.

During the first weeks the graft fixation construct is the most important load limiting factor. Patients with a BPTB graft fixed with interference screws can undergo an accelerated rehabilitation protocol [90, 97]. Early full weight bearing and unrestricted range of motion are possible. A brace can be avoided. After ACL reconstruction with a hamstring graft fixed indirectly with an endobutton and a suture disc or a post screw less aggressive rehabilitation seems to be appropriate. We place the patients in a hinged postoperative brace and start weight bearing not before 4 weeks after surgery.

Further aims during rehabilitation are to regain full range of motion, coordination, endurance and muscle strength. The patient is allowed to return to sports at 6 to 9 months.

Results

There is some debate about how to measure the result after ACL-replacement. ◻ Table 53-1 gives mid-term results after ACL replacement.

This metaanalysis shows that only 75% of the knees are normal or nearly normal in terms of the IKDC scores. It is not possible to restore the physiological laxity of the knee joint in all cases (side to side difference less than 3 mm). The mean side to side difference is 2 mm. Women seem to have a higher degree of laxity especially after the use of hamstring grafts [14,26]. The cause remains unknown at the moment.

However, the restitution of the »correct laxity« may be crucial with respect to the prevention of osteoarthritis.

It is not clear whether this goal is within the reach of ACL surgery. The initial trauma and the surgical procedure impair the homeostasis of the hyaline cartilage for at least 1 year [103]. Shelbourne und Gray [98] found a

Table 53-1. Results after ACL reconstruction

Author	Graft	FU [years]	n	IKDC A u. B [%]	KT 1000 <3 mm [%]	KT 1000 Side to side difference [mm]
Aglietti 1997 [5]	BPTB	5,4–8,6	89 [89%]	77	49	
Anderson 2001 [9]	BPTB	2	35 [100%]	100	71	2,1+/-2,0
Anderson 2001 [9]	STG	2	33 [94%]	91	52	3,1+/-2,3
Aune 2001 [11]	BPTB	2	29 [83%]			2,7+/-2,2
Aune 2001 [11]	STG	2	32 [86%]			2,7+/-2,1
Bach 1998 [12]	BPTB	5,5–9,4	97 [66%]	–	70	1
Corry 1999 [26]	BPTB	2	77 [85%]	86	91	1
Corry 1999 [26]	STG	2	77 [85%]	93	79	1,7
Deehan 2000 [27]	BPTB	5	80 [89%]	90	81	
Erikkson 2001 [27]	BPTB	2–4,9	80 [95%]	60	49	
Good 1994 [36]	BPTB	2	24 [100%]		54	2,0+/-2,3
Hamada 2001 [39]	STG	2	57 [66%]	93	93	0,9+/-1,8
Howell 1999 [48]	STG	2	67 [96%]	91	91	
Jäger 2001 [50]	BPTB	8,5–11	75 [82%]	83,7	79,8	2,0+/-1,2
Jomha 1999 [55]	BPTB	7	59 [74%]	76	64	1,7+/-1,8
Kartus 1999 [58]	BPTB	1,75–5,7	604 [95%]	74,5	72,9	1,5
Kleipool 1998 [61]	BPTB	3,5–6,2	26 [90%]	70	69	
O'Neil 1996 [79]	BPTB	2–5	45 [100%]	95	87	
Patel 2000 [81]	BPTB	>5	32 [72%]		87	
Ropke 2001 [86]	BPTB	2	20 [100%]	50		1,6
Ropke 2001 [86]	STG	2	20 [100%]	80		2,7
Rupp 2001 [94]	BPTB	3–6	51 [88%]	74	68	2,0+/-0,3
Shelbourne 1997 [98]	BPTB	2–9	806 [76%]	85		2,0+/-1,5

BPTB bone-patellar tendon-bone graft; *STG* semitendinosus-gracilis graft. *FU* follow-up (years); *n* number of patients (percentage of patients which were investigated at follow-up.

joint space narrowing in 94% of patients after ACL reconstruction for acute instability and in 89% of patients after ACL reconstruction for chronic instability 2 to 9 years after the index procedure. In contrary other authors described low rates of osteoarthritis at mid term follow-up [27,52]. Graft function and associated lesions with special emphasis on meniscal tears may have an important role [27,55].

Revision ACL Reconstruction

Revision ACL surgery becomes more important. Infection, persisting pain, restricted range of motion and residual or recurrent instability necessitate revision surgery in an increasing number of cases. The results after revision ACL reconstruction are inferior to the results after primary reconstruction.

Revision surgery needs a thorough analysis of the mechanism of failure. In most cases instability after ACL reconstruction is due to technical errors as mal-position of the tunnels, unstable primary fixation or insufficient tensioning of the graft. In addition, failure of graft remodeling or graft incorporation in the bone tunnels is possible. A rehabilitation which is too aggressive or high risk pivoting sports on an early stage after surgery may compromise graft function and lead to failure. A true traumatic re-rupture seems to be rare.

In most cases we see a giving way due to preexisting instability.

Planning and surgical technique are complex [64,78]. Graft selection and management of bone tunnels are crucial [64]. Revision surgery should be carried out by experienced knee surgeons

Future Directions

Expectations of patients and surgeons are high. However, with respect to knee function, objective stability and prevention of osteoarthritis results are not good enough. Further improvement of therapeutic concepts is necessary.

A relevant percentage of grafts is mal-positioned [63]. Computer-assisted drilling of the bone tunnels may improve graft position even in the hand of less experienced surgeons leading to better outcomes.

Improved techniques of graft fixation which allow for strong, rigid fixation on the joint level may improve the structural properties of the graft fixation construct.

Advances in molecular therapy, tissue engineering and gene therapy may offer options to accelerate and improve graft to tunnel healing and graft remodeling. However, routine clinical application of these techniques seems to be years away. In the near future improvement of results will come from optimizing of tunnel positions and graft fixation.

References

1. Abe S, Kurosaka M, Iguchi T, Yoshiya S, Hirohata K (1993) Light and electron microscopic study of remodeling and maturation process in autogenous graft for anterior cruciate ligament reconstruction. Arthroscopy 9: 394–405
2. Abrahams M (1967) Mechanical behaviour of tendon in vitro. Med Biol Eng 5: 433–443
3. Adam F, Pape D, Steimer O, Kohn D, Rupp S (2001) Biomechanische Eigenschaften der Interferenzverschraubung beim Ersatz des vorderen Kreuzbandes mit Patellar- und Hamstringtransplantaten. Orthopäde 30: 649–657
4. Aglietti P, Buzzi P, Zaccherotti G, Debiase P (1994) Patellar tendon versus doubled semitendinosus and gracilis tendons for anterior cruciate ligament reconstruction. Am J Sports Med 22: 211–218
5. Aglietti P, Buzzi R, Giron F, Simeone AJ, Zaccherotti G (1997) Arthroscopic-assisted anterior cruciate ligament reconstruction with the central third patellar tendon. A 5–8-year follow-up. Knee Surg Sports Traumatol Arthrosc 5: 138–44
6. Aichroth PM, Patel DV, Zorrilla P (2002) The natural history and treatment of rupture of the anterior cruciate ligament in children and adolescents. A prospective review. J Bone Joint Surg 84-B: 38–41
7. Amiel D, Kleiner JB, Roux RD, Harwood, FL, Akeson WH (1986) The phenomenon of »ligamentization«: anterior cruciate ligament reconstruction with autogenous patellar tendon. J Orthop Res 4: 162–172
8. Amis AA, Jakob RP (1998) Anterior cruciate ligament graft positioning, tensioning and twisting. Knee Surg Sports Traumatol Arthrosc 6 [Suppl 1]: S2–12
9. Anderson AF, Snyder RB, Lipscomb AB Jr (2001) Anterior cruciate ligament reconstruction. A prospective randomized study of three surgical methods Am J Sports Med 29: 272–279
10. Arnoczky SP, Tarvin GB, Marshall JL (1982) Anterior cruciate ligament replacement using patellar tendon. J Bone Joint Surg 64-A: 217–224
11. Aune AK, Holm I, Risberg MA, Jensen HK, Steen H (2001) Four-strand hamstring tendon autograft compared with patellar tendon-bone autograft for anterior cruciate ligament reconstruction. A randomized study with two-year follow-up. Am J Sports Med 29: 722–728
12. Bach BR Jr, Tradonsky S, Bojchuk J, Levy ME, Bush-Joseph CA, Khan NH (1998) Arthroscopically assisted anterior cruciate ligament reconstruction using patellar tendon autograft. Five- to nine-year follow-up evaluation. Am J Sports Med 26: 20–29
13. Ballock RT, Woo SL-Y, Lyon RM, Hollis JM, Akeson WH (1989) Use of patellar tendon autograft for anterior cruciate ligament reconstruction in the rabbit: a long term histological and biomechanical study. J Orthop Res 4: 474–485
14. Barrett GR, Noojin FK, Hartzog CW, Nash CR (2002) Reconstruction of the anterior cruciate ligament in females: A comparison of hamstring versus patellar tendon autograft. Arthroscopy 18: 46–54
15. Blevins FT, Hecker AT, Bigler GT, Boland AL, Hayes WC (1994) The effects of donor age and strain rate on the biomechanical properties of bone-patellar tendon-bone allografts. Am J Sports Med 22: 328–333
16. Boszotta H. (1997) Arthroscopic anterior cruciate ligament reconstruction using a patellar tendon graft in press-fit technique: surgical technique and follow-up. Arthroscopy 13: 332–339
17. Boszotta H, Anderl W (2001) Primary stability with tibial press-fit fixation of patellar ligament graft: An experimental study in ovine knees. Arthroscopy 17: 963–970
18. Brown CH, Hecker AT, Hipp JA, Myers ER, Hayes WC (1993) The biomechanics of interference screw fixation of patellar tendon anterior cruciate ligament grafts. Am J Sports Med 21: 880–886
19. Butler DL, Hulse DA, Kay MD, Grood ES, Shires PK, D`Ambrosia R, Shoji H (1983) Biomechanics of cranial cruciate ligament reconstruction in the dog: II. Mechanical properties. Vet Surg 12: 113–118
20. Butler DL, Grood ES, Noyes FR, Olmstead ML, Hohn RB, Arnoczky SP, Siegel MG (1989) Mechanical properties of primate vascularized vs. nonvascularized patellar tendon grafts; change over time. J Orthop Res 7: 68–79
21. Campbell JD (1998) The evolution and current treatment trends with anterior cruciate, posterior cruciate, and medial collateral ligament injuries. Am J Knee Surg 11: 128–135
22. Carter TR, Edinger S (1999) Isokinetic evaluation of anterior cruciate ligament reconstruction: hamstring versus patellar tendon. Arthroscopy 15: 169–72
23. Clancy WG, Narechania RG, Rosenberg TD, Gmeiner JG, Wisnefske DD, Lange TA (1981) Anterior and posterior cruciate ligament reconstruction in rhesus monkeys. J Bone Joint Surg 63-A: 1270–1284
24. Clatworthy MG, Annear P, Bulow JU, Bartlett RJ (1999) Tunnel widening in anterior cruciate ligament reconstruction: a prospective evaluation of hamstring and patella tendon grafts. Knee Surg Sports Traumatol Arthrosc 7: 138–145
25. Cooper DE, Deng XH, Burstein AL, Warren RF (1993) The strength of the central third patellar tendon graft. A biomechanical study. Am J Sports Med 21: 818–824

26. Corry IS, Webb JM, Clingeleffer AJ, Pinczewski LA (1999) Arthroscopic reconstruction of the anterior cruciate ligament. A comparison of patellar tendon autograft and four-strand hamstring tendon autograft. Am J Sports Med 27: 444–454

27. Deehan DJ, Salmon LJ, Webb VJ, Davies A, Pinczewski LA (2000) Endoscopic reconstruction of the anterior cruciate ligament with an ipsilateral patellar tendon autograft. A prospective longitudinal five-year study. J Bone Joint Surg Br 82: 984–991

28. Eriksson K, Anderberg P, Hamberg P, Löfgren AC, Bredenberg M, Westman I, Wredmark T (2001) A comparison of quadruple semitendinosus and patellar tendon grafts in reconstruction of the anterior cruciate ligament. J Bone Joint Surg 83-Br: 348–355

29. Fehnel DJ, Johnson R Anterior cruciate injuries in the skeletally immature athlete: a review of treatment outcomes. Sports Med 29: 51–63

30. Feller JA, Webster KE, Gavin B (2001) Early postoperative morbidity following anterior cruciate ligament reconstruction: patellar tendon versus hamstring graft. Knee Surg Sports Traumatol Arthrosc 9: 260–266

31. Fideler B, Vangsness C, Bin L, Orlando C, Moore T (1995) Gamma irradiation: effect on biomechanical properties of human bone-patellar tendobone allografts. Am J Sports Med 23: 643–646

32. Flahiff CM, Brooks AT, Hollis JM, Van der Schilden JL, Nicholas RW (1995) Biomechanical analysis of patellar tendon allografts as a function of donor age. Am J Sports Med 23: 354–358

33. Friederich NF (1993) Kniegelenksfunktion und Kreuzbänder: Biomechanische Grundlagen für Rekonstruktion und Rehabilitation. Orthopäde 22: 334–342

34. Friederich NF, O'Brien WR (1998) Functional anatomy of the cruciate ligaments. In: Jakob RP, Staubli HU (Hrsg) The knee and the cruciate ligaments. Springer, Berlin Heidelberg New York Tokyo

35. Fulkerson JP, Langeland R (1995) An alternative cruciate reconstruction graft: The central quadriceps tendon. Arthroscopy 11: 252–254

36. Good L, Odensten M, Gillquist J (1994) Sagittal knee stability after anterior cruciate ligament reconstruction with a patellar tendon strip. Am J Sports Med 22: 518–523

37. Goradia VK, Rochat MC, Kida M, Grana WA (2000) Natural history of a hamstring tendon autograft used for anterior cruciate ligament reconstruction in a sheep model. Am J Sports Med 28: 40–6

38. Haas N (2000) Kreuzbandchirurgie – Ein ewig aktuelles Thema (Editorial). Chirurg 71: 1023–1022

39. Hamada M, Shino K, Horibe S, Mitsuoka T, Miyama T, Shiozaki Y, Mae T (2001) Single- versus bi-socket anterior cruciate ligament reconstruction using autogenous multiple-stranded hamstring tendons with endoButton femoral fixation: A prospective study. Arthroscopy 17: 801–807

40. Hamner D, Brown C, Steiner M, Hecker A, Hayes W (1999) Hamstring tendon grafts for reconstruction of the anterior cruciate ligament: Biomechanical evaluation of the use of multiple strands and tensioning techniques. J Bone Joint Surg 81A: 549–557

41. Hefzy MS, Grood ES, Noyes FR (1989) Factors affecting the region of most isometric femoral attachments. Part II: The anterior cruciate ligament. Am J Sports Med 17: 208–215

42. Henche HR, Birkner W (1997) Die 8fach Plantarissehne. Eine neue Methode zur Kreuzbandrekonstruktion. Arthroskopie 10: 256–260

43. Hertel P (1997) Technik der offenen Ersatzplastik des vorderen Kreuzbandes mit autologer Patellarsehne. Anatomische Rekonstruktion in schraubenfreier Press-fit-Technik. Arthroskopie, 10: 240–245

44. Höher J, Scheffler SU, Withrow JD, Livesay GA, Debski RE, Fu FH, Woo SL (2000) Mechanical behavior of two hamstring graft constructs for reconstruction of the anterior cruciate ligament. J Orthop Res 18: 456–461

45. Howell SM, Taylor MA (1993) Failure of reconstruction of the anterior cruciate ligament due to impingement by the intercondylar roof. J Bone Joint Surg 75-A: 1044–1055

46. Howell SM, Barad SJ (1995) Knee extension and its relationship to the slope of the intercondylar roof. Implications for positioning the tibial tunnel in anterior cruciate ligament reconstructions. Am J Sports Med 23: 288–294

47. Howell SM (1998) Principles for placing the tibial tunnel and avoiding roof impingement during reconstruction of a torn anterior cruciate ligament. Knee Surg Sports Traumatol Arthrosc 6 [Suppl 1]: S49–55

48. Howell SM, Deutsch ML (1999) Comparison of endoscopic and two-incision techniques for reconstructing a torn anterior cruciate ligament using hamstring tendons. Arthroscopy 15: 594–606

49. Hulstyn M, Fadale PD, Abate J, Walsh WR (1993) Biomechanical evaluation of interference screw fixation in a bovine patellar bone-tendon-bone autograft complex for anterior cruciate ligament reconstruction. Arthroscopy 9: 417–424

50. Jäger A, Welsch F, Kappler C (2001) 10-Jahresergebnisse nach arthroskopischer vorderer Kreuzbandplastik mit dem Patellarsehnentransplantat. Vortrag Jahreskongress der DGOOC 2001, Berlin

51. Jansson KA, Harilainen A, Sandelin J, Karjalainen PT, Aronen HJ, Tallroth K (1999) Bone tunnel enlargement after anterior cruciate ligament reconstruction with the hamstring autograft and endobutton fixation technique. A clinical, radiographic and magnetic resonance imaging study with 2 years follow-up. Knee Surg Sports Traumatol Arthrosc 7: 290–295

52. Jarvela T, Kannus P, Jarvinen M (2001) Anterior cruciate ligament reconstruction in patients with or without accompanying injuries: A re-examination of subjects 5 to 9 years after reconstruction. Arthroscopy 17: 818–825

53. Jarvela T, Paakkala T, Kannus P, Jarvinen M (2001) The incidence of patellofemoral osteoarthritis and associated findings 7 years after anterior cruciate ligament reconstruction with a bone-patellar tendon-bone autograft. Am J Sports Med 29: 18–24

54. Jomha NM, Raso VJ, Leung P (1993) Effect of varying angles on the pull-out strength of interference screw fixation. Arthroscopy 9: 580–583

55. Jomha NM, Borton DC, Clingeleffer AJ, Pinczewski LA (1999) Long-term osteoarthritic changes in anterior cruciate ligament reconstructed knees. Clin Orthop 358: 188–193

56. Karlson JA, Steiner ME, Brown CH, Johnson J (1994) Anterior cruciate ligament reconstruction using gracilis and semitendinosus tendons. Comparioson of through the condyle and over the top graft placements. Am J Sports Med 22: 659–666

57. Kartus J, Stener S, Lindahl S, Engstrom B, Eriksson BI, Karlsson J (1997) Factors affecting donor-site morbidity after anterior cruciate ligament reconstruction using bone-patellar tendon-bone autografts. Knee Surg Sports Traumatol Arthrosc 5: 222–228

58. Kartus J, Magnusson L, Stener S, Brandsson S, Eriksson BI, Karlsson J (1999) Complications following arthroscopic anterior cruciate ligament reconstruction. A 2–5 year follow-up of 604 patients with special emphasis on anterior knee pain. Knee Surg Sports Traumatol Arthrosc 7: 2–8

59. Keays SL, Bullock-Saxton J, Keays AC (2000) Strength and function before and after anterior cruciate ligament reconstruction. Clin Orthop 373: 174–183

60. Keays SL, Bullock-Saxton J, Keays AC, Newcombe P (2001) Muscle strength and function before and after anterior cruciate ligament reconstruction using semitendonosus and gracilis. Knee 8: 229–234

61. Kleipool AE, Zijl JA, Willems WJ (1998) Arthroscopic anterior cruciate ligament reconstruction with bone-patellar tendon-bone allograft or autograft. A prospective study with an average follow up of 4 years. Knee Surg Sports Traumatol Arthrosc 6: 224–230

62. Kohn D, Rose C (1994) Primary stability of interference screw fixation. Influence of screw diameter and insertion torque. Am J Sports Med 22: 334–338

63. Kohn D, Busche T, Carls J (1998) Drill hole position in endoscopic anterior cruciate ligament reconstruction. Results of an advanced arthroscopy source. Knee Surg Sports Traumatol Arthrosc 6 [Suppl 1]: S13–15

64. Kohn D, Rupp S (2000) Strategien zu Revisionseingriffen bei fehlgeschlagener vorderer Kreuzbandrekonstruktion. Chirurg 71: 1055–1065

65. Kurosaka M, Yoshiya S, Andrish JT (1987) A biomechanical comparison of different surgical techniques of graft fixation in anterior cruciate ligament reconstruction. Am J Sports Med 15: 225–229

66. Lemos MJ, Jackson DW, Lee TQ, Simon TM (1995) Assessment of initial fixation of endoscopic interference femoral screws with divergent and parallel placement. Arthroscopy 11: 37–41

67. Lephart SM, Kocher MS, Harner CD, Fu FH (1993) Quadriceps strength and functional capacity after anterior cruciate ligament reconstruction. Patellar tendon autograft versus allograft Am J Sports Med 21: 738–743

68. Liao H, Belkoff SM (1999) A failure model for ligaments. J Biomech 32: 183–188

69. Liu SH, Panossian V, al-Shaikh R, Tomin E, Shepherd E, Finerman GA, Lane JM (1997) Morphology and matrix composition during early tendon to bone healing. Clin Orthop 339: 253–260

70. Morrison JB (1970) The mechanics of the knee joint in relation to normal walking. J Biomech 3: 51–61

71. Müller B. Rupp S, Seil R, Kohn D (2000) Entnahmestellenmorbidität nach VKB-Ersatzplastik mit dem Ligamentum-patellae-Transplantat. Unfallchirurg 103: 662–667

72. Müller W (1982) Das Knie. Springer, Berlin Heidelberg New York

73. Muneta T, Yamamoto H, Ishibashi T, Asahina S, Murakami S, Furuya K (1995) The effects of tibial tunnel placement and roof plasty on reconstructed anterior cruciate ligament knees. Arthroscopy 11: 57

74. Noyes FR, Grood ES (1976) The strength of the anterior cruciate ligament. Age and species related changes. J Bone Joint Surg 58-A: 1074–1082

75. Noyes FR, Butler DL, Grood ES, Zernicke RF, Hefzy MS (1984) Biomechanical analysis of human ligament grafts used in knee-ligament repairs and reconstructions. J Bone Joint Surg 66-A: 344–352

76. Noyes FR, Barber-Westin SD (1996) Reconstruction of the anterior cruciate ligament with human allograft. Comparison of early and later results. J Bone Joint Surg 78-A: 524–537

77. Odensten M, Gillquist J (1985) Functional anatomy of the anterior cruciate ligament and a rational for reconstruction. J Bone Joint Surg 67-A: 257–262

78. Oettel GM, Imhoff AB, (1998) Revisionschirurgie bei fehlgeschlagener vorderer Kreuzbandplastik. Zentralbl Chir 123: 1033

79. O'Neill DB (1996) Arthroscopically assisted reconstruction of the anterior cruciate ligament. A prospective randomized analysis of three techniques. J Bone Joint Surg 78-A: 803–13

80. Paschal SO, Seemann MD, Ashman RB, Allard RN, Montgomery JB (1994) Interference fixation versus postfixation of bone-patellar tendon-bone grafts for anterior cruciate ligament reconstruction. A biomechanical comparative study in porcine knees. Clin Orthop 300: 281–287

81. Patel JV, Church JS, Hall AJ (2000) Central third bone-patellar tendon-bone anterior cruciate ligament reconstruction: a 5-year follow-up. Arthroscopy 16: 67–70

82. Pierz K, Baltz M, Fulkerson J (1995) The effect of Kurosaka screw divergence on the holding strength of bone-tendon-bone grafts. Am J Sports Med 23: 332–335

83. Quapp KM, Weiss JA (1998) Material characterization of human medial collateral ligament. J Biomech Eng 120: 757–763

84. Rasmussen TJ, Feder SM, Butler DL, Noyes FR (1994) The effects of 4 mrad of gamma irradiation on the initial mechanical properties of bone patellar tendon bone grafts. Arthroscopy 10: 188–197

85. Rodeo SA, Arnoczky SP, Torzilli PA, Hidaka C, Warren RF (1993) Tendon-healing in a bone tunnel. A biomechanical and histological study in the dog. J Bone Joint Surg 75-A: 1795–1803

86. Ropke M, Becker R, Urbach D, Nebelung W (2001) Semitendinosussehne vs. Ligamentum patellae. Klinische Ergebnisse einer prospektiven randomisierten Studie nach vorderer Kreuzbandplastik. Unfallchirurg 104: 312–316

87. Rougraff B, Shelbourne KD, Gerth PK, Warner J (1993) Arthroscopic and histologic analysis of human patellar tendon autografts used for anterior cruciate ligament reconstruction. Am J Sports Med 21: 277–284

88. Rubinstein RA Jr, Shelbourne KD, VanMeter CD, McCarroll JC, Rettig AC (1994) Isolated autogenous bone-patellar tendon-bone graft site morbidity. Am J Sports Med 22: 324–327

89. Rupp S, Krauß P, Fritsch E (1997) Fixation strength of a biodegradable interference screw and a press-fit technique in anterior cruciate ligament reconstruction with a BPTB-graft. Arthroscopy 13: 61–65

90. Rupp S, Seil R, Müller B, Kohn D (1998) Biomechanische Grundlagen der Rehabilitation nach VKB-Ersatzplastik. Dt Zeitschr Sportmed 49, Sonderheft 1: 221–225

91. Rupp S, Seil R, Schneider A, Kohn D (1999) Initial fixation strength of three different types of biodegradable interference screws. J Biomed Mat Res 48: 70–74

92. Rupp S, Hopf T, Hess T, Seil R, Kohn D (1999) Resulting tensile forces in the human BPTB-graft – Direct force measurement in vitro. Arthroscopy 15: 179–184

93. Rupp S, Seil R, Kohn D, Müller B (2000) Influence of avascularity on tensile strength and viscoelastic properties of human bone-patellar tendon –bone grafts. J Bone Joint Surg 82-B: 1059–1064

94. Rupp S, Müller B, Seil R (2001) Knee laxity after ACL reconstruction with a BPTB-graft. Knee Surg Sports Traumatol Arthrosc 9: 72–76

95. Sgaglione NA, DelPizzo W, Fox JM, Friedman MJ (1993) Arthroscopically assisted anterior cruciate ligament reconstruction with the pes anserine tendons. Comparison of results in acute and chronic ligament deficiency. Am J Sports Med 21: 249–256

96. Shaffer BS, Tibone JE (1993) Patellar tendon length change after anterior cruciate ligament reconstruction using the midthird patellar tendon. Am J Sports Med 21: 449–454

97. Shelbourne KD, Nitz P (1990) Accelerated rehabilitation after anterior cruciate ligament reconstruction. Am J Sports Med 18: 292–299

98. Shelbourne KD, Gray T (1997) Anterior cruciate ligament reconstruction with autogenous patellar tendon graft followed by accelerated rehabilitation. A two- to nine-year followup. Am J Sports Med 25: 786–795

99. Sidles JA, Larson RV, Garbini JL, Downey DJ, Matsen FA (1988) Ligament length relationships in the moving knee. J Orthop Res 6: 593–610

100. Spicer DD, Blagg SE, Unwin AJ, Allum RL (2000) Anterior knee symptoms after four-strand hamstring tendon anterior cruciate ligament reconstruction. Knee Surg Sports Traumatol Arthrosc 8: 286–289

101. Stäubli HU (1992) Arthroscopically assisted ACL reconstruction using autologous quadriceps tendon. In: Jakob RP, Stäubli HU (eds) The Knee and the cruciate ligaments: anatomy, biomechanics, clinical aspects, reconstruction, complications, rehabilitation. Springer, Berlin Heidelberg New York Tokyo, S 443 ff

102. Südkamp NP, Haas NP (2000) Neue Wege in der Kreuzbandchirurgie. Chirurg 71: 1024–1033

103. Taskiran E, Taskiran D, Duran T, Lok V (1998) Articular cartilage homeostasis after anterior cruciate ligament reconstruction. Knee Surg Sports Traumatol Arthrosc 6: 93–98

104. Weiler A, Windhagen HJ, Raschke MJ, Laumeyer A, Hoffmann RF (1998) Biodegradable interference screw fixation exhibits pull-out force and stiffness similar to titanium screws. Am J Sports Med 26: 119–126

105. Werner S, Arvidsson H, Arvidsson I, Eriksson E (1993) Electrical stimulation of vastus medialis and stretching of lateral thigh muscles in patients with patello-femoral symptoms. Knee Surg Sports Traumatol Arthrosc 1: 85–92

106. Wilson T, Zafuta M, Zobitz M (1999) A biomechanical analysis of matched bone-patellar tendon-bone and double-looped semitendinous and gracilis tendon grafts. Am J Sports Med 27: 202–207

107. Yaru NC, Daniel DM, Penner D (1992) The effect of tibial attachment site on graft impingement in an anterior cruciate ligament reconstruction. Am J Sports Med 20: 217–220

108. Yoshiya S, Nagano M, Kurosaka M, Muratsu H, Mizuno K (2000) Graft healing in the bone tunnel in anterior cruciate ligament reconstruction. Clin Orthop 376: 278–286

109. Zavras TD, Race A, Bull AMJ (2001) A comparative study of »isometric« points for anterior cruciate ligament graft attachment. Knee Surg Sports Traumatol Arthrosc 9: 28–33

54 Image-Free Navigation in ACL Replacement with the *OrthoPilot* System

H.-J. Eichhorn

Introduction

In many areas of surgery, ever smaller approaches are being sought to reduce soft tissue traumatisation in minimally invasive operating techniques. This is associated with the danger that the surgeon will lose an overview of the topography of the structures as a whole. Computer-assisted navigation promises to remedy this. Computer-assisted surgery began in the 1990s with intracranial neurosurgical operations and the implantation of pedicle screws in spinal surgery, using CT and MRI imaging. Today however, there are other solutions which do not require pre- and intra-operative X-rays. One of these solutions is offered by the OrthoPilot navigation system (❑ Fig. 54-1).

One problem in cruciate ligament surgery has arisen because, whilst it is certainly true that the number of crucial ligament operations has substantially increased, there has at the same time been an over proportional rise in the number of surgeons performing these operations. In fact, approximately 70% of cruciate ligament operations are conducted by surgeons or orthopaedic surgeons who perform fewer than 20 cases a year, and who can thus gather relatively little experience. Responsible government departments and insurance companies are therefore now thinking out loud about establishing process and quality controls similar to those which exist for osteosynthesis. According to such a scheme, the operation may only be performed if the site of the tunnels, and therefore the site of the ACL replacement, is documented. Monitoring the tunnel site with an image converter is now being recommended at the various cruciate ligament congresses. However, there are problems associated with image converter monitoring: the patients are exposed to a not inconsiderable dose of radiation, and the position of the image converter must be altered several times in order to obtain an image in two planes.

The main problem in cruciate ligament surgery is correct tunnel placement. Computer-assisted navigation can represent a solution to this problem, as it can determine and document the tunnel site without CT scans or intraoperative X-rays.

For this reason, software was developed for OrthoPilot to allow the optimum tunnel sites to be defined by navigation.

The objectives for the OrthoPilot system are as follows:
- the additional operation time caused by navigation should be reduced to a minimum (max. 10–15 min);
- intraoperative X-raying of the patient should be avoided;
- the extremely time-consuming, CT- or MRI-based preoperative planning required by other navigation systems should not be necessary;

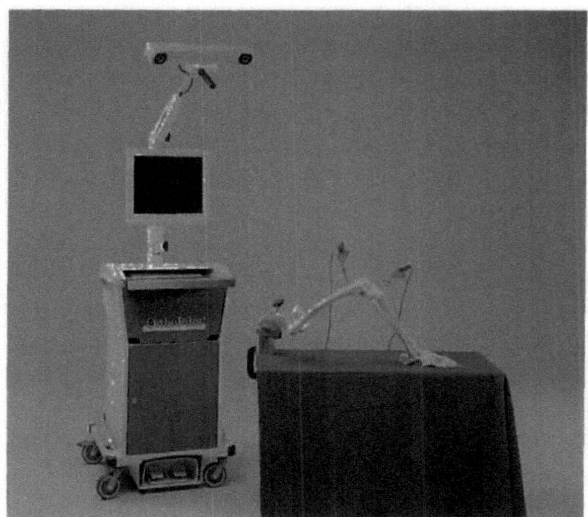

❑ Fig. 54-1. Setting up the OrthoPilot system

- fixing the sensors (rigid bodies) to record the anatomical landmarks in the knee and the knee kinematics should only be associated with minimal traumatisation for the patient;
- the entire system should be so user friendly that it can be operated by surgeons and theatre nurses without any problems.

Criteria for Tunnel Placement

The ACL navigation software contains the experiences and opinions of experts drawn from a great many publications in anatomical and surgical orthopaedics.

Criteria for anatomical placement of the tibial tunnel: The tibial exit point on the tibial plateau should satisfy the following criteria:

- 7 mm distance from the anterior margin of the posterior cruciate ligament with the knee joint in approx. 80° flexion,
- half way between the anterior horn of the external meniscus and the spine of the medial tibial tubercle,
- 44% of the coronary width of the tibial plateau beginning from the medial position.

If the navigation is being used for a double tunnel technique, only the anteromedial bundle is navigated. In this case the distance from the posterior cruciate ligament changes to 9 mm.

For tibial tunnel placement it is also important to project the silhouette of the intercondylar fossa in extension onto the tibial head, in order to show any possible impingement situation here.

If the intercondylar fossa overlaps the navigated, anatomically optimum target circle partially or completely, the surgeon has the alternative of either moving the tibial tunnel site in a dorsal direction or of performing a suitable notch plasty to avoid impingement.

Criteria for anatomical placement of the femoral tunnel: The femoral entry point in the notch should satisfy the following criteria:

- 3–5 mm distance from the posterior margin of the fossa,
- Placement of tunnel in
  - left knee: 12.30–01.30 o'clock position,
  - right knee: 10.30–11.30 o'clock position.

The main mistakes in planning the femoral tunnel occur through a placement which is too high (towards a 12 o'clock position) and/or too ventral. OrthoPilot shows a section between 10.30–11.30 o'clock for the right knee and 12.30–01.30 o'clock for the left knee during navigation. This is particularly important, since even slight distortion of the camera horizon can lead to a false interpretation of the fossa topography.

As the posterior margin of the fossa is palpated and recorded in the computer, OrthoPilot permanently displays the relation between the tip of the femoral pointer and the posterior outlet of the fossa. From this the surgeon can determine the distance according to the operating technique used.

Since OrthoPilot also records the kinematic data of the knee joint, the isometric relation between both selected target points (tibial exit point/femoral entry point) is given as useful additional information. Furthermore, an impingement check is conducted and recorded depending on the thickness of the graft across the entire flexion range of the knee up to extension.

Performing the Computer-Assisted, Image-Free Cruciate Ligament Operation

Preparing the Navigation

Firstly, the OrthoPilot is positioned next to the arthroscopy tower on the opposite side from the surgeon. Care must be taken to ensure that neither the arthroscopy tower nor any other instrumentation or people are standing in the camera's observation field. The ideal distance of the camera from the knee is 2 m ± 40 cm. The leg should be placed in a leg support.

After the leg has been washed and draped in a leg holder and the arthroscopy equipment has been made ready, arthroscopic joint revision is first performed. It is important to rectify any additional damage to the cartilage surfaces and the menisci before the rigid bodies are attached. If an obviously very narrow notch is found to exist before a secondary stabilization procedure, a notch plasty should already be performed at this point. The rigid bodies should only be fixed into position when these operation steps have been completed (◘ Fig. 54-2).

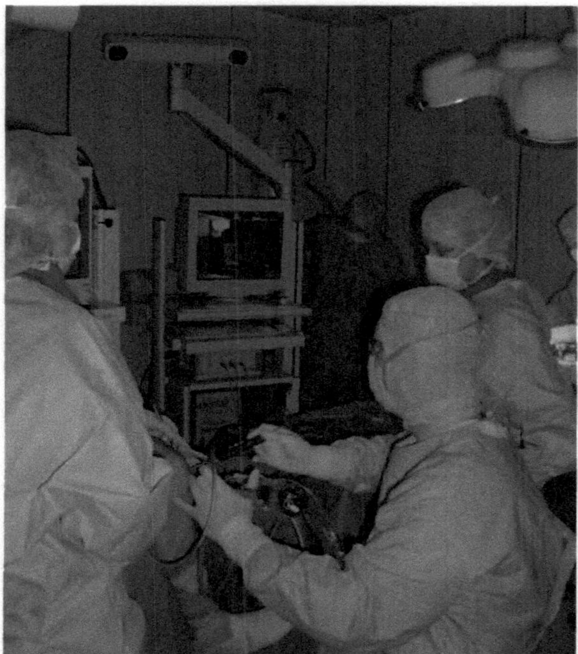

Fig. 54-2. Position of OrthoPilot during a cruciate ligament reconstruction

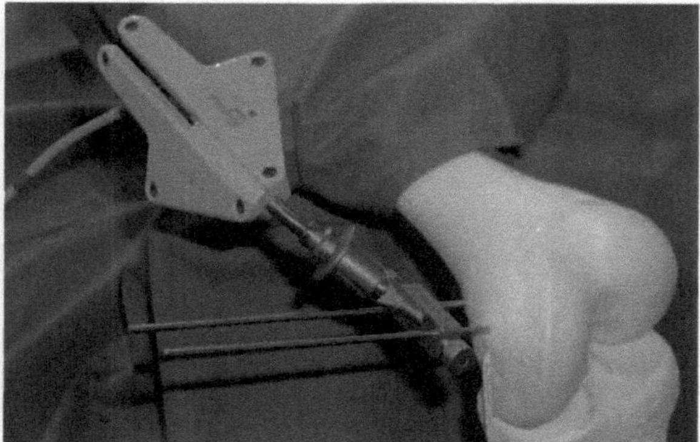

Fig. 54-3. Femoral rigid body fixation

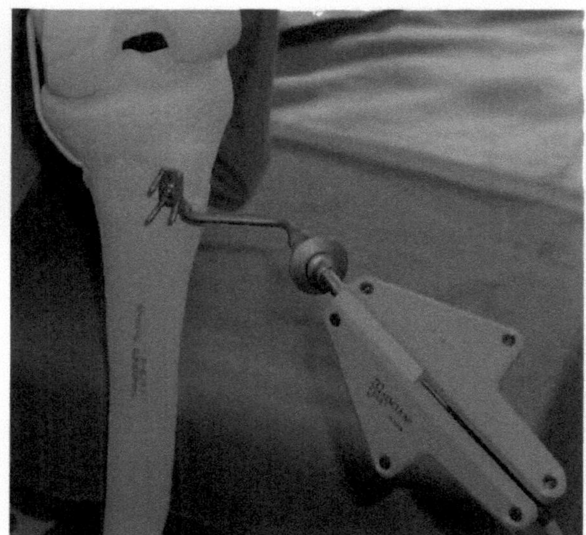

Fig. 54-4. Tibial rigid body fixation

Fixing the Rigid Bodies in Position

The peak of the medial epicondyle is palpated and a 2.5 mm Kirschner wire is inserted approx. 2 cm into the condyle. This site has been chosen because no nerves, vessels or sensitive capsule structures are injured with the knees in flexion. After the fixation has been put into place a second Kirschner wire is set somewhat proximally through the fixation.

Screwing the fixation tight just above the skin gives the Kirschner wires an overhang, which guarantees that the femoral rigid bodies are firmly fixed into position (**Fig. 54-3**).

The slightly angled holder for the tibial rigid body is fixed in the area of the tendon harvest site on the medial tibia head close up to the tuberosity. Here it has proved to be a good idea to predrill the setting hole for the central screw with a 2 mm drill. After this the appropriate thread is cut and the fixation plate is screwed on loosely. To achieve rotational stability, two further pins are inserted into the fixation plate. Before the fixation pins are hammered in, the site should be predrilled with a thin 0.6 mm Kirschner wire, since the cortex is extremely hard in this area and the pins could bend under the hammer (**Fig. 54-4**).

As an alternative to the fixation close to the tuberosity, the rigid body can be fixed approx. 10 cm distal from the tendon harvest site, as with the femoral fixation, with 2 Kirschner wires in the area of the ventral margin of the tibia (**Figs. 54-5 and 54-6**).

Instrument Calibration Check

Before the operation begins, the calibrated instruments should be checked to guarantee the accuracy of the navigation (**Fig. 54-7**).

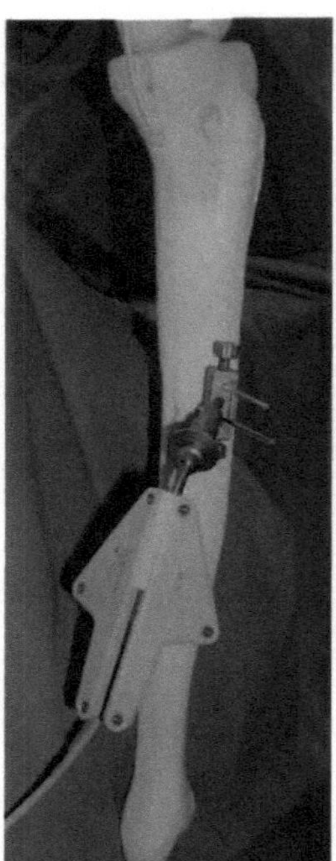

Fig. 54-5. Alternative tibial rigid body fixation

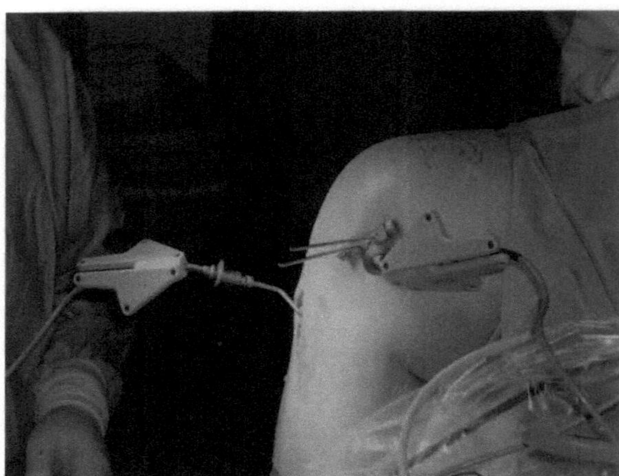

Fig. 54-6. Position of rigid body

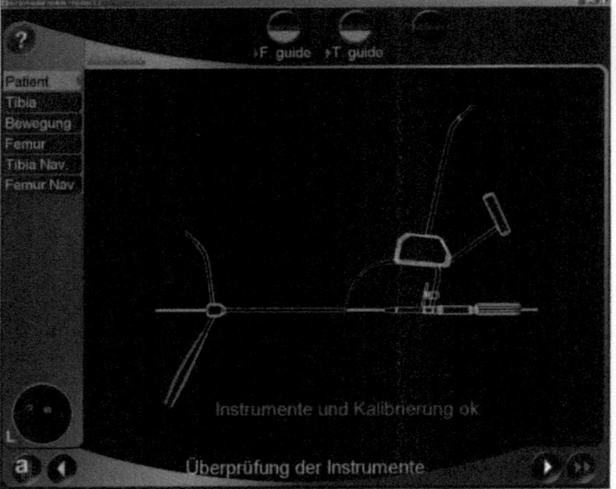

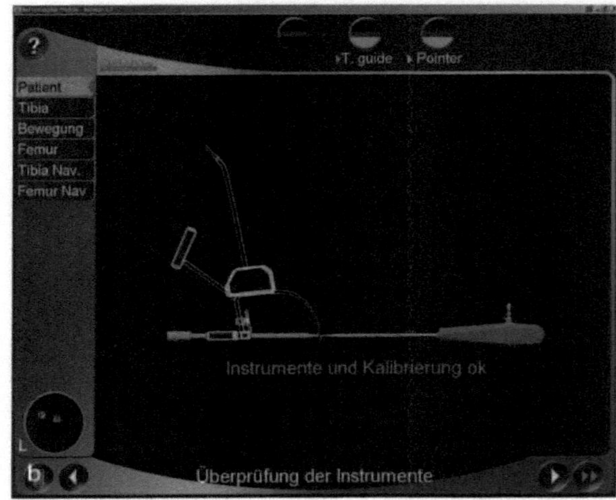

Fig. 54-7a,b. Instrument calibration check

Inputting Patient Data

The following data are subsequently input into the system: patient's name, the side of the operated knee joint, surgeon's name, graft thickness and desired distance from the posterior margin of the fossa (**Figs. 54-8 and 54-9).

Acquisition of Extraarticular Landmarks

The extraarticular reference points, tuberosity, ventral tibial margin, medial and lateral side of the tibial plateau are acquired using a navigated pointer (**Fig. 54-10).

Acquiring the Knee Kinematics

After the leg position has been established in 90° flexion and maximum extension, the kinematic data of the knee joint are recorded in the computer by letting the leg sink from the extension position to 90° flexion (**Fig. 54-11).

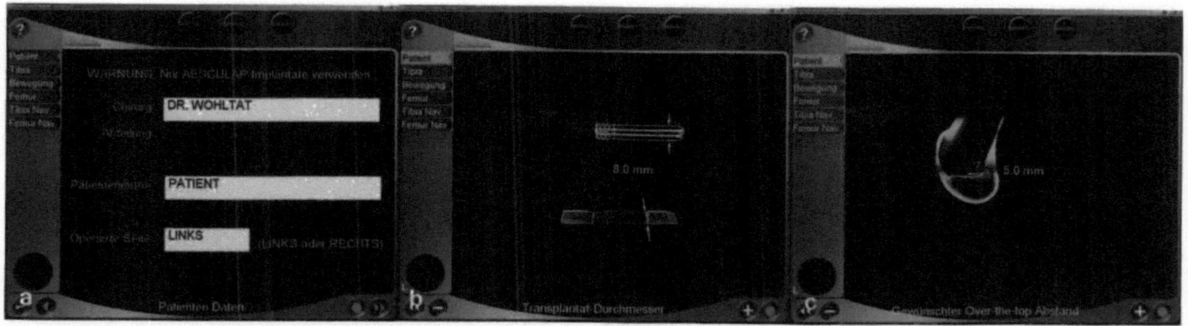

■ **Fig. 54-8a-c.** Data input, such as patient's name, graft thickness and desired distance from posterior margin of fossa

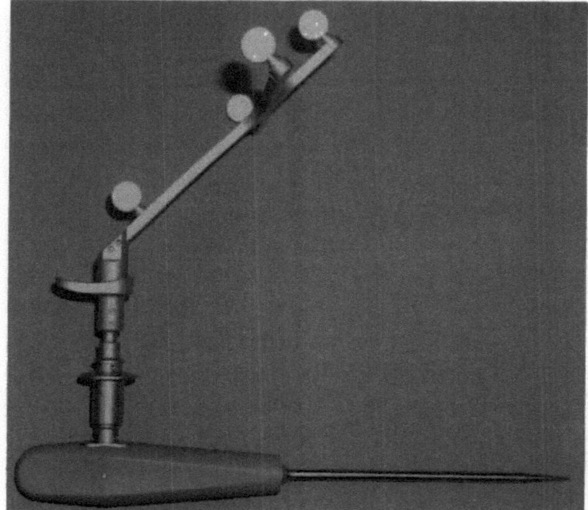

■ **Fig. 54-9.** Navigated pointer

Acquisition of Intraarticular Landmarks

After the extraarticular landmarks have been acquired, the arthroscope is inserted into the knee joint and the intraarticular reference points are recorded. To do this, the anterior margin of the posterior cruciate ligament, the anterior horn of the lateral meniscus, the transition to the transverse ligament and the medial spine of the intercondylar tubercle are first recorded (■ Fig. 54-12).

Acquisition of the notch data begins with palpation of the medial notch wall at 9 o'clock (left knee) or 3 o'clock (right knee) respectively. Following this, the contour of the ventral margin of the fossa is recorded with at least 10 points. This should be done starting from a medial position and moving to a lateral position. After the lateral notch wall has been acquired at 9 o'clock (left knee) or 3 o'clock (right knee), the wall is extensively palpated, also with at least 5 points (■ Figs. 54-13 and 54-14).

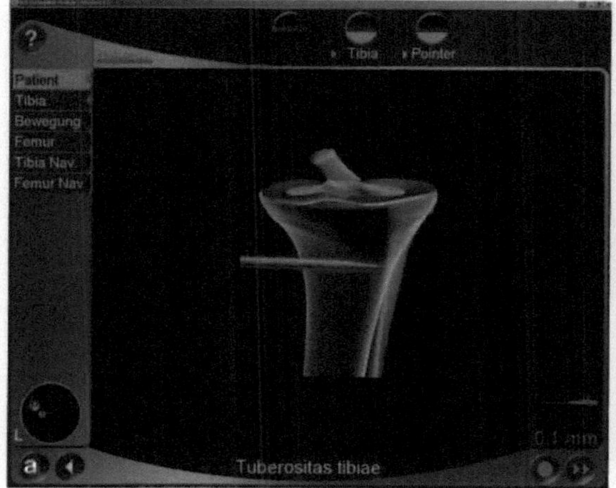

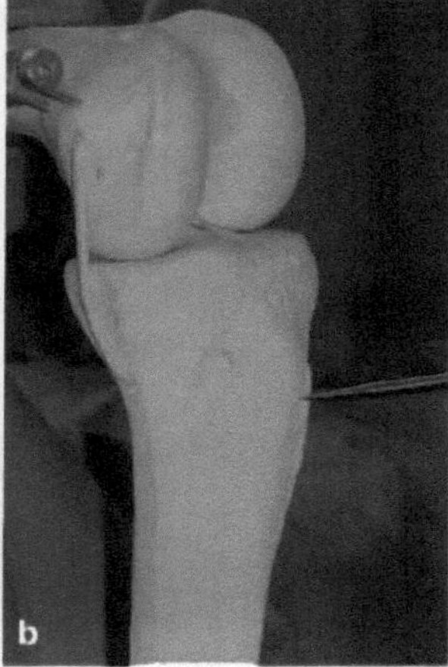

■ **Fig. 54-10a-b.** Palpation of extraarticular landmarks

The posterior margin of the fossa is then palpated. This is one of the most important and sensitive steps of the acquisition. The posterior margin must be fully freed from

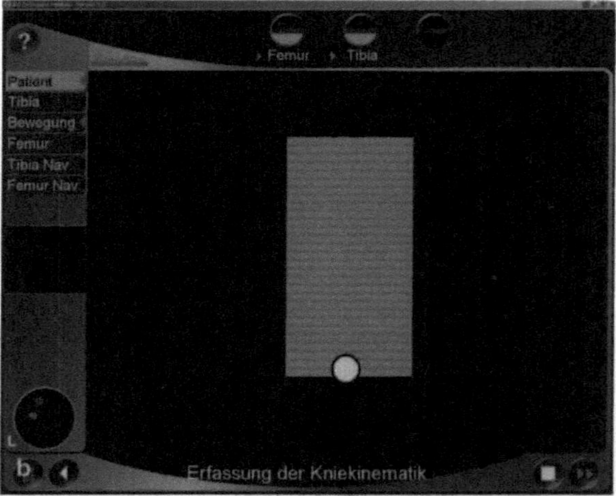

Fig. 54-11a,b. Recording the kinematics of the leg

soft tissue using the shaver and the curved raspatory if necessary, and well exposed to view.

The navigated hooked pointer must be carefully inserted, making sure that it sinks completely behind the fossa (**Fig. 54-15**). Now it is pulled very slowly in a ventral direction until the margin is palpated with the palpation hook. First of all the extreme cranial point (12 o'-clock »over the top« position) is palpated and recorded.

Subsequently the extreme lateral point (1.30 o'clock for the left knee and 10.30 o'clock for the right knee) is established in the same way.

Navigation of the Tibia

The tibial pointer fitted with the mobile rigid body is introduced through the medial port lying close alongside the patellar tendon. The navigation screen now displays the tibial plateau with the intercondylar fossa projected onto it in full knee extension.

The tip of the pointer is now moved backwards and forwards on the tibial plateau until the yellow circle, whose center represents the target point of the pointer, converges with the red circle (on the navigation screen; **Fig. 54-16**) and the colour changes to green. Now the distance from the posterior cruciate ligament and the coronary width distance (medial/lateral) is checked – here expressed in percentages. Thus OrthoPilot completes the missing dimension of the image and the incomplete overview of the entire topography which is a result of the tunnel vision of arthroscopy.

After the intraarticular target point has been fixed on the tibial plateau with the tip of the tibial pointer, it must be ensured that the extraarticular attachment on the medial

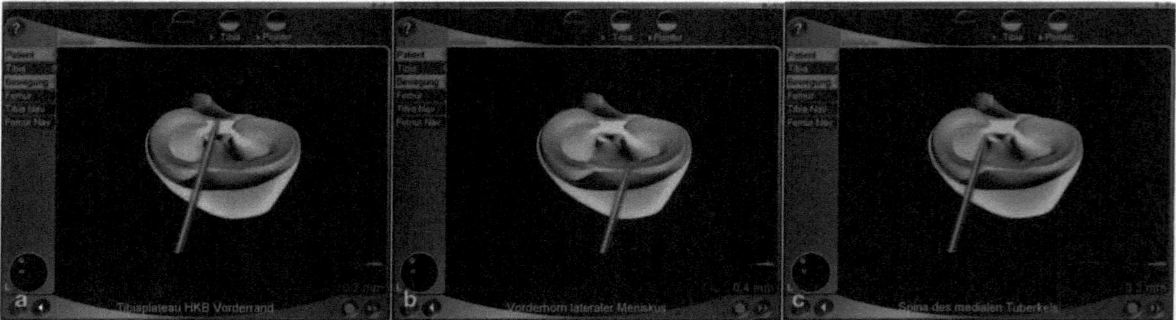

Fig. 54-12a-c. Acquisition of intraarticular landmarks

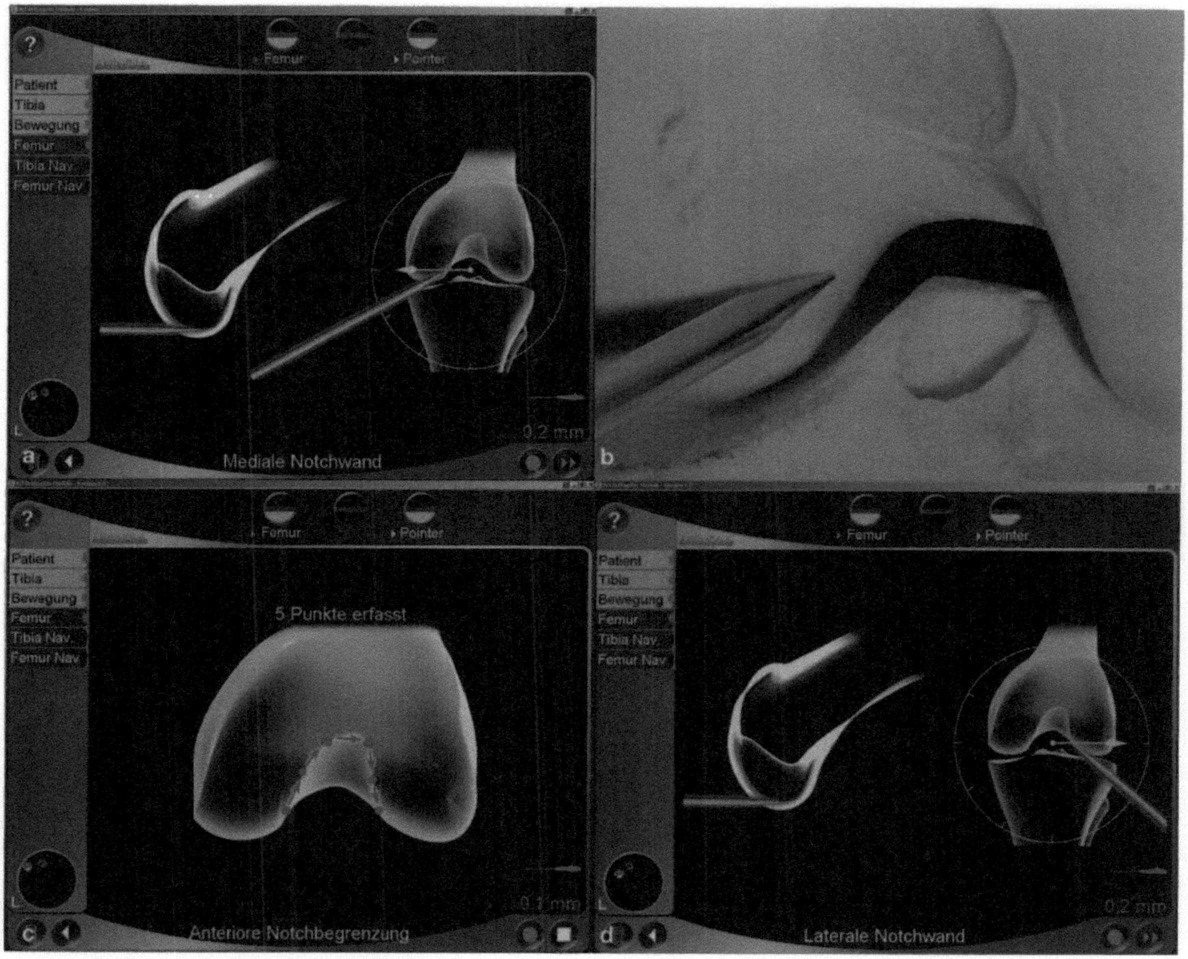

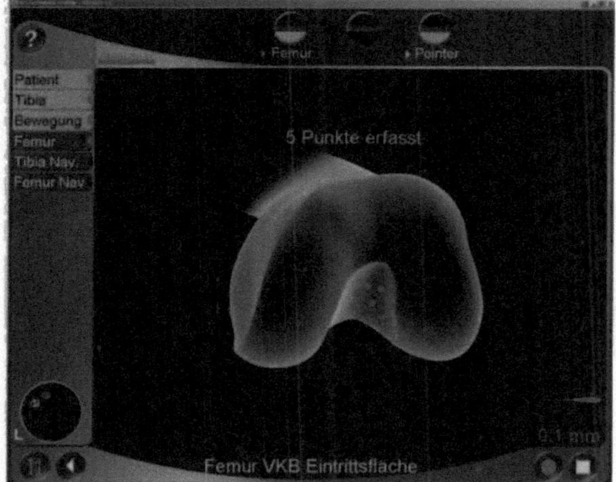

Fig. 54-13a-d. Acquisition of notch topography

Fig. 54-14. Fossa landmarks

tibia head is far enough away from the tuberosity. This guarantees that the pointer for femoral navigation can also reach the desired target points. Consequently an angle of between 25 and 30 degrees in the frontal plane should be chosen.

Once the target wire has been set, OrthoPilot records the data of this position. The guide wire is now overdrilled according to the size of the graft.

Explanatory Notes on the Tibia Navigation Screen

- The navigation target circle 1 (center of arrow head or center of green or yellow circle) corresponds to the point of intersection of the virtual axis of the K wire in the tibial target drill guide and the surface of the tibia plateau, and thus describes the tibial exit point on the tibial plateau.

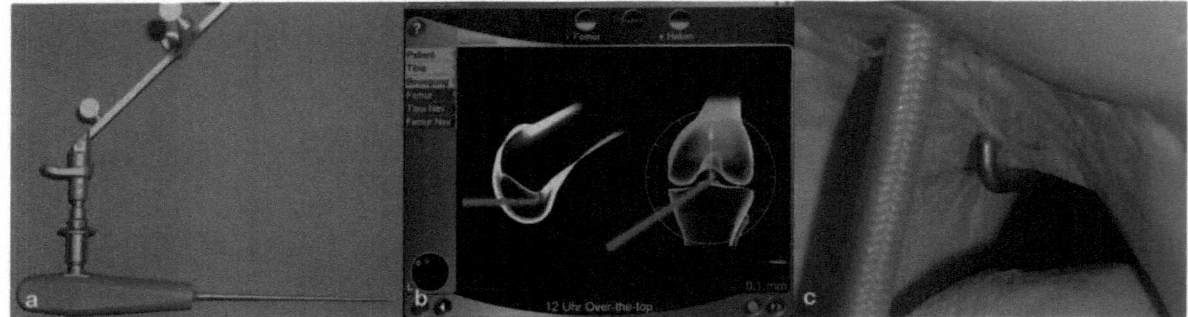

Fig. 54-15a-c. Navigated hooked pointer

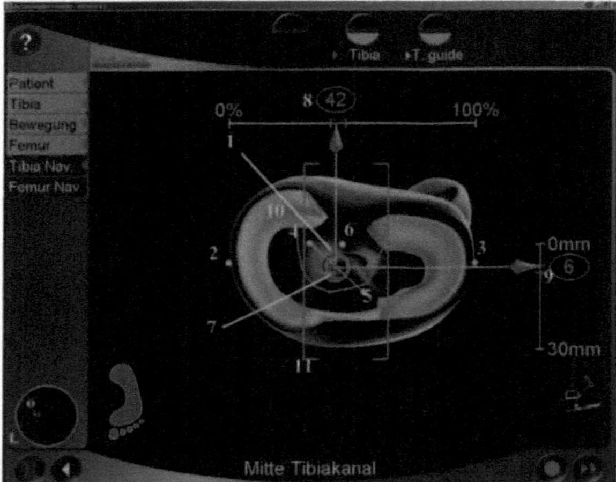

Fig. 54-16. Tibia navigation screen

- The scale **8** represents the width of the tibial plateau in the frontal plane beginning at 0% at the extreme medial point of the tibial plateau **2** and ending at 100% at the extreme lateral point **3**. The exit point for a correct tibial tunnel site in this plane should theoretically lie at around 44%.
- The scale **9** corresponds to the distance from the anterior margin of the PCL on the tibial plateau **7** in an anterior direction. The actual value of the distance from the PCL is shown in yellow outside the green area and in green inside it.
- The curve **10** and lines **11** correspond respectively to the recorded curve of the anterior notch margin, or of the points of the medial and lateral notch wall projected onto the tibial plateau in extension.

- If the tip of the tibial target drill guide is moved on the tibial plateau, this causes a simultaneous movement of the navigation target circle **1** on the screen. The diameter of the circle corresponds to the graft diameter which has been input.
- The yellow dot **2** corresponds to the medial point of the tibial plateau
- The yellow dot **3** corresponds to the lateral point of the tibial plateau
- The yellow dot **4** corresponds to the spine of the medial intercondylar tubercle
- The yellow dot **5** corresponds to the anterior horn of the lateral meniscus
- The yellow dot **6** corresponds to the anterior margin of the PCL on the tibial plateau
- The circle **7** shows the midpoint of the distance between the anterior horn of the lateral meniscus **5** and the spine of the medial intercondylar tubercle **4**.

Navigation of the Femur

The navigated femoral pointer is introduced transtibially. The insertion area registered previously is approached at approximately 90° flexion. During this procedure the navigation screen informs the surgeon permanently about the values of the position reached through the »clock position«, and about the distance from the posterior margin of the fossa. Isometric data and any threatening impingement situations are also given as additional information for every point palpated with the tip of the femoral pointer.

After the target point has been optimized, the pointed tip of the pointer is fixed into the bone with light hammer blows and the drilling wire is set. This position is also registered in the navigation system and thereby documented.

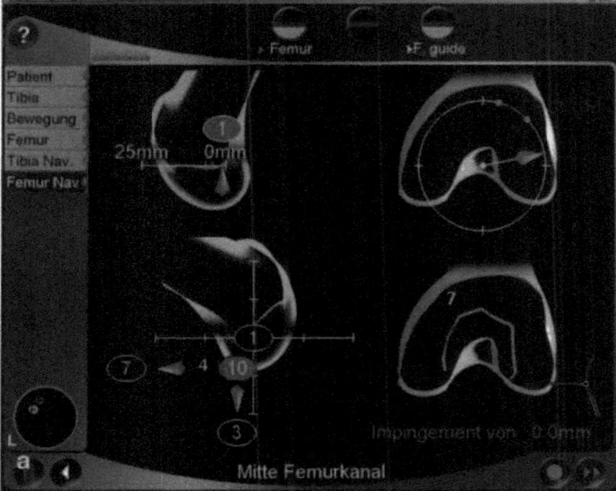

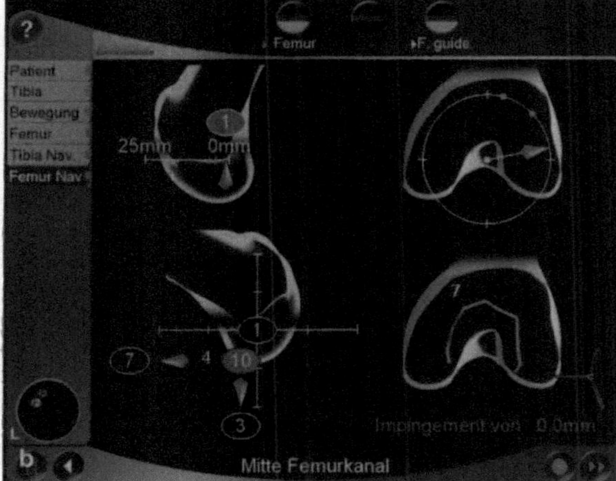

◘ Fig. 54-17a,b. Femur navigation screen

The drilling wires can be subsequently overdrilled according to the operating procedure selected. The tibial and femoral rigid body fixations are removed. After the tunnels have been set the operation is continued in the usual manner (◘ Fig. 54-17).

Explanatory Notes on the Femur Navigation Screen

— Area A shows the position of the femoral tunnel entry point relative to the over the top position. Point 1 corresponds to the over the top position. Scale 2 corresponds to the distance from the over the top posi-

tion on the notch surface in an anterior direction, beginning at point 1.
— Area **B** shows the position of the femoral tunnel entry point relative to the angle position in the notch area.
  - The compass dial 3 corresponds to the angle position in the notch area.
— Green area: 10.30 and 11.30 o'clock in the right knee.
— Green area: 12.30 and 01.30 o'clock in the left knee.
— Area **C** shows the isometrics chart of the ACL entry surface on the femur with regard to the tibial exit point recorded.
  - The cylinder 5 shows the virtual tip of the femoral target drilling guide and corresponds to the actual tip of the femoral drilling guide. The crosshair 4 shows in which direction the instrument tip must be moved in order to arrive at the point with the best isometrics. The yellow quarter circle 6 corresponds to the diameter of the graft and shows the anterior section of the transplant range.
— Area **D** shows any impingement of the graft occurring in respect of the tibial exit point recorded.
  - The region (notch roof or wall) in which an impingement occurs is represented in area **C** as a red segment on the anterior notch margin 7.

Summary

As a precondition for the safe use of ACL navigation it is necessary to master precise diagnostic arthroscopy and the precise use of the hooked pointer, since the result of the navigation depends crucially on the quality of the acquisition of anatomical landmarks.

During development the navigated points were checked with the Fluoroscope (C-Arm) and mechanical isometric measuring equipment (Isotac). A high level of accuracy and reproducibility of the navigation results was documented.

The experience gained has shown that the use of the computer assisted navigation system permits highly accurate placement of tunnels for cruciate ligament reconstruction and avoids tunnels placement errors, regarded as the main cause of graft failure.

Future prospects

Now that image-free navigation has proved its worth in anterior cruciate ligament surgery, we are working on further indications for which this technology can be used.

The next step is to adopt the navigated investigation of knee and ligament stability into the software. The investigation under anesthetic is performed preoperatively with the navigation equipment. This allows the Lachman test (corresponding to the KT 1000 test), the pivot shift phenomenon, and medial and posteromedial as well as lateral and posterolateral instability components to be documented. The same investigation is then repeated after the operation is completed, so that the improvement in stability achieved during the operation can be documented. Checks can also be made as to whether for instance a posterolateral additional instability component could be adequately reduced through the central stabilization, or whether an additional extracapsular operation is necessary.

In addition to this, work is also being done on surface mapping (anatomic fitting) of cartilage surfaces, which allows the surfaces to be treated by osteochrondral transplantation to be precisely defined, or the areas for autologous chondrocyte transplantation to be calculated. In future there will also be navigated surgical instruments; it will be possible for example to avoid divergent tunnel screw sites by using navigated screwdrivers. Retrograde drilling of an osteochondrosis dissecans in the condyle and talus will also be possible; these areas are often difficult to depict by image converter.

Computer-assisted reconstruction of the posterior cruciate ligament is also on the task list for the future.

Expanding the indications will mean that computer-assisted navigation in arthroscopic surgery will increasingly gain in significance.

55 Clinical Experiences for ACL-Repair with the *SurgiGATE* System

J. De Rycke

Navigation in orthopaedic surgery is often associated with the experimental environment of a university hospital. However, in our experience, the practical set-up is more frequently performed in regional hospitals.

The question if navigation is helpful in solving clinical issues in total joint and spine surgery has to be answered by those centers that have the capacity, both in men and material.

What we have to answer is: Are we able to add a complex but useful procedure to a common surgery without compromising our daily surgical routine?

We started using surgical navigation with the Surgi-GATE System (Medivision Oberdorf Switzerland) in early 2000 (■ Fig. 55-1).

Since then we performed about 300 total hip surgeries, navigation of the Trilogy cup (Zimmer Warsaw), with the help of this system. This navigation of the cup in total hip surgery was rather easy to use. A preoperative planning of the surgery is possible thanks to a preoperative CT scan. Indeed during surgery, cup position is checked with the preoperative done »virtual surgery« on the CT scan images. If this position matches the anatomy and the specific need for the patient, the cup is impacted accordingly.

Though we had a vast experience in total hip surgery, the indicated cup positions were sometimes surprising, but after checking the patients' position, and more precisely the position of the pelvis relative to the operating table, we had to admit that the system was often right, and better than our clinical experience.

Important, however is, that navigation is only a tool for improvement of the surgical result. It does **not** replace the surgeon, as is the case when a robot is used. Due to the intense preoperative planning, made possible on the CT scan, the surgery total time is not really influenced. In ligament surgery a preoperative CT scan is not very useful

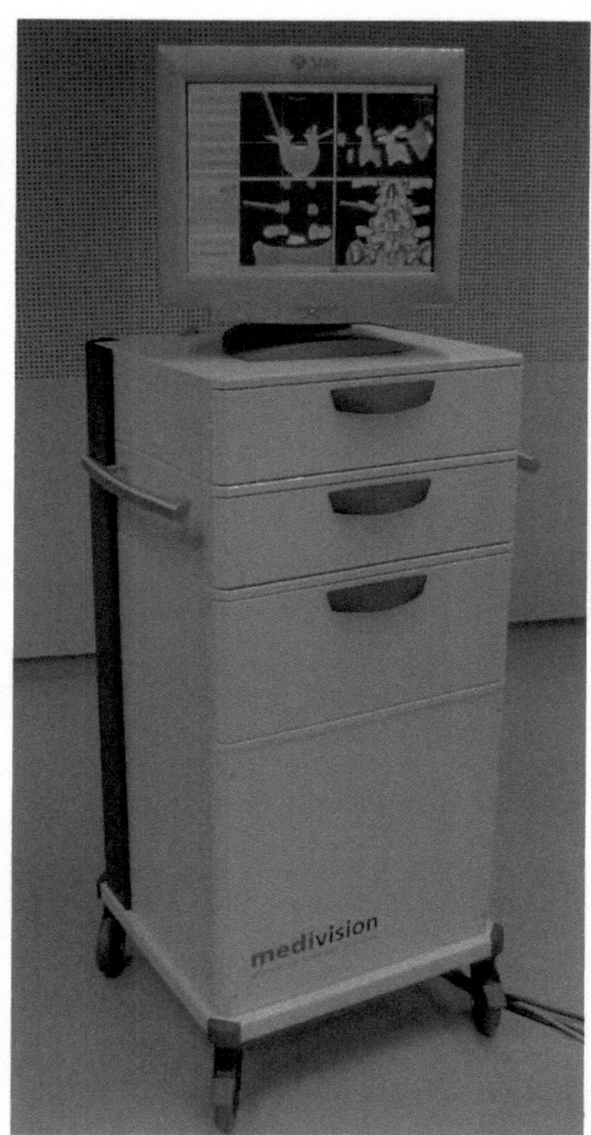

■ **Fig. 55-1.** Surgigate system Medivision

because the smooth structures of the knee are difficult to register. An ACL replacement is basically a soft tissue surgery.

On the other hand the »static« CT scan is not able to show changes such as notch plasty, as often performed in ACL reconstructions.

These are the main reasons for directly digitizing (»show« the knee to the computer system), without help of CT scan or fluoroscopic images during the surgery.

The **ACL module** makes it possible to simulate an ACL graft placement in the digitized knee during surgery, and check the properties of the future knee with graft, before having done any drilling.

For us most important answers to be provided by the system are:

1. Is impingement avoided?
2. What about isometric placement of the graft, and consequently if elongation is occurring, it has to be within acceptable limits.

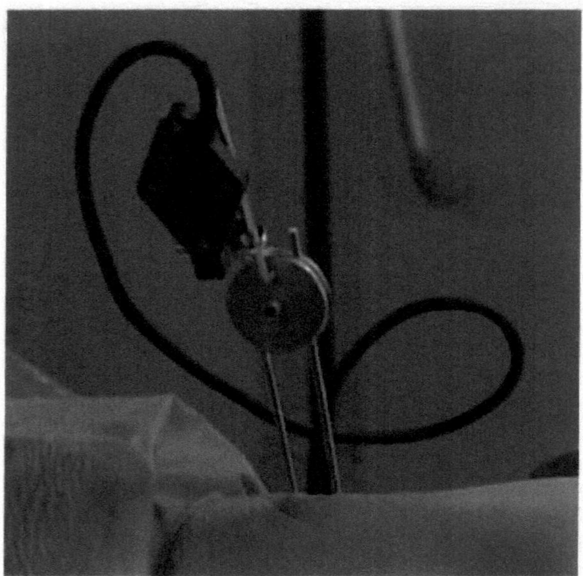

◘ Fig. 55-2. Double pin fixation of the shield

Those answers have to be provided, without adding too much time to the surgery. Unlike the hip surgery module, there is no preoperative planning through a CT scan in order to transfer the patients' knee anatomy to the computer.

Digitization of the knee anatomy automatically adds time to surgery. And of course, this time is limited because of the use of a tourniquet during the ACL surgery.

Description of our Procedure, Without Explaining the Basics of Navigation Principles

After starting up the system, both dynamic reference bases are fixed on the patients' anatomy, one for the tibia and one for the femur. Those dynamic reference bases (DRB) allow the computer to track relative motions between femur, tibia and instruments and also compensate for movements of camera and patient. For rigid fixation we use double pin (k-wires of 3 mm) fixation of the shields with 4 diodes (◘ Fig. 55-2).

It is of paramount importance that this fixation stays rigid during the procedure. In our experience, drilling of those pins percutaneous in femur and tibia didn't provoke postoperative problems for the patient.

After simple calibration of the free hook and pointer the digitization of the knees' anatomy can start. We here try to keep it as simple as possible, this means only digitize what is needed to answer both questions on impingement and isometry. To do so, one has to »understand« the navigation.

In order to digitize the knee, the interface asks for some anatomical landmarks. Those are:

1. proximal point of the femoral axis and middle of femoral condyles give the femoral axis,
2. middle of tibial plateau and middle of ankle results in tibial axis,
3. joint line.

Those axes are not important in an ACL replacement, they only help us recognize the structures on the computer screen. Due to the limitation of these landmarks, there is no loss of operation time.

4. Medial and lateral femoral condyles: following the preoperative prepared skin marks (not on the bone),
5. intercondylar roofline,
6. intercondylar notch: needs to be done carefully, because this will decide the presence of impingement,
7. potential femoral ligament insertion zone,
8. potential tibial ligament insertion zone.

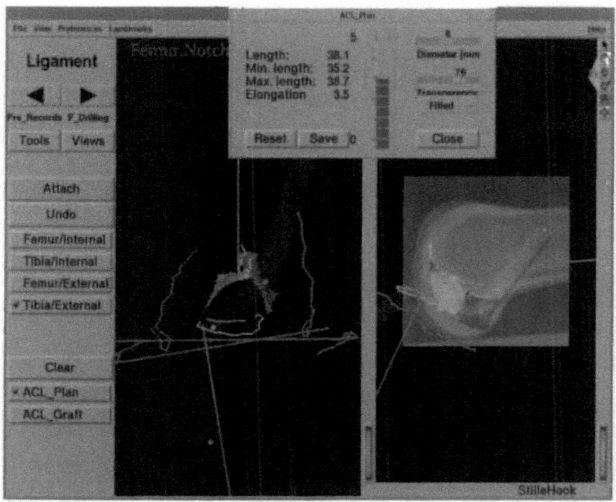

Fig. 55-3. Elongation of the virtual ligament

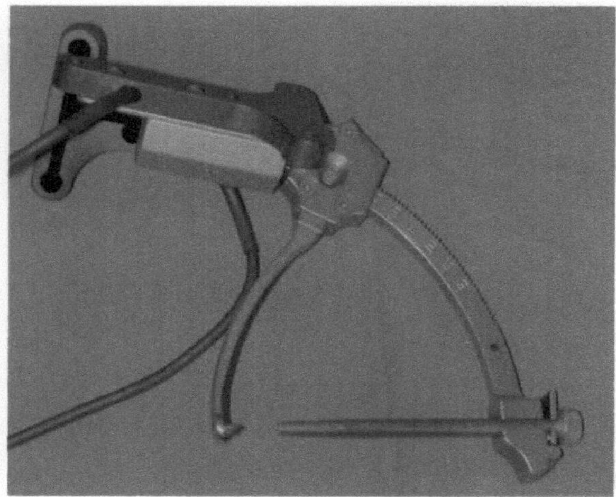

Fig. 55-4. Drill guide calibrated for navigation

Once the digitization of the knee complete, the system has enough information in order to start the simulation of graft implantation. To do so, we simply indicate the plan for ligament attachment, by pointing out 2 points for the supposed tibial and femoral attachment. The computer now shows a green virtual ligament on the screen, the diameter of that virtual graft has been adapted for the future real one. In this screen simulations can be made.

The leg is moved through the total range of motion, and on the screen the green virtual graft goes through or with or without touching the digitized intercondylar notch (impingement).

At the same moment the total virtual ligament elongation is showed on a diagram (**Fig. 55-3**).

By inadequate virtual graft position, new insertions can be tried. In order to facilitate this the systems suggests a better fixation zone both on tibia and femur. Once the ideal positioning of the graft is found, the bone tunnels can be drilled in order to fix the definitive graft just following the computer parameters

Normally the system is equipped with a navigated power tool. However we experienced some problems with the calibration of long and flexible drill bits. Therefore a drill guide is now calibrated for navigation (**Fig. 55-4**).

Align our drill bit with the proposed graft attachment is easily achieved.

Summary

In conclusion, we can positively answer our question about feasibility of complex navigation in the context of a regional hospital. Until now we navigated 91 ACL surgeries. The added surgery time for a standard ACL replacement is about 10 minutes.

The following remarks have to be made:
1. Learning curve is long.
2. The solutions proposed by the industry are not always adapted for use in a regional hospital, therefore, the exchange of ideas between surgeon and engineers is very important in order to develop useful tools.
3. Knee navigation is more complex than hip or spine navigation. One should not start his navigation experience in the knee.
4. We recently started navigation of the total knee arthroplasty (NexGen Zimmer). TKA navigation is more complex than ACL navigation. A big effort has to be done in order to develop well designed instruments.

56 Clinical Experience Using the *SurgiGATE* System

M. Wiese, A. Rosenthal, K. Bernsmann

Introduction

Anterior cruciate ligament (ACL) reconstruction occurs most commonly in the young and active patient [3,10,20]. The frequency of ACL injuries has increased because recreational activities and more risky sports became very popular. Frank and Jackson reported of 50,000 ACL reconstructions per annum in the USA in 1997. With the introduction of less invasive arthroscopic surgery in the 80s and 90s, ACL surgery is generally considered as a procedure with little risks. Open knee surgery becomes a method of the past lowering problems such as reduced proprioception and stability. When treated conservatively, knee joint instability after ACL tears has to be considered as a pre-arthritic condition leading to considerable cartilage and meniscus degeneration as reported by Schippinger et al. [18]. In a large follow-up study McDaniel and Dameron [12] recognized degenerative radiographic changes in over 80% of conservatively treated ACL injuries. Sutures of torn ACL show frustrating results with regards to blood supply and knee joint stability.

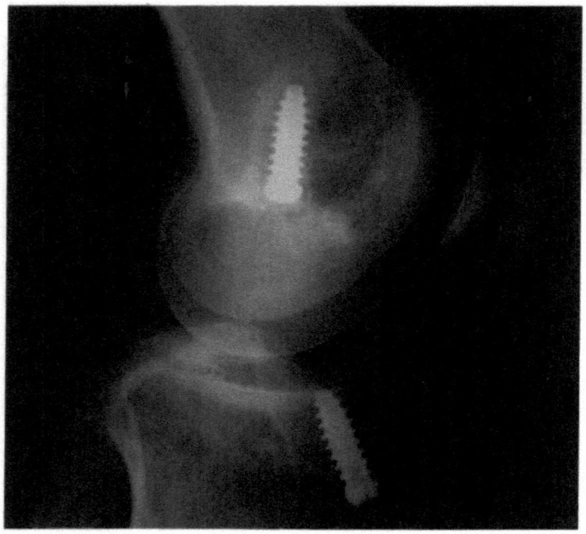

Most common choice for acute ACL reconstruction is autologous tendon tissue. Although drill guide instruments led to an increased precision of transplant position, inaccuracies are still possible. Mal-positioned ACL transplant lead to a variety of postoperative complications jeopardizing the outcome. The surgeon is responsible for correct graft placement and, therefore, one main source of error [4]. Important factors for graft placement include both tibial and femoral drill hole alignment.

ACL graft alignment influence both medium and long-term results [5, 9, 19] (◘ Fig. 56-1).

ACL mal-positioning may lead to notch impingement as shown by Watanabe and Howell [21]. Clinical outcome is poor in cases of 3 mm graft mal-position [14, 20] and leads to a 4-fold increase in tension within the ACL as shown by Friederich et al. [5]. Lengthening of the ACL below 5% is elastic, over 5% plastic [7, 17, 19]. Anterior placement of the ACL graft within the femur is the most common mistake and reason for graft failure. Poor clinical outcome post ACL surgery is reported between 5% to 52% [13].

◘ **Fig. 56-1.** Mal-positioning of the ACL with both the tibial and femoral canal placed to anterior within the notch. Entry points with suboptimal location

Methods

In order to enhance the outcome of ACL reconstruction computer-assisted surgery systems have been developed. The system utilized in this series was a by Sati modified CAS-System (Computer Assisted Surgery System, Medivision, Umkirch, Germany) from the M.E. Muller Institution

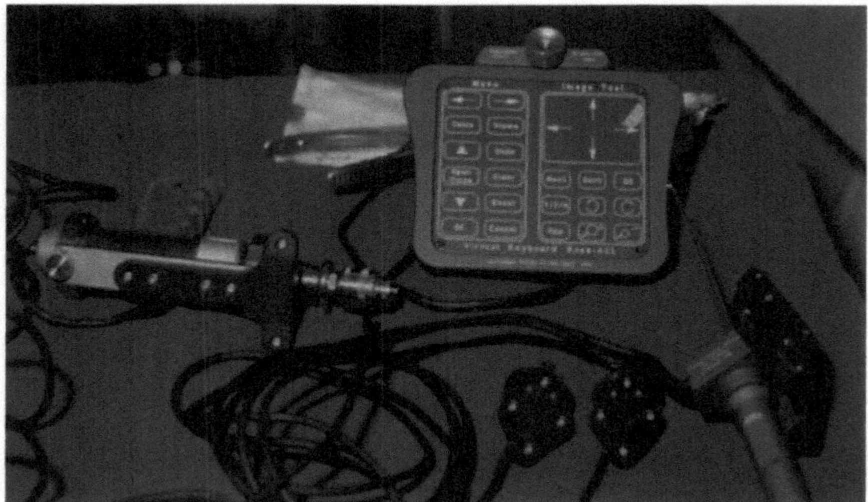

Fig. 56-2. Instruments with four active LED mounted on a shield

for Biomechanics in Bern, Switzerland. No CT or MRI data are required for this navigation system. A digitized radiograph of the knee joint in two planes is sufficient.

The navigation system has a computer (Ultra 10, SUN Microsystems) and works via an optoelectrical camera (Optotrak 3020, Northern Digital) tracing in a three-dimensional space. Four active markers are required in order to precisely identify the location of the instruments and markers attached the bones. The navigation system uses a set of standard arthroscopical instruments (**Fig. 56-2**). Additionally a special hook or pointer and a virtuell keyboard is used to digitize the patients' knee surface anatomy and to calculate a 3D image visible on the screen. The surgeon can use this virtual model as a reference for precise positioning of all instruments [2, 8, 17].

Information is needed for the motion in space of both femur and tibia in relation to all instruments. LED reference markers, which are traced by the camera, are pinned transcutaneously into femur and tibia with Kirschner wires (**Fig. 56-3**) and allow visualization of all instruments in relation to the knee anatomy.

With this system planning and identification of relevant structures of the operation are performed online during surgery using the standard approach. The surgeon identifies anatomical key structures by touching and digitizing them with the hook while pushing a foot paddle at the same time. The surface of the notch is digitized as a cloud and portrayed including notch roof, intercondylar line, and Blumensaat line from the posterior fossa to the

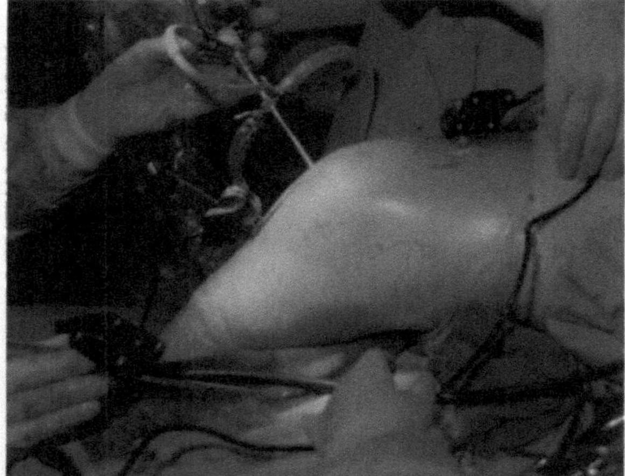

Fig. 56-3. Fixation of the reference base on tibia and femur using Kirschner wires

caudal aspect of the patellar groove. Additional reference points can be identified according to the surgeon's preferences. All acquired data are matched (overlay) with a digitized radiograph of the knee joint (**Fig. 56-4**). The digitized anatomical key structures have to show perfect rotation in order to match the radiograph without distortion. As shown in cadaver studies, a femoral rotation of 5 degrees equals 0.5 mm shortening of the Blumensaat line [1]. This allows exact positioning of the posterior femoral ACL insertion at the end of the intercondylar roof. Virtual graft placement and knee joint motion in

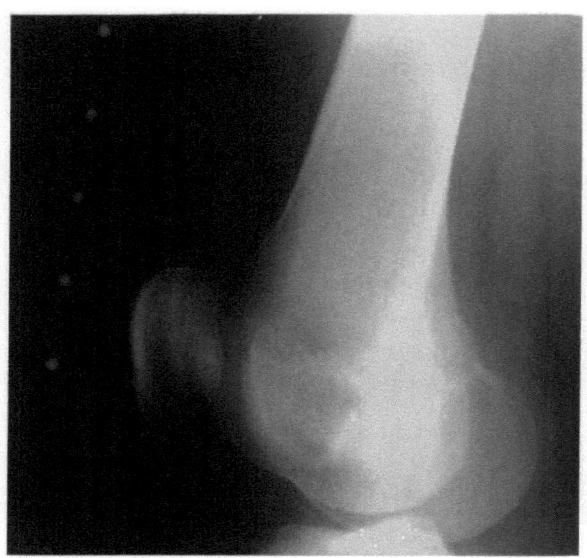

Fig. 56-4. Lateral view of a knee with a template attached to the anterior thigh. Moderate alterations of rotation are compensated

center is stored and graft elongation is checked at different locations. We recommend flexion from extension under posterior drawer stress during virtual ACL testing.

Drilling and placement of the bone canals are then guided by navigation and reference tools using simple overlay technique. The surgeon can choose and store different angles and standard views. The virtual knee is seen either from anterior or lateral through the notch and can be rotated allowing zooming in and out as well. The same navigation system provides alternative applications and interactions.

Results

flexion and extension will provide information of graft impingement or graft elongation. This maneuver is possible for all simulated graft sizes and insertions. Quantitative measures of graft deformity and isometric changes are listed on-line (**Figs. 56-5 and 56-6**). The insertion

A multicenter study tested successfully different surgical techniques included 20 cases with doubled quadriceps tendon, 12 cases with semitendinosus quadruple tendon and 40 cases with middle third patella tendons [1]. In a prospective study performed by the authors in Bochum, Germany, 100 ACL reconstructions were implanted utilizing the CAS system. Mean additional operating time was 15 min using a bone patellar tendon bone graft (BPTB). Lobbenhofer et al. In 1998 described this tech-

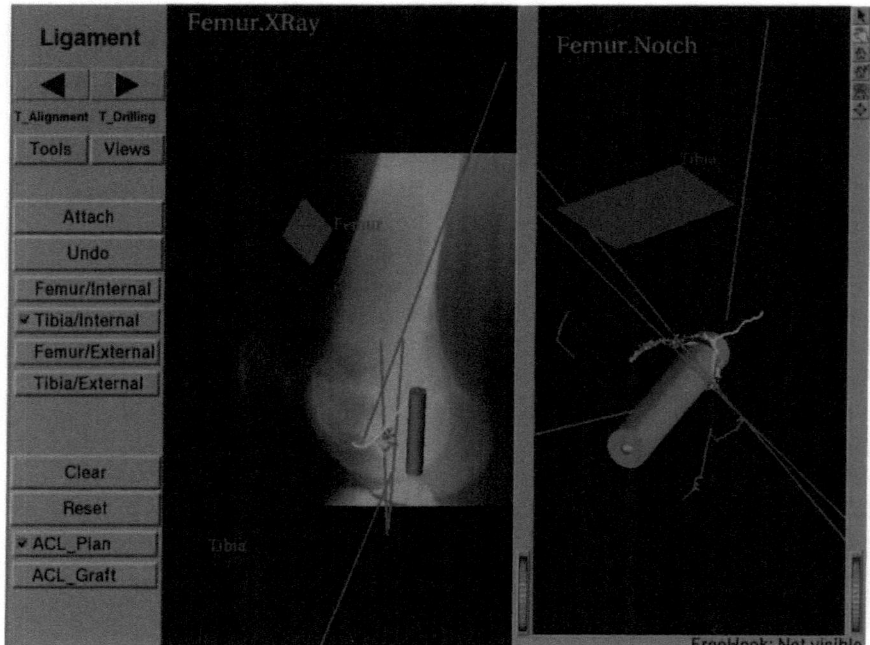

Fig. 56-5. Virtual placement of the ACL graft with impingement test prior to implantation

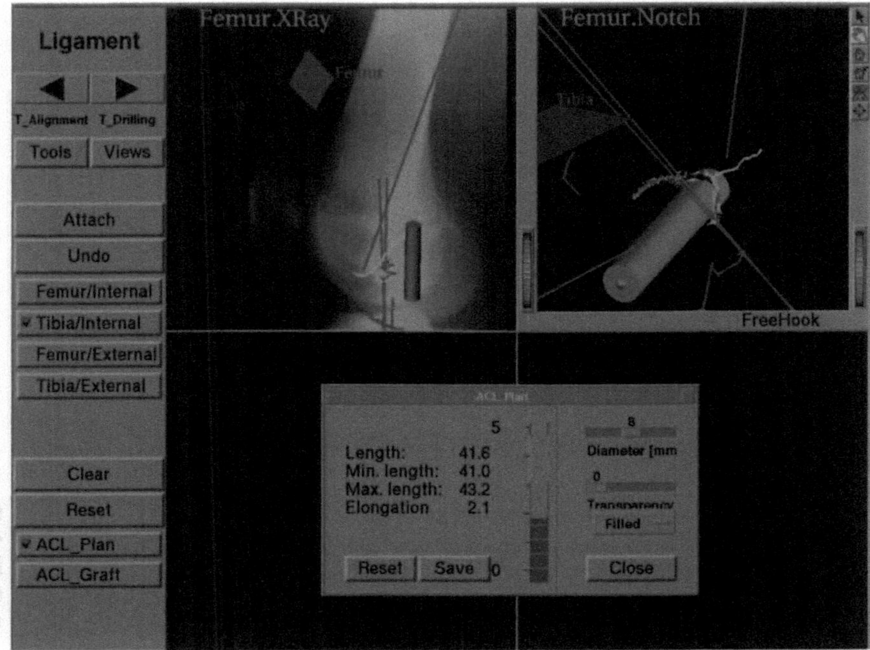

Fig. 56-6. Virtual check of isometric behavior of the ACL graft, again prior to implantation. The knee is flexed from full extension into 90 degrees with a posterior draw in order to avoiding anterior shift

nique due to its stable implantation with reference screws as the golden standard in ACL reconstruction.

Bone canal and K-wire drillings are guided by a LED tool (see Fig. 56.2). These additional temporary K-wires for dynamic reference bases (DRB) did not encounter for intra- or postoperative complications. All patients were treated with a full ROM orthosis (Promed). CPM therapy was used postoperatively for a couple of days. Full weight bearing was allowed when full extension was or less than 10 degrees flexion was achieved. Clinical follow-up included the Lysholm score and stability tests using ultrasound stability testing of the knee joint during anterolateral and anteromedial stress applying 150 Nm in 25 degrees of flexion. Gravitational forces are limited with the leg in side position [6]. Graft and canal positioning was measured on standardized lateral and anterior radiographs as recommended by Lemos et al. Early clinical results were comparable to not navigated ACL reconstruction, however, the ACL graft position was more accurate in the navigated group as measured on radiographs. Particularly femoral canal positioning at the posterior cortex showed a higher precision. Standard deviation was considerably lower in the navigated group ($p>0.05$).

Discussion

Computer assisted navigated ACL reconstruction surgery shows higher precision, accuracy and reproducibility than compared with conventional technique. We, therefore, recommend this modern technique particularly to avoid revision cases, where ACL graft failure is high and fixation is problematic as reported by Oettl and Imhoff [13]. ACL navigation surgery is beneficial both for the experienced surgeon and resident for training purposes. Operative outliers are avoided with navigation due to intraoperative feedback. The learing curve shortens. Documentation possibilities enhances quality control, which will become an important issue in the near future. Navigation systems are not routinely used in practice, although current systems meet the standards.

In our series of 100 CAS ACL reconstructions, this technique has proven its potential to become a routine procedure with minimal additional time consumption of so far 15 minutes, but increased accuracy of ACL graft positioning. There were no increased complications than compared with conventional procedures. We, therefore, consider CAS navigation in ACL reconstruction as a practical method, which enhances both accuracy and reproducibility.

References

1. Bernsmann K, Rosenthal A, Sati M, Stäubli HU, Cassens J, Menestrey J, Wiese M (2001) Multicentererfahrungen mit einem System zur computerassistierten vorderen Kreuzbandrekonstruktion. Orthopädische Praxis 37:1–5

2. Dessenne V, Lavallee S, Julliard R, Orti R, Martelli S, Cinquin P (1995) Computer-assisted knee anterior ligament reconstruction: First clinical tests. J Image Guid Surg 1:59–64

3. Diekstall P, Rauhut F (1999) Überlegungen zur Differentialindikation der vorderen Kreuzbandplastik. Ergebnisse nach Ersatz des vorderen Kreuzbandes im Vergleich zur Spontanprognose. Unfallchirurg 102: 173–181

4. Frank CB, Jackson DW (1997) The science of reconstruction of the anterior cruciate ligament. J Bone Joint Surg 79-A:1556–1569

5. Friederich NF, Müller W, O`Brien WR (1992) Klinische Anwendung biomechanischer und funktionell anatomischer Daten am Kniegelenk. Orthopäde 21:41–50

6. Grifka J, Bernsmann K, Hillen R (1993) Sonographische Stabilitätsdiagnostik des Kniegelenkes. Jahrbuch der Orthopädie: 143–83.

7. Grood ES (1992) Knee surgery, current practice. Aichroth PM, Cannon WD, Patel DV (eds) Martin Dunitz, London

8. Julliard R, Lavallee S, Dessenne V (1998) Computer assisted reconstruction of the anterior cruciate ligament. Clin Orthop 354:57–64

9. Khalfayan EE, Sharkey PF, Alexander AH, Bruckner JD, Bynum EB (1996) The relationship between tunnel placement and clinical results after anterior cruciate ligament reconstruction. Am J Sports Med 24:335–341

10. Klos TVS, Habets RJE, Banks AZ, Banks SA, Devilee RJJ, Cook F (1998) Computer assistance in arthroscopic anterior cruciate ligament reconstruction. Clin Orthop 354:65–69

11. Lobenhoffer P (1998) Golden Standard: Patellarsehnenplastik – Technik und postoperatives Komplikationsmanagement. Zentralbl Chir 123:981–993

12. McDaniel MJ, Dameron TB (1999) Long-term results of untreated anterior cruciate ligament rupture: a 28 year follow-up outcome study. AAOS Annual Meeting 1999; 4.–8. Feb. 1999, Anaheim, CA

13. Oettl GM, Imhoff AB (1998) Revisionschirurgie bei fehlgeschlagener vorderer Kreuzbandplastik. Zentralbl Chir 123:1033–1039

14. O`Meara PM, O'Brien WR, Henning CE (1992) Anterior cruciate ligament reconstruction stability with continuous passive motion – the role of isometric graft placement. Clin Orthop 277:201–209

15. Raunest J (1991) Application of a new positioning device for isometric replacement in anterior cruciate ligament repair and reconstruction. J Trauma 31:223–229

16. Sati M, deGuise JA, Drouin G (1997) Computer assisted knee surgery: diagnostics and planning of knee surgery. Computer Aided Surg 2: 108–123

17. Sati M, Bourquin Y, Stäubli H-U (1999) Flexible technology to consider both anatomical and functional factors in ACL replacement surgery. 4th International Symposium on Computer Assisted Orthopaedic Surgery 1999; March 17–19, 1999, Davos, Switzerland

18. Schippinger G, Passler JM, Seibert FJ, Schweighofer F (1997) Are complications in cruciate ligament replacement operations with patellar tendon transplantation dependent on surgical technique and surgical timing? Swiss Surg 3:154–159

19. Tomczak RJ, Hehl G, Mergo PJ, Merkle E, Rieber A, Brambs HJ (1997) Tunnel placement in anterior cruciate ligament reconstruction: MRI analysis as an important factor in the radiological report. Skeletal Radiol 26: 409–413

20. Vergis A, Gillquist J (1995) Current concepts. Graft failure in intra-articular anterior cruciate ligament reconstructions: a review of the literature. Arthroscopy 11:312–321

21. Watanabe BM, Howell SM (1995) Arthroscopic findings associated with roof impingement of an anterior cruciate ligament graft. Am J Sports Med 23:616–625

57 *ACL Surgetics:* An Efficient Computer-Assisted Technique for ACL Reconstruction

R. Julliard, S. Plaweski, S. Lavallée

Introduction

Background

Anterior cruciate ligament (ACL) rupture has become one of the most common knee injuries. Various surgical techniques have been proposed for its reconstruction, and one of the main difficulties is to determine an accurate placement of the ligament substitute, which has a predominant influence on the ACL reconstruction longevity [2, 8]. According to some publications, the rate of incorrectly placed ACL reconstructions may be as high as 40%. Thus, in a study performed in 24 cadaver knees, the results of the ACL grafts placements, only 4 of 24 were found to be correctly positioned [11]. This underlines the importance of graft placement at the anatomical insertion points of the native ACL. To meet this complex and challenging requirement, both technical points and anatomical features will need to be taken into consideration.

To address the issues of graft positioning, studies using computer-assisted surgery were conducted by our group in Grenoble starting in 1992. The work has been published in a number of papers. Ten years later, the most recent version of our computer-assisted surgery system (Surgetics Station) appears to be a significant help for the surgeon. This research period revealed that graft placement had to be based on three major criteria:

1. the ligament substitute must be positioned anatomically;
2. as isometrically as possible; and
3. avoiding impingement in the notch.

Femoral tunnel placement has been found to be essential for isometry, while tibial tunnel placement is essential in preventing graft-notch impingement [6].

The study presented below is based on the Surgetics navigation system of the PRAXIM Company.

This application to ACL reconstruction does not use any pre- or intraoperative imaging: no CT, no C-arm fluoroscopy, no radiography, no MRI. This technique of CT-less navigation for orthopaedics was developed, patented and published for the first time in 1993 [8]. The system processes data provided by optical sensors properly positioned on bones and instruments [10]. The tibia and the femur are represented in a reference coordinate system, which enables the articular kinematics of the lower limb to be measured, and the acquisition of anatomical reference points and surfaces to be performed accurately.

Criteria to Optimize: Anisometry and Notch Impingement

In ACL substitute placement, the optimal position of the femoral tunnel has not yet been determined: more often than not, it is placed deep and high in the notch, far from the center of the anatomical attachment site [1]. There is general agreement that the aim of ACL surgery is to obtain correct isometry and absence of impingement.

- Anisometry is defined as the maximal variation of distance between the tibial and femoral attachment

Acknowledgements: The authors wish to thank M. Bucki, M. Urbanek, P. Schnebelen, Prof P. Cinquin, and Prof J.P. Chirossel for their contributions to the work presented in this paper, and the French Ministry of Research for financial support (Research Grant NavPerop).

sites during flexion of the knee. We define positive anisometry as a pattern where this distance decreases from extension to flexion, and negative anisometry as a pattern where the distance increases with flexion. The anisometry profile is the curve of this distance with respect to the flexion angle.

- Impingement is defined as a contact of the graft with the notch in extension. A virtual straight cylinder is drawn between the insertion sites. If there is an impingement, the distance of penetration of this cylinder into the notch defines the impingement values.

The choice of the optimal values for those criteria is left entirely to the discretion of the surgeon.

The principle of the system resides in the interrelated and simultaneous choice of the tibial and femoral insertion point placements: the tibial placement depends on the femoral placement, and the femoral placement depends on the tibial placement The Surgetics system provides a visualization of those criteria: anisometry and notch impingement are shown for each pair of points selected by the surgeon. The system offers a passive help to ACL reconstruction; it is not an automated system which dictates the optimal position. It is like a GPS system rather than an automated pilot. Furthermore, since there is dis-

agreement concerning the need for a notch plasty, the computer appears to be an elegant solution to help the surgeon decide, in each individual case and in the light of the selected graft positions, on whether or not to perform a notch plasty.

Material and Step-by-Step Methods

Surgetics Station and Rigid Bodies

The system consists in positioning, in a reference coordinate system, two rigid bodies both on the femur and on the tibia. Retro-reflecting single-use markers are assembled on each rigid body. These markers are detected by an optical localization system, which measures the position and orientation of the rigid bodies in relation to a reference coordinate system. The F and T rigid bodies are to be fixed to the femur and to the tibia, respectively, on the side of the surgical approach, using minimally invasive external fixators with two pins. They are orientated in such a way as to make the markers point towards the optical localizer [9].

Set-up

The Surgetics ACL runs on the PRAXIM Surgetics Station, which is an open platform independent of implant companies (◼ Fig. 57-1). It is very versatile, simple to use, and compact. It is based on an accurate infrared optical tracking system. There is no keyboard or mouse; the main interaction is performed by the surgeon, pressing a blue footswitch to go forward and a yellow footswitch to go

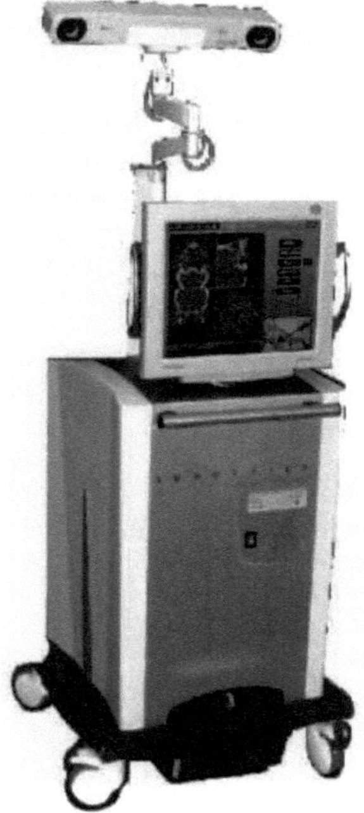

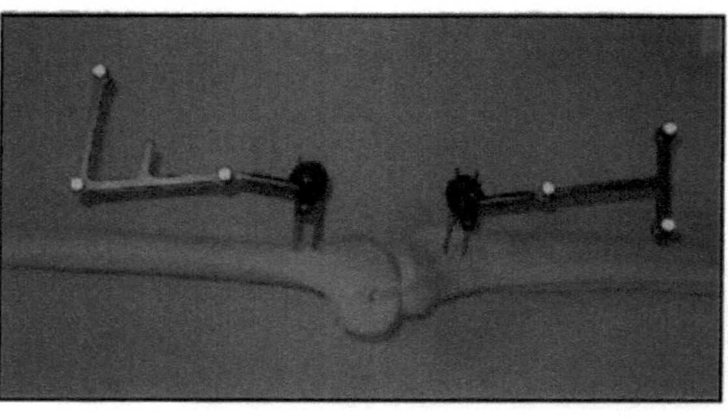

◼ **Fig. 57-1.** Surgetics Station of PRAXIM and positions of the F and T rigid bodies (illustration on sawbone)

backward. A touch screen is used to enter a few specific data. The Surgetics ACL can be started simply by inserting an appropriate CD-ROM, or by pressing the touch screen. Patient information can be recorded and stored in the intraoperative report on the individual patient's CD-ROM. The next stage consists in positioning the optical system, and then calibrating the position of the center of the spherical tip of the probe.

Data Acquisition

Anatomical Points

The 3D probe is used to acquire points under arthroscopy or on the patient skin.

- The center of the ankle is determined by computing a point half-way between the skin over the lateral and medial malleoli, in order to evaluate the flexion angle of the knee each time it will be necessary.
- The medial and lateral tibial spine points are acquired to constitute an anatomical reference.

Kinematic Data

The rigid bodies F and T on the bones are used to acquire the specific kinematics of the patient.

- A passive flexion-extension is performed by the surgeon. This measurement is aimed at calculating the anisometry values and profiles of the graft.
- Optionally, if requested by the surgeon, it is possible to acquire the center of the femoral head by performing a conic movement in order to calculate a true hip-knee-ankle angle in the sagittal plane.

3D Morphology

Bone Morphing consists in computing the accurate morphology of the patient's knee from a deformable statistical model, without use of CT, radiography, or fluoroscopy. Several hundred scattered points are acquired quickly by the surgeon, by »painting« the cartilage and bone surface with the probe. These points are matched with the statistical model using a 3D/3D registration algorithm. The bone model displayed on the screen is deformed in real time, to adapt to the knee of the patient [3].

- Tibial Bone Morphing consists in acquiring several points on the tibial bony surface in order to reconstruct the patient's anatomy from a tibial generic model. The procedure is straightforward and convenient, and consists in sliding the probe on the accessible zones of the tibia, i. e. the inter- and pre-spinal areas.
- Femoral Bone Morphing is based on the same features: three zones have to be covered – the anterior arch, the external notch wall, and the posterior notch close to the top.

Interactive Planning and Navigation with the Probe

The system computes and displays the anisometry and impingement criteria for any points selected. The surgeon navigates the pointer on the tibia and the femur, and interactively selects the insertion sites that best match the chosen values.

Building Anisometry Maps on the Femur

For any pair of insertion sites F and T selected by the surgeon on the femur and the tibia, the system computes and displays in real time the anisometry profile, based on the passive flexion that was performed at the beginning of the procedure. The maximum and minimum values of distance between F and T along the passive flexion-extension are shown as Max and Min, respectively. For a given tibial point, the Max-Min anisometry values are computed on each surface element of the femur, and a color is assigned. This provides anisometry color maps as illustrated in ◘Fig. 57-2. A favorable anisometry profile characterizes a fiber that loses tension during the flexion, whereas a non-favorable anisometry profile characterizes a fiber that stretches in flexion.

Building a Posterior Blumensaat Projection of the Femur on the Tibia

The radiological features of the tunnels are well known by the surgeons, and their positions are defined in relation to Blumensaat's line, which is a familiar radiological landmark for ligament placement [11]. The projection of the femoral notch on the tibia in the direction of Blumen-

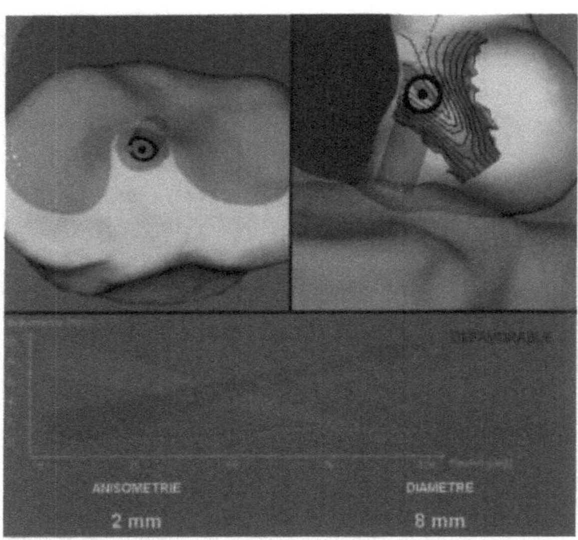

Fig. 57-2. Interactive planning on tibia and femur. The *blue circles* correspond to the insertion points of the tunnels – the *red area* on the tibia shows a potential impingement with the femoral notch – the anisometry map on the femur is colour-coded: *green* indicates an anisometry value of less than 2 mm; *yellow*, 2–4 mm; *orange*, 4–6 mm; and *red*, more than 6 mm. Blumensaat's line is represented by a *dotted line*. The anisometry curve is illustrated in *green*; it is computed in real time as the surgeon selects new insertion sites

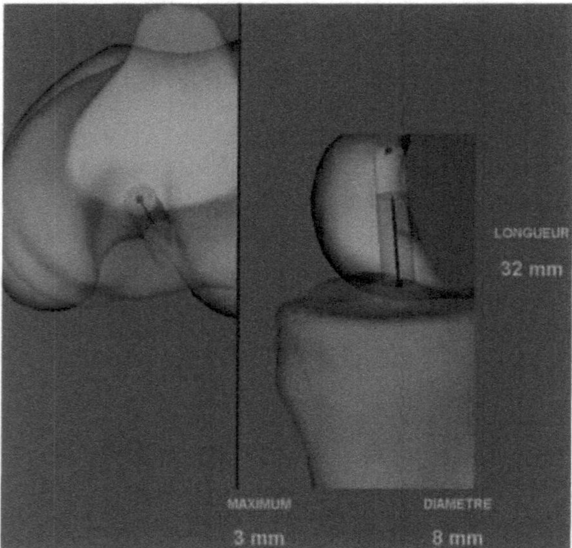

Fig. 57-3. Notch impingement testing. After the tibial and femoral tunnels have been planned, placing the knee in extension shows the potential impingement of the virtual graft with the arch of the notch – *area in red*

saat's line helps the surgeon to position the tibial tunnel as anteriorly as possible while avoiding notch impingement.

Simulating the Graft Envelope, and Notch Impingement Testing

The virtual ligament substitute is simulated by a cylindrical envelope. In the surgical technique, a cylindrical tunnel centered on points F and T is drilled virtually in the femoral and tibial surfaces: the intersection curves between the cylinder and the surfaces are generated. The line segments that link the intersection points on the femoral and the tibial surfaces, respectively, produce a representation of the external envelope of the graft that can be displayed for any flexion angle of the knee.

This stage consists in checking the position of the centers of the tunnels both on the femur and on the tibia, by dynamically viewing the potential impingement with the notch [5]. A red zone appearing on the femoral surface reveals the presence of a potential impingement between the cylinder and the notch. The displayed distance represents the maximum penetration distance of the virtual ligament inside the notch for all the flexion angles measured (**Fig. 57-3**).

A Possible Strategy for Planning

Two initial points are calculated by the system: the selected tibial point is the most anterior one positioned close to the notch of the arch projection, but with no significant impingement; the selected femoral point is the one which minimizes the anisometry. From those two initial points, the surgeon can adopt any strategy to select better points that suits his or her philosophy or surgical technique. The strategy described below (but not prescribed) by the authors is the most simple one:

1. The surgeon maintains the tibial point initially proposed by the computer.
2. The surgeon places a femoral point which is at the usual anatomical insertion of the ACL and which has the best anisometry: the anisometry must be positive and not too great. The maximum acceptable value of anisometry depends on the flexion angle which is used to tighten the graft. However, a high anisometry value should be avoided, since it would leave a laxity in flex-

ion that may be one of the causes of postoperative osteoarthritis.

3. The surgeon adjusts the tibial point to prevent any conflict for the given femoral point, and checks the corresponding new anisometry profile.

Other methods are possible.

Navigation of Tibial and Femoral Drill Guides

Using any standard instrumentation for drilling the tunnels, a rigid body is attached to the drill guide, and the system is calibrated. The operation then consists in navigating the tibial and femoral guides pointing at the planned points on the tibial and femoral surfaces [7]. The computer allows navigation with any kind of tunnel drilling, regardless of the drilling technique used. Thus, the femoral tunnel may be navigated and drilled inside-

out (through the medial arthroscopic portal or through the tibial tunnel) or outside-in (◨ Fig. 57-4).

Final Control on one Fiber of the Graft

The purpose of this stage is to view the insertion points thus determined and to calculate the anisometry of the ligament substitute model, whose central fiber is defined by these points. It is possible to check the position of a fiber on the graft's surface, by digitizing a single fiber on the graft and checking its anisometry as well as any potential impingement in the notch. The system displays the positions of the tunnels and all the associated data. The virtual fiber is digitized from the tibial tunnel to the femoral tunnel. The value of the length of this fiber is displayed for each angle of flexion, so that its anisometry can be checked. Positioning the knee in extension enables the surgeon to check the presence of impingement between this fiber and the notch. This process is primarily applied to the most anterior fiber of the graft.

CD-ROM

At the application end, the system allows to write the intraoperative data onto a CD-ROM. This information is contained in an html report. The advantages are that the data can be analyzed postoperatively, and that the patient information is entered on the CD-ROM. This constitutes an important point in terms of audit and traceability.

Results

One of the major challenges of computer-assisted surgery is the collection of clinical data including long-term patient follow-up in larges series of patients and involving different clinical centers, in order to assess the clinical benefits of the technique. However, some first results can be presented.

Results in Patients with a Prototype

Results have been published about the comparison between conventional and computerized methods for ACL

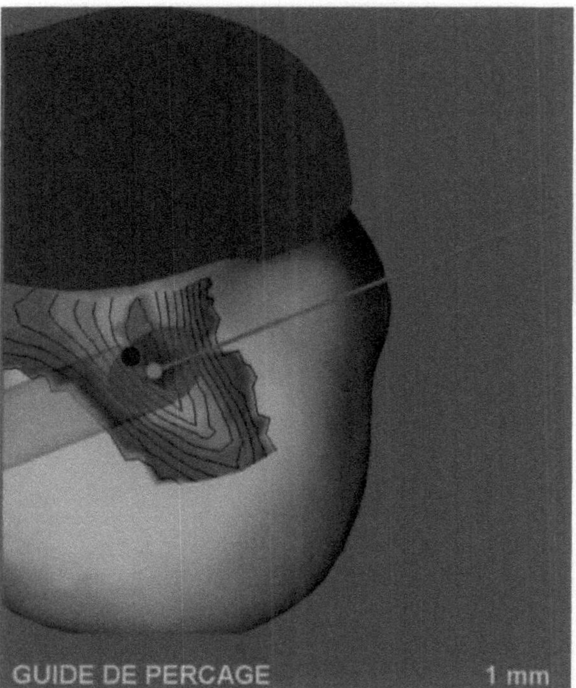

◨ **Fig. 57-4.** Navigation of drill guide on femur. Once the drill guide has been calibrated, the surgeon adjusts the guide – light blue cylinder displayed – by pointing on the screen the planned point – dark blue point on the screen – until the light and dark blue points coincide

reconstruction: twenty-three patients' knees underwent an ACL reconstruction using a standard technique. Central graft fiber isometry was measured using the computer, and found to be 5 mm on average. Computer-assisted surgery was then carried out in the laboratory: the navigation simulation showed that the surgeon could have obtained more isometric results: the average central graft fiber value measured with the computer was found to be 2.3 mm. The clinical utility of the computer-assisted method was thus demonstrated [4, 5].

Results in Specimens

The most recent studies were performed in seven knee specimens. The results are presented in ◼ Table 57-1.

The comparison of the values obtained for different ways of positioning a drill guide on a tibial or a femoral surface shows that there was no major difference between the figures. The values tend to be fairly similar, which suggests that the use of the system enables points to be placed significantly closely to the usual positions that would be used by surgeons experienced in ACL reconstruction. This proves the reliability of the navigation system for placing the substitute ACL in as accurate as possible a site, both in the femur and in the tibia.

Conclusion

The Surgetics navigation system as described above is a passive system that provides data and efficient help to the surgeon. It is like a »third eye« that allows the surgeon to achieve accuracy, safety, reliability, and precision, and allows him or her to adjust the technique and customize the parameters to suit the individual patient's pattern.

The computer is not a solution in itself: the surgeon's opinion and experience remain essential [2]. The system is versatile, in that it has proved itself adaptable to the different drill guides in current use. Indeed, when the current instrumentation is used according to the traditional surgical technique, it appears not to be accurate enough to provide entry points at their expected position: Navigation enables to use adequate instruments and compare their relative efficiency [4].

The system is also very easy to use and efficient: the linear protocol, the visual aids, the 3D views obtained by Bone Morphing, the wireless instruments combined with the absence of the need for pre- and intraoperative imaging, make it well-suited for routine use in the clinical setting. Another benefit is the automated generation of a report on CD-ROM, which should be of major importance in terms of audit, medicolegal issues, and ease of patient record management. These features enable

◼ **Table 57-1.** Synthesis of the distances calculated between the planned point and the drilled points performed with navigation/with a drilling guide 1/with a drilling guide 2

	Distance between the planned point and the point actually drilled using navigation	Distance between the planned point and the point obtained with conventional method – Drill guide 1	Distance between the planned point and the point obtained with conventional method – Drill guide 2
x-, y-, z- axis	Average for 7 knees [mm]	Average for 7 knees [mm]	Average for 7 knees [mm]
Tibia T0-T [mm]			
Distal/Proximal	–0,15	0,75	–0,21
Medial/Lateral	–0,35	–0,70	–1,66
Anterior/Posterior	–1,32	0,97	1,90
Femur F0-F [mm]			
Distal/Proximal	–1,34	–2,05	–0,33
Medial/Lateral	0,30	1,83	–1,02
Anterior/Posterior	–1,13	–3,60	–2,76

T0 is the barycenter of the outline of the insertion point of the anatomical ACL ligament on the tibia; *T* corresponds to the planned, the drilled, or the navigated point on the tibia; *F0* is the barycenter of the outline of the insertion point of the anatomical ACL ligament on the femur; *F* corresponds to the planned, the drilled, or the navigated point on the femur

the navigation system to be used for teaching purposes as well [6].

References

1. Arnold MP, Kooloos J, van Kampen A (2001) Single-incision technique misses the anatomical femoral anterior cruciate ligament insertion: a cadaver study. Knee Surg Sports Traumatol Arthrosc 9: 194–199

2. Dessenne V, Lavallée S, Julliard R, Orti R, Martelli S, Cinquin P (1995) Computer-assisted knee anterior cruciate ligament reconstruction: first clinical tests. J Image Guided Surg 1: 59–64

3. Fleute M (2001) Shape reconstruction for computer-assisted surgery based on non-rigid registration of statistical models with intraoperative point data and X-ray images. TIMC IMAG Laboratory

4. Julliard R, Lavallée S, Dessenne V (1998) Computer-assisted reconstruction of the Anterior Cruciate Ligament. Clin Orthop 354, pp 57–64

5. Julliard R, Plaweski S, Merloz Ph Cinquin P (2002) La navigation sans imagerie du ligament croisé antérieur (NASALCA). Anterior cruciate ligament navigation. SURGETICA, Grenoble. Troccaz J, Merloz Ph (ed). Sauramps medical: pp 254-262

6. Julliard R, Plaweski S, Merloz P, Moyen B, Nizard R, Perrier JP Computer-assisted anterior cruciate ligament reconstruction.

7. Lavallée S, Julliard R, Orti R, Cinquin P, Carpentier E (1993) Anterior cruciate ligament reconstruction: computer-assisted determination of the most isometric femoral attachment point. Orthop Traumatol 3: 87–92

8. Orti R, Lavallée S, Julliard R, Cinquin Ph, Carpentier E (1993) Computer-assisted Knee Ligament Reconstruction – IEEE EMBS Conference, Paris, pp 963-964

9. Picard F, DiGioia AM, Moody J (2001) Accuracy in tunnel placement for ACL reconstruction. Comparison of traditional arthroscopic and computer-assisted navigation techniques. Comp Aided Surg 6: 279–289

10. Sati M, Bourquin Y, Säubli H-U, Nolte L-P (2000) Considering anatomic and functional factors in ACL reconstruction: new technology. CAOS, USA

11. Sati M, Stäubli H-U, Bourquin Y, Kunz M, Nolte L-P (2002) Real-time computerized in situ guidance system for ACL graft placement. Comp Aided Surg 7: 25–40

58 Clinical Experience with *CASPAR*-Assisted ACL Reconstruction

L. Gotzen, A. Pashmineh-Azar, E. Ziring

Introduction

The causes and reasons for unsatisfactory results and failures after replacement of the anterior cruciate ligament (ACL) are numerous and diverse. However, irrespective of what material is used for replacement, the incorrect position of the transplant plays the leading role. According to the consensus conference of the International Knee Society, more than 40% of all ACL transplants are incorrectly positioned. It has been documented many times in the literature that there is a close correlation between the position of a transplant and the clinical outcome [e.g. 1, 5–8]. Revision operations after ACL reconstruction are based on transplant mal-positioning in 70% to 80% [loc. cit. 9].

In order to be able to carry out an anatomical, almost isometric and impingement-free positioning of the transplant with the greatest possible and most reproducible accuracy, the CASPAR system from Ortho Maquet was integrated into anterior cruciate ligament reconstruction. Almost two years of development and testing were required before the system appeared to be suitable for computer planning and robot implementation of the transplant tunnels in terms of software and hardware. From April 1999 to October 2000, 92 ACL replacement operations were carried out using the CASPAR system.

Problems and Changes in the Application Phase

Most problems which became manifest in clinical application could be rapidly eliminated. The following important amendments were made and optimization measures undertaken:

Reduction of the Fiducials from Four to Two Bone Screws

In the beginning, two voluminous registration screws were introduced into the distal femur and the proximal tibia for referencing purposes. This elaborate procedure which traumatizes soft tissues and is a burden to the patient was replaced by the application of a thin carrier screw on the tibial and femoral side. Registration crosses are mounted on the carrier screws for referencing purposes.

Improvement of Knee Fixation

Fully constraining immobilization of the knee joints is required during the process of milling the transplant tunnels with the robot. In the first operations, the robot stopped repeatedly because of movements. A more stable knee clamp which only grips the femoral condyles and a special ground plate were then developed. The knee clamp and the ground plate were connected to the robot via articulated arms.

Installation of Water Cooling for the Diamond Hollow Burr

Without cooling, the hollow burr caused substantial heat damage in the transplant tunnel in milling. The thermal damage to the bone tissue could be prevented completely with continuous water cooling.

Hand Guidance of the Hollow Burr up to the Bone Surface Before Starting the Milling

After referencing, the robot arm automatically assumes the planned milling trajectory. The robot carried out the milling process, initially without the possibility of external intervention. The hollow burr not uncommonly encountered the patellar ligament in creating the femoral tunnel or collided with the inferior pole of the patella. Afterwards, the procedure was changed in such a way that the hollow burr was guided by hand up to the bone surface after taking up the start position. Any obstacle detected in the milling trajectory can be eliminated by altering the knee flexion.

Graduated Regulation of the Milling Speed

A further problem that was noted in the initial phase was that the hollow burr slipped off when it impinged obliquely on the bone surface. This caused it to deviate from the planned milling trajectories. The slippage resulted from a too rapid feed rate of the hollow burr and was eliminated by graduated regulation of the milling speed. Until the hollow burr has penetrated a short distance into the bone, it is advanced at a very low speed and the rate of forward movement is only raised afterwards.

Description of the CASPAR-Assisted ACL Replacement

Implantation of the Carrier Screws and Computer Tomography

The implementation of the planning for the surgical operation is achieved using registration crosses which are measured both in the CT and by the robot. Special bone screws serve as mounting platforms for the registration crosses. A carrier screw is introduced by a stab incision from lateral into the distal femur and anteromedially into the proximal tibia mostly on the day before the operation and usually under 3-in-one block analgesia.

The physiological positional situation of the intact knee joint in full extension is taken as the basis for planning in order to eliminate the pathological extension, translation and rotation conditions in the injured knee that are caused by the instability. A CT of both knee joints is therefore taken. For this purpose, the legs are arranged in parallel in the extended position and fixed in a special foot holding device with freely dangling knee joints (◘ Fig. 58-1). Before taking the CT, the registration crosses must be screwed on the carrier screws. The CT data set is transferred online to the planning station.

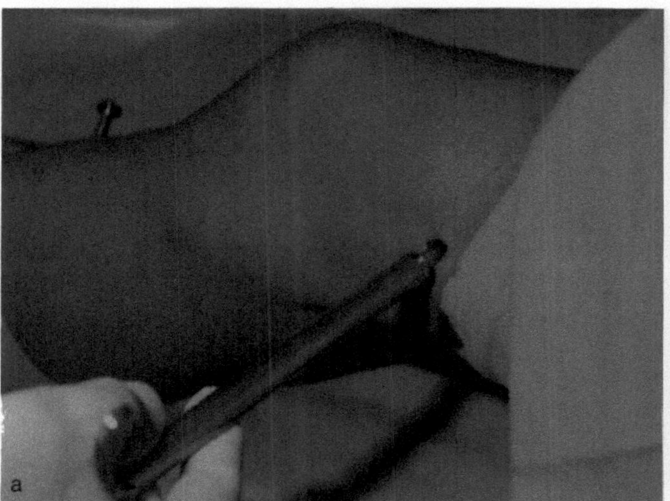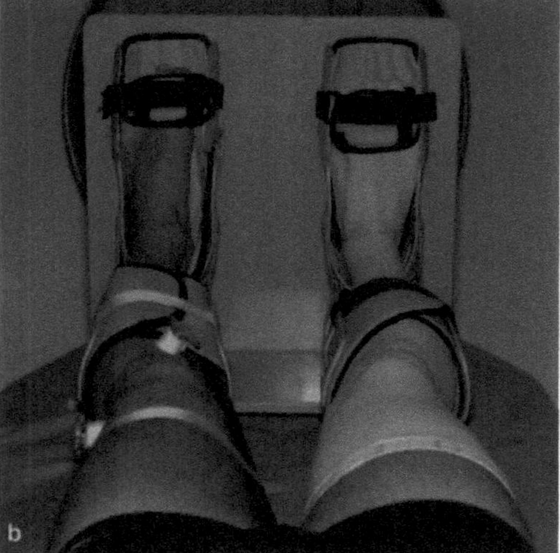

◘ **Fig. 58-1a,b. a** Percutaneous implantation of the carrier screws: into the tibia from anteromedial and into the femur from lateral. **b.** Symmetrical positioning of both legs with loosely hanging knee joints with a special foot clamping device to take the CT. The registration crosses are mounted on to the vector screws

Planning of the Transplant Tunnels

The transplant tunnels can be planned in two ways that are fundamentally different. On the one hand, the surgeon can determine the position of the tunnels entirely without constraints by free navigation in the 3D CT data set on the basis of his own position criteria. Alternatively, the tunnel placement can be established using specified parameters. All the intermediate strategies between these approaches are feasible if the planning parameters are restricted to a greater or lesser extent.

The planning takes place in four steps: **standardization, matching, femoral and tibial tunnel planning.**

In standardization, the femur of the unstable knee joint is brought into a standard position in all three planes interactively using an orientation tool that is visible in the three orthogonal planes.

In interactive matching, the difference in position in the tibia on the unstable side and that on the intact side is determined in relation to the standardized femur. With the translatable matching tool, at first the femur of the unstable knee represented in the CT in blue shades is matched with the femur of the contralateral knee in the CT represented in green shades. Matching of the tibiae then follows. After adaptation, the two superimposed femora and tibiae appear in a blue-green mixed shade. The result of matching is the transformation, which describes the difference in position between the tibiae relative to the femur coordinate system. The further planning takes place in the unstable knee, but under the positional conditions of the intact knee in physiological extension.

In the femoral planning, the tunnel entry center is emplaced in the sagittal plane in the rectangle inaugurated by Bernard and Hertel [3]. This rectangle is placed at Blumensaat's line and adjusted to match the lateral condyle by navigating through the CT and looking for the maximal condyle size. The position of the tunnel entry center within the rectangle is laid down in percentage distance values along and perpendicular to Blumensaat's line. Whereas Amis and Jacob [2] have suggested 38% along and 20% perpendicular to Blumensaat's line, Bernard and Hertel [3] recommend 25% in both cases. Different percentage values are used by the various surgeons of our own institution. However, these were largely within the range of the values suggested above. In the third dimension, the tunnel entry center is laid down interactively according to individual positional criteria in the transverse section. Starting from the tunnel entry center that has been laid down, the further planning of the tunnel axis is car-

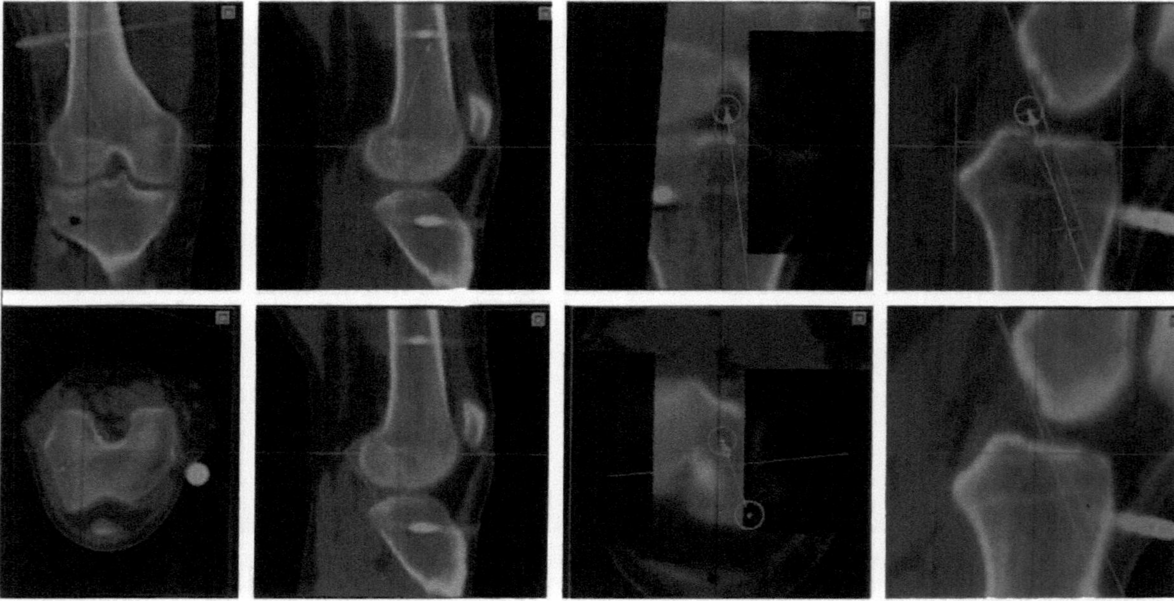

Fig. 58-2. Femoral and tibial tunnel planning in the CT of a patient

ried out by free navigation. This is laid down in such a way that there is no intraoperative collision of the hollow burr with the medial femoral condyle.

In the planning of the tibial tunnel in the frontal plane, the medial margin of the intraarticular tunnel opening is placed on the tip of the medial intercondylar tubercle and the tunnel axis is lined up with that of the femoral tunnel. For planning the tunnel in the sagittal plane, our own procedure published in 1990 [4] was largely integrated into the CASPAR software. The point of intersection of the transformed Blumensaat's line with the tibial plateau marks the position of the anterior tunnel margin intraarticularly. In the prolongation to distal, the transformed Blumensaat's line forms the anterior tunnel wall in the tibia.

An example of a plan of the transplant tunnels is shown in ◘ Fig. 58-2.

After completion of planning, the planning data are stored on a PC card.

Preparation of the Robot for the Surgical Operation

The transfer card with the planning data is inserted into the disk drive of the control unit in the operating theater. The control unit provides the planning data and the control signals for the robot. When the control signal is turned on, the operating system is installed and a self-test is carried out. Afterwards, the robot arm is brought into the start position for application of the tool using the hand-operating device. The robot is then covered with a sterile transparent plastic sheet (◘ Fig. 58-3). A sterile plastic tube is pulled over the hand-operated device and the cable connection to the control unit. Special attention must be paid to the covering and close collaboration between the sterile and non-sterile surgical staff is necessary in order to maintain aseptic conditions. Afterwards, the sterile instrument column is fixed on the robot and the tool is calibrated.

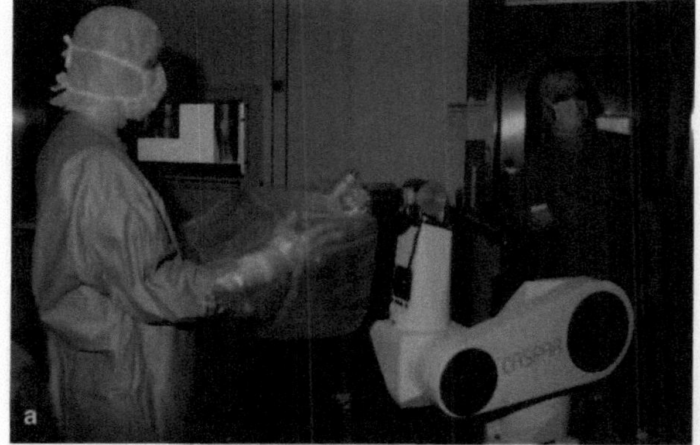
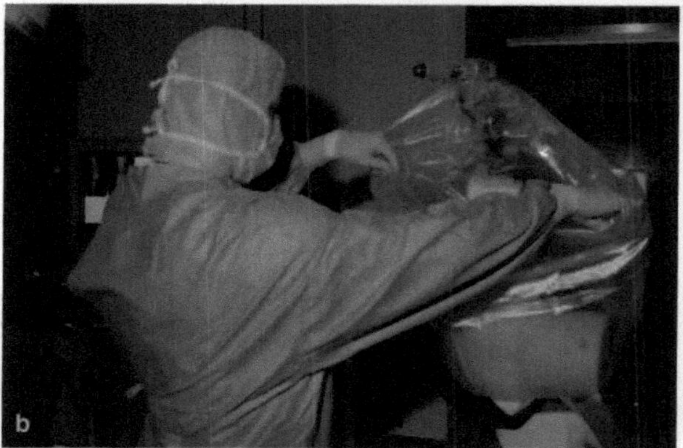
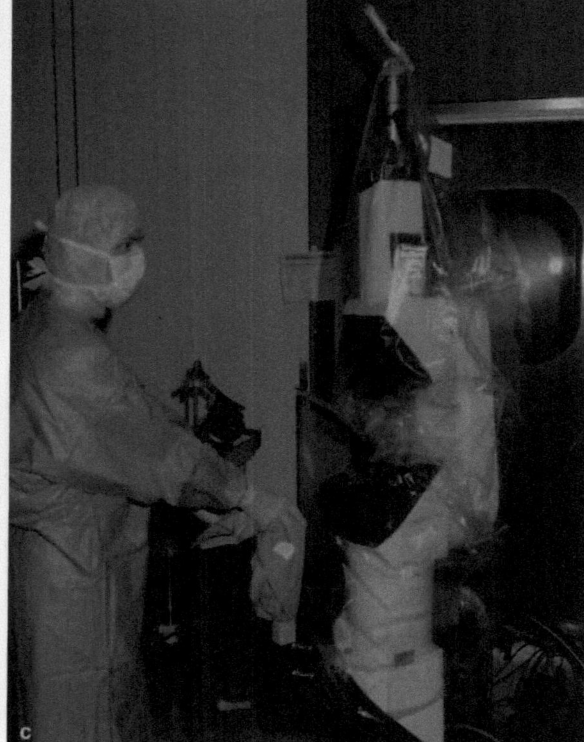

◘ **Fig. 58-3.** Covering the robot with sterile plastic sheet

Surgical Procedure

After arthroscopy of the knee and graft harvesting, a foot support is first of all fastened on to immobilize the knee and then the leg is placed with the foot support into a special ground plate with knee flexion of about 100–120° and the knee clamp is applied. In addition, an articulated arm is mounted between the ground plate and the knee clamp. The robot is moved up to the operating table and lowered and afterwards also connected to the ground plate and to the knee clamp via articulated arms. To monitor the complete immobilization of the knee joint, rigid bodies are fixed to the knee clamp onto which an infrared camera connected to the control unit of the robot is focused. Afterwards, sterile fidcucial registration crosses are mounted onto the carrier screws (◘ Fig. 58-4).

Initially, the referencing is carried out on the tibial side. At the fiducial cross, four measurement points are targeted with the measurement tip fixed in the tool. The tibial carrier screw is then removed. After the robot has automatically taken up its start position for creation of the tibial tunnel, the hollow burr is guided manually above the access incision to take the transplant or via a separate stab incision to the anterior medial surface of the tibia. Now, the tibial tunnel is milled by the robot with continuous water cooling and initially with low feed rate.

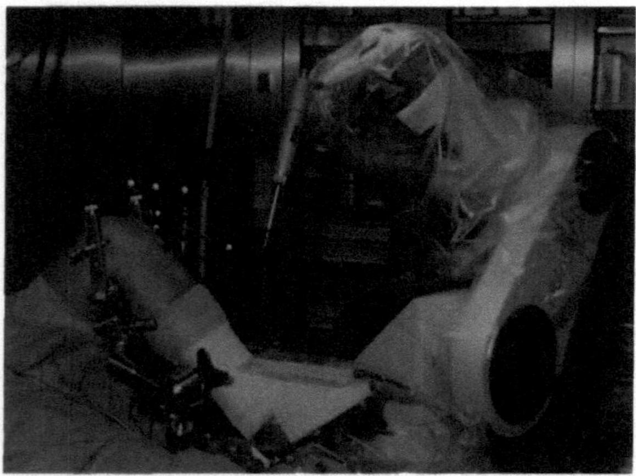

◘ **Fig. 58-4.** Knee and robot prepared for setting up the tunnels. Knee bent about 110° degrees, leg fixed into the ground plate with the foot support, knee clamp applied, robot with sterile covering on the operation table and lowered, articulated arms between the ground plate and the knee clamp and the robot, infrared camera focused on the rigid bodies at the knee clamp, measurement tips inserted into the tool for registration

In planning the tibial tunnel, the length of the milling trajectory is set in such a way that the hollow burr penetrates about 7 mm into the joint, so that the bone cylinder remains within it when the hollow burr is drawn back automatically.

Afterwards, the referencing is carried out on the femoral side. After adopting the start position, the hollow burr is introduced by hand into the joint and into the notch up to bone contact via a parapatellar medial mini-arthrotomy or via the anteromedial arthroscopy portal. If it is shown that the milling trajectory is obstructed, mostly due to a collision of the hollow burr with the inferior pole of the patella, the knee flexion must be altered. However, fresh referencing registration is necessary after this. The carrier screw is therefore initially left in the femur and only removed during the milling process. The femoral tunnel is set up as a continuous mill channel so that the bone cylinder inside is pulled back with the hollow burr, as on the tibial side.

◘ Figure 58-5 shows the robot in milling of the tunnels.

After creating the tunnels, the robot is disconnected from the ground plate and from the knee clamp and moved away from the operating table. The knee clamp is removed and the operation is continued in the usual way.

Time Required for Integration of the CASPAR System into ACL Replacement

The time required to integrate the CASPAR system into cruciate ligament replacement in the last of the 25 of the 92 operations was analyzed. On average, 30 min were necessary for analgesia and subsequent implantation of the carrier screws. The CT positioning of the knees and taking the CT took an average of 20 min, and subsequent data calculation 30 min. The planning averaged 25 min. Preparation of the robot, switching it on and reading in the planning data, mounting of the tool and sterile covering and calibration of the tool could be completed in 20 min. On average, a further 10 min were required to apply the knee clamp and fix the leg on the ground plate and to mount the articulated arms between the robot and the clamping device. The registration and milling of the transplant tunnel took an average of 15 min. Overall, an increased time requirement of about 2.5 h thus resulted for employment of the CASPAR system. This time limit

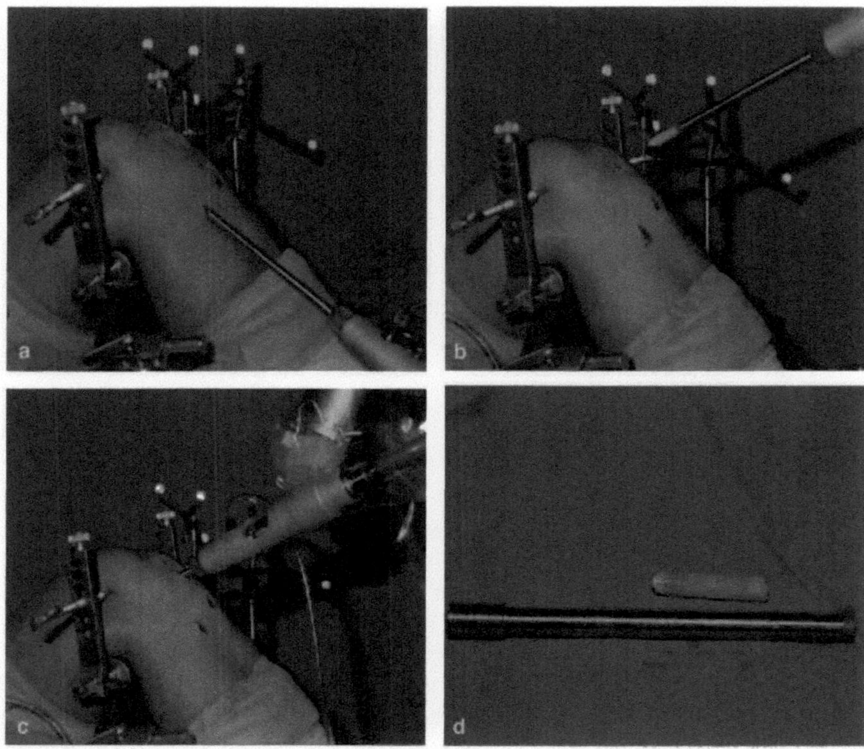

Fig. 58-5a-d. Robot in the process of milling the tibial and femoral tunnel

can only be met when no problems occur, and when all those participating are well-versed and cooperate smoothly.

Analysis of Results and Conclusions

In our own patients, it could not be demonstrated that ACL replacement assisted by the CASPAR system leads to better results than those attained in our conventional technique. Forty-three patients with isolated ACL replacement in whom the CASPAR operation had been carried out at least one year previously were followed up. A group of 151 patients with isolated and conventionally operated ACL reconstruction served for comparison; however, they had a follow-up time of at least two years. According to the IKDC score, rating A was found in 39.1% and rating B in 47.0% of the conventionally operated patients. In the CASPAR-operated patients, the rating was A in 23.3% and B in 65.1% (□ Table 58-1). A lower rate of impingement was found radiologically in the CASPAR knees (□ Table 58-2). According to the Marburg classification, the degree of

Table 58-1. Appraisal of the results in accordance with the IKD score in isolated ACL replacement with creation of the transplant tunnels in the conventional technique and with the CASPAR system

	Conventional (n=151)	CASPAR (n=43)
A Normal	59 (39.1%)	10 (23.2%)
B Almost normal	71 (47.0%)	28 (65.1%)
C Abnormal	20 (13.2%)	4 (9.3%)
D Highly abnormal	1 (0.6%)	1 (2.3%)

Table 58-2. Roof impingement in creation of a tibial tunnel in conventional Marburg technique [4] and with the CASPAR system

	Conventional (n=151)	CASPAR (n=43)
Degree of impingement 0	71 (47.0%)	29 (65.4%)
Degree of impingement I	65 (43.0%)	13 (30.2%)
Degree of impingement II	13 (8.6%)	1 (2.3%)
Degree of impingement III	2 (1.4%)	

Table 58-3. Stability results in isolated ACL replacement with creation of the transplant tunnels in conventional technique and with the CASPAR system (KT1000 measurement in maximum anterior drawer; difference in millimeters between the knee operated on and the contralateral knee)

	Conventional (n=151)	CASPAR (n=43)
0–1 mm	75 (49.7%)	17 (39.5%)
2–3 mm	58 (38.4%)	16 (37.2%)
4–5 mm	16 (10.6%)	6 (13.9%)
>5 mm	2 (1.2%)	4 (9.3%)

impingement was 0–I in 90% and a degree of impingement from II–III in 10%, whereas the CASPAR knee showed 0–I in 97.3% and a degree of impingement of II in 2.3%. This is a clear indication that a roof impingement is avoided with greater certainty using the CASPAR system. However, it was also demonstrated that the degree of severity I has neither a subjective nor an objective disadvantageous effect. In the KT1000 measurement, better stability values than for the CASPAR knees were determined for the knees that had undergone conventional operation (Table 58-3). The reason for this is that no anatomically and isometrically validated parameters were available in particular for planning of the femoral tunnel and the position of the tunnel was planned by various surgeons with largely free navigation according to their own subjective positional criteria. This procedure evidently did not lead to the same precision and constancy in placement of the tunnel as that reached with the over-the-top targeting device used in the conventional technique. Mainly for this reason, use of the CASPAR system ceased in October 2000. The entire planning strategy was reconsidered as well as being checked anatomically and isometrically on knee preparations using the CASPAR system.

Anatomically and Isometrically Validated Standard Planning

In a superimposition-free lateral X-ray of the distal femur, the bony structures are marked and reference lines that are used for planning the femoral tunnel in the sagittal plane are drawn in (Fig. 58-6). This was the roof of the

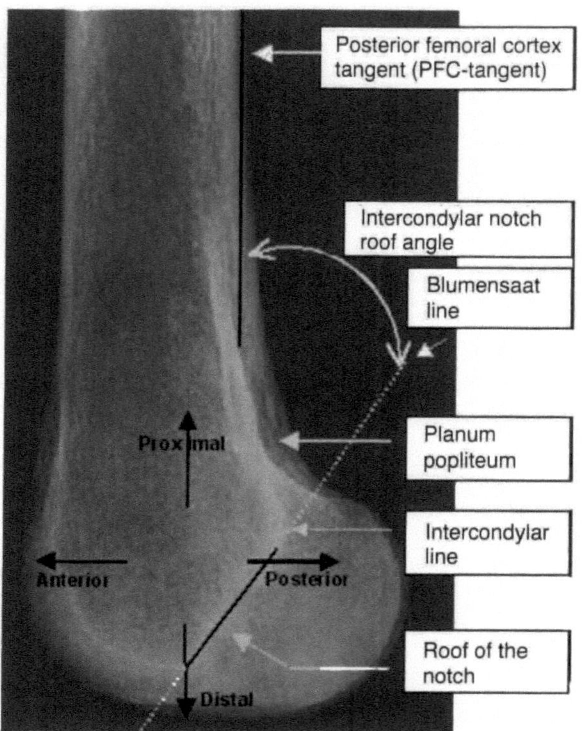

Fig. 58-6. Lateral X ray of the distal femur with marking of the roof of the notch, the intercondylar line and the popliteal plane. Blumensaat's line and the tangent to the posterior cortex of the femur (PFC tangent) between which the intercondylar notch roof angle is measured are drawn in

notch and Blumensaat's line, the tangent to the posterior femur cortex (PFC tangent), the intercondylar line and the popliteal plane.

In order to determine the position of the femoral ACL insertion area in relation to Blumensaat's line and the intercondylar line, this was marked circumferentially with titanium beads on femur preparations. It was observed that the roof of the notch forms the anterior boundary and the intercondylar line forms the proximal boundary of the area of insertion. The roof of the notch can be exactly identified in the CT. In order to be able to locate the intercondylar line which constitutes the boundary between the intercondylar sulcus and the popliteal plane with great precision and reproducibly in the CT, the intercondylar line was marked with a titanium bead in the middle of the roof of the notch in femur preparations. As can be seen in Fig. 58-7, the position of the bead corresponds to a pointed overhang aligned in the direction of

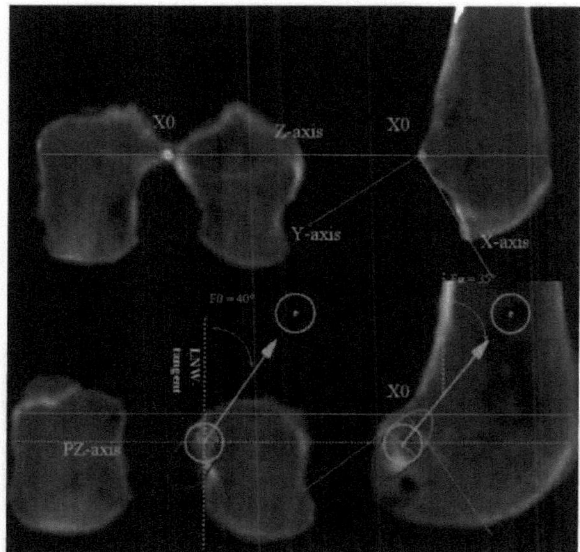

Fig. 58-7. CT of a distal femur preparation. Intercondylar line *(upper part of the picture)* marked with a titanium bead in the middle of the roof of the notch. The condylar edges are seen which project to the titanium bead and via which the position of the intercondylar line can be determined exactly in the frontal CT. In the sagittal CT, the x-axis and the y-axis of the three-dimensional coordinate system in relation to the femur with the 0 point at the intersection of the x-axis with the intercondylar line are drawn in. The z-axis is the transverse axis trough the 0 point and passes exactly through the titanium bead which marks the intercondylar line in the frontal CT. In the *lower part of the picture*, the standard femoral planning is shown. In the sagittal plane, the anterior tunnel margin is located on the x-axis and the proximal tunnel margin on the y-axis, sagittal tunnel angle Fα = 40°. In the frontal plane, the tunnel entrance center is placed at the intersection between the tangent to the lateral notch wall (LNW tangent) and the pz-axis, which passes as an axis in parallel to the z-axis through the center of the tunnel entrance established in the sagittal plane. Frontal tunnel angle Fα = 35°

the roof at the medial and lateral femoral condyles in the frontal CT. The intercondylar line can be determined precisely from these condylar edges.

To plan the entrance of the femoral tunnel, a three-dimensional coordinate system was established in which Blumensaat's line represents the x-axis. The point of intersection of the x-axis with the intercondylar line corresponds to the 0 point. The posterior perpendicular on the x-axis through the 0 point forms the y-axis. The z-axis is the transverse axis through the 0 point.

The entrance to the femoral tunnel in the sagittal plane is planned in the coordinate system in such a way that the anterior margin is on the x-axis and the proximal margin on the y-axis. The pz-axis which passes in parallel to the z-axis through the center of the tunnel entrance established in the sagittal plane is used for anatomically correct positioning of the tunnel entrance in the transverse and frontal plane. The lateral notch wall tangent (LNW tangent) was created as a further reference line. In the frontal CT, the LNW tangent passes through the pz-axis. The point of intersection F between the LNW tangent and the pz-axis is the fixed point for placing the center of the tunnel entrance in the frontal and transverse plane.

The tunnel entrance which is manifested as a circle in the planning steps described up to now takes up an oval form when the tunnel trajectory itself is planned. The extent and direction of the oval extension of the tunnel entrance into the lateral notch wall, the roof of the notch and the popliteal plane depend on the angles between which the tunnel is planned. In order to be able to establish the angular direction of the tunnel precisely, the sagittal tunnel angle was defined as angle Fα between the PFC tangent and the tunnel axis. Furthermore, the frontal tunnel angle was defined as angle Fβ between the perpendicular on the condylar plane and the tunnel axis.

On the basis of the described planning of the tunnel entrance, the tunnel of 10 mm diameter was milled on isolated femur preparations with the robot under different Fα and Fβ angles. Before this, the ACL insertion area was stained. The results indicated that for several reasons an angle Fα of 35° and an angle Fβ of 40° was the most favorable for standard femoral planning.

1. The tunnel entrance does not pass beyond the physiological site of insertion of the ACL to distal.
2. The oval extent of the tunnel chiefly extends to posterior into the area of ACL insertion.
3. To proximal, the tunnel only passes a few millimeters beyond the intercondylar line and a sufficiently thick back wall remains.
4. The planning values can be implemented intraoperatively without any problems.

The standard planning for the femoral tunnel in the CT of a femoral preparation is shown in the lower part of Figure 58-7. A CT of a knee preparation is shown in **Fig. 58-8.**

For the standard planning of the tibial tunnel in the frontal plane, from the anatomical studies the medial intercondylar tubercle was determined to be an important

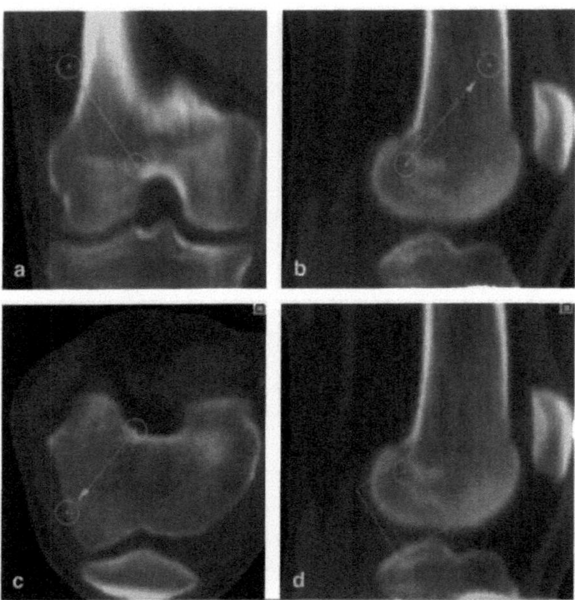

Fig. 58-8a-d. Femoral standard planning in the CT of a knee preparation

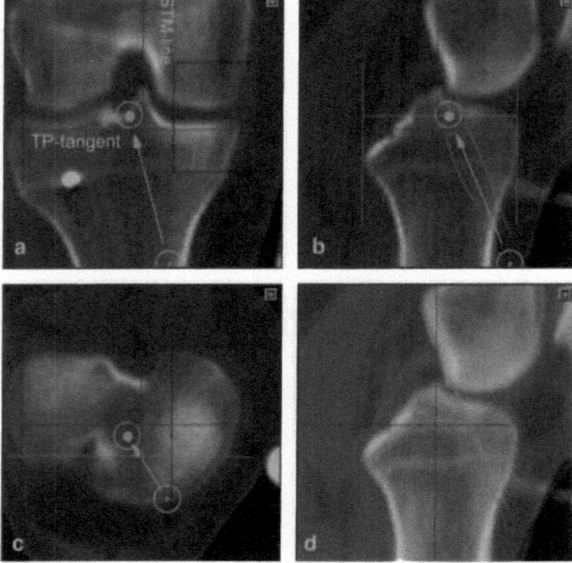

Fig. 58-9a-d. Standard tibial planning in the CT of a knee preparation. In the frontal CT, the medial margin of the intraarticular tunnel opening is placed on the intersection between the PMT line (*green*) and the TP tangent (*violet*). The frontal tunnel angle Tβ is planned with 20°. In the sagittal CT, the anterior margin of the intraarticular tunnel opening is placed on the intersection of the prolonged x-axis with the tibial plateau and the x-axis forms the anterior tunnel wall in the further course to distal

landmark. The perpendicular through the tip of the medial tubercle, which is abbreviated as the PMT line, exactly marks the medial boundary of the area of tibial insertion of the ACL. A tangent at the tibial plateau (TP tangent) serves as a further reference line for correct placement of the tibial tunnel. As can be seen from **◻** Fig. 58-9, the crossing point T between the PMT line and the TP tangent corresponds to the fixed point at which the medial tunnel margin is placed interarticularly. In the sagittal plane, the anterior tunnel margin is defined over the point of intersection of the prolonged x-axis with the tibial plateau at complete knee extension. In the further course to distal, the x-axis also forms the anterior boundary of the tunnel in the tibia and determines the sagittal tibial tunnel angle Tα. This is measured between the prolonged x-axis and the tangent to the posterior tibial cortex bone (PTC tangent). Under real-life conditions, its size depends on the intercondylar notch roof angle and the degree of physiological overextension of the contralateral intact knee joint. The frontal tibial tunnel angle is the angle between the perpendicular to the TP tangent and the tunnel axis. A value of 15–25° is taken as the basis for angle Tβ in standard planning.

Knee preparations without arthrotic lesions and with intact capsule ligament apparatus were used for isometric validation of the described planning. These were suspended in a fixture under complete extension, registration crosses were applied and a CT was taken.

At the planning station, the position of the transplant tunnel is planned according to the parameters presented. In the laboratory, the knee joints were firmly fixed in accordance with the procedure in the operating theater and the anterior cruciate ligament was dissected via a parapatellar medial approach route. After referencing, the transplant tunnels were milled with a diameter of 10 mm by the robot in accordance with the plan. For replacement of the ACL, a BTB transplant from the middle third of the patellar tendon was used. An inductive distance gauge transducer was connected on the tibial side to the transplants fixed on the femoral side. With an initial tension of 60 N, the tibiofemoral distance changes between the sites of insertion were measured with the relative shift of the transplant in the tibial tunnel over a movement radius varying from 0° extension to 120° flexion. For simultaneous registration of the femorotibial distance changes in relation to the degree of flexion, an electronic goniometer was fixed in addition to the knee preparations (◘ Fig. 58-10). The isometry study was carried out on eight knee preparations. As can be seen from ◘Fig. 58-11, the femorotibial distance changes average 1 mm without exceeding the threshold value of 2 mm in the standard deviation.

It can be inferred from the investigations and the results that the standard planning presented leads to an anatomical, almost isometric and impingement-free transplant positioning and thus fulfils the criteria for a validated planning strategy.

Concluding Commentary

Whether a transplant can take on the function of a natural ACL completely and permanently is crucially dependent on its positioning in the knee joint. The rate of misplacement is high, so that it is a clinically relevant problem. Integration of innovative technologies into anterior cruciate ligament reconstruction with the objective of correct anatomically and isometrically reproducible placement is hence intrinsically a good thing. However, it is only justified if it enables better results to be obtained than with the conventional techniques. This could not be demonstrated for the CASPAR system in our patients, mainly because an anatomically and isometrically validated standard planning was not available. Free navigation in the planning of the tunnel is the least suitable strategy for correct and reproducible planning of the tunnel, as our own experience has shown. It takes a lot of time and entails a high error potential even for the experienced knee surgeon. The CASPAR system was no longer used clinically, although reliable planning parameters were available after the new conception of the planning strategy and its isometric and anatomical validation. The reasons

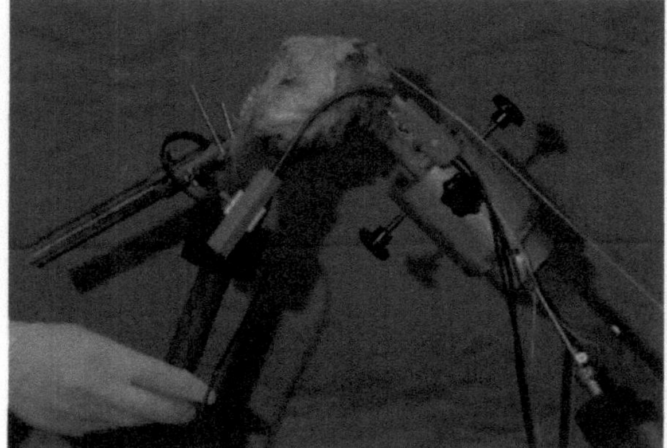

◘ Fig. 58-10. Experimental design for isometric validation of the standard planning on the knee preparation

for this are the high requirements in terms of logistics, instruments, apparatus, staff and time that the system entails. Its integration into a fully running surgery unit is therefore particularly difficult. The considerable financial burdens this system entails are also not to be neglected, since the costs are not covered by the paying agencies. Furthermore, it is a disadvantage that the system restricts flexibility in the surgical techniques; this rules out certain procedures, such as transtibial creation of the femoral tunnel from the start.

The requirement for improved technical solutions in order to achieve reproducible transplant positioning that is anatomical, almost isometrical and impingement-free continues to exist in ACL replacement. However, this should be achieved using more flexible, lower-scaled, less time-consuming and expensive CAS systems specifically designed for cruciate ligament reconstruction. The insights and results attained in the laboratory study provide an important foundation for this.

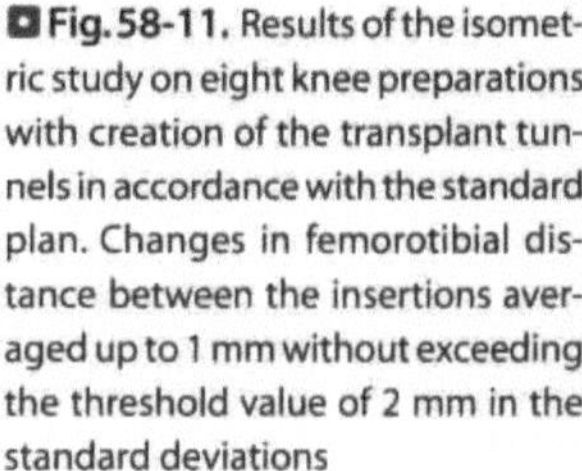

◘ **Fig. 58-11.** Results of the isometric study on eight knee preparations with creation of the transplant tunnels in accordance with the standard plan. Changes in femorotibial distance between the insertions averaged up to 1 mm without exceeding the threshold value of 2 mm in the standard deviations

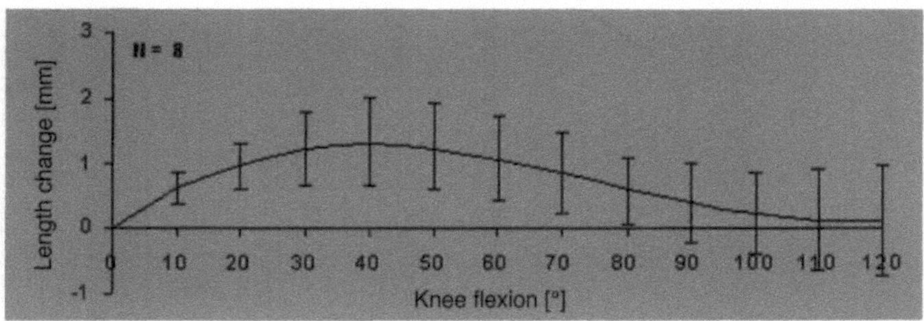

References

1. Aglietti P, Zaccherotti G, Menchetti PM et al. (1995) A comparison of clinical and radiological parameters with two arthroscopic techniques. Knee Surg Sports Traumatol Arthrosc 3: 2–8
2. Amis A, Jacob RP (1998) Anterior cruciate ligament graft positioning, tensioning and twisting. Knee Surg Sports Traumatol Arthrosc 6 [Suppl 1]: 2–12
3. Bernard M, Hertel P, Hornung H, Cierpinski T (1997) Femoral insertion of the ACL. Radiographic quadrant method. Am J Knee Surg 10: 14–22
4. Gotzen L, Petermann J (1994) Rupture of the anterior cruciate ligament in athletes. Chirurg 65: 910–919
5. Howell SM, Taylor MA (1993) Failure of reconstruction of the anterior cruciate ligament due to impingement by the intercondylar roof. J Bone Joint Surg 75A: 1044–1055
6. Khalfayan EE, Sharkey PF, Alexander AH et al. (1996) The relationship between tunnel placement and clinical results after anterior cruciate ligament reconstruction. Am J Sports Med 3: 335–341
7. Romano VM, Graf BK, Keene JS, Lange RH (1993) Anterior cruciate ligament reconstruction. Am J Sports Med 3: 415–418
8. Sommer C, Friederich NF, Müller W (2000) Improperly placed anterior cruciate ligament grafts: correlation between radiological parameters and clinical results. Knee Surg Sports Traumatol Arthrosc 8: 207–213
9. Wetzler MJ, Getelman MH, Friedman MJ, Bartolozzi AR (1998) Revision anterior cruciate ligament surgery: Etiology of failures. Oper Tech Sports Med 2: 64–70

59 ACL-Reconstruction with the *Navitrack System*
Critical Analysis of Navigation in ACL-Surgery

A. Ellermann, R. Siebold

Introduction

Decisive for successful surgical stabilization of the knee-joint following rupture of the anterior cruciate ligament is the correct anatomical positioning of the cruciate-ligament graft. Even though anatomically the differentiation is made between an anteromedial and a posterolateral fascicle and there is thus a superficial insertion onto the femur and the tibia, there is however a general consensus regarding the position of the tibial and femoral insertion points and of the drilled tunnels for the reconstruction of the anterior cruciate ligament [4, 7, 13].

The arthroscopic identification of the insertion points often presents difficulties however, even for the experienced surgeon. Sati et al., for example, were able to show that in a group of patients studied by them after anterior cruciate ligament reconstruction surgery there was incorrect placement of the insertion points in about 40% of the cases. Other authors describe poor results after anterior cruciate ligament replacement in between 10 and 29% of the cases [1].

In 2002 we operated over 1000 cases of anterior cruciate ligament injuries. Almost 30% of these were revision cases in whom a second operation was carried out due to incorrect placement of the tibial tunnels.

With the increase in the surgical treatment of ruptures of the anterior cruciate ligament, worldwide, various computer-assisted surgical systems were developed, also for the field of anterior cruciate ligament replacement [5, 6, 10, 11, 13].

The Navitrack system (Centerpulse Orthopedics, Switzerland), which was already well known in the field of spinal surgery, became available to us for the computer-assisted reconstruction of the anterior cruciate ligament for the first time in October 1999.

Description of the System and Surgical Procedure

The first software version is based on an electromagnetic application. With this, starting with a transmitter (3D coil), a cylindrical 600 mG magnetic field is created in a expansion of 750×600 mm. The instruments and references are fitted with a receiver and are connected with the system by cable. If the receivers are now moved within the magnetic field, the position of the instruments in space can be calculated from the change in the magnetic waves. For this procedure ferromagnetic influences on the magnetic field should be excluded, and these can be prevented by an optional field-monitoring system.

On the day of the operation, firstly a nuclear-spin tomography of the injured knee-joint with a layer-thickness of 1.5 mm is carried out. The data in Dicom-3 format that are obtained in this way are transferred by means of a CD-ROM to an external calculation unit of the Navitrack system and, within a segmentation module, by separation of the individual grey values of the bone and soft-tissue contours, they are converted into an accurate 3D model of the injured knee-joint.

The accuracy obtained with the 3D model of the electromagnetic application was checked by means of cadaver-bone and artificial-bone tests by the firm Orthosoft in Montreal, Canada. The surfaces of the dissected knee-joints were measured with a laser and compared with the reconstructed 3D model of the Navitrack system. By this procedure, with a nuclear-spin-tomographic layer thickness of 1.5 mm a femoral and tibial 3D inaccuracy of less than 1 mm could be demonstrated [2, 9].

The representation of the notch roof (flower-seed line) which is necessary for correct identification of the tunnels is made possible by integration of the whole 3D

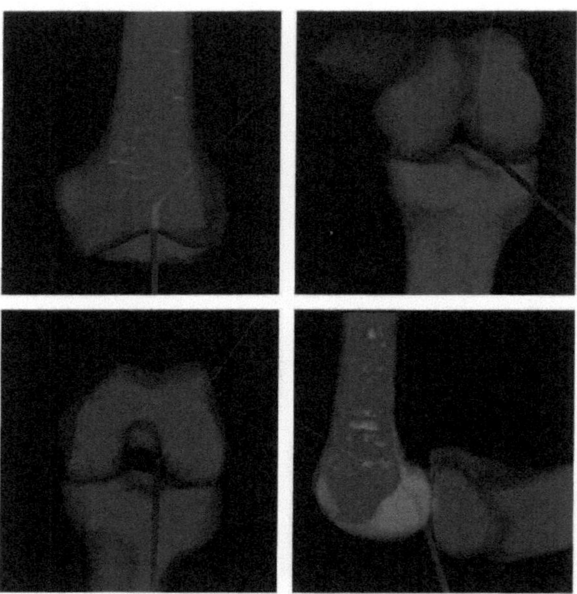

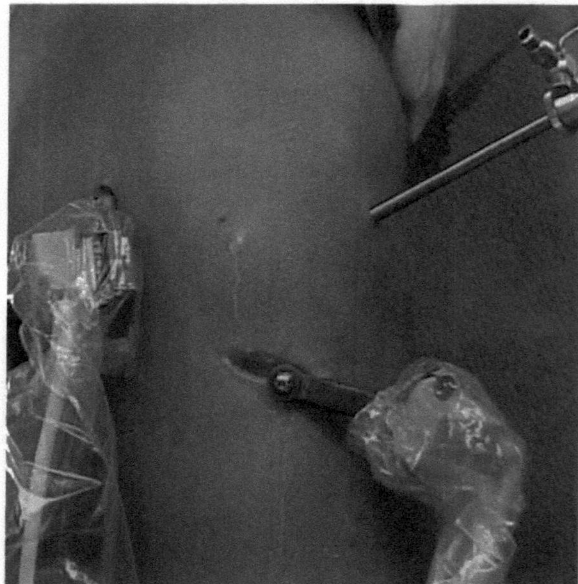

Fig. 59-1. 3D model with transparency effect to show the flower-seed line and a surgical instrument

Fig. 59-2. Fixing of sensors on the femur and the tibia

data set and is represented by a transparency effect of the 3D model. This time-consuming way of calculation of the 3D model through a three-dimensional data cube (polygonization of the 3D voxel) allows the visualization of various different surgical instruments introduced into the knee-joint at the same time (**Fig. 59-1**). In the electromagnetic application, the instruments usually used in arthroscopy (probe hooks, screwdrivers, arthroscopic aiming device) are provided with sensors in order for them to be recognized in the electromagnetic field that is created by the 3D coil which is positioned close to the knee-joint. By means of a calibrating block an alignment is made by the surgeon between the instrument being used and the magnetic field, whereby the length and axis of the instrument are calculated as a function of a reference sensor on the calibrating block.

For the intraoperative visualization, additional sensors must be fixed to the femur and the tibia, close to the joint. The femoral sensor is fixed through a small incision on the medial epicondyle. The tibial sensor is fixed in the region of the site of removal of the tibial graft, so that a further incision can be avoided. These temporary sensors must be stably anchored, but fixation with one relatively short cortical screw would seem to be sufficient (**Fig. 59-2**). Simultaneously with these system-dependent surgical

steps, the usual removal and preparation of the graft is carried out.

In order to create a real-time synchronization between the knee that is to be operated and the 3D model, before the operation five points each have to be defined on the femoral and tibial surfaces of the model and then identified in the patient's knee by arthroscopy, using the probe hook (so-called »matching«; **Fig. 59-3**).

After successful matching, the femoral and tibial insertion points are defined, with simultaneous arthro-

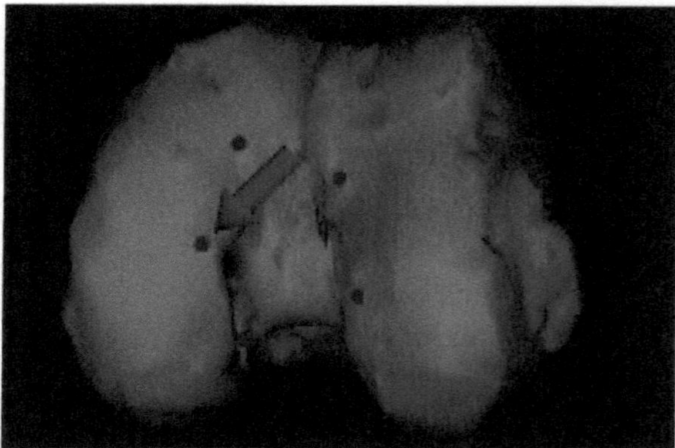

Fig. 59-3. Five-point identification for matching between the model and the patient's knee

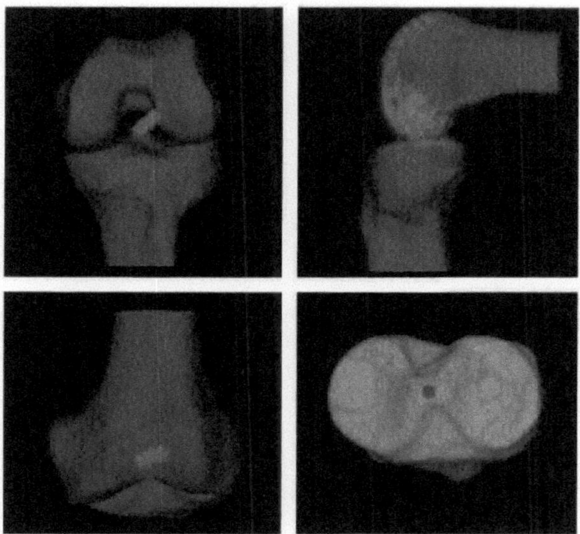

Fig. 59-4. Presentation of the virtual anterior cruciate ligament graft

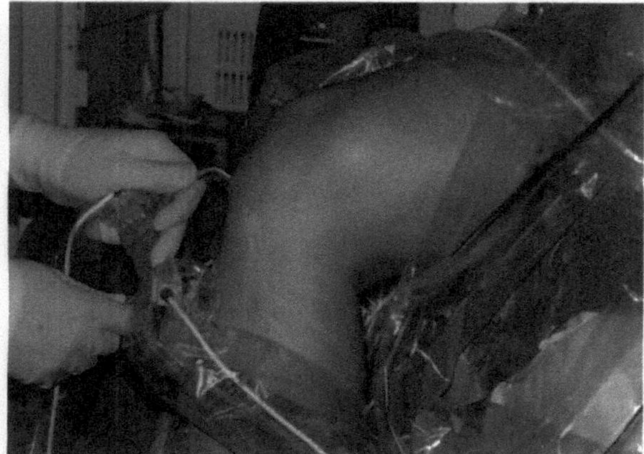

Fig. 59-5. Aiming device for placement of the tibial tunnel

scopic control and by means of the flower-seed line represented in the 3D model. For this, methods of identification for the tibia according to Howell [7] and Stäubli [13] and for the femur according to Bernhard and Hertel [4] are used, in the sense of intraoperative planning. Then the insertion points in the 3D model are linked with a virtual graft, the diameter of which corresponds to that of the original graft (**Fig. 59-4**).

The patient's knee, on which up till now no drilling or fixation has been carried out, is now flexed and the virtually reconstructed anterior cruciate ligament on the 3D model is subjected to dynamic isometry testing and impingement testing. The system calculates the isometry as the difference between the longest and the shortest extension of the graft and signals an impingement both acoustically and visually on the screen.

Although it is known that the anatomical anterior cruciate ligament is not an absolutely isometric structure, this test nevertheless helps to detect fluctuations.

The same applies for the impingement testing at the cranial and lateral limits of the notch: even if the test is carried out on a patient's knee with a defective anterior cruciate ligament, the acoustic signal given by the system helps to prevent a disturbing impingement on the roof or the lateral wall of the notch.

At this point it may not be forgotten that the system is testing a virtual ligament in an unstable knee. This matter will be discussed later.

If the positioning is correct, the operation is continued with placement of the tibial tunnel. Its position and length and its position in relation to the tibial plateau are fixed by means of the navigating positioning device in such a way that it is possible for the surgeon, if necessary, to place the femoral tunnel transtibially (**Fig. 59-5**).

Besides the conventional drilling procedures, the use of the Navitrack system also allows manual impaction of the tunnels (in contrast to the robot-assisted systems). With pure ligament grafts this ensures an improved healing process [14]. An intraoperative image-converter control to take into account the very great variation in the notch-roof angle then becomes superfluous.

Clinical Experience

Between October 1999 and March 2001 sixteen anterior cruciate ligament reconstructions were carried out with the electromagnetic first version, whereby ten operations were performed successfully with the navigation procedure.

In one case there was a complete breakdown of the system, and in the other five cases we did not succeed in achieving a match between the 3D model and the patient's knee (five-point method) which would have ensured sufficient accuracy. In our opinion the reason for this was an insufficiently accurate reconstruction of the surfaces in the 3D model, based on insufficiently accurate nuclear-spin tomographic data. However, all six cruciate-ligament reconstructions could be operated, in good time and without further problems, by the conventional method.

The ten patients who were operated completely by the navigation method underwent a full postoperative examination, with an extensive previous history, a clinical examination, manual measurement of the maximum KT-1000 and standardized radiograms to assess the placement of the tunnels in the operated knee-joint. The clinical examination showed stable knee-joints with unrestricted mobility. Measured on the IKDC score, all the knee-joints could be classified as good to very good. Radiologically, all the patients also showed correct placement of the tunnels, measured according to the above mentioned radiological parameters.

No peri-operative complications appeared. Thus in no case were there postoperative infections or problems of wound healing, vascular or neural damage or deep-vein thrombosis in the legs.

Taking an average of 90 min, the preoperative reconstruction of the nuclear-spin tomographic data is very time-consuming. However, this is largely responsible for the picture quality obtained with nuclear-spin tomography. In the patients successfully operated by the navigation procedure, the time taken to perform the operation was prolonged by about 30 min, but this time lag decreased with the increasing number of operations performed. However, it will not be possible, in the medium term, to achieve an operation time as short as that which is customary for operations carried out by the conventional method. In the following overview, the times for the various steps, based on our experiences with the electromagnetic version, are presented:

> **Data on Times for the Procedure Based on Experience with the Electromagnetic Version**
>
> - Preoperative
>   - MRT: 20 min
>   - Processing of the data: 60 min
>   - Data transfer: 10 min
> - Intraoperative
>   - Preparation of the patient
>   - Start of the ASK (with care of concomitant injuries and preparation of the notch area)
>   - Calibration of the arthroscopic instruments: 5 min
>   - Removal and preparation of the graft
>   - Fixing of the reference sensors: 5 min
>   - Matching of tibia and femur: 10 min
>   - Navigated definition of the femoral and tibial insertion points: 5 min
>   - Impingement and isometry testing of the virtual graft: 5 min
>   - Navigated placement of the tunnels: 5 min

The intraoperative procedure was not significantly impaired by the additional sensor cables on the surgical instruments. All the operations performed by the navigation procedure were minimally invasive, i. e. they were carried out by arthroscopy. An arthroscopic check of various steps in the navigation procedure was possible at any time.

Consequences and Modifications

Since December 2001 a second revised software version, with optoelectronic navigation, has been available. With this variant, infra-red light is emitted by a positioning sensor (Polaris camera) by means of LEDs. The field of vision of the camera describes a cylindrical geometry of 1 meter diameter. The position of instruments or references that are held at a distance of 1.4–2.4 m within this geometry, and which bear spherical, reflecting surface markers, can be determined from the reflected infra-red light by means of a control unit – the so-called tool-interface unit.

Improved with this new version were especially the reconstruction of the 3D model and the synchronization (matching) between the patient's knee and the 3D model. While with the first version, supported by nuclear-spin tomography, the surface of the cartilage was completely reconstructed, with the second, CT-supported version the developers concentrated on the cartilage-free area of the notch and the tibial plateau. It is exclusively these areas that are decisive for identification of the insertion points.

The reconstruction of the other parts of the joint is however continued, in order to make orientation over the whole three-dimensional model of the knee-joint easier for the user.

The thickness of the CT layer in the area of the condyles is 1 mm. As in the first version, the reference sensors are fixed to the tibia and the femur during the oper-

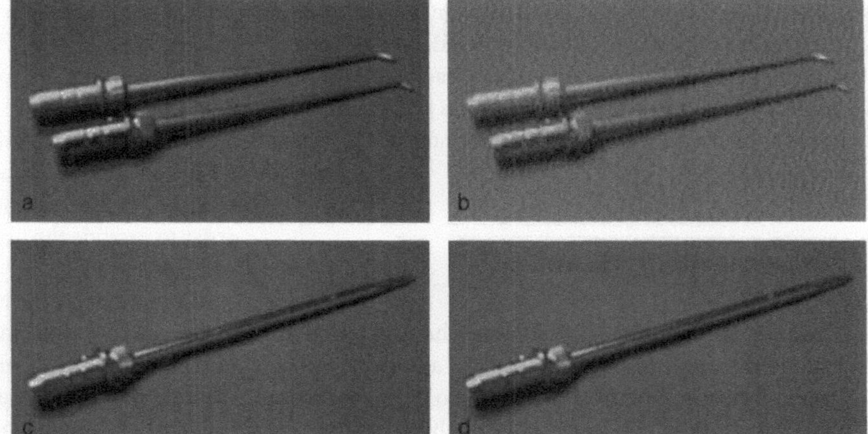

Fig. 59-6a-d. a Universal handle with passively reflecting markers and easily exchangeable instrument fitments. **b** Probe hooks, **c** tibial aiming device, **d** impactor,

ation with so-called passively reflecting markers. The procedure is made significantly easier by the universal handle, which can be calibrated in a few seconds and on which the different surgical instruments can be fixed as required (**□** Fig. 59-6). Using the probe-hook, surface matching is now also possible within a matter of minutes, whereby 15 points can be callipered anywhere in the region of the notch and the intercondylar eminence. The time-consuming identification of previously defined points (five-point method) is no longer necessary with the present version. In addition, for the clear identification of the different insertion points, graphic aids can be blended in on the screen. These correspond, for the femur, to the »quadrant method« described by Bernard and Hertel [4], and, for the tibia, to the »43% method« according to Stäubli et al. [13] (**□** Fig. 59-7 and 59-8). In each stage of the operation, the diagrams for the intraoperative planning can be blended in or faded out on the screen as re-

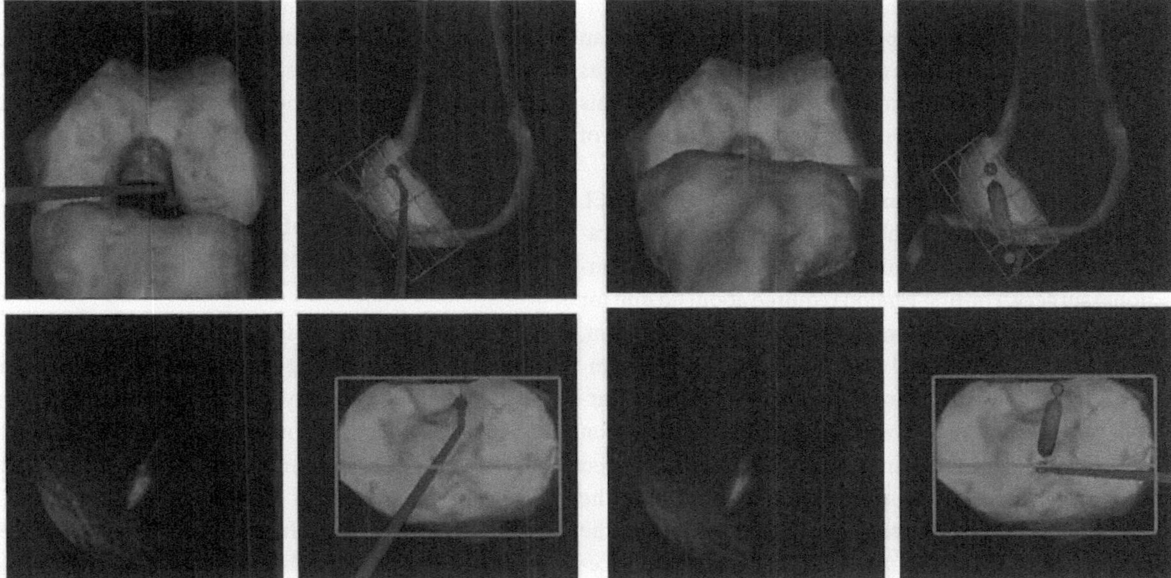

□ Fig. 59-7. Reference diagram according to Bernard and Hertel [4] for identification of the femoral insertion point (*upper right*)

□ Fig. 59-8. Reference diagram according to Stäubli [13] for identification of the tibial insertion point (*lower right*)

quired. Also, the arthroscopic picture can be displayed on the monitor situated in the lower left window of the screen.

This second version, which greatly facilitates the procedure, was also first tested on cadavers and on artificial bone. It was first used clinically in our hospital in February 2002.

Discussion and Summary

The basis for the physiological biomechanical functioning and the correct remodelling of the anterior cruciate ligament graft is the approximately anatomical placement of the femoral and tibial tunnels. Wrongly placed tunnels, with relevant anisometry or an impingement in the region of the notch are the main reasons for the failure of anterior cruciate ligament reconstruction surgery.

As the number of anterior cruciate ligament reconstructions is constantly increasing, the question of the intraoperative checking of the placement of the tunnels arises. An intraoperative image-converter method for checking of the placement of the tunnels was therefore promoted by experienced surgeons [3].

For this particular problem the Navitrack system of Centerpulse Orthopedics in its first versions has proved to be promising instrument for the future. This system creates a virtual 3D model of the bone surface of the injured knee-joint with a possible 3D error of less than 1 mm. The handling of the navigated surgical instruments is comparable to that of conventional instruments. This allows accurate, arthroscopically controlled placement of the tunnels.

However, the routine use of any navigation aid in ACL surgery is still a questionable procedure since the operation itself is time consuming in comparison to conventional surgery. The first version required about 90 min for reconstruction of the 3D model of the injured knee-joint. The good quality of the 3D model is the basis for problem-free intraoperative matching. As a function of the nuclear-spin tomography, in this way the time for the operation was prolonged by 20–30 min. After this time was passed we stopped the surgical navigation and performed the operation in the conventional way. In no case in which the patient was operated completely by the navigation procedure did the period of partial deprivation of the blood supply exceed 2 h.

The second version of the Navitrack system leads to a considerable saving of time both before and during the operation. With this present version the bone reconstruction of the of the limits of the notch and the eminence is carried out with CT support, which is sufficient for the navigation of the insertion points. However, a 3D model of the whole knee-joint is deliberately created in order to provide the user with support in his orientation within the system.

To summarize, the Navitrack system represents a step that is aimed at reducing the variability of the placement of the tunnels, with minimally invasive methods. The accurate preoperative and intraoperative virtual reconstruction of the anterior cruciate ligament with dynamic isometry and impingement testing allows active but controlled placement of the tunnels. According to our experience with the Navitrack system up till now, it can be hoped that in the future this method will lead to greater reliability and accuracy in regard to the positioning of the tunnels. The preoperative 3D reconstruction of the knee-joint takes time and the quality of the reconstruction determines the success of the navigation procedure. In the ideal case, the duration of the anesthesia and the time taken to perform the operation are not significantly prolonged. The graft and the fixation technique can be chosen freely. In the case of a successful navigation procedure, the intraoperative image-converter check becomes superfluous. The system needs further improvement and the pre- or peri-operative imaging has to be modified to provide a more user-friendly environment and make the system a routine tool.

Critical Analysis of Present ACL Navigation and Visions

Looking at different navigation techniques it seems an advantage that we are not only able to identify anatomic insertion points correctly, but also restore proper knee kinematics by using impingement- and isometry-tests. It has been forgotten to mention so far that we are testing kinematic parameters of a virtual ligament in an ACL-insufficient knee. Until further investigation has been made it seems doubtful that this data is valid enough especially in cases with increasing instability which we see in revision situations. As a consequence we should for the moment focus on the correct identification of the insertion points alone which we will determine with the help of our virtual models. These models should ideally represent patients anatomy with millimetric accuracy.

This leads to another question: What is the ideal tool to create a valid model of the patients knee?

MRI data might not be accurate enough since it is quite difficult to differentiate between bony and soft tissue structures. CT scans provide high accuracy, but similar to MRI it is a time consuming procedure at the moment. Furthermore, there is a rather high radiation exposure to the patient. It has to be further proved that procedures based on plain X-rays or image-less information will provide an acceptable accuracy of the model since the combination with kinematic information might not be valid. »Painting«-techniques seem promising, but only in areas with solid structures like cartilage or bone. Other than in open knee surgery we have very limited access to bony structures in arthroscopic surgery to correctly identify the dimensions of the knee joint. Especially the a.p. dimensions will be hard to determine and a »matching« of the model with the patients knee will be very difficult because it cannot be desirable to remove important soft tissue structures: if we focus on the intercondylar area alone a »painting« of the interesting femoral part with the lateral notch area seems possible, but to correctly identify the tibial dimensions one would have to remove parts of the fat pad and most of the tibial stump of the former ACL (which can be considered a biologically important structure for the ACL graft) not to mention the distal insertion area of the PCL.

High quality fluoroscopy based on three dimensional data could be a promising tool if it proves to be accurate enough. This might even allow the surgeon to rather easily obtain kinematic data from the uninjured knee which then could be converted to the injured one. Ultrasound features combined with arthroscopic instruments could be another option for future minimally invasive data acquisition.

Performing rather high numbers of conventional ACL surgeries we believe that, despite all problems that occur at the moment and the fact that navigation or robotics in ACL surgery have not proven to be superior to conventional procedures, navigation will help to improve the outcome of cruciate ligament surgery in the future. This will hopefully be true for primary reconstructions but certainly for revision and PCL surgery.

References

1. Almekinders LC, Chiavetta JB, Clarke JP (1998) Radiographic evaluation of anterior cruciate ligament graft failure with special reference to tibial tunnel placement. Arthroscopy 14: 206–211
2. Amiot LP (1999) Computer assisted ACL-reconstruction: A feasibility study. Presentation 2nd ACL-Symposium: State of the Art 2000, March 25–27, Heidelberg, Germany
3. Amis AA, Jakob RP (1998) Anterior cruciate ligament graft positioning, tensioning and twisting. Knee Surg Sports Traumatol Arthrosc 6 [Suppl 1]: 2–12
4. Bernard M, Hertel P, Hornung H, Cierpinski T (1997) Femoral insertion of the ACL. Radiographic quadrant method. Am J Knee Surg 10: 14–21
5. Bernsmann K, Rosenthal A, Sati M (1999) Use of CAS system for »standard« patellar-tendon acl reconstruction. Presentation 4th Int Symposium on Computer Assisted Orthop Surg, March 17–19, Davos, Switzerland
6. Fleute M, Lavallee S, Julliard R (1999) Computer assisted ACL Reconstruction: Incorporating a Statistical Shape Model of the Femur for 3D Visualization. Presentation 4th Int Symposium on Computer Assisted Orthop Surg, March 17–19, Davos, Switzerland
7. Howell SM, Barad SJ (1995) Knee extension and its relationship to the slope of the intercondylar roof. Implications for positioning the tibial tunnel in anterior cruciate ligament reconstructions. Am J Sports Med 23: 288–294
8. Lyle Cain E, Phillips BB, Charlebois SJ, Daniels AU, Azar FM (1999) Effect of tibial tunnel dilatation on pullout strength of quadrupled semi-tendinosus/gracilis autograft in ACL reconstruction secured with bioabsorbable interference screws. Unpublished data, University of Ta.-Camphell Clinic, Dep. Orthop Surg, Memphis, Tennessee
9. Milne AD, Chess DG, Johnson JA, King GJW (1996) Accuracy of an electromagnetic tracking device: A study of the optimal operating range and metal interference. J Biomech 29: 791–793
10. Petermann J, Schierl M, Pashimeh-Azar A, Gotzen L (2000) Computer and roboter assisted ACL reconstruction with Caspar system. Presentation 9th Congress of the European Society of Sports Traumatology, Knee Surgery and Arthroscopy, London, GB
11. Rosenthal A, Bernsmann K, Ansari B, Sati M (2000) Navigierte Ersatzplastik des vorderen Kreuzbandes (VKB). Z Orthop [Suppl] 138: 63
12. Sati M, Bourquin Y, Stäubli HU, Müller ME (1999) Flexible technology to consider both anatomical and functional factors in ACL replacement surgery. Presentation 4th Int Symposium on Computer-Assisted Orthop Surg, March 17–19, Davos, Switzerland
13. Stäubli HU, Käsermann S, Sati M (1999) Inter-operator variance of ligament placement: Endoscopic versus CAS. Presentation 4th Int Symposium on Computer-Assisted Orthop Surg, March 17–19, Davos, Switzerland
14. Weiler A, Windhagen HJ, Raschke MJ, Laumeyer A, Hoffmann RFG (1998) Biodegradable interference screw fixation exhibits pull-out force and stiffness similar to titanium screws. Am J Sports Med 26: 119–128

V Navigation: Pelvic and Lower Extremity

60 High Tibial Osteotomy – Use of Navigation System

J. Hassenpflug, M. Prymka

In patients suffering from gonarthrosis, which is limited to the medial aspect of the knee joint, high tibial valgisation osteotomy appears to be an appropriate alternative to knee arthroplasty [6,9]. In 1958, Jackson described this procedure for axis correction of the proximal tibia [8] for the first time. This operation was modified 1965 by Coventry [3]. At first, it was used mainly for correction of valgus deformities. According to the knee baseline in valgus deformity, distal femur osteotomy may be recommended [1,7]. For a long time the indication for high tibial osteotomy was not subject to discussion [2]. Within the last years high tibial osteotomy was performed more and more seldom and seemed to be replaced by uni- or bicondulary knee arthroplasty. Taking into account the biomechanical basics and the very positive long-time results, which were achieved by the traditional osteotomy technique this change of treatment does not seem to be adequate.

The aims of a high tibial osteotomy are:

- correction of the joint deformity to release the loading of the medial joint compartment,
- pain reduction and improvement of the joint function,
- possibility of a biological joint healing with additional intraarticular procedures to enhance regeneration of the joint surface.

With correction of the deformity weight-bearing of the affected medial part of the joint could be reduced significantly. Even partial regeneration of the cartilage is possible [4,10]. With an additional intraarticular cartilage reconstruction, the biological joint resurfacing could be significantly improved, so that perhaps one day we can speak of a »bio-prosthesis«, which could allow preservation of function and reduction of pain for a longer time. In total, high-tibial valgisation osteotomy for varus gonarthrosis still is frequently performed at our hospital. Long time

follow-up studies have demonstrated positive outcome. Follow-ups between 5 and 17 years of several authors presented an improvement of pain and joint function in more than 3/4 of the operated patients [11,12]. In our first long time study we reported on 177 patients [5], which were operated between 1974 and 1983. In the 10-year follow-up of 74% of the patients subjectiveley were very satisfied. During the follow-up period the presumption that the patients needed knee alloplasty was less than 5%. The complication rate was very low. In a not yet published study 226 high tibial osteotomies between 1984 and 1993 were evaluated. There were similarly good clinical results as compared to the first study. Coherent with the first study, the complication-rate revealed only a few affections of the peroneus nerve, but we saw more cases of disturbed healing of bone. In 8 cases this could be treated by plaster cast, further 8 patients had to be treated with an external fixator. Also loosenings of the Coventry clamps in 7 cases less than 4 weeks after the operation were found. In 3 patients we observed an overcorrection, which had to be revised. One fracture of the tibial plateau and one deep and six skin-near infections could be documented.

The principle of the high tibial osteotomy seems to be easy, but for this operation precise planning and an exact intraoperative transformation of the planning is required. Therefore, this operation is not an operation for beginners. The failure analysis leads to the assumption, that the results of high tibial osteotomies could be predicted better by means of a navigation system, moreover the use of a navigation system could decrease major and minor failures of the operation. In cooperation with Aesculap (Tuttlingen, Germany) we developed a software program to perform high tibial osteotomies with the help of a navigation system (»OrthoPilot«) computer-assisted. Now the software package is commercially available. By means of this system the conventional preoperative planning, using X-ray templates, could be transformated intraoperatively with eye exactness and without intraoperative X-ray control. The positioning of the saw jigs was also performed with the help of the navigation system as was the size and position of the osteotomy wedge. The navigation system is used for the orientation of the saw jigs and to navigate the sawing procedure itself. For the development of the system and the intraoperative transformation several pre-requisitions have to be fulfilled:

— **Stable fixing of the saw-jig:** After the navigated positioning of the jig it must not be moved. The stability of the jigs could be improved with the help of specially designed self-cutting spongious screws.
— **Rigidly stable saw-blade:** The saw blade is not allowed to flex during the cutting procedure, because the calibration relatively to the rigid body at the corpus of the saw would not remain exact and therefore a control during the cutting-procedure would not be possible. This problem could be solved with the help of specially designed saw blades. Therefore, visual control of the cutting procedure is possible.
— **Intraoperative control of the leg axis:** It is necessary to mark the position of the upper leg. This is possible with the help of a 2nd reference marker at the distal femur and additional definition of the hip centre.

Before the procedure, the planning data, which were achieved by X-ray, are loaded into the computer into the Orthopilot system (■ Fig. 60-1). The correction angle is required as well as the exact width and depth of the tibial plateau. The operation starts in a classical style after exposure of the peroneal nerve with a shortening osteotomy of the fibula (■ Fig. 60-2). Then the lateral tibial metaphysis is prepared for the osteotomy, the first reference marker (rigid body) is fixed 10 centimeters below the joint space (■ Fig. 60-3a). This marker has to be fixed so stable, that it does not move during the whole operation. An additional marker is fixated at the distal femur. By moving of hip, knee and ankle joint the joint centers and the leg axis are determined exactly by the system. After that, the

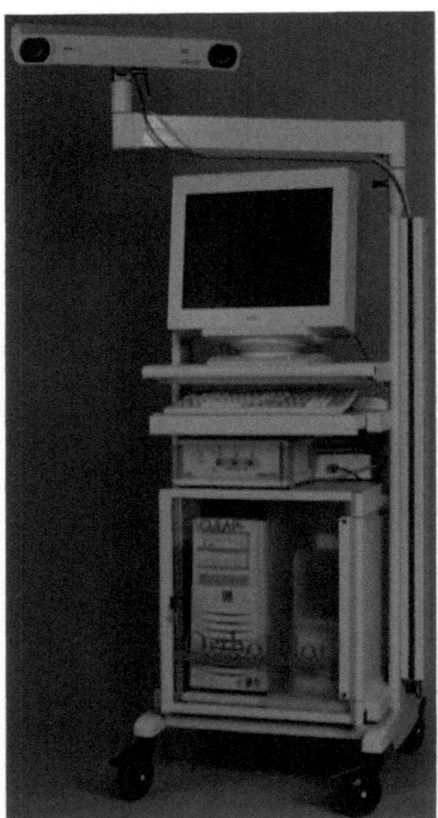

■ **Fig. 60-1.** The navigation system OrthoPilot

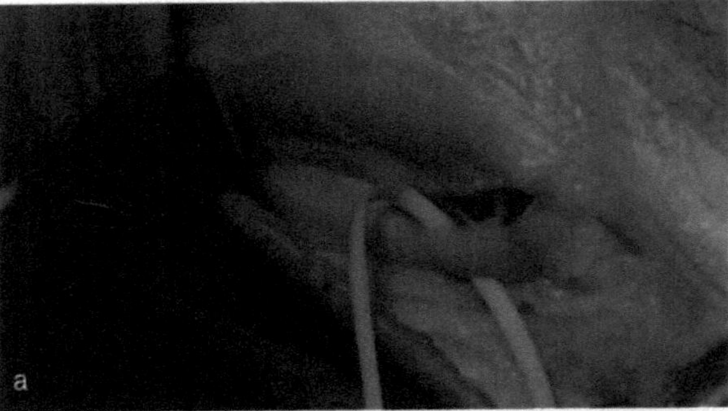

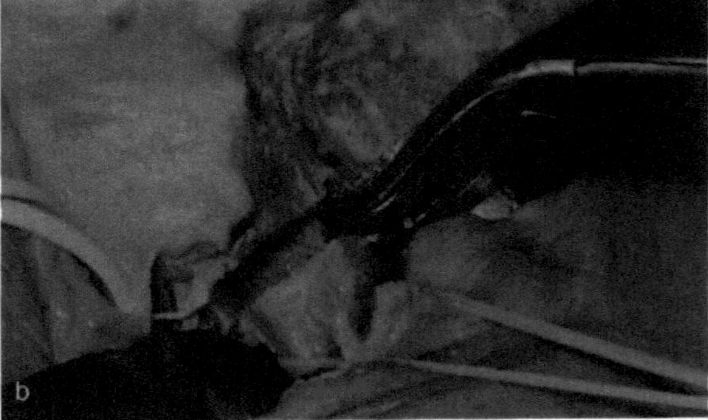

■ **Fig. 60-2a, b.** Standard preparation: **a** exposition of the peroneal nerve and **b** shortening osteotomy of the fibula

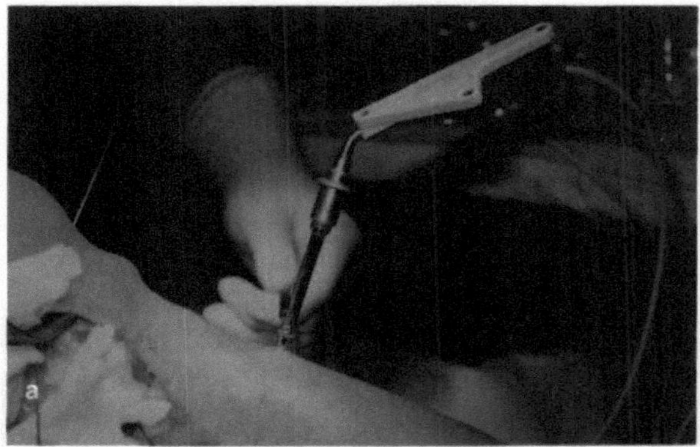

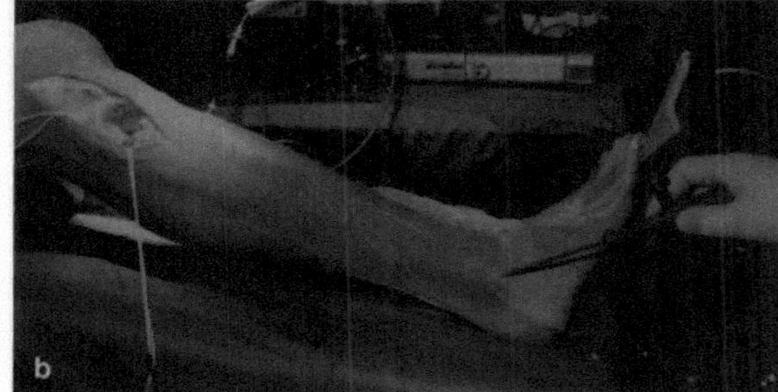

Fig. 60-3a, b. **a** Fixing of the rigid body in the tibiae, referencation, palpation of the lower leg, here of the lateral malleolus (**b**)

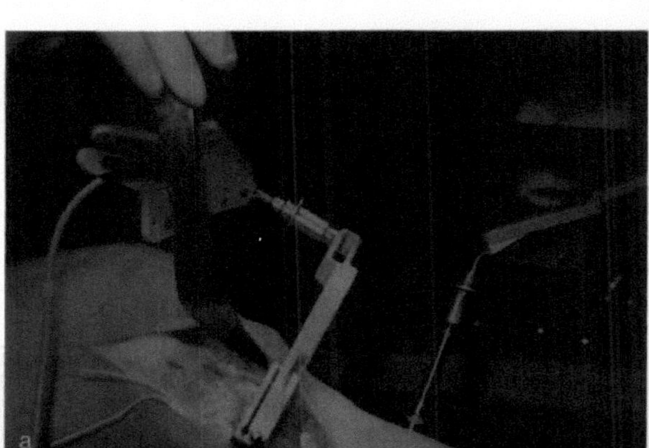

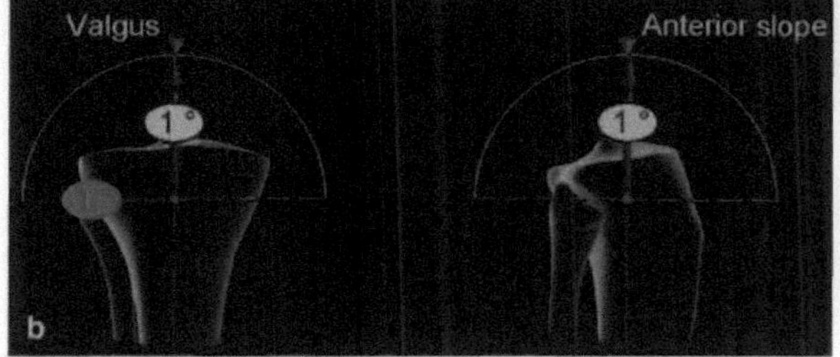

Fig. 60-4a, b. **a** Jig for the first osteotomy, **b** picture of the monitor

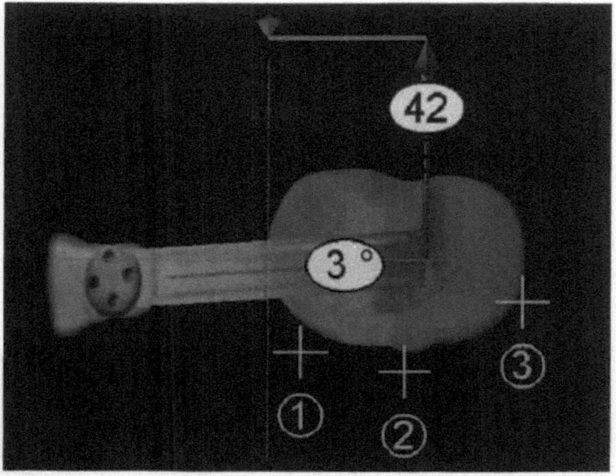

Fig. 60-5. Monitor view of the first osteotomy (cutting procedure)

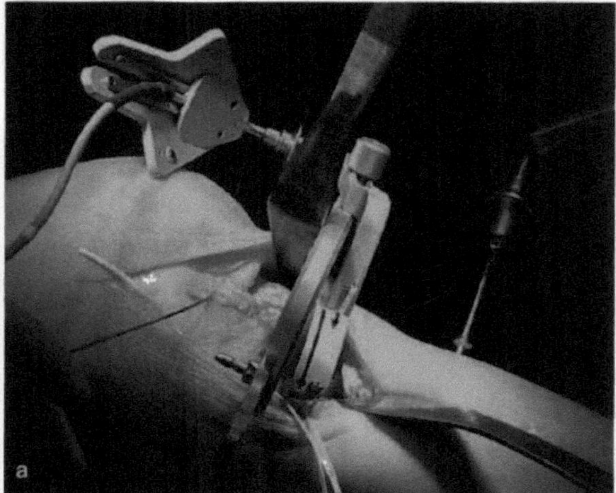

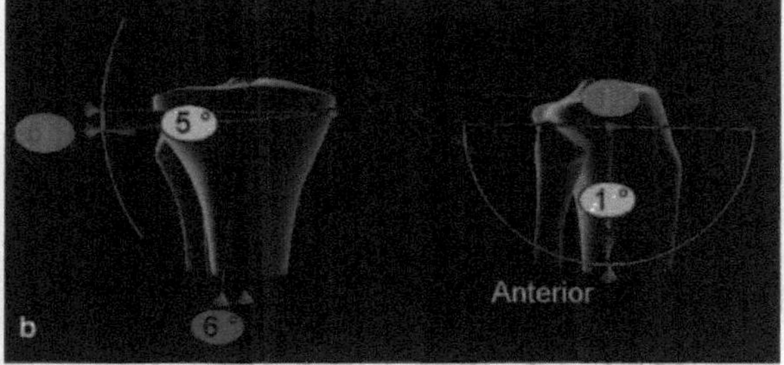

Fig. 60-6a, b. **a** Check-blade pivoted saw-jig for the 2nd osteotomy, **b** monitor view

geometry of the lower leg is calibrated with the system by palpating exact defined points at the lower leg (◘ Fig. 60-3b). For this palpation we use a special measurement tool with optoelectronical reference.

By means of the navigation system the saw jig for the first horizontal osteotomy can be positioned exactly according to the preoperative planning (◘ Fig. 60-4). The surgeon can control this positioning on the system monitor with the help of two virtual horizons for the a.p. and

sagittal view. Now the cutting procedure is performed. During the cutting procedure the positioning of the saw blade and the distance between the tip of the saw blade and the medial cortex of the tibia can be controlled on the monitor (◘ Fig. 60-5). With a check blade, where also reference markers are fixed, the osteotomy surface can be checked on the monitor. At this stage the pivoting point of the osteotomy is determined. After fixing of the 2nd saw jig, which is pivoted with the help of the navigation

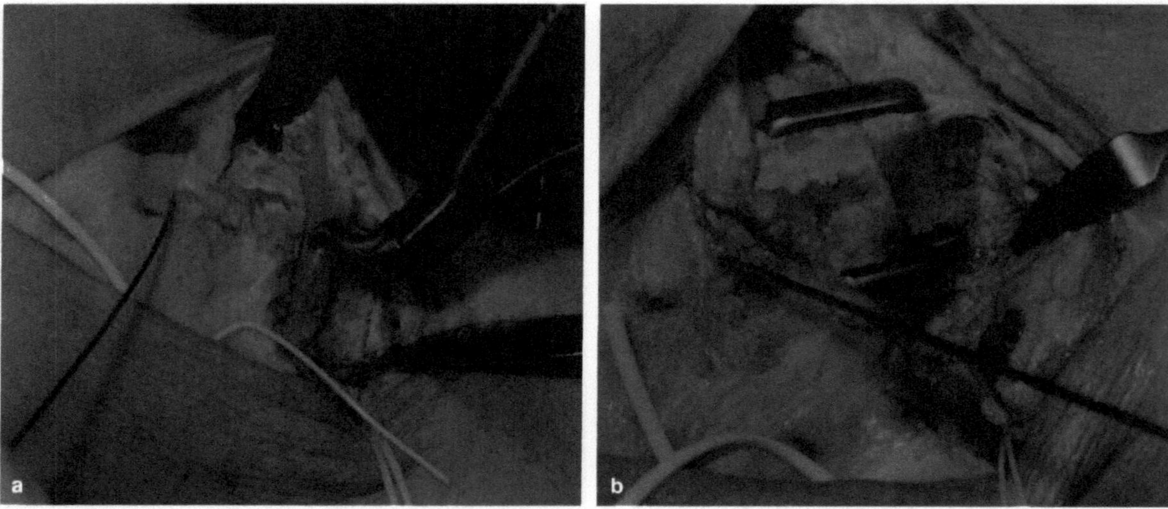

◘ **Fig. 60-7a, b. a** Removal of the bone-wedge; **b** closing ot the osteotomy, osteosynthesis with Coventry clamps

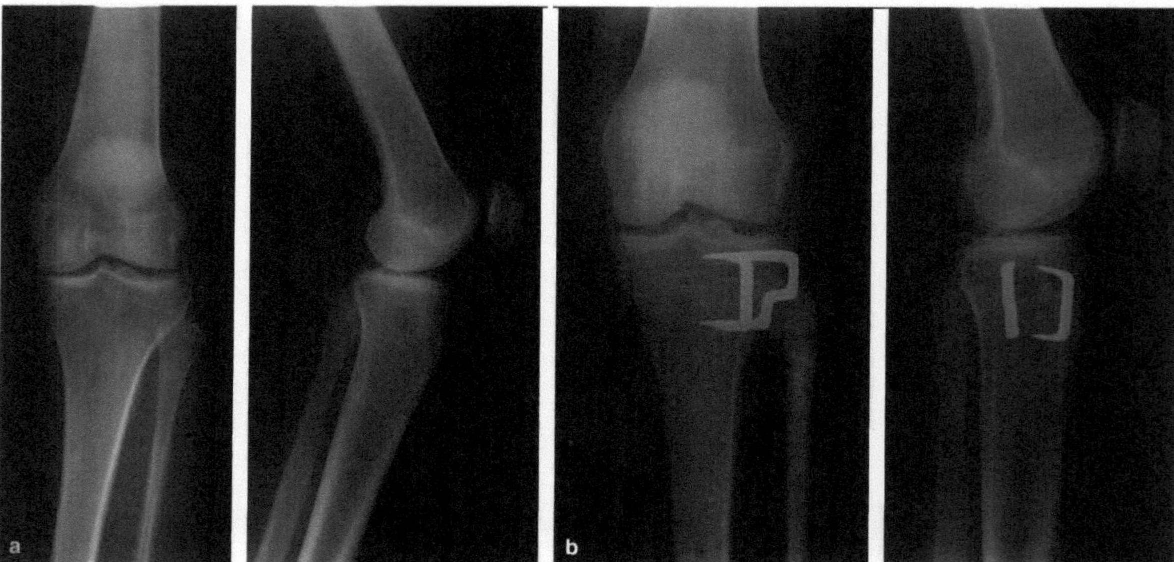

◘ **Fig. 60-8a, b.** Case: female 28 y., **a** preoperative; **b** 7 weeks postoperative

system around the check blade (◘ Fig. 60-6) the 2nd osteotomy can be performed. After removal of the lateral based bone wedge the osteosynthesis can be performed with Coventry clamps (◘ Fig. 60-7). The ◘ Figure 60-8 showed the pre- and postoperative X-rays of a 20 year old female sport student, which was operated because of a symptomatic varus knee deformity.

Perspective

The use of a navigation system in high tibial osteotomy ensures exact intraoperative orientation without X-ray-control. The size of the wedge and its position can be chosen optimally. Smoother osteotomy surfaces could lead to enhanced healing and rehabilitation. We expect decrease of the operation-associated complication rate. The described system is nowadays used at the Orthopaedic Department of the University of Kiel and is now developed with Aesculap for commercial use. In addition to the described subtractive technique, additive techniques are also possible to perform with the Orthopilot system.

References

1. Blauth W, Schuchardt E (1986) Orthopädisch-chirurgische Operationen am Knie. Thieme, Stuttgart New York, S 19.42–19.51
2. Blauth W, Stünitz B, Hassenpflug J (1993) Die interligamentäre valgisierende Tibiakopfosteotomie bei Varusgonarthrose. Oper Orthop Traumatol 5: 1–15
3. Coventry M (1965) Osteotomy of the upper portion of the for degenerative arthritis of the knee. J Bone Joint Surg 47A: 984–990
4. Coventry M (1985) Upper tibial osteotomy for osteoarthritis. J Bone Joint Surg 67A: 1136–1140
5. Hassenpflug J, Haugwitz V, Hahne A (1998) Langfristige Ergebnisse nach Tibiakopfosteotomie. Z Orthop 136: 154–161
6. Hassenpflug J, Plötz GMJ (2000) Alternativen zur Endoprothetik. In Eulert J, Hassenpflug J (Hrsg) Praxis der Knieendoprothetik. Springer, Berlin Heidelberg New York Tokyo, S 7–18
7. Healy WL, Anglen JO, Wasilewski SA, Krackow KA (1988) Distal femoral varus osteotomy. J Bone Joint Surg 70A: 102
8. Jackson JP (1958) Osteotomy for osteoarthritis of the knee. J Bone Joint Surg 40B: 826
9. Jerosch J, Heisel J (1999) Knieendoprothetik. Springer, Berlin Heidelberg New York Tokyo, S 38–41
10. Maquet PGJ (1984) Biomechanics of the knee. Springer, Berlin Heidelberg New York Tokyo, S 9–74
11. Naudie D, Bourne RB, Rorabeck CH, Bourne TJ (1999) Survivorship of high tibial valgus osteotomy – a 10 to 22 year follow up study. Clin Orthop 367: 18–27
12. Rinonapoli E, Mancini GB, Corvaglia A, Musiello S (1998) Tibial osteotomy for varus gonarthrosis. Clin Orthop 353: 185–193

61 Navigated Correction Operations of the Pelvis

T. Hüfner, J. Geerling, U. Berlemann, T. Pohlemann, T. Gösling, A. Sott, C. Krettek

Introduction

Nonunions or clinical relevant posttraumatic malunions of the pelvis are rare entities due to the application of standardized treatment protocols. However, also with an optimal primary treatment these problems may occur [8,10].

Tile gives an estimation of about 5% post-traumatically malunions of the pelvis after unstable pelvic ring fractures type B and C [12]. Other authors report 55% to 75% nonunions and mal-unions after nonoperative treatment of pelvic C type fractures [3,4,9].

The indications for a correction operation of the pelvis are pain, instabilities and persistent and relevant problems during daily activities.

When these patients present with the post-traumatic nonunion or malunion a thorough analysis and numerous diagnostic procedures must be done prior to a correction operation.

Diagnostics

The most frequent symptom is pain, which is related to the instability or the displacement within the sacroiliacal region [11]. However also after a correction operation of a malunited pelvic fracture the pain within the posterior pelvic ring can be reduced significantly [7]. The clinical diagnosis of a pelvic ring fracture may be quite visible in severe instabilities; the diagnosis of a nonunion is very difficult with clinical examination only.

Frequently, the examiner cannot provoke an instability with compression of the pelvic ring. Weight-bearing radiographs with left or right leg standing may be helpful in documenting instability.

In our own experience, a fluoroscopy-controlled infiltration with local anesthesia of painful regions of the pelvic ring may help also for a more precise diagnosis.

Besides the pain, limping or sitting incongruencies are typical symptoms. Frequently, cranial or posterior displacements and rotational displacements are seen according to the initial pelvis ring fracture [7]. These displacements can be diagnosed with the initial clinical examination. Another typical symptom is sitting incongruencies as the patient complains about having pain while sitting or lying on their back. The reason therefore is an internal rotation of one hemipelvis leading to external rotation of the spina iliaca posterior superior becoming more prominent. If one hemipelvis is shifted cranially, the sacrum or coccygeum might be prominent as well and may lead to pain while sitting.

Limping is due to a cranial displacement of the hemipelvis, which leads to functional shortening of the leg. In the literature, leg differences from 3 to 6 cm have been measured [7].

Internal or external displacements may lead to limping, too.

Radiological Evaluation

The radiological standard examination includes the AP, inlet and outlet views and with acetabular involvements the Judet views as well. These conventional radiographs allow an initial quantitative analysis of the displacement. In the a.p. view the cranial displacement is visible and posterior displacements are diagnosed best with the inlet view.

The spiral computertomography (CT) is the most important examination for further thorough analysis. The three-dimensional views provide the surgeon with an excellent whole overview of the problem. The reconstruction in axial, sagittal, and coronal planes allow an excellent analysis in all planes. The software allows measurements of angles and distances within one millimeter. In special cases a model of the pelvis (»rapid prototyping«) may be helpful.

Further Examinations

To exclude other problems a thorough neurological examination is essential according to fresh pelvic ring injuries. Huittinen found 50% neurological lesions with unstable pelvic fractures [2]. The nerve roots L5 and S1 are most frequently damaged. However, other sacral roots may be involved. After the neurological examination further neurophysiological examinations as EMG and ENG may be necessary.

Also, a urological examination should be done in conservatively treated complex injuries, since the original injury may have involved the urogenitary tract [1].

Operation Planning

Correction operations of the pelvis require extensive planning.

After the above-mentioned examinations have been done further examinations are necessary. There is the need of acknowledgement of previous operations (operation report), prior incisions and possible infections (antibiogram).

Operation

The procedure itself must be planned preoperatively in detail. Letournel reports three steps of the operation to achieve a high correction potential [6]. According to the displacement, the patient is first in the prone and then in supine and then again in prone position. However, this can be changed according to the displacement.

The first operation step is the osteotomy of pelvic or liberating of a non-union. Step two is the mobilization of the hemipelvis and the reduction are done. The third step is the definitive stabilization is performed.

Osteotomies should be done within the old fracture line. In cases of the cranial displacement of a hemipelvis the dissection of a sacrotuberal and sacroiliac ligaments must be done first since this is necessary to mobilize the hemipelvis.

Navigated Pelvic Correction Operations

Contrary to the preoperative excellent visualization the intraoperative visualization is limited in conventional pelvic correction operations. The direct visualization is limited with extended approaches and the intraoperative fluoroscopy does not reflect the complex three-dimensional displacement.

With the following case report the advantages and limitations of a navigated correction operation of a malhealed pelvic fracture are discussed.

Case Report

A 22-year old patient presents 4 months after a motorcycle accident. At an outside institution an isolated transiliac pelvic ring fracture type C1 21 [9] was operated using an ilioinguinal approach, and an incomplete reduction was performed using a plate osteosynthesis. At admission the patient presented with pain while walking and required a crutch for walking with full-weight bearing. Conventional radiographs and a CT showed the malpositioning and partial non- union as well (■ Fig. 61-1 and Fig. 61-2). Neurological examination revealed a partial lesion of the sciatic nerve. The operation was planned to be done with navigation. The CT dataset was loaded into the navigation system (SurgiGATE, Medivision, Oberdorf, Switzerland).

The operation was planned in three steps:

1. Prone position: dissection of the sacrotuberal ligaments for mobilization of the right hemipelvis. Suturing was done immediately.
2. Prone position: Using the Kocher-Langenbeck approach, initially a neurolysis of the sciatic nerve was performed. Using navigation (Medivision, Oberdorf, Switzerland), a partial osteotomy within the primary fracture line was done using the module spine and navigated chisels (■ Fig. 61-3). After this the wound was closed up.

3. Supine position: In a first step, two dynamic reference bases (DRB) were fixed to the pelvis and the later fragment. Registration was performed after the ilioinguinal approach was completed. The module developed for periacetabular osteotomies was used [5] The implants were removed and the osteotomy, again navigated, was completed from anterior. Afterwards the navigated reduction was performed. The reduc-

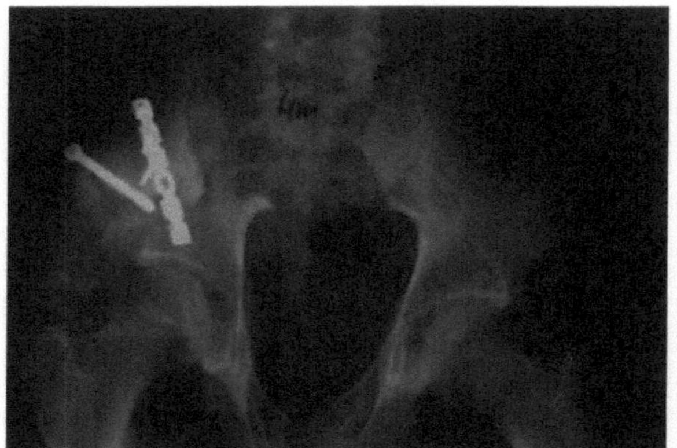

Fig. 61-1. Malreduced transiliac pelvic ring fracture. X-ray taken 4 months postoperatively. This transiliac pelvic ring fracture (C type, AO/OTA) was left malreduced at the referring center. This X-ray taken on admission to our unit shows delayed union. Clinically, there is pain as well as seating imbalance

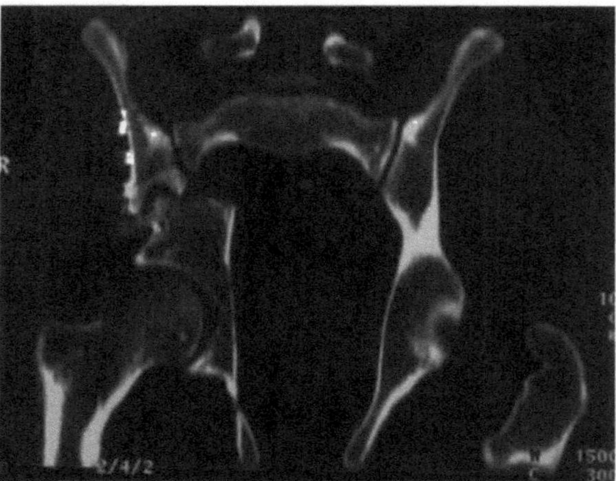

Fig. 61-2. CT view: Malunited pelvic ring fracture. CT cuts clearly show significant malunion with medialization and malposition in external rotation.

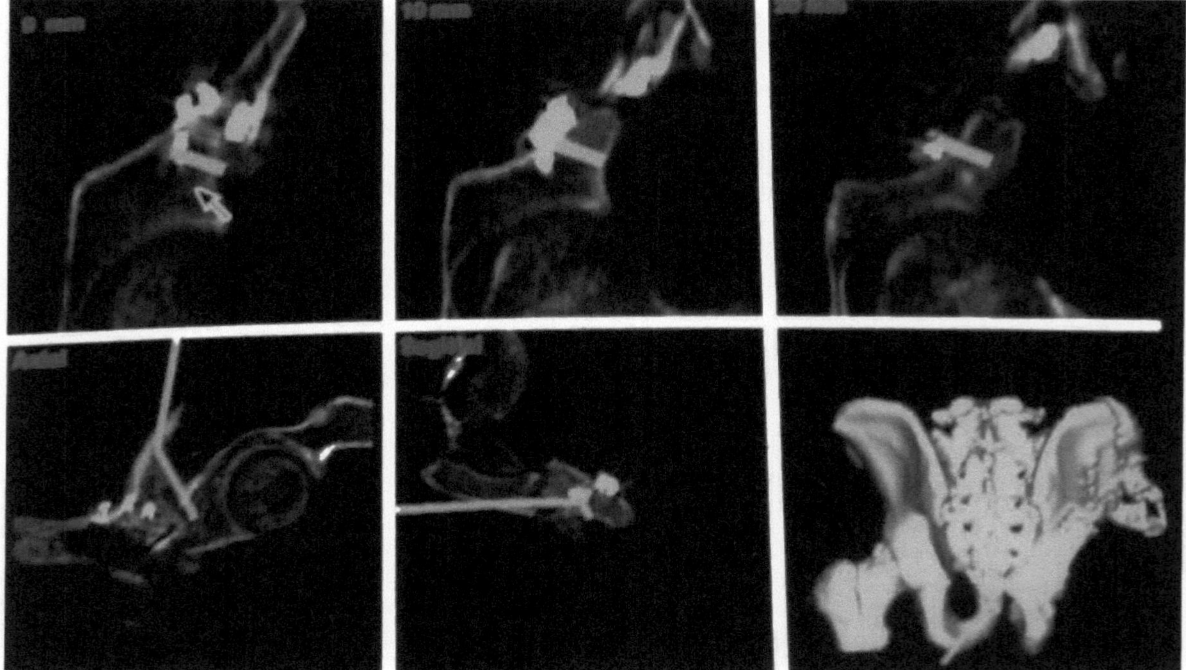

Fig. 61-3. Intraoperative view: Navigated dorsal partial osteotomy. The monitor shows the localization of the osteotomy in relation to the pelvis. Registration has already been completed: *PPR* on posterior superior iliac spine, ischial spine and ischial tuberosity. Surface registration carried out via exposed bone through K-L approach

tion was controlled in real-time on the monitor screen (■ Fig. 61-4). Unfortunately, the DRB placed nearby the symphysis was loosening at the end of the reduction maneuver. Another registration was not possible due to a changed situation compared to the initial CT dataset. The operation was completed in conventional manner.

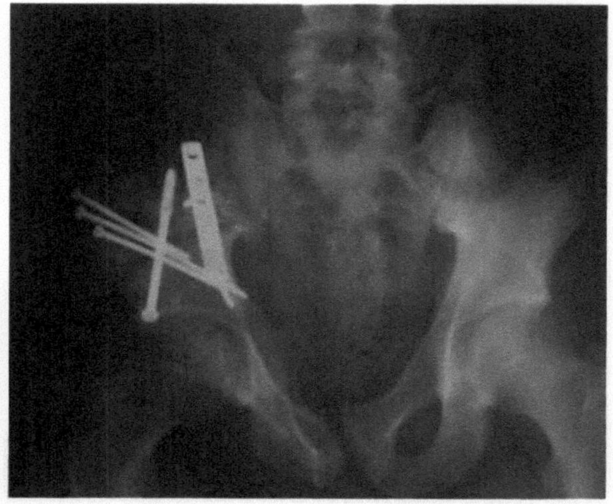

■ **Fig. 61-5.** Radiograph 4 months postoperatively. Four months after this procedure the patient is now fully weight-bearing. The fracture continues to unite well

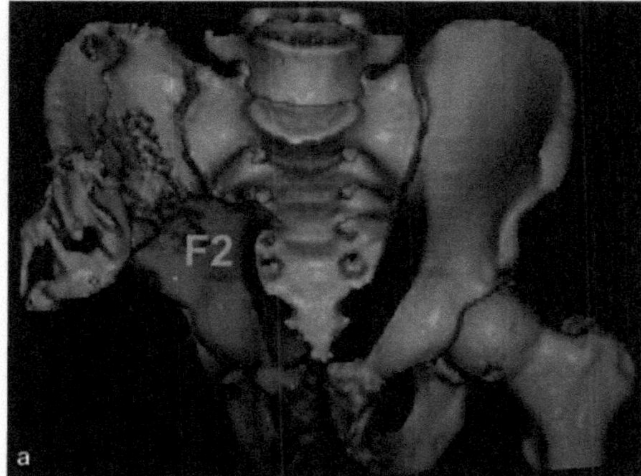

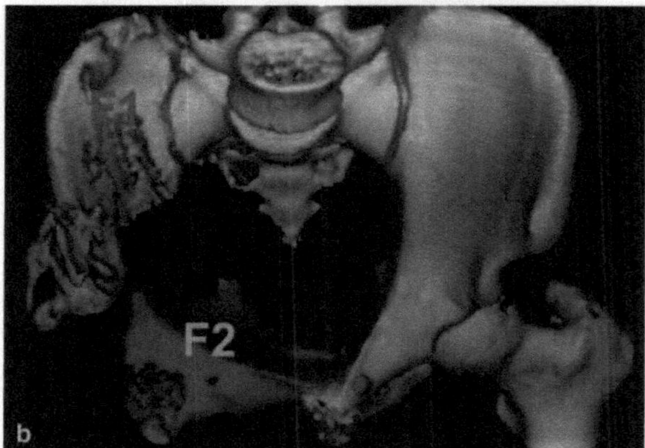

■ **Fig. 61-4a,b.** Intraoperative view: Navigated control of fracture reduction. After registration the osteosynthesis plate was removed and the osteotomy was completed from ventral. The virtual image still displays the plate. It is yet impossible to update the virtual data accordingly. The preoperatively defined fragments F1 and F2 have already been set up with their DRB. **a** Before reduction: intraoperative control of reduction, i. e. rotation of the ventral fragment (F2 *red*). **b** After reduction: At this stage, just prior to completion, the connection between DRB and fragment F2 became loose and reduction was completed via the conventional route under image intensifier control (II inlet view). The apparent defect of the right iliac bone is a result of the virtual planning of the osteotomy which was carried out preoperatively on a three-dimensional object

Radiographs done postoperative and after follow-up revealed an almost anatomical reduction (■ Fig. 61-5).

Discussion

Correction operations of the pelvic ring are rare, usually last long and are patient-loading operations. The intraoperative control of the reduction is done through the approaches supported by fluoroscopic control. For a three-dimensional analysis, fluoroscopic control should be performed after each reduction at least within three planes (AP, in- and outlet). This procedure is time-consuming and the radiation exposure for the patient as well as for the surgeon has to be mentioned. Implants or retractors can be a limiting factor for visualization using intraoperative fluoroscopy as well.

Using extended approaches for better visualization the morbidity for the patient increases. A prospective study from the pelvis study group of the German Traumatology Society revealed an increased blood loss of 1392 ml (700–3000 ml) using extended approaches compared to 680 ml (200–7600 ml) using simple approaches (ilioinguinal, Kocher-Langenbeck).

Navigation could be the solution for improved results of these operations. It is based on CT datasets providing excellent images. If the registration procedure is done correctly, the accuracy is excellent. The surgeon has the three-dimensional images displayed on the monitor screen during the critical steps, at osteotomy and reduction. Additionally, virtual instruments are displayed in relationship to the patient's anatomy.

This is crucial for perfect cuts and improved reduction and reduced radiation exposure.

With the PAO module the osteotomy is planned on the intact pelvis. Cuts can be done only on the three-dimensional model and not using reformations (axial, sagittal and coronal plane). During the operation the chisels are not displayed in relationship to the planned cuts. The surgeon must perform the cuts according to the preoperative planning, because an intraoperative deviation of the osteotomy can not be registered by this system.

Also, a loosing of the DRB during the reduction manuever is a potential pitfall. If not recognized, the information displayed on the monitor is incorrect.

Conclusion

Navigation was very helpful for pelvic correction operations. The preoperative planning increases the three-dimensional knowledge of the surgeon. intraoperatively, the increased visualization improves the quality of the cuts and the reduction.

Further improvements as an improved planning station, repeated registration also after reduction has commenced will further improve this technology.

References

1. Bosch U, Pohlemann T, Haas N, Tscherne H (1992) Klassifikation und Management des komplexen Beckentraumas. Unfallchirurg 95:189–196
2. Huittinen V, Slätis P (1972) Nerve injury in double vertical pelvic fractures. Acta Chir Scand 138:571–575
3. Hundley J (1966) Ununited unstable fractures of the pelvis. J Bone Joint Surg 48-A:1025
4. Kellam J (1989) The role of external fixation in pelvic disruptions. Clin Orthop 241:66–82
5. Langlotz F, Bächler R, Berlemann U, Nolte LP, Ganz R (1998) Computer assistance for pelvic osteotomies. Clin Orthop 354:92–102
6. Letournel E (1993) Open reduction internal fixation of acetabular fractures: long term results and analysis of 1040 cases. 1st International Symposium on surgical treatment of acetabular fractures, May 10–11, Paris
7. Matta, J., Dickson, K., and Markovich, G., Surgical treatment of pelvic nonunions and malunions. Clin Orthop, 1996. 329: p. 199–206.
8. Matta J, Saucedo T (1989) Internal fixation of pelvic ring fractures. Clin Orthop 242:83–97
9. Orthopedic Trauma Association Committee for Coding and Classification (1996) Fracture and dislocation compendium. J Orthop Trauma 10 [Suppl 1]:V–IX
10. Pennal G, Massiah K (1980) Nonunion and delayed union of fractures of the pelvis. Clin Orthop 151:124–129
11. Semba R, Yasukawa K, Gustillo R (1983) Critical analysis of results 53 Malgaigne fractures of the pelvis. J Trauma 23:535–537
12. Tile M (1988) Pelvic ring fractures: should they be fixed? J Bone Joint Surg 70-B: p 1–12

62 Computer-Based Drilling of Osteochondral Lesions of the Talus (OLT) with an Aiming Device

R. E. Rosenberger, Ch. Hoser, Ch. Fink, R. J. Bale

Introduction

The complex anatomic location and the resulting difficult access path often causes problems in surgical treatment of symptomatic osteochondral talus lesions (OLTs) [13, 17]. While anterolateral lesions are amenable to arthroscopic treatment, those located dorsomedially are much less accessible arthroscopically [7,18]. In open surgical interventions, these lesions are only accessible via osteotomy of the inner malleolus. Although arthroscopic and open surgical interventions differ in detail, the underlying principle of therapy is very similar [12]. On the one hand they consist of debriding the chondritic part, on the other hand they support and promote revascularization of the necrotic bony areas by for example drilling into the subchondral zone. Direct anterograde drilling of osteochondral lesions, however, is sometimes technically impossible, true especially for the dorsomedially located lesions. Transmalleolar drilling [20] or the use of curved drill bits [6] have been described as a possible approach. However, a disadvantage of anterograde drill techniques is that, should the chondral surface over the lesions still be intact, it gets damaged. The transmalleolar drill technique also damages the malleolar joint cartilage [16].

Due to these problems, some authors favor retrograde drilling techniques [7, 18]. However, because of the complex anatomy of the talus, exact retrograde drilling becomes a technical challenge and misplaced drill attempts are common, even under fluoroscopy. Aiming devices, similar to those used in tunnel placement during anterior cruciate ligament grafting, are useful, but, since the lesions are at times difficult to locate arthroscopically, such devices are not always applicable.

The method of computer-assisted drilling presented below should be seen as a furtherance to already existing techniques. The aim is to place a drill precisely in the centre of a lesion. A hollow drill can then be guided over the initial drill to then fill the defect with spongiosa [18] or, using a parallel template as guide, insert further drills into the necrotic bone lesion.

Materials and Methods

A pre-requisite for use of computer-assisted navigation systems is precise superposition (co-registration) of planning-CT/MRI data with the real patient. For this purpose, external CT/MRI markers are applied during initial imaging which later allows the user to later co-register the pre- and intraoperative datasets using the navigation system. Since markers attached to the skin did not grant the desired precision [21] the markers for such orthopaedic/surgical interventions are usually screwed into bone allowing accurate registration however at the cost of an additional invasive procedure [8, 9, 14, 20]. In an attempt to spare the patient this procedure, a special fixation technique was developed at our hospital which combines both non-invasiveness and repositioning accuracy [1]. Another objective was to decrease intraoperative complexity. This could be realized thanks to the development of two special adjustable aiming devices which reduce the use of the navigation system to the preoperative planning phase [1, 3].

The following detailed description of the process from fixation right to the actual drilling is summarized in ◘ Fig. 62-1.

Acknowledgements: The present study was generously supported by the »Lorenz-Boehler Society – for the support of research in trauma surgery« (Proj. 2/99). Reinhart A. Sweeney, M.D. assisted in manuscript preparation.

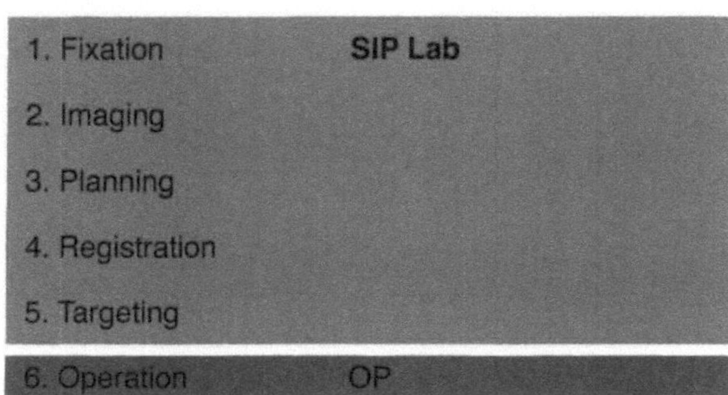

Fig. 62-1. SIP-Lab Innsbruck concept: Steps 1–5 occur preoperatively, Steps 3–5 are performed in the patients absence in the planning laboratory

Non-Invasive Fixation of the Ankle Joint

The fixation device (FISCOFIX cast) serves both to reproducibly fixate the ankle-joint and as rigid external structure onto which the external markers are pasted. It is based on individually fitted elastic fiberglass material (STS Copy-Sock, Götz GmbH & Co, Göppingen, Germany), which is pulled over the foot like a stocking after which it hardens. After this hardened stocking is removed in a quick and simple procedure, it is externally reinforced by multiple layers of Scotchcast (3 M Health Care, St. Paul, MN, USA). Plexiglas connectors to the baseplate are also integrated in this cast granting a precisely defined relationship of the cast to the baseplate. After the Scotchcast material has hardened, the cast is cut in two by use of an oscillating saw. Radiodense fiducial markers (Philips Medical Systems, Best, Netherlands) are asymmetrically glued to the surface of the cast over the area of the lesion.

During both the imaging and surgical phases, the two halves are clamped together over the patients foot with Velcro straps as they are during the planning phase (without patient) in the SIP-Lab.

Imaging (CT)

A computed tomography (CT) data-set is obtained with the patient immobilized in the FISCOFIX cast (1 mm slice thickness). The CT dataset is transferred to the navigation system in the SIP-Lab via local network.

3D- Reconstruction und Planning of the Path

For this study, a navigation system based on an optical positioning measurement system (OPMS) was used (*StealthStation*, Medtronic, Minneapolis, MN, USA) [15, 21]. Coronal, sagittal and axial slices as well as a 3D reconstructed object as well as up to 400% zoom capability allows precise definition of target and entry-points of the planned drilling intervention.

Registration

In the stereotactic planning laboratory the closed FISCOFIX cast is repositioned on the base plate in its defined position. In the following registration procedure, the data-set »ankle joint + FISCOFIX cast« is registered to the real object »FISCOFIX cast« by co-referencing the external markers on the surface of the cast (Fig. 62-2).

Adjusting the Aiming Device

For frameless stereotactic targeting we have developed a targeting device (Vertek) in collaboration with Medical Intelligence Inc. (Schwabmünchen, Germany) and Med-

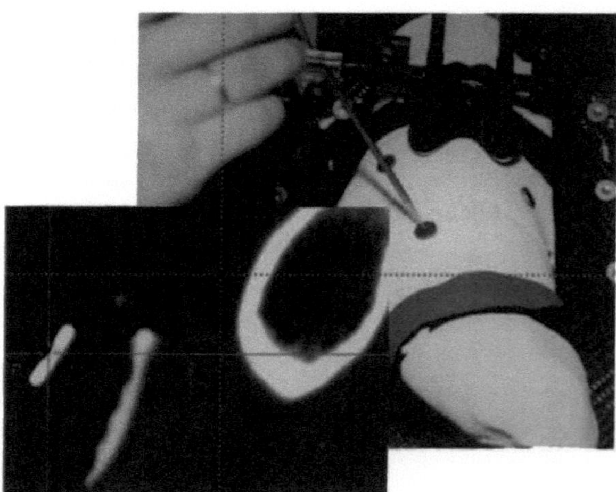

Fig. 62-2. The respective marker chosen on the CT data set is registered to the real marker on the cast with the tip of a registration wand, itself registered automatically by the navigation system. Three or more markers thus allow co-registration using the optical positioning capability of the navigation system

tronic Inc. (Minneapolis, MN, USA) [3]. The Vertek device consists of an articulating support arm which is mounted to the baseplate of the FISCOFIX via a connector, the aiming device, a guide frame and a reducing tube.

The multiple joints of the articulated arm allow for convenient and versatile positioning. All pivots on the arm lock in place by turning the locking handle. The guide frame has a LED tracking device to enable the Stealth Station to detect its spatial position. The reducing tube reduces the inner diameter of the guide frame to accommodate the required drill bits. Two independent pivot joints enable precise alignment of the guide frame (and thus drill) with the planned surgical path.

The identical relationship of the aiming device to the FISCOFIX cast is given by their connection to the base plate. After calibration of the guide frame, the arm is positioned such that the guide frame assembly is located above the entry point for the drilling procedure. The target aim is assessed by using the trajectory views and guidance views of the navigation system software. First the tip of the guide frame is arranged on the line which extends through the predefined entrance position and the target position (i. e. alignment line). Then the longitudinal axis of the aiming device is aligned with the virtual path. When the correct alignment with the trajectory is found and verified, all joints are tightened. The depth of the biopsy needle insertion is also calculated using the navigation system.

In the region of the planned entry point of the drill over the skin, an area of 3 cm in diameter is cut out of the cast. The now rigid aiming device/mechanical arm unit and the FISCOFIX cast are disconnected and gas-sterilized together with the base plate, the mounting screws as well as the Velcro straps.

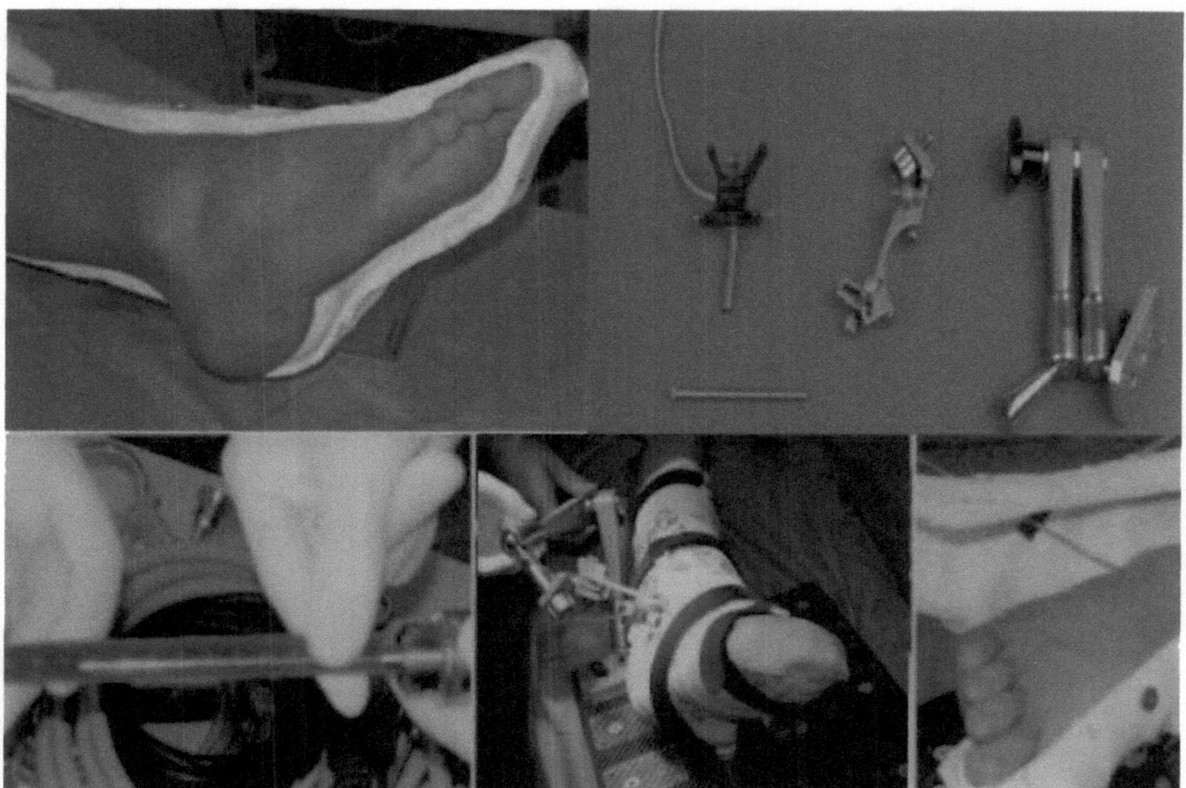

Fig. 62-3. Operation steps (from upper left to lower right). After sterile washing and draping, the FISCOFIX cast is assembled. Cast and aiming device are reproducibly tightened to the carbon fiber base plate. The drill bit is then tightened into the drill chuck at the pre-determined depth. After insertion through the aiming device, the drilling is begun. Then cast and aiming device are removed

Drilling

Before initiating general anesthesia, the patient is repositioned in the FISCOFIX cast in a sterile environment. The FISCOFIX cast and the previously adjusted aiming device are connected to the base plate in the correct relationship (◘ Fig. 62-3).

To ensure correct drill depth, the drill is tightened into the chuck according to the calculated distance »Aiming-device → target point«. The mechanical stop prevents drilling too deeply/overshooting the lesion. After drilling, the chuck is opened and the drill and the aiming device are removed, leaving the drill-bit in place, Its correct position is verified under fluoroscopy before performing a talocrural (upper ankle-joint) arthroscopy to analyze the condition of the joints cartilage and for intraarticular verification of correct drill placement.

Depending on the lesions characteristics, either additional drillings into the osteonecrotic zone are made using a parallel drill template or the drill bit is overdrilled using a cannulated (hollow) 3.5–5 mm drill bit followed by a retrograde spongiosa filling as described by Conti et al. [7]. After cleaning the lesion with a curette, the channel can be filled with a spongiosa cylinder from the calcaneous or tibial metaphysis (◘ Fig. 62-4). This method seems especially effective in cystic lesions.

Results

From December 1999 to January 2002, 17 patients with OLTs were treated by computer-assisted drilling in our department.

Accuracy of Drilling

As could be shown on post-operative CT scans in the first 7 patients with a percutaneous retrograde approach from a lateral direction, the tip of the preoperatively planned drill bit could be placed with an accuracy of 2.5±1.2 mm. The center of the osteochondral lesions was hit in all 17 cases, as seen by intraoperative fluoroscopy. Furthermore, arthroscopy verified that no drill bit damaged the talar chondral surfaces.

Time Requirements for Preparation and Operation

After the period of initial development, the FISCOFIX cast took about 30 min to make. CT, data transfer and navigation (planning) took 45–60 min. The patients, however, need only be present for production of the initial stocking cast (about 10 min) as well as imaging (including positioning in the cast (about 10 min).

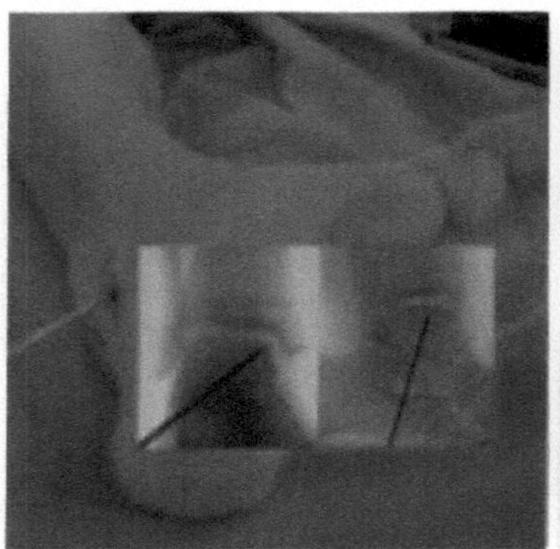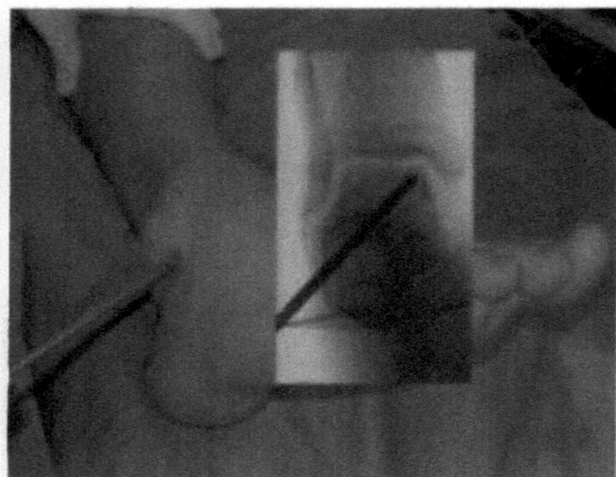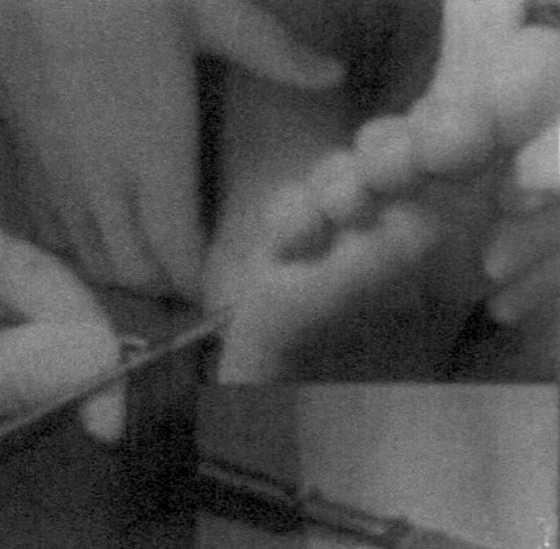

◘ **Fig. 62-4.** The drill-bit position is checked under fluoroscopy, then more complex operative procedures (such as curettage of the necrotic bone lesion, parallel drillings or insertion of a spongiosa cylinder taken from the calcaneus) can be performed

In the OR, mounting the cast and setting up the aiming device takes 3–5 min, however, this can be done prior to initiating anesthesia. The actual drill process including removal of the cast takes another 2–5 min.

Clinical Results and Complications

No intra or post-operative complications occurred in any case. Mean hospital admittance of this procedure was 1.6±0.8 days (1 to 3 days).

Due to the short follow-up period, we cannot report any relevant clinical results at this point. It can, however, be expected that they are at least in the range of the results described in conventional retrograde techniques [18].

Discussion

Computer-assisted retrograde drilling of osteochondral talus lesions has shown to be a safe and efficient method. The combination of a stereotactic navigation system with a non-invasive fixation method (FISCOFIX cast) allows preoperative adjustment of an aiming device according to the ideal planned operative trajectory. Thanks to this accurate, preoperative planning and the increased precision, the effective operating time and intraoperative radiation exposure can be reduced and misses avoided altogether. The technical extravagance inside the OR is reduced since the navigation system need not be present for the actual drilling process. This aspect is greatly appreciated by the surgical staff. In treating OLTs, the chosen technique depends mainly on localization, extent and size of the necrotic bone and on the condition of the cartilaginous surface [4, 5, 19]. While anterograde drill techniques seem to be an adequate method for many lesions leading to good clinical results [12], retrograde drill techniques offer the advantage of easier access to dorsally located lesions and allow sparing of possibly still intact chondral surfaces [7, 18]. They also serve as a good therapeutic alternative in cases of extended necrotic or cystic bone lesions by allowing placement of a retrograde spongiosaplasty [18].

This study was, however, not intended to compare techniques but rather to simplify and increase the precision of retrograde OLT-drilling. Building on the positive experiences with this computer-assisted method, similar applications may be possible in the near future, such as a modification of the method of transplanting osteochondral cylinders from the knee joint to treat OLTs as described by Hongody et al. [11]. Retrograde implantation of osteochondral cylinders to reestablish the chondral contour of the talar ridge, whereby both removal and implantation could be planned preoperatively in this computer-assisted manner, is another possibility. Initial in vitro experiments are currently being conducted at our clinic in this regard. For all computer-assisted surgical interventions, the best equipment cannot replace intense and constructive cooperation between radiologists, technical staff and surgeons. The common goal should always be to recognize a complex surgical challenge and to then find a solution which represents an acceptable compromise between additional procedures with their related costs and increased precision without increased risk to the patient. For computer-assisted retrograde drilling of OLTs (and given the appropriate teamwork), the surgeons only preoperative part should be to define target and entry points of the drill trajectory. Thanks to the non-invasive nature of fixation, this aspect does not additionally burden the patient, but does allow a precise result. The currently still somewhat extravagant process of creating the individualized fixation cast (FISCOFIX cast) might in the future be significantly reduced by using a reusable, vacuum-based fixation method [2].

Conclusion

Computer-assisted retrograde drilling of OLTs has shown to be a safe and efficient method. Planning the intervention using 3D datasets (CT/MR) allow a direct transfer of diagnostic information to the intraoperative situation. The additional workload required in the preoperative planning process is more than compensated for by the accurate drilling process and reduced operation times. It is also quite likely that these technical possibilities will in the future allow even more complex surgical techniques in therapy of OLTs (such as retrograde osteochondral transplantation).

Due, however, to the high technical and equipment prerequisites, computer-assisted drilling of osteochondral talus lesions is currently restricted to specialized centers

References

1. Bale RJ, Hoser C, Rosenberger R, Rieger M, Benedetto KP, Fink C (2001) Initial experiences with Computer-assisted retrograde drilling of osteochondral lesions of the talus – feasibility and accuracy. Radiology 218: 278–282
2. Bale RJ, Vogele M, Rieger M, Buchberger W, Lukas P, Jaschke W (1999) A new vacuum device for extremity immobilization. Am J Roentgenol 4: 1093–1094
3. Bale RJ, Vogele M, Lang T et al. (2002): A novel vacuum immobilization device and a novel targeting device for computer-assisted interventional procedures. In: Lemke HU et al. (eds). Computer-assisted radiology and surgery. Elsevier, Amsterdam New York, pp 92–97
4. Berndt AL, Harty M (1959) Transchondral fractures of the talus. J Bone Joint Surg Am 41: 988–1020
5. Bruns J, Behrens P (1998) Osteochondrosis dissecans. Arthroskopie 11: 166–176
6. Bryant DD, Siegel MG (1993) Osteochondritis dissecans of the talus: a new technique for arthroscopic drilling. Arthroscopy 9: 238–241
7. Conti SF, Taranow WF (1996) Transtalar retrograd drilling of medial osteochondral lesions of the talar dome. Oper Tech Orthop 6: 226–230
8. Dessenne V, Lavallèe S, Juillard R, Orti R, Martelli S, Cinquin P (1995) Computer-assisted knee anterior cruciate ligament reconstruction: First clinical tests. J Image Guided Surg 1: 59–64
9. DiGioia AM III, Jaramez B, Colgan BD (1998) Computer-assisted orthopaedic surgery. Clin Orthop 354: 8–16
10. Ferkel RD, Scranton PE (1993) Current concepts review: arthroscopy of the foot and ankle. J Bone Joint Surg Am 75: 1233–1242
11. Hongody L, Kish G, Zarpati Z, Szerb I, Eberhardt R (1997) Treatment of osteochondritis dissecans of the talus: use of the mosaicplasty technique: a preliminary report. Foot Ankle Int 18: 623–634
12. Kumai T, Takakura Y, Higashiyama I, Tamai S (1999) Arthroscopic drilling for the treatment of osteochondral lesions of the talus. J Bone Joint Surg Am 81: 1229–1235
13. Lahm A, Erggelet C, Steinwachs M, Reichelt A (1998) Arthroskopische Therapie der Osteochondrosis dissecans des Talus – Nachuntersuchung mit einem neuen »Ankle-Score«. Sportverl Sportschad 12: 107–113
14. Macunias RJ, Galloway RL, Latimer JW (1994) The application accuracy of stereotactic frames. Neurosurgery 35: 682–694
15. Maurer CR, Fitzpatrick MJ, Wang MY, Galloway RL, Maciunas RJ, Allen GS (1997) Registration of head volume images using implantible fiducial markers. IEEE Transactions on Medical Imaging 16: 447–462
16. Morgan CD (1991) Gross and arthroscopic anatomy of the ankle. In: McGinty JB (ed) Operative arthroscopy. Raven Press, New York, pp 677–694
17. Ritzler T, van Dijk CN (1998) Arthroskopische Behandlung der Osteochondrosis dissecans der Talusrolle. Arthroskopie 11: 187–192
18. Taranow WS, Bisignani GA, Towers JD, Conti SF (1999) Retrograde drilling of osteochondral lesions of the medial talar dome. Foot Ankle Int 20: 474–480
19. Van Buecken K, Barrack RL, Alexander AH, Ertl JP (1989) Arthoscopic treatment of transchondral talar dome fractures. Am J Sports Med 17: 350–355
20. Vannier MW, Marsh JL (1996) Three-dimensional imaging, surgical planning and image-guided therapy. Radiol Clin North Am 34: 545–563
21. Zinreich SJ, Tebo SA, Long DM et al. (1993) Frameless stereotatic integration of CT imaging data: accuracy and initial applications. Radiology 1888: 735–742

63 Computer-Assisted Osteosynthesis of Long Bone Fractures

P.A. Grützner, G. Zheng, B. Vock, C. Keil, L.P. Nolte, A. Wentzensen

Introduction

Image intensifiers (C arms) are the most common and most used medical device for image acquisition in the trauma operating room. The image intensifier is an important device for intraoperative diagnosis of results of actual fracture reductions, for monitoring the actual position of surgical instruments drill bits, and also for checking the correct position of materials for an osteosynthesis, and of other implants. In the last decades, techniques in trauma surgery have changed tremendously. In former times, fractures were treated with large incisions and stabilized with plates in similar dimensions. Today we know that the technique of minimally invasive osteosynthesis, with a reduction of the trauma by minimizing the incision and the related soft-tissue damage, is an essential benefit for the patient, not only because of the cosmetic result but also for speed of recovery and functional results.

The challenge with minimally invasive techniques is that the surgeon has no direct view of the position of the implant relative to the bone, and of the actual result of the fracture reduction. Thus, the use of the image intensifier is much more demanding and thus causes a significant radiation exposure for both the patient and the OR-team. The imaging with an image intensifier is also limited [6]. The image is a two-dimensional composite image and, as there is only one C arm in the OR, not more than one plane can be displayed simultaneously. During the image acquisition, the C arm is over the operating field and may disturb the surgical actions. Using surgical navigation techniques, some of these problems could be totally or partly solved [1, 4, 5, 8].

Computer-assisted operation techniques in trauma surgery are becoming more and more widespread, developing from a stage of experimental and scientific approach to increasingly routine use. The principle is the combination of medical images with intraoperative instrument and implant positions. The medical images can be generated preoperatively, e.g. CT or MRI, but also intraoperatively with the use of a conventional image intensifier. The system presented here is based on the principle of passive navigation, meaning the surgeon uses instruments and guiding implants freehand. The optical information is combined with the tactile information gathered during the intervention. Without navigation, this combination of highly complex image data with the position of the instrument is performed in the surgeon's head.

The System

The core of each navigation system is the detector, which is able to precisely track surgical instruments and implants, as well as the position of the patient in three-dimensional space. Usually, this detector is an infrared camera (Optotrack, Northern Digital Inc. Canada), which tracks up to 20 objects simultaneously with a precision <0.3 mm in a FOV (field of view) of about 1 m^3. A high performance workstation processes this information about instrument position with the information of the medical images (SurgiGATE Medivision, Switzerland). These highly complex calculations are processed in real-time.

For the use with navigation, the surgical instruments, mostly standard instruments, have to be equipped with »markershields«, small infrared light emitting diodes (LED). A calibration of the instruments is also mandatory. The accuracy of the navigated intervention depends on the calibration and the rigidity of those instruments.

In order to compensate the relative motions of the bones operated on in relation to the instrument positions, both must be monitored by the camera. A major part of the processing time of the system is used to compensate these relative motions in real-time. A dynamic reference base (DRB) must therefore be affixed on the bone which is to be operated on. This DRB registers all movements of the bone due to manipulation by the surgeon, breathing or the use of instruments. Navigation is thus completely independent of movements of the camera or the patient on the OR table (frameless navigation). The rigid and stable fixation of the dynamic reference base on the bone is extremely important. The DRB must be in the »field of view« during the image acquisition as well as during the navigation, but it should not interfere with the surgical procedure. The relative position between DRB and bone is in principle not important. The handling of the navigation system is performed under sterile conditions with a »virtual keyboard«. The camera also monitors the position of the virtual keyboard in relation to the tip of an instrument. A surgeon can thus use the computer under sterile conditions, no additional personnel is required for system handling.

Registration-Free Navigation, Virtual Fluoroscopy

Using C-arm images in different planes, it is possible to visualize the instrument position in relation to the patient's anatomy in different planes simultaneously. Displaying the instrument position dynamically in real-time and in different planes simultaneously is the key function of fluoroscopy-based navigation. With virtual fluoroscopy, up to four C-arm images can be displayed as a kind of simultaneous virtual constant radiography, providing this optical information to the surgeons.

There are three essential criteria necessary to enable navigation in images of a C arm. Firstly, C-arm images are, due to physical properties, distorted (cushion effect) and they have to be geometrically corrected/undistorted by use of a mathematical algorithm. In addition, the distortion depends on the actual position of the C arm. Further, the distortion is different for each single C arm, so each C arm has to be calibrated for navigational use [1, 3, 4, 5, 7, 8]. Secondly, the navigation system and the tracking of the different instruments, have to combine the anatomical situation with the image information. In the last step, the instrument position is combined with the

image information. Usually, this is done by displaying two-dimensional linear graphics, which is sufficient for the visualization of the drilling processes and implant positioning in two dimensional virtual X-rays.

At the beginning of the intervention, after the fixation of the dynamic reference base, the image intensifier images are taken. Then the C arm can be removed from the operating field.

For the use of the system, no preoperative data such as CT or MRI is required. The image data will be generated in the OR, appropriate to the individual situation. A preoperative planning in the sense of working on CT data or definition of special landmarks, which have to be reproduced intraoperatively, is not required. The system works registration-free, meaning that the procedure to match the preoperative image data with the intraoperatively found anatomical situation is not necessary. A further decisive advantage of the virtual fluoroscopy is the feature that images can be regained after modification of the anatomy by fracture reduction maneuvers. With this feature, updates of the actual situation are possible at any time, in sharp contrast to CT-based navigation.

Up to nine images can be transferred to the navigation system which are then geometrically corrected and stored in a library. Using the virtual keyboard, the surgeon can change magnification and contrast under sterile conditions. Different calibrated instruments, e. g. drill, screw driver, pedicle awl etc., are connected to the system. Calibration of the instruments is also checked under sterile conditions. During navigation, the image data of the C arm is combined with the position of the instruments by projecting the instrument into the images.

The decisive feature is the correct shooting of the X-ray projections. The navigation system features a special guiding mode (alignment) in which the required position of the C-arm can be defined and stored. The image intensifier will be navigated exactly in this axis. This algorithm allows standardized shooting of the images, so improving quality and decreasing radiation exposure.

Reality Enhancement

The substantial disadvantages of intraoperative image-intensifier-supported navigation currently in use are the linear, two-dimensional representation of implants and instruments as well as the inability to show modified anatomy without the additional use of X-rays.

In the project presented, we would like to show the widening of the use of image intensifiers. Goals of the development were the dynamisation of conventional C-arm pictures in different levels at the same time, i. e. referencing through various fragment types and by dynamisation of X-rays to produce a realistic check of the positioning in the virtual X-ray. A further goal was to visualize the instruments and implants used (i. e. osteosynthesis plates and nails) with the help of CAD data as true to live three-dimensional structures in the graphic data of more complex pictures.

The dynamisation of X-rays is the result of the so-called concept of virtual cylinders. Here the individual bone fragments in the two-dimensional figures are formed relative to the three-dimensional cylinder model. Using at least two 2D pictures taken from different positions, we reconstructed a three-dimensional structure with this cylinder model. This structure, a virtual representation of the genuine bone structure, can, after further handling and outlining, be separated into two sections which can then be reset in relation to the virtual X-rays. So it is possible to show spatial changes in the position of the bone structures as a modification in the two-dimensional pictures (□ Fig. 63-1).

The repositioning of the fragsments can so be controlled radiation-free and followed in real-time. A further step to approximate virtual fluoroscopy to the realistic is the representation of three-dimensional implants as three-dimensional in two-dimensional figures mentioned earlier. For this purpose, a virtual 3D representation based on the virtual X-ray is created. Using information from the two-dimensional level, the position of the radiation source and the image amplifier, a virtual space is created, in which the surgical object, i. e. the bone structure is shown, and the position of the instruments and implants is determined in relation to it [2].

Dynamisation of C-Arm Pictures

After the development of this software module and the implementation of the instruments and different implants as three-dimensional structures, the module was first tested on plastic models (Synbone). The fractures were, as a standard, created at the transition from the middle to the distal third of a tibia model. In the first step, a reference base with LED markers was affixed under the intraoperative site in the proximal and distal fragment. Single C-arm pictures were taken in 2 planes each, proximally, distally and in the fracture zone. The pictures were loaded into the navigation system and, depending to the mode chosen, cylinders were formed around the bone structures semi automatically segmented at the fracture region on the computer monitor.

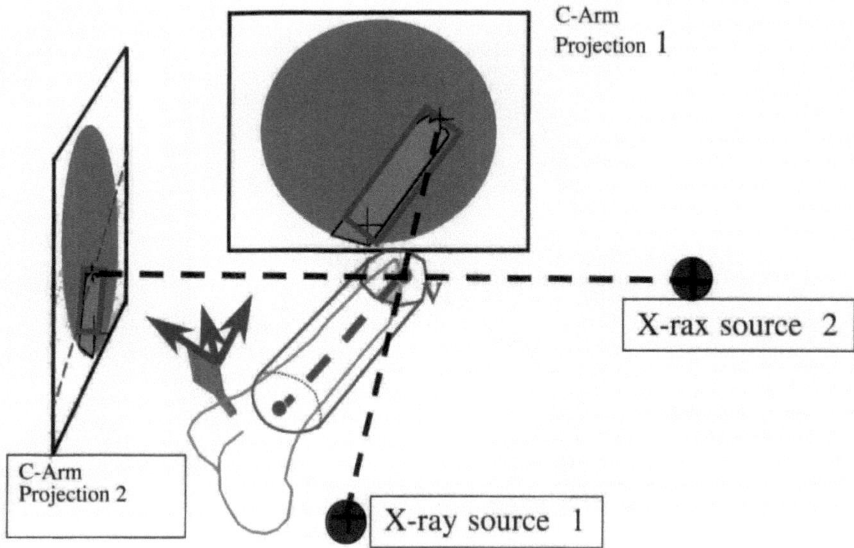

□ **Fig. 63-1.** Virtual three-dimensional space from 2D X-ray projections

First, the fracture reduction was visually checked by the so achieved dynamisation of the X-rays using the representation of the virtual reduction and dynamisation of the pictures. In the next step, the tests were repeated with foam-encased models and the fractures stabilized by a virtually controlled osteosynthesis with plates passed through under the foam coating. Here the trials of the entire reduction maneuver could be carried out under navigation conditions without further radiation. To check the accuracy at the end of the test phase, a series of C-arm shots with still affixed reference bases were taken and loaded into the system. So it was directly possible to check the result between X-ray projections of the implant, the dynamic reduction and the actual result of reduction. The plastic foam was subsequently removed for further visual examination [2] (□ Fig. 63-2).

Measurement of the Real Femur Antetorsion Angle

Due to the accurate mathematical relationship of the registered fluoroscopy images in three-dimensional space, geometrical analysis to this imaging information is possible. This is clinically relevant for defining angle degrees in torsion measurement. CT-based measurement has established itself as a standard method for determining the femur torsion angle. The high radiation dose and the lack of intraoperative availability are unfavorable factors for osteosynthesis or derotating osteotomies. Using referenced, calibrated C-arm pictures it is possible to define anatomical landmarks in bone structures. The navigation system can measure the angle between two defined lines in these pictures with a mathematical algorithm.

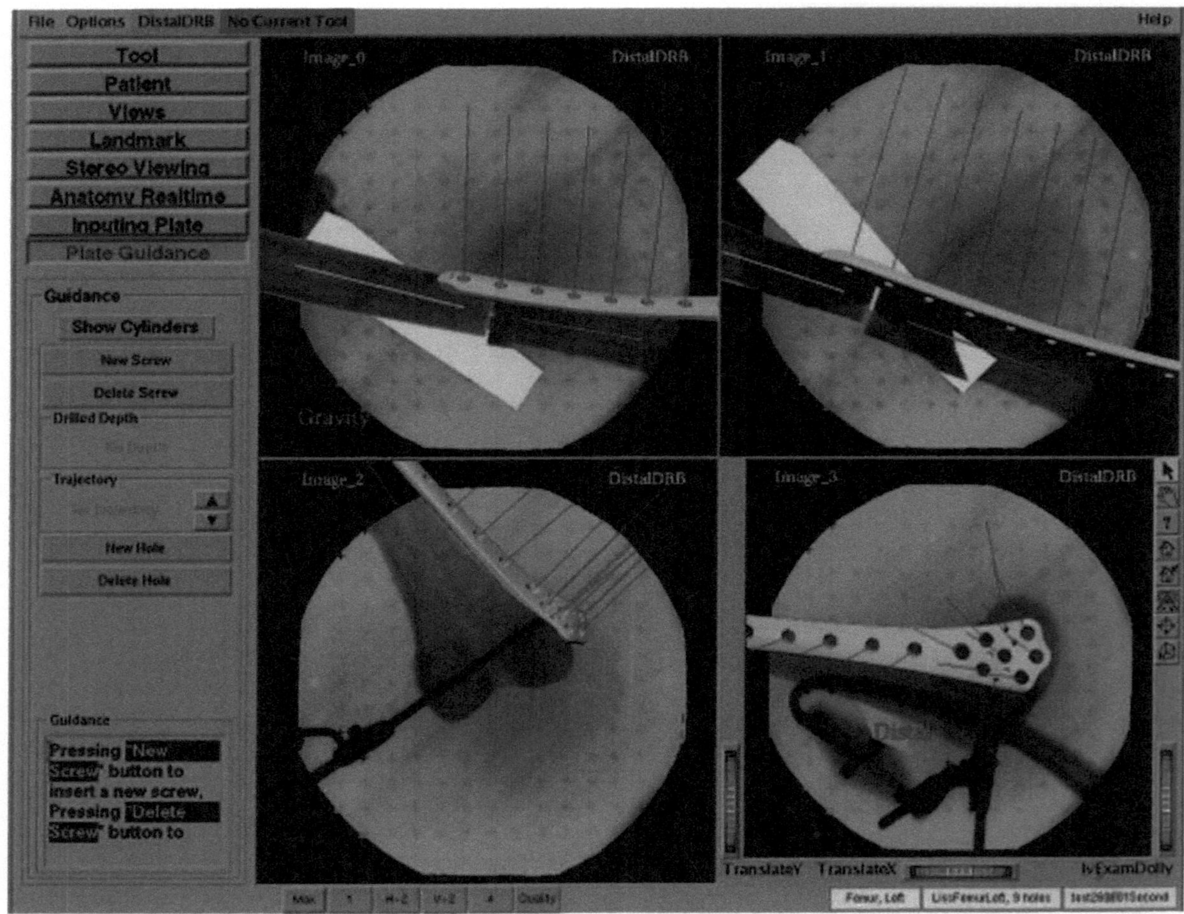

□ **Fig. 63-2.** User interface with representation of the X-ray dynamisation and three-dimensional visualization of the implant

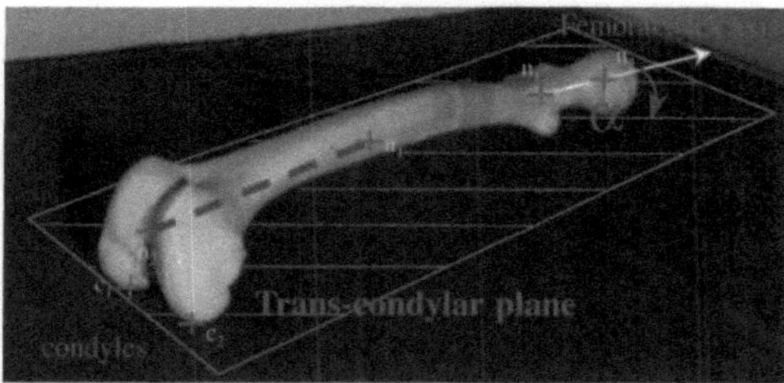

◘ Fig. 63-3. Measuring points for the determination of the real femur antetorsion angle

The fluoroscopy-based, navigated determination of the femur antetorsion angle is a statistically significant reproducible method of measurement. The reproducibility on models corresponds to that of conventional CT measurements. With this method it is possible to check intraoperatively both corrective osteotomies and osteosynthesis of the femur in regard to antetorsion and to compare results with the healthy side (◘ Fig. 63-3).

Clinical Use

With LISS, we have an osteosynthesis procedure, which allows a minimally invasive stabilization of the fragments with **metaphyseal** problem fractures. LISS is best compared to an internal fixator. The problem lies in the need for an accurate operation technology with minimal room for error and does not permit conventional »buttressing reduction by the plate«, but allows the implant to lie perfectly in the convexivity of the bone. The goals of the development of the LISS navigation were on the one hand the X-ray-free check of the reduction process in navigated C-arm pictures (virtual fluoroscopy), on the other hand the three-dimensional representation of instruments and implants in these pictures with a reduction in the size of the problems specified above.

After successful laboratory testing, the module could be implemented into the existing navigation system. This technology with LISS was first clinically used in the BG Trauma Centre for osteosynthesis. In a first step, one reference base with LED markers was affixed on both the proximal and distal main fragments. After acquisition of C-arm pictures in 2 planes each proximally, distally and within the fracture area, a reduction of the fracture and

stabilization of the bone was carried out. With the help of the virtual cylinders from different X-rays, a structure with similar bone volume was created. The X-rays can be dynamized and the reduction process can thus be checked without further radiation.

The implants, including the LISS plates, screws and instruments, are compared three-dimensionally to virtual X-rays, realistically adjusted and represented in real-time. Both the insertion of the plate as well as the fixation with screws including the drilling process and linear measurement could be navigated. As an accuracy check, C-arm pictures were taken of the fracture area in two planes and stored in the system, taking care to leave the reference bases still affixed at the bone and the plate. Thus we could ensure the alignment between X-ray shadows and the implant position as visualized by the navigation system. All 4 navigated interventions displayed the correct reduction of the fracture and positioning of the plate at first attempt. A disadvantage would be the unfamiliar operation of the software and the need for an additional operator at the navigation system.

Summary

Navigation systems are spreading rapidly in trauma and orthopedic operating rooms. This technology does not make an inexperienced surgeon an expert, but gives the experienced surgeon a helpful instrument to improve both the procedure and the quality of results and to reduce in particular the possibility of outliers. The experience in our hospital shows that only the consistent use of navigation, in complex and standard cases, leads to an increasing acceptance and a broader application of this system with increasing confidence and safety in its technical execution. Only the future will show whether a direct profit for the patient can be obtained using this technology, and also whether a socioeconomic effect can be achieved by a decrease of the complication rate.

The navigation systems themselves and their software applications are subject to rapid growth with the goal of improved user interfaces, minimal changes in existing operating room flow and, of course, by the development of more economical systems, in finding a broader application.

The goals of the improvements are the simplification of the intraoperative setup, the improvement of the image quality and the adaptation of the instruments to the navigation technology. The potential of these techniques appears enormous and already proves to possess advantages such a decrease in the intraoperative radiation dose, more precise operation techniques and thus more safety for the patients.

By way of the navigated LISS osteosynthesis, the disadvantages of the minimally invasive procedure could be crucially reduced by visualization, the repositioning, the placement and the adjustment of the implant.

References

1. Foley KT, Simon DA, Rampersaud YR (2001) Virtual fluoroscopy: computer-assisted fluoroscopic navigation. Spine 26: 347–351
2. Grützner PA, Vock B, Zheng G, Kowal J, Nolte L, Wentzensen A (2001) Minimal invasive, computerassistierte Plattenosteosynthese bei Frakturen langer Röhrenknochen. Unfallchirurg 283: 160
3. Hofstetter R, Slomczykowski M, Krettek C, Koppen G, Sati M, Nolte LP (1999) Computer-assisted fluoroscopy-based reduction of femoral fractures and antetorsion correction. Comput Aided Surg 5: 311–325
4. Hofstetter R, Slomczykowski M, Sati M, Nolte LP (1999) Fluoroscopy as an imaging means for computer-assisted surgical navigation. Comput Aided Surg 4: 65–76
5. Nolte LP, Slomczykowski MA, Berlemann U et al. (2000) A new approach to computer-aided spine surgery: fluoroscopy-based surgical navigation. Eur Spine J 9 [Suppl 1]: S78–S88
6. Rampersaud YR, Foley KT, Shen AC, Williams S, Solomito M (2000) Radiation exposure to the spine surgeon during fluoroscopically assisted pedicle screw insertion. Spine 25: 2637–2645
7. Slomczykowski M, Hofstetter R, Burquin I, Nolte LP, Synder M (1998) The method of computer-assisted orthopedic surgery based on two-dimensional fluoroscopy: the principles of action. Chir Narzadow Ruchu Ortop Pol 63: 443–450
8. Slomczykowski MA, Hofstetter R, Sati M, Krettek C, Nolte LP (2001) Novel computer-assisted fluoroscopy system for intraoperative guidance: feasibility study for distal locking of femoral nails. J Orthop Trauma 15: 122–131

64 Pelvic Osteotomy with Template Navigation

H.-W. Staudte, E. Schkommodau, M. Honscha, F. Portheine, K. Radermacher

Introduction

Various surgical techniques are used for the treatment of hip dysplasia in young people and adults. In contrast to acetabuloplasty in children, the position of the complete acetabulum is corrected. The repositioning serves to enlarge the weight bearing zone of the dysplastic acetabulum covering the femoral head, in order to reduce pressure on this area to physiological levels. The major goals of this therapy are relief from pain as well as preventing premature osteoarthritis with the necessity for artificial hip replacement. The basics of the biomechanics as well as diagnosis and indications are described and discussed in detail elsewhere [9, 11]. Apart from the triple osteotomy according to Tönnis, practiced by our clinic since more than 15 years, particular mention should be made of the periacetabular osteotomy technique described by Ganz [3]. In contrast, the spherical osteotomy procedure of Wagner [12] has not become established due to the danger of acetabular necrosis.

Following the procedures of Tönnis, the acetabulum is mobilized by three pelvic osteotomies that must be performed in defined positions and orientations in relation to the acetabulum. Too short a distance from the acetabulum leads to an increased risk of avascular necrosis, but if the acetabulum fragment becomes too large it impedes the free rotation necessary for repositioning. Moreover, the inclination of the cut planes influences the ability to freely rotate the fragment in a specific direction. This also applies, if the situation arises, to a desired translation particularly in the medial direction (see [11]). According to Tönnis, as a measure for the surface coverage of the femur head, LCE (lateral center edge) and ACE (anterior center edge) angles should be close to 30–35°. The additional use of CT image data is also recommended since it enables more accurate and reliable assessment of the individual anatomical and biomechanical conditions [1, 2, 4, 5, 6, 11].

Operative Procedure

The operative procedure closely follows the technique described by Tönnis and Kalchschmidt. The ischial osteotomy is performed via a dorsal approach with the patient in lateral position. It must proceed at a distance of ca. 10–20 mm from the acetabulum, starting from the ischiadic sulcus from the dorsolateral basis of the ischiadic spine, cranial to the sacrospinal ligaments, while preserving the sciatic nerve, to the obturator foramen below the posterior obturator tubercle. After closing the wound, the patient is laid in supine position. The lateral position in contrast to the earlier prone position of the patient allows faster repositioning of the patient without complete renewal of sterile covers.

The pubic osteotomy is carried out via a ventral approach at a distance of about 14–20 mm from the acetabulum. It is a relatively short and simple to perform osteotomy running transversal to the obturator foramen, whereby preserving the blood vessels/nerve fibers the inclination must also be adjusted in two planes in order to enable a medialisation of the joint if necessary. This inclination as well as the possibilities of fixation using screws and/or plates can be determined and checked in the planning, however, in general the precision when performing this osteotomy is less critical.

The iliac osteotomy is the longest and most difficult osteotomy and has the greatest effect on the rotational mobility of the acetabular fragment and the initial stability of the fixation. For manipulation and repositioning of the acetabulum a Schanz screw has to be fixed as a »handle« on the acetabular fragment, whereby the screw axis must be placed parallel to the iliac osteotomy at a defined distance (ca. 7–10 mm) from the acetabular fragment and osteotomy plane. Thin Kirschner wires are placed parallel and vertical to the Schanz screw (parallel to the osteotomy plane) in the fixed part of the iliac and serve as a reference for the repositioning of the acetabular fragment.

Following the recommendations of Kalchschmidt/Dortmund, Germany, release of the M. glutaeus medius from the lateral pelvic wall has to be avoided the iliac osteotomy is carried out from medial [11]. The osteotomy is planned and carried out between the inferior and superior iliac spine and positioned at a minimal distance of 20 mm from the acetabulum running towards the ischial notch, whereby the inclination (i. e. descending slightly in a medial direction) must take the planned repositioning and fixation into consideration. The necessary inclination particularly in the sagittal direction varies considerably in individual cases and can be optimally defined using 3D planning taking into consideration the boundary conditions mentioned above (see below).

After carrying out the osteotomies the acetabular fragment is rotated according to the planned angles. The angle measurement between the reference wires and the Schanz screw is carried out using a simple goniometer. Subsequently, a bone fragment is removed from the iliac crest as an autologous transplant and inserted between the ilium and the acetabular fragment. Fixation is achieved with 4–5 Kirschner wires or with screws. After an X-ray control, withdrawal and closing of the wound follow.

Computer-Assisted Planning

For the computer-based planning CT-image sequences are prepared using a standard protocol with 30–40 images and slice distances of 3–4 mm, including one anteroposterior (a.p.) topogram (»pilotscan«). The images are transferred from the radiology department through a DICOM interface, via ISDN, network or CD-ROM to the planning PC-workstation[1].

[1] Minimum requirements: PC-Pentium II or higher with 450 MHz, 128 MB RAM, Windows NT 4.0 or 2000 or XP, 1024x768 resolution 64 k color graphics, color inkjet printer

The computer-based planning session starts with the selection of the patient's data set. The three-dimensional reconstruction of the bone structure is generated automatically. It can be checked by the surgeon with reference to the sectional images and 3D views and modified if necessary. Image analysis and measurement functions are available at all times as additional options.

After selecting the type of intervention (here triple repositioning osteotomy according to Tönnis) and the affected hip (left/right), the user is guided step by step through the surgical planning session according to established surgical guidelines. Additional instructions and explanations provide information about each required entry or action. An entire planning session normally lasts a maximum of 5 min. The user can scroll forwards or backwards through the planning process on demand allowing previous actions and settings to be checked or corrected if necessary in the case of complex anatomical or pathological situations.

Since the measurements given by Tönnis for lateral center edge and anterior center edge angles represent a standard reference, LCE and ACE angles are also included here as comparison values. In the first step integral projections of the affected hip in a.p. and faux-profile planes are automatically reconstructed by the system from the CT data. Using these artificial biplanar X-ray images, the center and radius of the femoral head and acetabulum as well as the ACE and LCE angles are determined using predefined virtual measuring tools (◘ Fig. 64-1). Here, the eccentricity of the femur head can also be evaluated, which if extreme can present a contraindication for a triple osteotomy.

In the next step the system presents a 3D frontal view and a lateral control view on demand. The user can alter the direction of the view as required. The operator can now set a safety margin for which the system automatically defines a corresponding spherical safety zone and automatically generates osteotomy planes tangential to this sphere (◘ Fig. 64-2). Apart from the protection of the acetabulum, this guarantees optimal rotational mobility.

Following this the surgeon can adjust the inclination of the osteotomy in transverse and sagittal planes and can control this osteotomy in various 3D views as well as through a secondary CT grey level cut plane corresponding to the osteotomy plane.

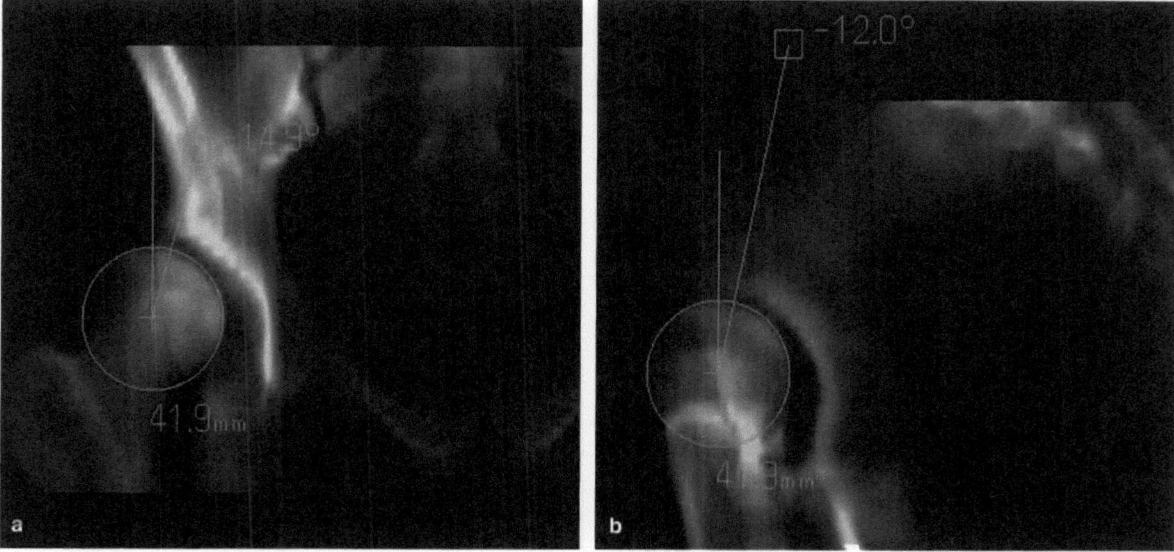

Fig. 64-1a,b. Measurement of **a** LCE and **b** ACE angle on reconstructed integral projections

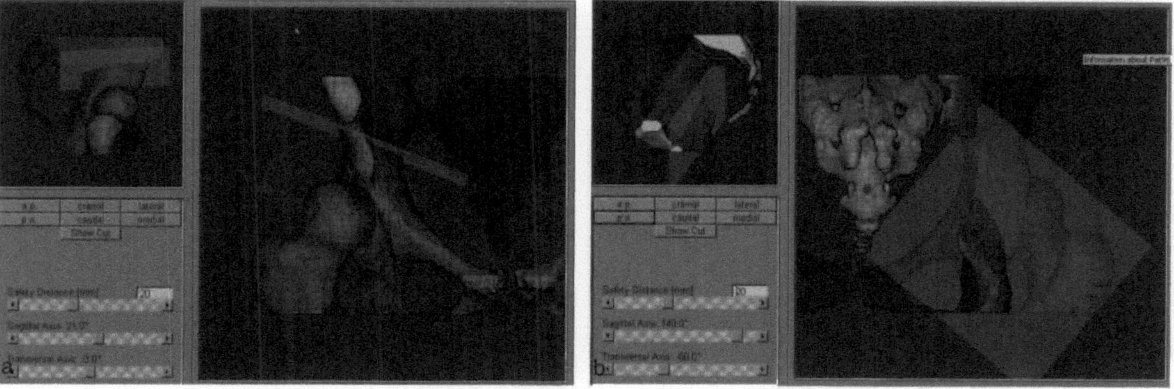

Fig. 64-2a,b. The osteotomy planes (**a** ilium, **b** ischium) are automatically defined as tangential planes of a sphere at a safe distance from the acetabulum. The safety zone and inclination of the osteotomy planes can be adjusted by the user

The planning of the pubic and ischial osteotomy is carried out in the same way, whereby in each case the system provides the optimal 3D views as well as standardized pre-positioned osteotomy planes based on statistical case data that are then adjusted by the planning surgeon to the individual anatomical situation.

Interactive manipulation of the acetabular fragment can be simulated by the surgeon in the transverse and sagittal planes (**Fig. 64-3**). The resulting LCE and ACE angles are calculated and displayed automatically. In addition, the original starting values calculated from the artificial X-ray images are shown and can be com-pared with the corrected values. Planning sessions carried out together with orthopedic surgeons showed that due to the complex spatial structure of the bony acetabular rim, both angles cannot be independently defined by rotation around single axis. The corresponding study concerning the influence of the manipulation angle on the resulting LCE and ACE angle was published by our group elsewhere [6]. Taking these facts into consideration, planning based on biplanar X-ray images alone is in practice almost impossible. In contrast, CT-image-based 3D planning allows spatial analysis of the individual situation.

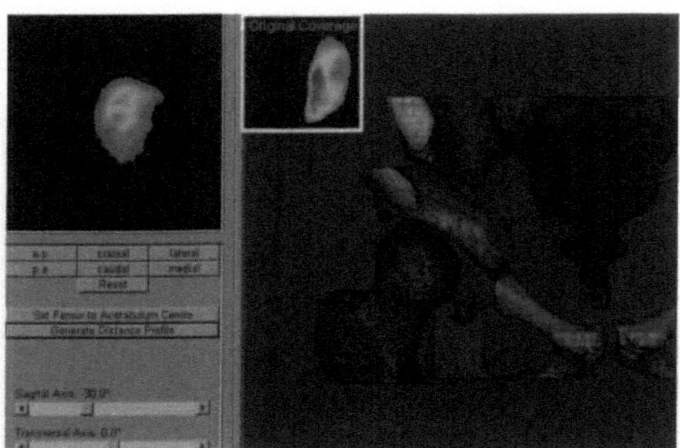

Fig. 64-3. Simulation of the repositioning and the resulting coverage of the femoral head (*above left*) vs. the original coverage (*insert at the right*); automatic calculation of LCE and ACE angles resulting from the repositioning

The resulting ACE and LCE angle correction as well as the intraoperative correction angles to be adjusted in transversal and sagittal planes are automatically documented by the system. Moreover, potential collisions between bone fragments that may possibly impede rotation are analyzed. Also, fixation options for the bone fragments in the area of the iliac and pubic cut can be checked and strategically planned accordingly using freely selected 3D views. The planning and simulation on the 3D data set decisively supports any possible cut optimization that might be necessary. Changes of leg lengths resulting from the repositioning and manipulation can also be simulated. Biomechanical need for a medialisation of the joint can be checked beforehand.

In the last planning step the surgeon decides for which cuts they will prepare an individual template. For the pubic cut planning and simulation of the cut inclination with 3D data is very helpful, however, intraoperative implementation requires no precise guidance using a template. With respect to the ischial osteotomy analyses using anatomical preparations as well as initial clinical studies have also shown here that 3D planning and checking of the osteotomies' position and orientation together with the identification of corresponding anatomical landmarks on the individual 3D model provide the major support. The optimal adjustment for carrying out the osteotomy is generally represented by the shortest connecting line between the sulcus ischiadicus and the foramen obturatorium, parallel to the S. ischiadicus. This assumption is verified in the 3D planning and can then be implement-

ed during the operation using an optimal adjustment of Homann hooks inserted at the obturator foramen. A universal cut guide has also been developed for the corresponding alignment of this osteotomy (Radermacher 1999).

The iliac osteotomy is, as already mentioned, the longest, and due to the large variation in individual anatomy, also the most difficult osteotomy with the greatest effect on the mobility of the acetabular fragment. Therefore, here we always use an individual template. The type and size of a suitable template can be selected from a database. The system automatically aligns the chosen template to the osteotomy plane so that the user only has to slide the template along the osteotomy plane to the desired position. For the iliac cut it has been shown that the choice of contact surfaces in the upper front area of the ilium (spina iliaca anterior superior) from the medial side and above the cutting plane allows a reliable and safe referencing through a minimal surgical access.

The contact surfaces (»impression or molded area«) of the template on the bone are indicated semi-transparent (green) so that the user can check the positioning area of the template on the 3D model (**Fig. 64-4**).

In order to be able to place this template exactly in this planned position on the bone during the intervention, at the press of a button an exact fit of this 3D impression of the contact surfaces is automatically milled in a blank template of polycarbonate within 5–10 min. Similar to a 3D printer, this is done by a 3D desktop milling device connected to the DISOS system (Radermacher 1999). The customized templates are subsequently autoclaved for 5–20 min (134 °C) and are then available for surgery. A protocol of the entire planning session is produced automatically and the documentation together with the corresponding images can be saved and optionally printed out at the end of the planning session.

Intraoperative Approach Using Individual Templates

Intraoperatively, no cameras or computer systems are necessary. Thus, there is no adjustment of cameras, fixing of reference frames and referencing of bone structures as necessary in the case of conventional freehand navigation system. The patient and instruments are prepared in the usual way. In addition to the planning information stored

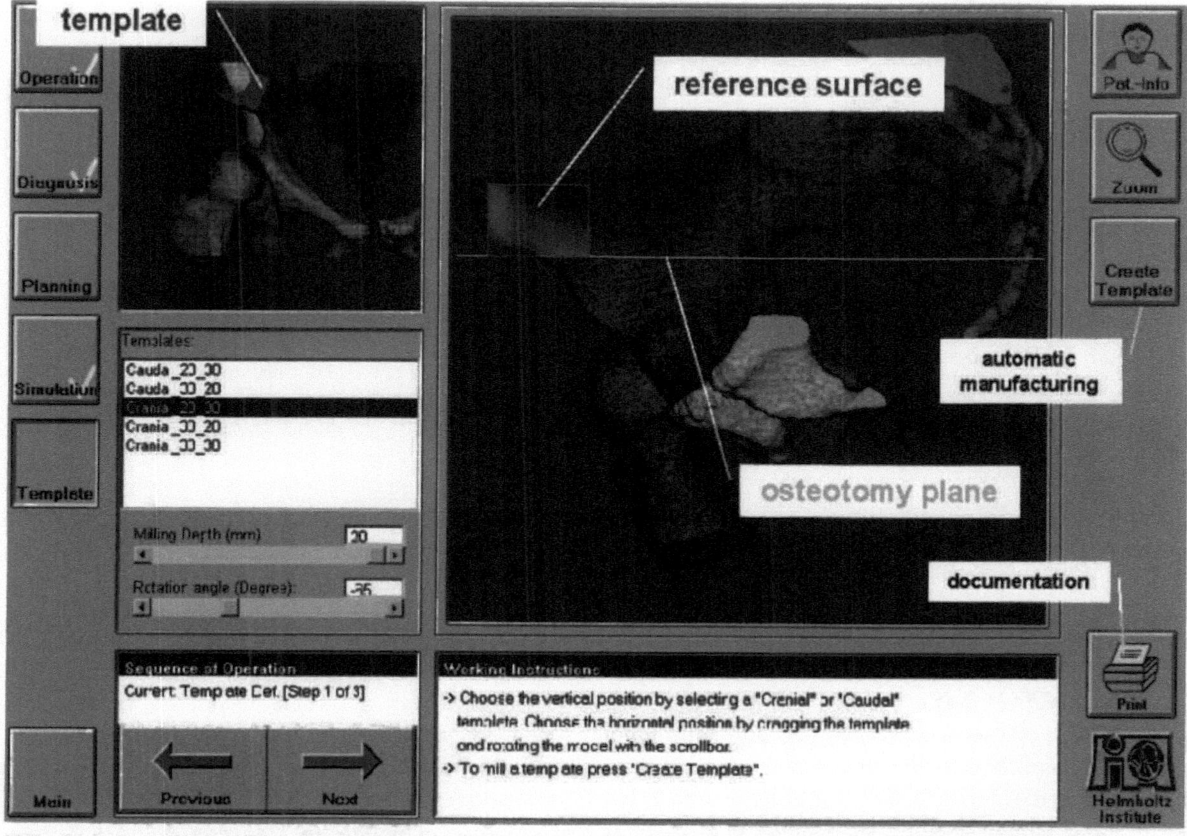

Fig. 64-4. Determination of template position and reference plane at the inner iliac crest

in the template, optional color printouts are also available as planning documentation with 3D views of the positioning, orientation and correct angles to be adjusted in transversal and sagittal planes.

The ischial and pubic osteotomies are carried out in the conventional manner described, if necessary with additional help from the 3D planning images. A template for the ischial cut is generally not required. Also access to the ilium in the osteotomy area is achieved from the medial side in a conventional manner. The individually fitting ilium template is placed on the selected area from the medial direction on the bone. The unambiguous fit of the individual contact surface generated during the preoperative planning session ensures that the established position and orientation can be found again in an intuitive way, in other words the template can be adjusted to the precise pre-defined position due to the perfect fit of the »3D impression«.

The template is optionally fixed with a bone pin. The tool guide can also be mounted or changed with the inserted bone pin. Using these references, instruments, osteotomies or bone fragments can be aligned exactly in the operating site without further computerized aids or loss of time. After fixing the template the Schanz screw as well as the Kirschner wires are introduced parallel to the reference plane defined by the template. Following an optional X-ray control, the osteotomy is carried out using a jigsaw along the cutting guide of the template. The last third of the osteotomy is completed if necessary with a chisel, again along the template guide. The repositioning is performed in the conventional way, whereby the planned and documented positioning angle is checked using a simple goniometer in the sagittal and transversal plane with respect to the Kirschner wires. Following another control X-ray and fixing of the acetabular fragment the surgeon withdraws and closes the wound(Fig. 64-5).

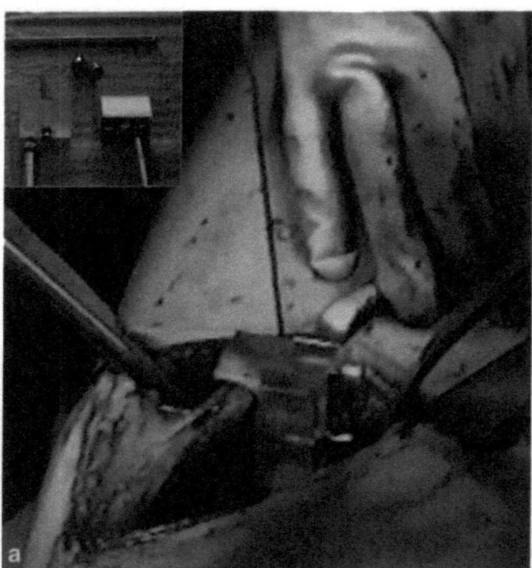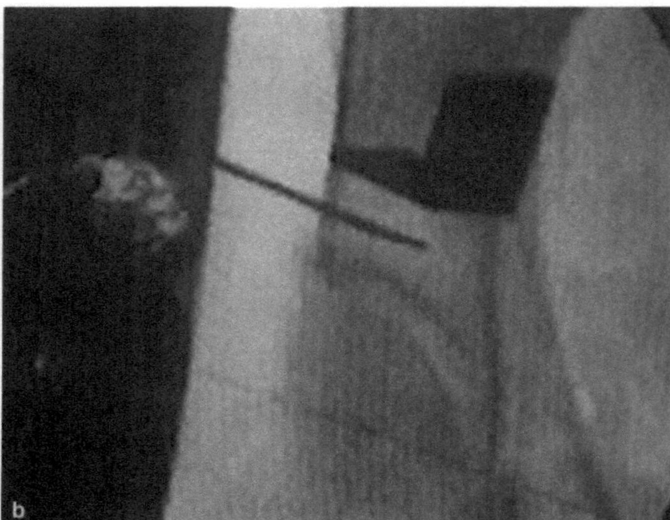

◘ Fig. 64-5a,b. Intraoperative guidance. **a** Sterile instrument set with individual template made out of polycarbonate, optional bone pins and screw-on guiding plates (*above left*); the positioned template shows the osteotomy plane; **b** control X-ray image.

Clinical Results

In a retrospective study a total of 34 triple repositioning osteotomies, carried out between 1997 and 2001 under the same conditions, were completely documented and reinvestigated. This particularly concerned a uniform lateral/supine patient position, the reduced medial access to the ilium as well as the use of a new jig saw, conditions that – to our experience – also considerably influenced the operation time. Neither the planning system nor the template blanks used for the computer-assisted cases were further modified functionally in the time period under observation. In contrast to previously reported analyses, the amount of experience – one surgeon had over 15 years of specific operating experience (>150 interventions), and two were less experienced (<30 interventions) – was taken into account in this type of operation. 10 operations were carried out in a conventional manner (K group) and 24 operations with computer-assisted preoperative planning and preparation of individual ilium templates (C group). These cases included a total of 32 female and 2 male patients between the ages of 11 and 49 (K: 13–36 vs. C: 11–49). The average body mass index (BMI) in both groups was about 22–23 and showed no significant differences. However, retrospectively we found a significant age difference (K: Ø 19 years old, vs. C: Ø 31 years old) between the groups ($p<0.05$). From a retro-

spective point of view this situation most likely resulted from the fact that the indication for CT imaging with young patients was initially more diffident and restricted to more complex cases. From today's standpoint we recommend the general use of CT imaging with modern multi-layer spiral CTs due to the advantages of a computer-supported planning and guided positioning. The age difference was analyzed further in the evaluation of the results. This showed no significant dependence on age concerning the investigated criteria (OP-time, hospital stay, etc., see below). Therefore the age difference between the groups could be neglected in the further evaluation of the operative technique.

In addition to the Harris hip score and the score according to Merle d'Aubigné, the clinical investigations included the operation time, the intraoperative X-ray exposure time and loss of blood as well as the length of hospitalization. The results are summarized in ◘ Table 64-1.

Comparisons show that the use of individual templates can achieve a highly significant reduction in the average operation time of over 23% ($p<0.005$). Whereas the reduction in operation time was highly significant regardless of the experience level of the surgeon, the X-ray time of the **experienced** surgeons was significantly reduced, almost by 70% (40.7 s vs. 13.5 s; $p<0.05$). The reasons for this are improved preoperative planning and planning documentation of all osteotomies, optimal

Table 64-1. Comparison between conventional and computer-assisted procedures

	Conventional (K); (n=10)	Computer- and template-supported (C); (n=24)
Duration of operation [min]	150.9	115.8
Intraoperative X-ray time [s]	30.9	21.4
Loss of blood [ml]	783.3	641.3
Hospital stay [days]	22.9	18.4

positioning of the ilium osteotomy plane at the first attempt with a single X-ray control, and consistent use of the individual template as a reference for further working steps as well as in searching for better mobility of the acetabulum. In contrast, the less experienced surgeons needed an unchanged, high number of control X-rays, particularly for carrying out of the ischiadic cut, so perhaps for less experienced surgeons an individual template for this osteotomy would also be helpful. Therefore, reduced X-ray time independent of experience (see Table 64.1) amounted to only 30% and was not significant ($p>0.05$). Blood loss was independent of experience and with the computer-supported planning and template guidance was marginally, although not significantly reduced. Similarly independent of the surgeon's experience was the reduction in the time spent in hospital by the computer and template-supported patients in comparison with the conventional group by about 19% (ca. 4 days; $p<0.05$). Since uniform criteria concerning the general conditions and mobility of the patient were the basis for release from hospital, retrospectively establishing reasons for this observed reduction in hospital stay required further investigation. First, one cause may relate to the fact that a slightly larger entry area was chosen in the conventional technique, with greater detachment of the adductor muscles for a better overview in situ, which could influence the postoperative pain situation of the patients. A second suggestion is that improved planning achieves improved mobility and also refixing of the acetabular fragment. The evaluation of post-operative X-ray images hints at improved primary fixation. However, these hypotheses must be re-examined by further investigations.

The clinical follow-up of the patients after about 6 months (due to organizational reasons retrospective cases were also partially examined later) showed no significant differences between the two groups. However, for the experienced surgeon in group C a tendency towards a clear improvement in the Harris hip score as well as the Merle d'Aubigne score could be seen ($p>0.05$).

Discussion

Investigations with orthopedic and medical students with no specific technical pre-knowledge or experience with the work concept involved in the planning and production system DISOS[2] showed that following an introduction lasting on average 15 min all the test persons could use the planning system completely autonomously. The planning possibilities using three-dimensional reconstruction of CT data allowed a better overview of the individual anatomical situation, improved planning of osteotomies for which no template were produced, planning and simulation of the required repositioning, as well as evaluation of the fixation options for the acetabular fragment. In general, a planning session lasts about 2–5 min. The option of autonomously producing the template with the integrated milling device corresponds in complexity to printing out a document, and after positioning the blank it runs fully automatically even in the absence of the user (in about 5–20 min – according to each template type and number, for TKE/triple/pedicle). Very little effort is involved in this »navigation option« and during the operation absolutely no changes in conventional procedures are necessary.

According to our own experiences, although involving considerably higher intraoperative effort compared to the template technique, freehand X-ray-based navigation systems, particularly in traumatology and especially vertebrae surgery, offer several advantages with respect to flexibility of intraoperative planning as well as percutaneous applications. In orthopedics, no percutaneous applications are possible with the template technique. However, interventions which can be planned such as the triple osteotomy with a need for three-dimensional analysis and optimization of the individual strategies and biome-

____

[2] Desktop Imageprocessing System for Orthopaedic Surgery (DISOS)

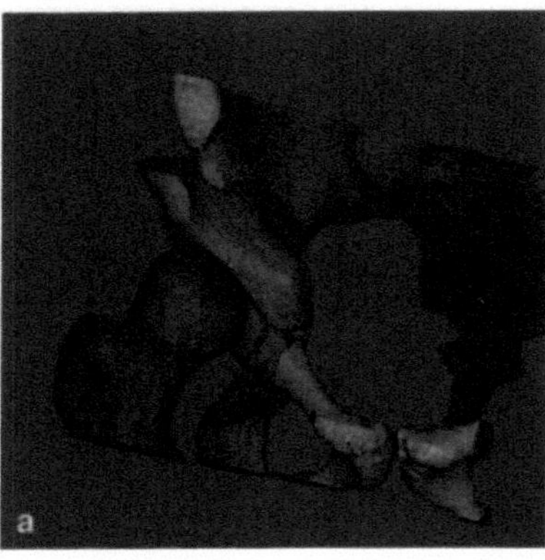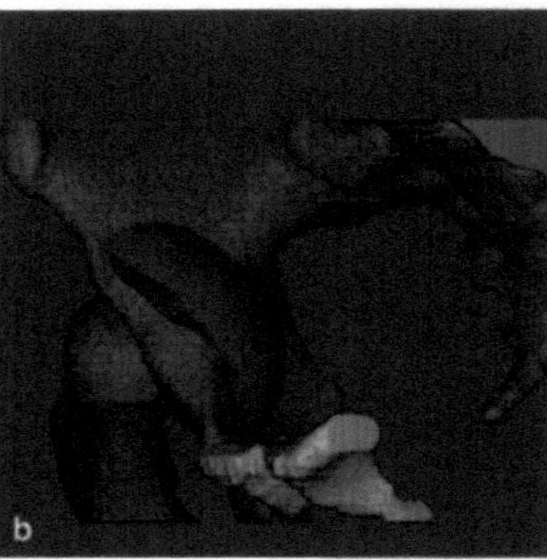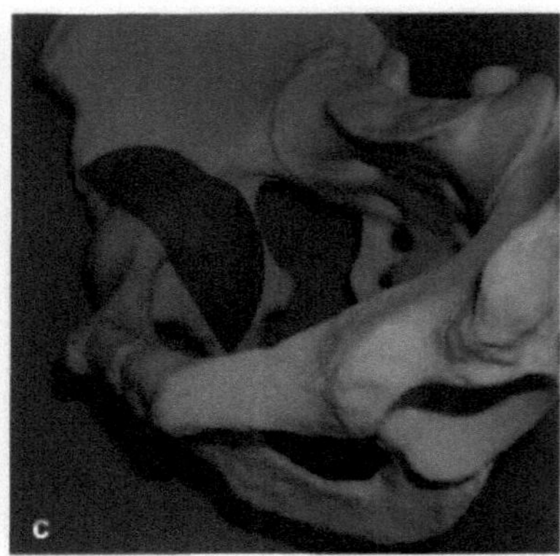

Fig. 64-6a-c. Study for a novel spherical repositioning osteotomy: (from left to right) Simulation of the repositioning according to a spherical osteotomy concentric to the acetabulum center; definition of a spherical individual template positioned concentric to the acetabulum (a dorsal bony pillar is preserved); laboratory model of a spherical template automatically produced in a rapid prototyping process (the center of the sphere is located at the center of the acetabulum, the radius is 16 mm larger than the related radius of the acetabulum)

chanics, particularly in the case of deformities deviating from the normal case, the CT-based 3D planning represents an extremely important and highly recommendable alternative or complementary method. An extended 3D biometry option is in preparation. Planning requires a standard desktop computer. The optional template can be produced autonomously by a connected computer controlled milling unit, or alternatively if required, requested via network or floppy disc from a service provider. The fixed costs are minimal, and costs per operation pay for themselves through savings in operation time alone, which also clearly benefits the patients. Furthermore, the reduction in intraoperative X-ray time and the related irradiation load on the operating team must be taken into consideration (Radermacher 1999). We think, that CT imaging with modern spiral CT systems together with the improved planning and implementation options, in comparison to the conventional operation-associated risks, can be fully justified and highly recommended.

Perspectives

Future perspectives suggest the possibility of investigating new osteotomy concepts. Figure 64-6 shows a study of a spherical osteotomy, where the osteotomies are carried out from the medial direction at a safe distance from the acetabulum, comparable to a Tönnis or Ganz osteotomy, with a flat or small spherical chisel (alternatively also a

special saw). In contrast to a Wagner osteotomy, only a thin bone layer needs to be cut from the medial side and the osteotomy is located at a safe distance from the acetabulum. With LCE and ACE angles >0° and no necessity for medialisation, this osteotomy could be carried out through a single surgical access. It would offer the advantage of an optimal mobilization, pure compression load (no primary shear stresses) in the osteotomy surfaces in the area of the ilium and ischium, and a potential corresponding simplification of refixation and primary stability. This concept should be thoroughly investigated in the future. Based on our experience to date, this new type of osteotomy potentially could be optimally applied using the computer assisted planning and individual template technique.

References

1. Abel MF, Sutherland DH, Wenger DR et al. (1994) Evaluation of CT scans and 3D reformatted images for quantitative assessment of the hip. J Pediatric Orthop 14: 48–53
2. Brunner R, Robb J (1996) Inaccuracy of the migration percentage and center-edge angle in predicting femoral head displacement in cerebral palsy. J Pediatr Orthop 5: 239–241
3. Ganz R, Klaue K, Vinh TS, Mast JW (1988) A new periacetabular osteotomy for the treatment of hip dysplasia. Technique and preliminary results. Clin Orthop 232: 26–36
4. Klaue K, Wallin A, Ganz R (1988) CT-Evaluation of coverage and congruency of the hip prior to osteotomy. Clin Orthop 232: 15–25
5. Millis MB, Murphy SB (1992) Use of computed tomographic reconstruction in planning osteotomies of the hip. Clin Orthop 274: 154–159

6. Portheine F, Radermacher K, Staudte H-W (2000) Potentiale der CT-basierten Planung und schablonengestützten Ausführung in der Hüft- und Kniechirurgie. Orthop Praxis 12: 786–791

7. Radermacher K, Portheine F, Anton M et al. (1998) Computer assisted orthopaedic surgery with image-based individual templates. Clin Orthop 354: 28–38

8. Radermacher K (1999) Computerunterstützte Operationsplanung und -ausführung mittels individueller Bearbeitungsschablonen in der Orthopädie. Berichte aus der Biomedizinischen Technik, Bd 7. Shaker, Aachen

9. Tönnis D (1984) Die angeborene Hüfdysplasie und Hüftluxation im Kindes und Erwachsenenalter. Springer, Berlin Heidelberg New York Tokyo

10. Tönnis D, Arning A, Bloch M, Heinecke A, Kalchschmidt K (1994) Triple pelvic osteotomy. J Pediatr Orthop 3: 54–67

11. Tönnis D, Kalchschmidt K, Heinecke A (1999) Die Hüftpfannenschwenkung durch Dreifachosteotomie des Beckens – Stellenwert und Indikation in der Vielfalt operativer Korrekturen der Dysplasiehüfte. Orthop Praxis 10: 607–620

12. Wagner H, Wagner M (1984) Rekonstruktive Operationen an der Hüfte. In: Bauer R, Kerschbaumer F, Poisel S (Hrsg) Orthopädische Operationslehre, Bd. II/1. Thieme, Stuttgart New York

VI Navigation: Spinal Surgery

65 Fundamentals in Spinal Surgery

R. Rao, M. Singrakhia

The past thirty years have seen an evolution of spine surgery from limited decompressive procedures to extensive spinal reconstruction, involving multilevel decompressions, fusions, and instrumentation. With a better understanding of spinal anatomy, pathology and the biomechanics of the spine and instrumentation systems, surgical options in the spine are constantly growing. The aim of this chapter is to review the essential concepts in spine surgery, and evaluate conventional surgical techniques.

Anatomic Basis of Spine Surgery

An understanding of the anatomy of the spinal column and neural structures facilitates surgical decision-making, improves techniques, and reduces complications. This section deals with the relevant anatomy in commonly used surgical approaches to the spine, with an emphasis on anatomic concerns in these regions.

Cervical Spine

The anterior approach to the cervical spine is through the plane between the sternocleidomastoid muscle and the carotid sheath laterally and the strap muscles with tracheoesophageal viscera on the medial side. The approach follows fascial planes, and is generally safe. The recurrent laryngeal nerve is more variable in its course, and hence more likely to be injured on the right side. The vertebral arteries course up the cervical spinal column within the transverse foramina, and are prone to injury during anterior procedures that extend too far laterally. The sympathetic trunk may be more vulnerable to damage during lower cervical approaches, as it is more medially located within the longus colli muscle at the C6 level than it is at C3.

Posterior approaches to the cervical spine attempt to preserve the midline ligamentous structures where possible to avoid the development of adjacent segment instability. In the occipitocervical region the bony landmarks are the external occipital protuberance, superior and inferior nuchal lines, and the external occipital crest, which extends from the protuberance to the foramen magnum. The occipital bone is thicker in the area of the external protuberance and crest, allowing better screw purchase in the midline here. The transverse venous sinus courses intracranially 7 mm superolateral to the external occipital protuberance, and instrumentation should be avoided here [3].

Instrumentation in the subaxial cervical spine is either anteriorly with a plate, posteriorly with pedicle screws, lateral mass screws, wires or laminar hooks. Anterior plates are being increasingly used to provide immediate stability and avoid the need for rigid and prolonged postoperative immobilization. The plates are low profile, with locking screws that are not likely to pull out from the plate and erode through the esophageal wall. Posterior pedicle screw instrumentation is challenging in the cervical spine because of the small size of the pedicles (widths 5–6 mm, heights 7–8 mm) [8]. The lateral mass provides an alternative site for posterior instrumentation, and is bounded by the inferior edges of the inferior facets above and below, medially by a sulcus at the junction with the lamina, and laterally by the lateral edge of the bone. Screws are directed laterally about 20° to avoid the vertebral artery, and superiorly to avoid the exiting nerve root. The lateral mass at C7 is thin, and at this level the pedicle provides a more reliable posterior fixation site. The C2 pedicle is morphologically unique and forms a good anchor for occipitocervical and atlantoaxial operations. Xu et al suggest the C2 pedicle screw be started 5 mm inferior to the superior border of the lamina and

7 mm lateral to the lateral border of the spinal canal. The screw is directed about 35° medially and 20° superiorly. Interspinous wiring is simple, relatively safe, and provides adequate stability for most cases [17].

Thoracic and Lumbar Spine

Anterior access to the upper thoracic spine is generally through a right thoracotomy, to avoid the aortic arch and great vessels. Alternative approaches to the T1–T4 levels include low cervical approaches with resection of the medial clavicle, detachment of the sternal muscles, and partial or complete sternotomy. Anterior exposure of the mid and lower thoracic spine can be achieved through either left or right approaches. Using the left sided approach avoids having to retract the liver or mobilize the large veins. Radicular arteries are ligated close to the aorta when necessary to prevent ischemic injury to the cord. The artery of Adamkiewicz is a large radicular feeder to the spinal cord, and generally lies between T8 and T12 on the left. Ligation of this vessel may result in ischemic cord injury.

Anterior exposure to the lumbar spine is either through a flank or anterior incision. The flank incision lends itself to a left-sided retroperitoneal approach. The peritoneum is gently retracted from the posterior abdominal wall and the lower pole of the left kidney. The aorta, iliac vessels, and segmental vessels are then mobilized to expose the ventrolateral surface of vertebral bodies. Using this approach from the right side requires mobilization of the inferior vena cava, which has a thinner wall and is more difficult to repair in the event of injury. Retroperitoneal access to the lumbar spine can also be obtained through a transverse or vertical anterior incision. The posterior rectus fascia/transversalis fascia is incised to expose the peritoneum, which is then mobilized off the lateral abdominal wall to visualize the retroperitoneal structures. Transperitoneal approaches are usually utilized for lower lumbar and lumbosacral access. Primary concerns with the anterior approaches are potential injury to the large vessels, and injury to the sympathetic chain or hypogastric plexus, which is minimized by careful dissection and avoiding unipolar cautery use. Posteriorly, the lumbar spine can be approached through the traditional midline muscle splitting approach. This approach is familiar to spine surgeons, and allows decompression,

fusion and instrumentation. For limited decompression or fusion, the use of a microscope allows smaller incisions, better visualization and illumination.

Minimally invasive spine surgery is being increasingly carried out as a means to minimize muscle stripping, and allow faster rehabilitation. For posterior visualization of the lumbar spine, a 1–2 cm incision is made directly over the level of surgery. Blunt spreading of the muscle fibers is carried out by insertion of sequentially larger rods, until a working cannula can be inserted through the space. Laminotomy, discectomy, posterior lateral fusion and pedicle instrumentation can be carried out through this portal. The long-term benefits of this type of minimally invasive approach are still unclear, and the benefits of decreased incision length and muscle stripping must be weighed against the potential risks of diminished visualization or inadequate decompression.

Anterior transperitoneal laparascopic exposure is frequently used for surgery at L5- S1. Laparoscopic discectomy with cage insertion is generally feasible at this level, but difficult at other levels because of the vascular anatomy of the region. Multiple abdominal portals are necessary, and most surgeons have gravitated to a mini-open approach where specially designed retractors allow easier working in the depth and retraction of the large vessels.

Common Disorders of the Spine

Most spinal disorders are successfully managed with non-operative measures. Degenerative changes are frequently present in asymptomatic patients, and must not automatically be assumed to be the source of symptoms. Anti-inflammatory agents, analgesics, education, proper body mechanics, physical therapy and occasional cortisone injections relieve symptoms in the vast majority of patients. Failure of non-operative measures, significant neurological deficit, or a structurally unstable spinal column necessitates surgical intervention.

Disorders of the intervertebral disc or degenerative spinal stenosis may result in axial pain, radiculopathy or myelopathy. Neurologic findings with nerve root or spinal cord compromise may be present. Most patients are treated successfully with anti-inflammatory medications, analgesics, physical therapy and epidural injections. As a rule, the results of surgery are more reliable when performed for radicular manifestations, and less reliable when performed solely for axial symptoms. Decompression of the nerve root or spinal cord through a laminotomy or laminectomy relieves the neurologic symptoms. Fusion may be carried out when a significant component of axial symptoms are present, or for potential instability from the extent of decompression.

Spondylolisthesis and spondylolysis are common causes of back and radicular pain in both the pediatric and adult population, with L5 the most common site of involvement. Treatment varies depending on type of pain, degree of slip, and segmental instability, and begins with lumbar stabilization exercises and bracing. Surgical decompression and fusion are the mainstays for advanced disease. Scoliosis represents another potential cause of back pain in adults. Although the exact pain etiology is unclear, back pain is present in 86% of lumbar scoliotics. Surgical intervention is reserved for larger curves, progressive deformity, radicular pain, instability and neurologic deficit.

Spinal column infections can present as discitis, vertebral osteomyelitis, or epidural abscess. The presence of an epidural abscess mandates surgical evacuation and debridement. In the absence of a significant soft tissue abscess spinal infections can generally be treated with antibiotic treatment and bracing. Potential instability necessitates surgical stabilization.

Pain at rest or nocturnal pain is characteristic of neoplastic lesions of the vertebral body. Metastatic lesions are 25–40 times more common than primary lesions and can result in neural deficit from epidural compression. Primary or metastatic malignant lesions usually affect the vertebral body while benign lesions tend to involve the posterior elements. Operative intervention is directed at pain relief, stabilization, debulking of tumor, and relief of neurologic compromise. The overall prognosis depends on the type of neoplasm, spinal location and extent of systemic spread.

Rheumatoid arthritis can present in the cervical spine as atlantoaxial subluxation (40%), basilar invagination (20%), or subaxial subluxation (7–29%) [4]. Indications for surgery in RA of the cervical spine are significant bony destruction, ligamentous laxity and potential for neural compression. Stabilization after successful arthrodeses has shown to decrease chronic grannulomatous pannus

and thus restricting the pathogenesis of the disease. Ankylosing spondylitis presents with a stiff kyphotic spine. An inability to look straight ahead may necessitate extension osteotomy, carried out either at the cervicothoracic junction or in the mid-lumbar spine.

Minor spine trauma can usually be managed satisfactorily with an orthosis. More significant trauma frequently necessitates surgical intervention to decompress neural structures and optimize recovery of spinal cord injury, stabilize an unstable spinal column, and allow early rehabilitation. Instability of the spinal column results from either bone or ligament injury. The approach is either anterior or posterior depending on the area of pathology, area of spinal cord compression, time since injury, and fixation options.

Common Surgical Techniques

Surgery on the spine generally involves a combination of decompression of neurologic structures, bone graft fusion when stabilization of a motion segment is felt to be beneficial to eliminate a source of pain, and instrumentation to increase fusion rates and facilitate faster rehabilitation. Anterior or posterior approaches are used depending on the location of pathology. Segmental instability, destruction of bone, or gross deformity requires reconstruction of the spinal column, usually carried out with bone graft and metallic implants.

Cervical Spine

Anterior cervical spine surgery is usually carried out through the Smith-Robinson approach, with the plane of dissection between the sternocleidomastoid and carotid sheath laterally and the strap muscles and tracheoesophageal structures on the medial side. This approach is used for anterior cervical discectomy, vertebrectomy, fusion and instrumentation. For discectomy, the anterior annulus is incised, and a complete discectomy carried out with the help of pituitary rongeurs, curettes and kerrison rongeurs. The lateral annulus is left intact. Gentle distraction of the disc space allows good visualization of the posterior annulus. Resection of the posterior longitudinal ligament is generally not necessary, but is indicated when

65

a free fragment exists dorsal to this ligament. The uncovertebral joints delineate the posterior-lateral aspects of the disc space, and are resected in cases of severe foraminal nerve impingement. The vertebral artery lays 2 mm lateral to the margin of the vertebral body from C3–C6, and must be avoided during lateral dissection. Sharp teeth on retractors, or prolonged retraction may cause esophageal injury, or injury to the laryngeal nerves. Fusion following anterior discectomy is frequently carried out using autologous iliac crest bone graft. A tricortical structural graft is harvested from the anterior ilium, measured and cut to the depth and height of the recipient disc space, and inserted into the disc space with the cortical portion anterior. Allograft iliac crest bone provides equivalent fusion rates when used at one level, but may have a slightly higher incidence of graft resorption and collapse.

Laminectomy and laminaplasty are posterior options typically used for multilevel decompression of the cervical spinal canal, or posterior approaches to the dura for removal of intradural pathology. A posterior approach may be indicated when cervical myelopathy exists with cervical lordosis still maintained. Laminectomy allows good decompression, but is usually supplemented with posterior instrumentation to prevent the subsequent development of instability. Laminaplasty was introduced in Japan to decompress ossification of the posterior longitudinal ligament without resulting in postoperative instability, and thus obviating the need for fusion or instrumentation. As introduced by Hirabayashi, the lamina is detached on one side at its attachment to the lateral mass, and manipulated posteriorly through a partially osteotomized lamina/lateral mass on the contralateral side.

Instrumentation of the cervical spine is occasionally carried out in addition to a decompression or fusion procedure. The use of instrumentation offers a degree of immediate stability to the spine, obviates the need for a halo in some cases, increases fusion rates, and allows earlier mobilization. Anterior cervical plating is now a common procedure, and allows earlier mobilization following an anterior cervical fusion. The locked plates used nowadays allow unicortical screw insertion, and have a lower incidence of the screw backing out and impinging on the esophagus.

Posterior instrumentation of the cervical spine has traditionally been with interspinous or oblique facet

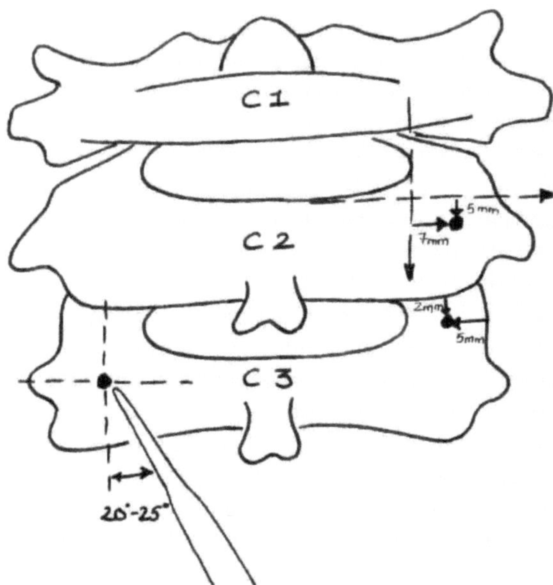

Fig. 65-1. Posterior screw insertion in the cervical spine. On the left is the direction of lateral mass screw insertion from C3–6. On the right are shown starting points for pedicle screw insertion at C2 and C3

wiring, which continues to be simple, safe and efficacious procedures in some clinical situations. Posterior plating with lateral mass screws or pedicle screws are biomechanically superior, but have a steep learning curve even for experienced spine surgeons, and carry significant potential risks. The lateral mass is well developed from C3 to C6, and screws are generally inserted beginning just medial to the midpoint of the lateral mass and angled superiorly and laterally, to avoid the exiting nerve root and vertebral artery (**Fig. 65-1**). The pedicles of the cervical vertebrae are small, and inaccurate placement of pedicle screws could lead to spinal cord injury. Pedicle screws are generally medially directed 30–45°, beginning 2–3 mm inferior to the superior articular process, lateral to the midpoint of the lateral mass (see Fig. 65.1). A laminotomy may allow palpation of the pedicle and decrease the incidence of cortical breakthrough. Pedicle screws are frequently used at C2 and C7 because the pedicles at these levels are larger.

Thoracic and Lumbar Spine

Anterior column surgery in the thoracic spine is carried out commonly through a thoracotomy. This provides the most direct approach to the middle and lower thoracic vertebral bodies. After entering the chest cavity, the lung is deflated and the pleura incised longitudinally, exposing the segmental vessels, vertebral bodies and discs. The segmentals are ligated if necessary. Excision of the vertebral body or disc is carried out as necessary, followed by reconstruction of the defect with bone graft or metallic cages. Anterior instrumentation is easily carried out, and may preclude the need for subsequent posterior stabilization. Limited access to the anterior column is also possible through a posterior-lateral approach. Resection of the pedicle, transverse process and rib head allows varying access to the vertebral body, disc and paraspinal tissues.

Lumbar laminotomy and laminectomy are among the most commonly performed spinal procedures. Through a midline posterior incision the interlaminar window and posterior elements are exposed unilaterally or bilaterally. Resection of the ligamentum flavum and posterior elements allows exposure of the dural sac and nerve roots. Removal of protruded disc relieves anterior pressure, and resection of hypertrophic articular process and facet joint capsule decompresses the lateral recess. The decompression extends laterally to the medial wall of the pedicle, and at the end of the procedure the traversing nerve root is mobile and free of pressure. Preservation of 50% of the facet joint preserves motion segment stability, and avoids the need for a simultaneous fusion.

Traditional lumbar motion segment fusion is carried out in the posterior-lateral gutters. The fusion mass involves the transverse processes, facet joint and pars region. The native bone is decorticated, and autogenous bone graft is laid down. Anterior and posterior interbody fusion techniques are an alternative to the posterior lateral fusion. The advantages are the broader surface area for fusion, anterior column structural support, and the higher rates of fusion. In cases where the pain is felt to be from the disc, the anterior discectomy and fusion theoretically removes the source of the pain.

Anterior lumbar interbody fusion (ALIF) involves an open or laparoscopic approach to the anterior disc space. After discectomy, distraction of the disc space is carried out to restore the height of the disc space and foramina.

Metallic or other manufactured dowel or block supports are inserted into the disc space. The drawback with this approach is that stenosis of the lateral recess or spinal canal cannot be addressed at the same time. Posterior or transforaminal lumbar interbody fusion (PLIF/TLIF) is performed in conjunction with a posterior decompressive procedure. Through a window in the posterior annulus disc material is excised, end plates of the vertebrae decorticated, and structural support inserted into the disc space. The shortcomings of a PLIF/TLIF are the risks of dural injury from manipulation of the thecal sac, and the potential for greater epidural scarring.

Posterior instrumentation of the lumbar spine helps with restoration of lumbar spinal stability, and promotes increased fusion rates. Pedicle screws are most frequently used. They allow maintenance of lumbar lordosis, while providing greater biomechanical strength than hooks or sublaminar wires. Pedicle screws are inserted under fluoroscopic control, typically angling 5–25° medially in the lumbar spine (◘ Fig. 65-2). Anterior instrumentation is usually a single or dual screw construct passing through the vertebral bodies from side to side, the different levels being connected with rods or plates. Anterior instrumentation is difficult at the L5 level because of the bulk of the psoas muscle. Metallic or bony threaded bone cages are frequently used to maintain disc height in an interbody fusion. The cages should be placed centrally, again

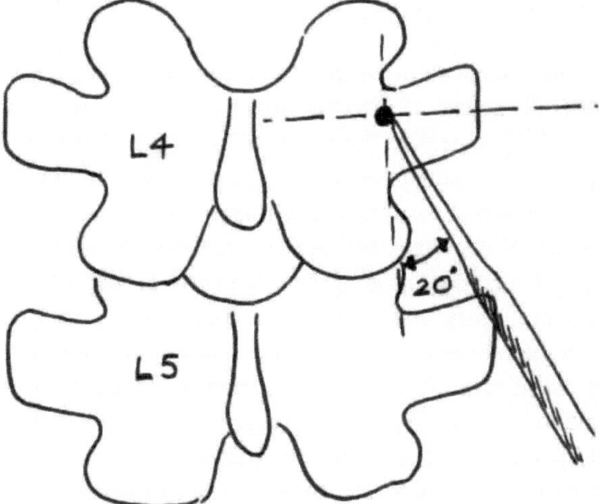

◘ **Fig. 65-2.** The starting point for pedicle screw insertion in the lumbar spine is generally at the intersection of the middle of the transverse process and the base of the superior process

under fluoroscopic control, ensuring that the canal or foramen are not violated.

Complications

Complications are frequently related to the position of the patient during surgery, and can be easily avoided by meticulous positioning technique. Peripheral nerves and bony prominences must be well padded. Obese patients are particularly prone to injury, and extra precautions are taken in these individuals. For posterior cervical operations in the prone position, a Mayfield clamp head holder is preferred to a horseshoe shaped headrest, to avoid pressure on the eyes. If using a knee chest position for lumbar operations, care must be taken to avoid excessive pressure on the tibial crest, or development of compartment syndrome in the leg. Ensuring the abdomen is free of pressure will decrease intraoperative bleeding.

Inadvertent durotomy occurs relatively frequently during spine surgery. Wang et al in their five-year study of 641 consecutive patients had a 14% incidence of durotomy [15]. Dural tears and cerebrospinal fistulas can be prevented with good illumination, using diamond tip burs in the vicinity of the dura, and remembering that the posterior longitudinal ligament thins laterally. Tears recognized intraoperatively are repaired, and can be reinforced with a fat graft. Large defects may require dural or fascial grafts. Persistent CSF leaks are treated with a subarachnoid drain.

Neurological injury in the course of spine surgery is generally a result of direct trauma from surgery, traction from realignment of the spinal column, or ischemic injury. Direct trauma results from misplaced instruments or implants. If recognized, the implants should be removed immediately, and intravenous steroids administered. Instrumentation of the spine carries a higher risk of nerve injury, and should be carried out by surgeons with a good understanding of the anatomy, who are proficient in spine surgery. In particular, sublaminar wires have been associated with neurological deficit. Reduction of a spondylolisthesis can result in injury to the L5 nerve root or cauda equina. The spine should be allowed to fall back to its unreduced position, and the foramina and central canal explored to ensure there is no mechanical compression. Ischemia can occur with extensive anterior pos-

terior operations, especially in patients with tenuous pre-existing blood supply to the spinal cord. Intraoperative hypotension can contribute to this ischemic insult.

Anterior lumbar spine surgery must protect the vessels and viscera within the abdominal cavity. Laceration of the large abdominal or iliac vessels occasionally occurs during anterior lumbar procedures. Early identification of the vessels and using deep retractors that keep the vessels out of the way diminish the incidence of this complication. Deep vein thrombosis can occur as a result of prolonged retraction of the large veins. In revision surgery or in cases of malignancy the ureters can be tethered and shrouded in scar tissue, and are prone to injury. Preoperative ureteral stents must be placed to diminish the risk of injury in these patients. Injury to the superior hypogastric plexus occurs during anterior dissection over the lower lumbar spine. This can cause retrograde ejaculation and/or sterility in men, and bladder dysfunction in women. This complication is prevented by avoidance of monopolar electrocautery or excessive dissection in this area.

During an anterior cervical approach the carotid artery and the internal jugular vein are prone to injury, and can be protected by staying medial to the carotid sheath, and placing deep retractor blades below the longus colli muscles. Vertebral artery injury from the use of cutting burrs in the lateral extent of the dissection is seen in 1% of all anterior cervical approaches. This is avoided by staying oriented to the midline at all times, identifying the lateral margins of dissection at the uncovertebral articulations, and preoperative evaluation for vertebral anomalies. Prolonged retraction of the esophagus and trachea during anterior cervical surgery can result in injury to these structures. Self-retaining retractors should be placed below the longus colli muscle belly, released frequently, and a thorough search for injury carried out prior to closure. Extension of lower anterior cervical dissection laterally can result in injury to the sympathetic chain, presenting as an ipsilateral Horner's syndrome.

Outcomes of Current Surgical Procedures

Surgery for Degenerative Cervical Disc Disease

Anterior cervical discectomy and fusion provides good pain relief over the long term, with recurrent symptoms related to adjacent segment deterioration. A 21-year retrospective study of 50 patients who underwent anterior cervical discectomy and fusion showed 64% of patients continued to remain asymptomatic, while 32% developed recurrent pain at an average of 7.2 years after surgery. Only half of this symptomatic group required revision surgery for adjacent segment disc disease [6]. With posterior decompression, late development of deformity remains a potential concern. After multiple level cervical laminectomies Kato et al found that 47% of patients developed cervical kyphosis. These changes did not affect neurological status of the patients [9]. Laminaplasty was developed to counter the instability seen with laminectomy. Kawai et al in their 130 patients who had undergone Z-laminoplasties for cervical compressive myelopathy followed up on an average period of 2 years and reported stable and favorable results with persistent enlargement of the spinal canal, which was demonstrated, on follow-up radiograms [10]. Wada et al felt that pseudarthrosis was the major concern after corpectomy, while stiffness and axial neck pain were the main complaints of patients after laminaplasty [14]. Chiba et al in a 14-year follow-up of patients treated with either anterior decompression and fusion or posterior laminoplasty found degenerative adjacent disc disease in 57% of patients with anterior surgery as compared to 7% with laminaplasty. They further noticed the deterioration of the alignment of the anteriorly operated cervical spines and required a salvage posterior surgery in 10% [20].

Surgery for Degenerative Lumbar-Sacral Disc Disease

Weber in his prospective, controlled study with ten years of observation compared the outcome between the surgically treated and the conservatively managed patients for lumbar disc herniation. At one year follow-up he found that the surgically treated patients did statistically better than those treated conservatively; the results became similar in both groups at four and ten years [16]. The study has some limitations, but the results are widely quoted and may, for the most part, be fairly accurate. In the lumbar spine following discectomy for disc herniation Yorimitsu et al felt that poor results following lumbar discectomy were correlated with age at presentation <35 years, recurrent back pain, advanced disc degeneration with decreased disc height [18]. Atlas et al found in their prospective study of 5 years that patients with moderate or severe sciatica did better with surgical treatment than those who were treated non-operatively. Improvement from surgery was less in patients who continued receiving disability compensation benefits [1]. Decompressive laminectomy for spinal stenosis provides good relief of radicular/claudication symptoms. Ten years following decompressive laminectomy more than half the patients had good or excellent functional outcome [7]. Fusion following decompression may be indicated with sagittal or coronal listhesis, deformity, or wide decompression.

Turner et al performed a meta-analysis of patient outcome following all types of lumbar fusion. They found an average 68% satisfactory results, with 61% of these having good or excellent pain relief. The studies showed 10.8% graft donor site complications, 7.3% instrumentation failure, 3.7% pulmonary embolism and 2.2% neural injury. They concluded that the results did not support the superiority of any single lumbar fusion procedure over the others [13]. The role of instrumentation is not entirely clear. While the addition of pedicle screws may increase immediate pain relief, and improve fusion rates, the long term benefits are unknown. A two-year prospective randomized study to determine the difference in the outcome between instrumented and non-instrumented posterolateral fusion concluded that supplementary transpedicular instrumentation does not add to the fusion rate or improve the clinical outcome [12]. Fischgrund et al [5] felt that instrumentation following decompression and fusion for degenerative spondylolisthesis improved fusion rates, but did not affect the clinical outcome.

Both anterior and posterior interbody fusions have shown good to excellent results with proper surgical technique. Kuslich and colleagues in their prospective study of lumbar fusion with cages on 196 patients at the end of 4 years follow-up concluded that early pain relief and functional improvement following the lumbar fusion with cages were persisted at 4 years. The fusion rates were 95.1% and around 62.7% patients were able to get back to gainful employment. The complications such as secondary operations were present in 8.7% and were indistinctly related to the cages [11]. Poor results following interbody cage fusion appear to be related to: a) undersized cages leading to inadequate vertebral distraction, b) subsidence of the implant in poor quality bone, c) failure of fusion from segmental instability, poor implant-host bone contact or multilevel arthrodesis, d) use of anterior stand-alone cages in tall disc spaces and e) technical errors such as improper placement, excessive end plate removal and lack of adequate bone grafts [19].

Future Directions in Spine Surgery

Minimally Invasive Techniques

In keeping with a general trend in surgical specialties, the future of spine surgery may lie in minimally invasive techniques. Endoscopic techniques are being increasingly used in the thoracic and lumbar spine. The use of a fiberoptic scope and light source allows the visualization and magnification necessary to carry out therapeutic interventions through small percutaneous portals, causing minimal harm to the surrounding normal tissues. Long-term studies will determine whether clinical success through these approaches equals that seen with a more conventional wider incision.

Minimally invasive lumbar surgery permits percutaneous endoscopic disc removal and fusion. Instrumentation systems have been developed that allow for percutaneous transpedicular fixation through an endoscopic approach. Endoscopic retroperitoneal or laparascopic transperitoneal approaches are utilized to carry out complete anterior discectomy, and simultaneously replace the disc with a variety of devices (threaded cylinders, disc spacers, allograft rings) to regain native height and facilitate fusion.

Video-assisted thoracoscopic surgery (VATS) is utilized for a variety of procedures like sympathectomy, lung resection, and mediastinal tumor excision. It has been used for thoracic disc herniation, anterior transthoracic releases, corpectomy for vertebral body tumor and osteotomies for deformity correction. The initial investigators using this approach have reported anterior instrumentation through the working portals. Getting used to the monocular video-assisted vision and the lack of tactile feedback associated with long-handled instruments create a steep learning curve for the technique.

Disc Replacement

Recurrent symptoms following a spinal fusion result in many cases from adjacent segment deterioration. It is commonly believed that the stiffening of a motion segment results in increased wear at the adjacent segment. This has led to the concept of intervertebral disc replacement, as a means to preserve segmental motion. Replacement of the nucleus pulposus, or a total disc replacement with a shock-absorbing polymer between metal end plates are two lumbar disc replacement techniques undergoing clinical trials in the United States. Early European studies with cervical disc replacement have shown good results in the short term. The preoperative condition of the posterior elements may determine the success of these prostheses in the long term.

Instrumentation

Lumbar pedicle screws are widely used, and outside of minor variations between manufacturers, their design is for the most part uniform. Accumulation of wear debris from spinal instrumentation may become a more significant issue in the future, as we obtain long-term follow up on these patients. Instrumentation systems to allow insertion of these pedicle screws percutaneously or through minimal incisions are already on the market. Future developments may include the design of bioresorbable screws, and varying rigidity of the spinal fixation device. Pedicle screws are being increasingly used for fixation of the cervical and thoracic spine, but still carry significant risk due to the small size of these pedicles. Translaminar lumbar facet screws can be inserted through small incisions and may provide additional stability when used in conjunction with anterior fusion.

Anterior cervical instrumentation has made little progress since the development of plate systems with locked screws. Newer plates have a lower profile, and allow some degree of dynamization of the construct to allow the instrumented disc space to settle on the graft. The greatest difficulty with anterior lumbar fusion using metallic interbody cages has been reliable evaluation of fusion status. Radiolucent devices that allow better determination of fusion while still maintaining stability of the construct are currently being evaluated.

Osteoporotic Vertebral Body Augmentation

The injection of methylmethacrylate into the vertebral body has been shown to reduce or eliminate fracture pain, prevent further collapse and rapid return to activity in osteoporotic and osteolytic compression fractures. Restoration of vertebral body height prior to cement stabilization is desirable. This is either carried out through extension positioning on the operating table, or with an inflatable tamp. These procedures provide excellent pain relief and restoration of function in these elderly patients, through a minimally invasive approach. Long-term analysis of the benefits or potential side effects of these procedures is still lacking. Bone substitutes such as calcium phosphate, calcium carbonate, hydroxyapatite and coral granules have been tried as alternatives to the methacrylate, and may prove to be more biocompatible and have less stiffening effect at the injected segment.

Bone Graft Substitutes for Fusion

Bone graft is a vital component of spinal reconstruction, providing the impetus for a fusion between spinal motion segments. Traditionally, autologous bone graft is used in anterior and spinal fusion. Autograft bone harvesting is associated with significant morbidity, and over the past few years a concerted effort has been made to find alternative sources of osteoinduction that are biocompatible.

Various agents have been used to stimulate the differentiation of mesenchymal stem cells into bone forming osteoblasts. Demineralized bone matrix (DBM) was initially used by Urist in 1965 to stimulate ectopic bone formation in a rabbit muscle. Bone morphogenetic proteins (BMP) 2 through 9, which are a component of DBM, are felt to be involved with bone growth. Synthetic recombinant BMP-2 and BMP-7 have been extensively investigated, and are currently being used to augment spinal fusion procedures. Collagen sponges, hydroxyapatite, or tricalcium phosphate are all being used to carry the BMP. The use of these synthetic products allows decreased operating time, decreases blood loss, and avoids the morbidity of bone graft harvest, and allows some procedures to be carried out in a minimally invasive fashion. Other agents that have been used to stimulate bone formation include platelet-derived growth factors, transforming growth factor (TGF) and vascular endothelial growth factor [2].

Biologic Innovations in Spine Surgery

Using genetic engineering, segments of DNA can be modified to produce recombinant protein products. Recombinant BMP is an example of how biologic developments are beginning to play a major role in spine surgery. Researchers are now attempting to halt the degenerative process at the disc level. Degenerative changes at the disc result from a loss of proteoglycan content within the nucleus pulposus. TGF is felt to be one of the genes involved in the production of proteoglycans in the nucleus. Human chondrocytes transfected with a vector that carries the gene for TGF have been shown to increase the production of proteoglycans, thereby restoring some of the biomechanical properties of the intervertebral disc.

Gene therapy may also play a role in spinal fusion. BMP genes in an adenovirus vector have induced bone formation in experimental models. An intracellular signaling protein named LIM mineralization protein-1, transfected into harvested marrow cells and subsequently implanted into an experimental posterolateral fusion, has also shown promise in inducing bone formation.

Image Guidance/Computer Assistance

Computerized-tomography-based image-guidance systems are used preoperatively to reconstruct three-dimensional topographic views of the bony anatomy. By linking known landmarks in surgery to the preoperatively obtained images, the position of any instrument can be tracked during surgery. The use of this technology has expanded from lumbar pedicle screw insertion to cervical and thoracic pedicle screw placement, transarticular screws at C1-C2, and other anterior cervical surgery. Further development of this technology may provide three-dimensional imaging intraoperatively with the use of two-dimensional fluoroscopy. The benefits of being able to locate and »visualize« difficult anatomic regions intraoperatively ensure that spine surgeons will increasingly adopt this technology.

References

1. Atlas SJ, Keller RB, Chang Y, Deyo RA, Singer DE (2001) Surgical and non-surgical management of sciatica secondary to a lumbar disc herniation: five-year outcomes from the Maine Lumbar Spine Study. Spine 26: 1179–1187

2. Boden SD, Titus L, Hair G et al. (1998) Lumbar spine fusion by local gene therapy with a cDNA encoding a novel osteoinductive protein [LMP-1]. Spine 23: 2486–2492

3. Ebraheim NA, Lu J, Biyani A et al. (1996) An anatomic study of the thickness of the occipital bone. Spine 21: 1725–1730

4. Frymoyer JW et al. (1991) The adult spine: principles and practice. Lippincott-Raven, Philadelphia

5. Fischgrund JS, Mackay M, Herkowitz HN, Brower R, Montgomery DM, Kurz LT (1997) Volvo Award winner in clinical studies. Degenerative lumbar spondylolisthesis with spinal stenosis: a prospective, randomized study comparing decompressive laminectomy and arthrodesis with and without spinal instrumentation. Spine 22: 2807–2812

6. Gore DR, Sepic SB (1998) Anterior discectomy and fusion for painful cervical disc disease. A report of 50 patients with an average follow-up of 21 years. Spine 23: 2047–2051

7. Iguchi T, Kurihara A, Nakayama J, Sato K, Kurosaka M, Yamasaki K (2000) Minimum 10-year outcome of decompressive laminectomy for degenerative lumbar spinal stenosis. Spine 25: 1754–1759

8. Karaikovic EE, Daubs MD, Madsen RW, Gaines RW (1997) Morphologic characteristics of human cervical pedicles. Spine 22: 493–500

9. Kato Y, Iwasaki M, Fuji T, Yonenobu K, Ochi T (1998) Long-term follow-up results of laminectomy for cervical myelopathy caused by ossification of the posterior longitudinal ligament. J Neurosurg 89: 217–223

10. Kawai S et al. (1988) Cervical laminoplasty (Hattori's method). Procedure and follow-up results. Spine 13: 1245

11. Kuslich SD, Danielson G, Dowdle JD, Sherman J, Fredrickson B, Yuan H, Griffith SL (2000) Four-year follow-up results of lumbar spine arthrodesis using the Bagby and Kuslich lumbar fusion cage. Spine 25: 2656–2662

12. Moller H, Hedlund R (2000) Instrumented and noninstrumented posterolateral fusion in adult spondylolisthesis – a prospective randomized study: part 2. Spine 25: 1716–1721

13. Turner JA, Ersek M, Herron L, Haselkorn J, Kent D, Ciol MA, Deyo R (1992) Patient outcomes after lumbar spinal fusions. JAMA 268: 907–911

14. Wada E, Suzuki S, Kanazawa A, Matsuoka T, Miyamoto S, Yonenobu K (2001) Subtotal corpectomy versus laminoplasty for multilevel cervical spondylotic myelopathy: a long-term follow-up study over 10 years. Spine 26: 1443–1447; discussion 1448

15. Wang JC, Bohlman HH, Riew KD (1998) Dural tears secondary to operations on the lumbar spine. Management and results after a two-year-minimum follow-up of eighty-eight patients. J Bone Joint Surg Am 80: 1728–1732

16. Weber H (1983) Lumbar disc herniation. A controlled, prospective study with ten years of observation. Spine 8: 131–140

17. Xu R, Nadaud MC, Ebraheim NA, Yeasting RA (1995) Morphology of the second cervical vertebra and the posterior projection of the C2 pedicle axis. Spine 20: 259–263

18. Yorimitsu E, Chiba K, Toyama Y, Hirabayashi K (2000) Long-term outcomes of standard discectomy for lumbar disc herniation: a follow-up study of more than 10 years. Spine 25: 1754–1759

19. Zigler JE, Anderson PA, Bridwell K, Vaccaro A (2001) What's new in spine surgery? J Bone Joint Surg Am 83-A: 1285–1292

20. Zigler JE, Boden S, Anderson PA, Bridwell K, Vaccaro A. (2002) What's new in spine surgery? J Bone Joint Surg Am 84-A: 1282–1288

66 Navigation in Cervical Spine Surgery

A. Weidner

Introduction

In general there is no difference in stabilization techniques of the cervical spine compared with the lumbar spine: screws are inserted into the spine and connected with rods (posterior) and a plate (anterior) to achieve primary stability. Transarticular screw fixation is introduced by Magerl for C1/C2. Judet described another fixation technique for fracture of the pars interarticularis of C2 in which a screw bridges the both fracture parts.

Landmarks in the operating field include facet joints and transverse processes, which serve for identification of the screw's entry point. Because drilling direction and screw length is difficult to judge precisely, intraoperative fluoroscopic examination is required. The main difference between lumbar and cervical spine is the different size of anatomical structures. Therefore, manual feed back while drilling into a pedicle is less helpful in the cervical spine, where additionally important structures are nearby and thus at risk: vertebral artery, spinal nerve, or spinal cord. Cervical spine surgery has a lower frequency as compared with lumbar spinal surgery, a fact that leads to a limited amount of relevant clinical studies.

Intraoperative navigation promises preoperative planning of screw alignment and intraoperative transfer of these data for optimal screw positioning. Due to the fact that cervical anatomy is more complex higher precision standards and reliability are demanded for surgical navigation tools.

Cervical Spine Navigation: Intraoperative Techniques

Two different navigation techniques are available, which differ in the type of digital data sets loaded into the work station: CT scan data provide three-dimensional reconstruction in comparison with intraoperative fluoroscopy, which delivers two-dimensional images only.

CT-Based Navigation

CT-based navigation requires a special CT protocol preoperatively. Consecutive axial images of 1.5 mm thickness are mandatory for precise screw placement planning. Screw entry point and screw direction are calculated preoperatively by navigational software in order to minimize potential risks of damaging vital structures including spinal cord, spinal nerve and vertebral artery. Also screw length and diameter are determined preoperatively.

Preoperative planning is transferred intraoperatively into the surgical field, provided that the virtual anatomy can be matched with intraoperative land-marks, a process referred to as »registration«. Surgical instruments equipped with light emitting diodes (LEDs) are linked with the navigation system via an optoelectrical camera tracing them in a three-dimensional space, thus identifying the location of the instruments in the virtual field. The surgeon can use this virtual field as a reference for precise positioning of all instruments. The reference frame, also equipped with LEDs linked by the camera to the work station, traces also excursion of the thorax caused by breathing or manipulation by the surgeon from the surgical to the virtual field. The surgeon identifies spinal landmarks touching and digitizing them. All acquired data are matched with the digitized CT scan. The entry points of screws are identified and matched with the virtual image on the screen for optimal placement.

Fluoroscopy-Based Navigation

With this technique the computer is loaded intraoperatively with a number of two-dimensional fluoroscopic views of the cervical spine. The image intensifier is equipped with LEDs feeding continuously information to the navigation computer. When fluoroscopic views are taken, the position of the image intensifier is known, so matching of virtual and surgical field is not necessary. LED-equipped tools are calculated into the two-dimensional fluorographs. However, the third dimension (depth) has to be added by the imagination and experience of the surgeon.

Cervical Spine Applications

Transarticular Screw Fixation C1/C2 (Magerl Technique)

A 1.5 mm CT scan is required for this technique. Dorsal flexion of the neck during scanning provides reduction of the altlantodental subluxation. This set of data is transferred into the computer for optimal screw alignment planning (■ Fig. 66-1). First the centerpoint in the interarticular part of C2 has to be identified where the vertebral artery has the closest contact to C2. With a diameter of less than 6 mm a safe transarticular screw placement is impossible. From this centerpoint the cranial direction of the screw is determined: On the sagittal plane the screw must cross the C1/C2 joint at the dorsal or middle third of the joint and should be anchored at least 10 mm into the lateral mass of C1. On the coronal plane the screw should be placed in the middle third of C1/C2 (see Fig. 66-1 and Fig. 66-2b).

The screw tip will not be monitored correctly in the virtual field because C1 is not matched with the surgical field. Position of C1 must be evaluated via the fluorographs after positioning of the patient. Intraoperative atlantodental distance should be nearly similar to the distance during data acquisition of the CT, so that conclusions can be drawn from this virtual surgical field with regards to screw placement within the first vertebra. The screws were inserted according to preoperative planning.

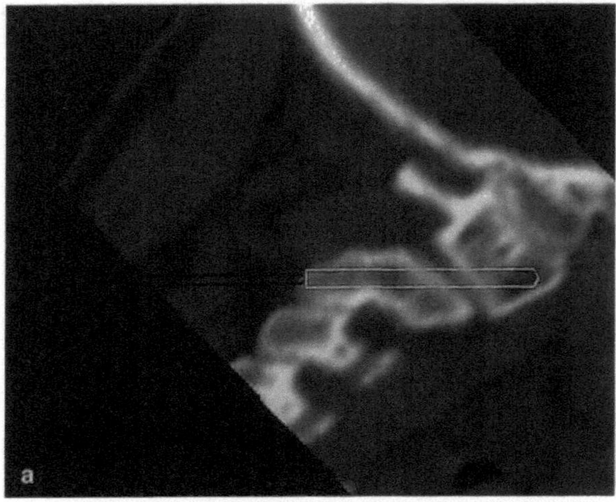

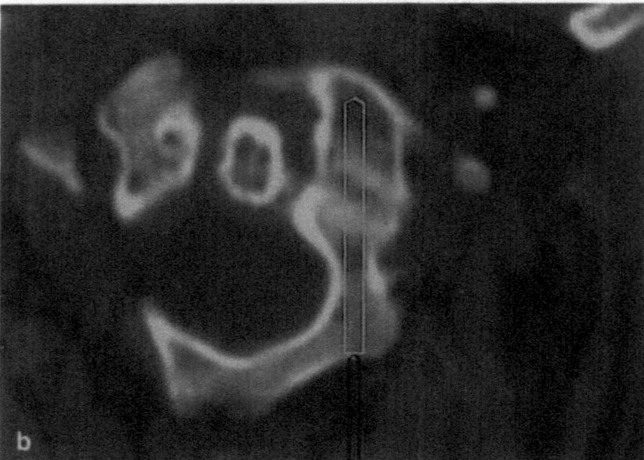

■ **Fig. 66-1a,b.** Preoperative planning CT scan for C1/C2 transarticular screw fixation. **a** Sagittal, **b** axial screw direction

In our own reported series of 115 patients (108 suffering from rheumatoid arthritis) transarticular screw fixation was performed because of atlantodental subluxation [10]. In 37 cases the screws were inserted utilizing CT-based navigation, in a control group of 78 cases the conventional technique based on anatomical landmarks and intraoperative fluoroscopy was utilized.

Out of 230 theoretical screw placements 228 screws could actually be implanted. In two patients one screw could not be inserted. There were no infections or injuries of the dura or neurological structures. One female patient from the control group died in consequence of a vertebral artery injury by a screw; the screw was biomechanically placed correctly, yet the vertebral artery showed an anatomical variation, which was not detected prior to surgery.

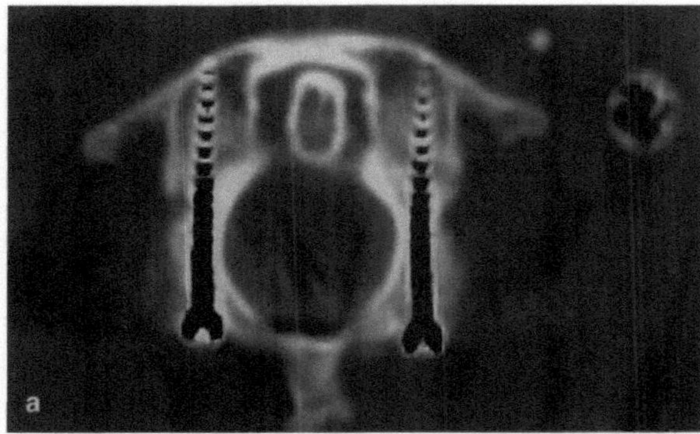

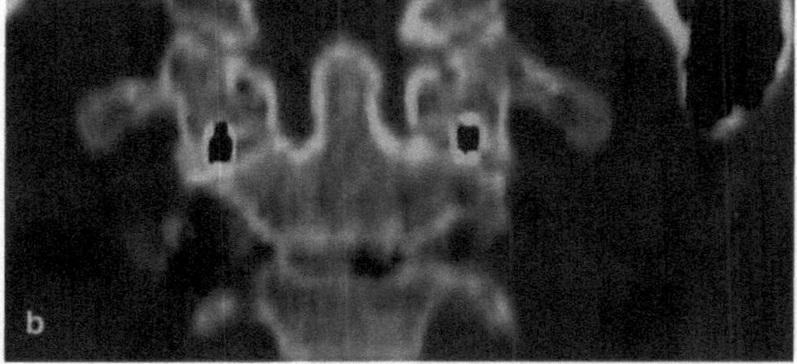

Fig. 66-2a,b. Postoperative CT follow up of transarticular screw fixation of C1/C2. **a** The axial, and **b** coronal view, are perpendicular to the screw direction at the level of the C1/C2 joints

Screw placement was evaluated by the classification of Madawi [6]: Correct screw position includes a more than 5 mm screw insertion into C1, protrusion of the screw tip over the anterior arch of C1 of less than 5 mm on the lateral radiograph (see Fig. 66-1a). Furthermore, the screw tip should be projected in the middle third of the C1/C2 joint seen on an anteroposterior radiograph (Fig. 66-1b, **Fig. 66-2b**). Deviation exists, if the screw is not placed in this middle third, but still within the interarticular part of C2. The screw is malpositioned if medially and laterally outside of the interarticular part of C2.

Lateral deviation was most commonly observed. In the navigation group four screws only were deviating into the lateral third. Lateral deviation was significantly higher in the control group, where 23 screws deviated. There were no screws malpositioned in the navigation group compared to eight screws in the control group, without any clinical consequences. That number was too little for drawing statistically significant conclusions.

Transpedicular C2 Screw Fixation

In Hangman's fractures (fracture of pars interarticularis of C2) direct screw fixation of both fragments can prevent spinal fusion and therefore neck mobility is not impaired by surgery. Arand et al. [1] reported two cases that were treated with such a technique (Judet's fixation) performed with the aid of CT-based navigation. All screws could be inserted through the fracture cleft fully covered by bone inside of the interarticular part of C2. We were able to perform this technique in four patients with a minimally invasive approach by stab incision guided by CT-based navigation. Postoperative follow-up revealed correct position of all screws.

Navigation in Anterior Cervical Spine Surgery

CT-based navigation of anterior cervical spine surgery is possible, but identification of anatomical landmarks in this area is unequally more difficult for matching than at the dorsal aspect of the craniovertebral junction. Bolger et al. [2] reported 40 surgeries in which the navigation could not be executed in the first seven because of landmark identification problems. The following five had considerably prolonged surgery time; however, in the final 28 a precision of 0.74 mm ± 0.4 mm could be achieved without delay. We performed this technology in few cases of tumors only. Often a conventional radiograph is sufficient for intraoperative orientation. For anterior cervical spine osteosynthesis, computer-navigation technique has no major advantage over conventional technique, because the screw entry point is clearly visible and modern screw design allows monocortical purchase. Neither two-dimensional conventional fluoroscopy (because of accuracy of the fluorograph) nor three-dimensional CT-based navigation technology (because after inserting a bone graft the position of the vertebral body is changed compared to the preoperative image) is currently capable of imaging the posterior cortex of the vertebral body.

Navigation in Posterior Cervical Spine Surgery

During a posterior approach in cervical spine surgery screws are inserted either into the lateral mass or into the pedicle. Nerve root or vertebral artery injuries are reported. Richter et al. [8] found that in 92% of all pedicle screws inserted with navigation a perforation of the pedicle wall did not occur. In another study, in 36 cases the pedicle screw was reportedly inserted correctly [4]. Lateral mass screws, however, can be inserted safely without navigation in cervical spine surgery. The direction of the screw is parallel to the facet joint plane and the screw is directed 20 degrees anterolaterally. This procedure is monitored easily by direct observation.

Discussion

Intraoperative navigation in spine surgery increases precision. This has been demonstrated to be true for the lumbar spine in a randomized prospective clinical study [5]. However, no clinical advantage could be established so far [9]. Few studies are published for cervical spine surgery. We were able to show a significantly improved screw position with the use of navigation, however, this does not directly indicate a decreased incidence of vertebral artery injuries [10].

The most important factor of a new technology has to include clinical improvement and outcome: This would be a decreased incidence of pseudarthrosis in this group of patients. However, there are no data currently available supporting this to be the result of navigation. Developing pseudarthrosis is multifactorial and therefore it is difficult to apply a reduced rate of pseudarthrosis to navigation alone, particularly in a disease where radiographic findings and clinical symptoms do not necessarily correlate.

Therefore, CT-based navigation at present should not be considered as standard and always superior to conventional techniques. This would be the case, if prospective randomized and controlled studies would demonstrate significantly improved outcomes. Additional radiation (CT scan) is another issue of concern, particularly taking the fact into account that only few patients' first CT scans are precise enough for making it relevant for navigation. Only improved clinical results would justify the costs of this technology.

However, navigation may be indicated in complex anatomical situations, such as malformations, or in revision surgeries. CT navigation makes sense for screw fixation of C1/C2 instability and for C2 fractures (Hangman's), as well as for surgeries where it is difficult to obtain intraoperative images, e.g. the craniocervical and cervicothoracic regions. The latter is not routinely performed in most centers due to difficult registration.

For insertion of multiple cervical pedicle screws at several levels, each vertebra would have to be registered and matched individually – a procedure that is time consuming and impossible after laminectomies, because no reference frame can be attached. Insertion of lateral mass screws can be safely monitored by the surgeon.

Matching of preoperative CT scan and intraoperative radiographs will certainly open new ways for minimally invasive methods in cervical spine surgery, but this should be associated with the development of entirely new surgical techniques to get more benefits from the advantages of navigation.

References

1. Arand M, Hartwig E, Kinzl L, Gebhard F (2001) Spinal navigation in cervical fractures – a preliminary clinical study on Judet-osteosynthesis of the axis. Comput Aided Surg 6: 170–175
2. Bolger C, Wigfield C, Melkent T, Smith K (1999) Frameless stereotaxy and anterior cervical surgery. Comput Aided Surg 4: 322–327
3. Foley K, Smith M (1996) Image-guided spine surgery. Neurosurg Clin N Am 7: 171–186
4. Kamimura M, Ebara S, Itoh H, Tateiwa Y, Kinoshita T, Takaoka K (2000) Cervical pedicle screw insertion: assessment of safety and accuracy with computer-assisted image guidance. J Spinal Disord 13: 218–224
5. Laine T, Lund T, Ylikoski M, Lohikoski J, Schlenzka D (2000) Accuracy of pedicle screw insertion with and without computer assistance: a randomised controlled clinical study in 100 consecutive patients. Eur Spine J 9: 235–40; discussion 241
6. Madawi AA, Casey AT, Solanki GA, Tuite G, Veres R, Crockard HA (1997) Radiological and anatomical evaluation of the atlantoaxial transarticular screw fixation technique. J Neurosurg 86: 961–968
7. Nolte LP, Zamorano L, Visarius H, Berlemann U, Langlotz F, Arm E, Schwarzenbach O (1995) Clinical evaluation of a system for precision enhancement in spine surgery. Clin Biomech 10: 293–303
8. Richter M, Amiot LP, Neller S, Kluger P, Puhl W (2000) Computer-assisted surgery in posterior instrumentation of the cervical spine: an in-vitro feasibility study. Eur Spine J 9 [Suppl 1]: S65–70
9. Schulze CJ, Munzinger E, Weber U (1998) Clinical relevance of accuracy of pedicle screw placement – a computed tomographic-supported analysis. Spine 23(20): 2215–2221
10. Weidner A, Wahler M, Chiu ST, Ullrich CG (2000) Modification of C1-C2 transarticular screw fixation by image-guided surgery. Spine 25: 2668–2673; discussion 2674

67 Pedicle Screw Placement

J. Geerling, U. Berlemann, B. Frericks, M. Kfuri, T. Hüfner, C. Krettek

Introduction

During the last two decades transpedicular fixation systems became standard for stabilization in thoracal and lumbar spine surgery [15]. For example, the number of fusions operations, especially for lumbar and lumbosacral degenerative diseases, has increased during that period [36]. In trauma spine surgery it is common to use these implants as well. In a multicenter study of the »Spine Study Group« of the German Trauma Society, the posterior instrumentation is the standard procedure in vertebral fractures of the thoracic and lumbar spine [25].

Several biomechanical studies showed the potential of stabilization for transpedicular implants especially for flexion, extension and lateral bending [27]. The biomechanical stability for torsion is less stable [31]. However the transpedicular screw placement is one of the most stable fixation method of one vertebra segment.

Pedicle screws should be placed within the axis of a pedicle, ideally, and should use the whole diameter of the isthmus of the pedicle [43]. The anatomy, size, and orientation of the pedicle have been analyzed in numerous studies, as well as anatomical [26, 30] and in CT-datasets [8]. The variability within one segment and in the whole spine is enormous. The smallest diameter of the isthmus of the pedicle, oval in cross section, is the critical size. This determines the maximal size of the screw, perforations are frequently in the range of the isthmus. The smallest pedicles can be expected in the segment of T4, sometimes the diameter is smaller than 4 mm [39, 46]. The size is increasing the more caudal the pedicle is. Lumbar pedicles measure up to 10 mm in diameter [26]. For orientation, the inclination of the pedicle is another important issue which is within the thoracolumbar spine 0° and increasing cranial and caudal [33, 43].

Anatomical studies showed the narrow relationship of neural structures and the pedicle. Nerve roots are medial and inferior to the bony structure [3]. These anatomical relationship requires a precise pedicle screw placement to preserve these neural structures.

Drilling and Placement

For a perfect placement of the pedicle screws the insertion point at the posterior cortex must be correct. The pedicular canal should be in a trajectory straight through the pedicle. The canal should be placed to the anterior cortex, not penetrating it. Due to this facts, several authors described several techniques for the pedicle screw placement [35].

Pedicle screws should be placed according to anatomical landmarks and with fluoroscopy control, most of the time with the lateral beam for the sagittal orientation of the screw [4]. With about 20 seconds per screw, X-ray exposure for the patient as well as for the surgeon is enormous [20]. There are some descriptions for technical aiming devices, like a special drill sleeve [44]. But it is hardly imaginable that a rigid advice can take care for the variability of the pedicle.

Misplacements

A CT-scan with reconstructions should be performed postoperatively to evaluate the screw placement [5, 45]. A review of the literature of the rates of the misplacements is shown in ◘ Table 67-1. In some cases even a placement through the cauda equina is described [12].

The placement of the screws is the more difficult, the more the anatomy varies. In surgery of scoliosis the insertion at the apex of the spine is a challenge due to the maximal rotation of the vertebra. Papin [34] pointed

67

Table 67-1. Data within the literature concerning misplacement rates of pedicle screws placed without navigation

Author	Number of screws	Misplacement rate [%]	2–4 mm [%]	>4 mm [%]
Gertzbein 1990 [16]	167	28,1	9,0	6,6
Sim 1993 [40]	200	8,0	3,0	3,0
Sjöström 1993 [41]	82	20,0	k.A	k.A
Güven 1994 [19]	379	10,0	k.A.	k.A.
Castro 1996 [10]	131	40,0	5,3	6,9
Odgers 1996 [32]	238	10,1	2,9	0,8
Haaker 1997 [21]	141	8,5	(b)	0
Schulze 1998 [37]	244	41,0	11,6	9,0
Merloz 1999 [29]	64	46,9	20,3	3,1 (d)
Laine 2000 [28]	277	13,4	2,5	1,4
Amiot 2000 [2]	544	15,0	1,8	0,9

Consequences

The rate of clinical relevant misplacement is rated up to 2–5% [14]. Multicenter studies from the early 90´s reveal a rate of transient neuropraxies up to 2,4% and a rate of permanent neurological disorders ranging from 0,6 to 2,6% [11, 13].

But also from the biomechanical point of view it is useful to hit the pedicle as precise as possible. The better the screw fills the pedicle, the higher is the fixation strength [9]. This effect is higher with a screw as long as possible.

Principles of Computer-Assisted Pedicle Screw Insertion

out this dangerous issue and presented a case of a scoliosis correction operation with misplacements at vertebra T 8 and 10 with a setoff of 4 mm and consecutive neurological symptomatic. Especially within the range of the thoracic spine due to the small pedicles, screws should only be placed by experienced surgeons. This is demonstrated in an in vitro study by Vaccaro, showing that 41% of the pedicle screws perforated the cortex and 21% of the implants were placed into the spinal canal [42].

In computer-assisted surgery (CAS) it is necessary to differ between CT-based and fluoroscopy-based systems. In both the vertebra is the »therapeutical object« The position of the instrument to operate is controlled by the »navigator«. The navigator connects the surgical and the virtual object on the monitor geometrically. The virtual object is either the reconstruction of the CT dataset of the vertebra or the intraoperative fluoroscan. The navigator theoretically can use either magnetic, acoustic, or optical signals [1]. The most precise system theoretically is the

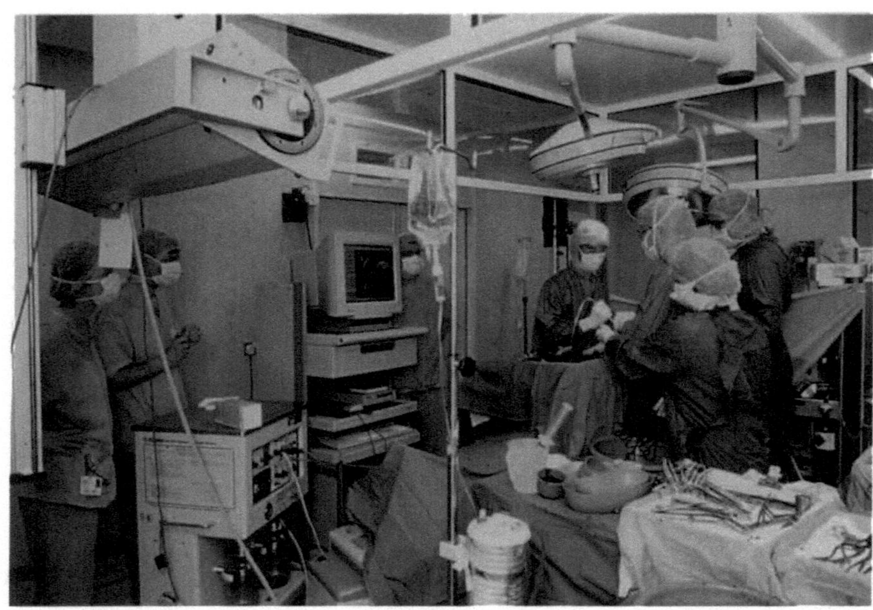

Fig. 67-1. Intraoperative use of the navigation system: During the operation the pedicle screw is placed using the navigation system. The control is done with the monitor view. Left handed there is the optoelectronical camera, receiving the signals of the navigated instruments

optoelectronic system using infrared LED marked instruments to localize the orientation in space (◫ Fig. 67-1.).

Details of the theoretical basics are described in other capital in detail. In this text just the principle steps will be discussed.

Calibration of the Instruments

Registration – Referencing (Matching) of the Therapeutical Object

The registration, also called »matching« is the most important step in CT-based navigation. There are two different kind of procedures.

1. Pair-point-registration: At least three, due to own experience up to five points, not on a straight line, are identified on the surface as well as on the therapeutical as on the virtual object. Preoperatively these points are marked on the virtual object at the navigation system. These points should have an as large distance as possible and should be on different levels. intraoperatively the corresponding points are localized on the therapeutical object. These points are digitalized with an instrument recognized by the navigation system, the so called »pointer«. Due to the pairs of the corresponding points the computer can calculate the position of both coordinate systems, the virtual and the real one, and overlay both.

2. Surface registration: Using this registration technique, a three-dimensional model of the bony surface of the CT dataset is calculated preoperatively. Intraoperatively a cloud of several points is digitalized on the real bony surface. The computer calculates this points to the surface of the model. This points should be as symmetric as possible on the posterior cortex of the vertebra, including the posterior process (◫ Fig. 67-2).

In most navigation systems both registration forms are used to increase the accuracy. Each vertebra should be registrated on its own due to the flexibility of the spine. The CT scan is performed on the back, operation in prone position. This can change the position and relationship between the segments, as well as intraoperative movements. The single vertebra itself is a rigid body. Therefore, the registration for

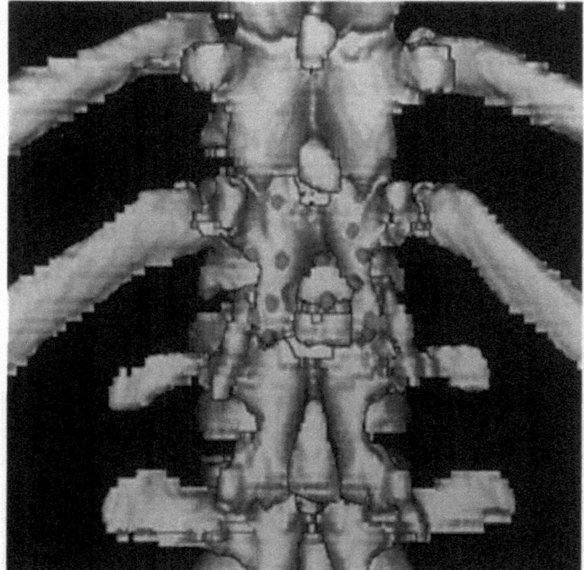

◫ **Fig. 67-2.** On the calculated spine on the navigation system the red marked points are for pair-point-matching. The green ones are the surface matching points registrated on the vertebra. Those should be as symmetric as possible

each vertebra can be performed independent from the positioning of the spine. The DRB has to be placed to each vertebra that is operated on at the posterior process.

CT-Scan Protocol

Within the lower thoracic and the lumbar spine at least three segments should be scanned, the injured and one above and one below. Within this region the spinosus process is almost in a perpendicular angle to the vertebral body. Within the upper thoracic spine, the posterior process is bent caudal. Therefore it is necessary to scan at least two, sometimes three segments below the injured vertebra. These circumstances should be mentioned to the radiological department, avoiding problems during the operation or to avoid a new CT scan.

Intraoperative Problems

One mistake is the right definition of the vertebra to operate on. The correct localization must be defined by the surgeon. Within the lumbar spine this is easy, but it is still necessary to use a fluoroscope to verify the correct level. Within the thoracic spine a fluoroscope is essential to localize the right spinosus process of the navigated vertebra.

Another pitfall is related to the navigation system itself. While calculating the surface of the vertebra the surface might not be calculated correctly due to osteoporotic bone or other artifacts. This might lead to dangerous mistakes. With an incorrect surface calculation the registration will not be correct and the position of the vertebra might be calculated incorrect. This might lead to the mistake that the pedicle screw is displayed on the correct position on the monitor screen but is wrong in reality. The same mistake can happen for the registration itself. In a case of osteoporotic bone the pointer might sink into the cortex. In this case the calculation might be with an geometrical non-overlapping. The same effect can happen if there is to much soft tissue on the dorsal cortex. The registrated surface seems lifted, and a tilt within the calculation might follow.

In Vitro Evaluation

Several groups evaluated the navigation of pedicle screw insertion. During 1994–1996 the first results of the laboratory experiments were published, with small numbers of trials. Amiot reported in 1995 the navigated preparation of six pedicles with a deviation of the navigated to the planned trajectory of 4.5 mm ± 1.1 mm and 1.6° ± 1.2°. This was confirmed by Glossop in 1996 with 1,2 mm (accuracy of the entrance point) and 6° within 8 pedicle preparations. In an own evaluation with 100 pedicle screw placements the precision was between 1.0 and 1.9 mm at the isthmus. The deviation of the axis was between 3.3 and 5.3° [5].

But the accuracy in computer-assisted pedicle screw placement is dependent on the experience of the user because there is a learning curve. In an actual *in vitro* study with human thoracic spines 120 pedicle screws were placed. The placement was evaluated with a CT scan as well as by direct visualization. Pedicle perforations were found in 19.2%. 9.5% were classified as »severe«. In the same study an improvement of the results was found over the time. Within the first experiments 37,5% penetrations were found in contrast to 4,2% at the last cases [24].

Evaluation *in Vivo*

Following the promising results in the laboratories the navigation systems were approved for the clinical use. One of the first works is published by Kalfas in 1995 [22]. He reports navigated pedicle screw placement in 150 cases with »satisfactory« results, however, without any distances. Table ◨ 67-2 gives an overview of the actual literature of navigated pedicle screw insertions. In contrast to Table 67-1 the clearly reduced number of misplacements is remarkable. In a prospective randomized study Laine [28] showed a significant reduced misplacement with computer navigated pedicle screw placement.

There is no doubt that the pedicle screw placement with the use of computer-assisted navigation is more precise than the insertion in conventional manner (◨ Fig. 67-3).

Pitfalls

Potential pitfalls should be mentioned. This might be an incomplete CT dataset or a wrong preoperative CT [38]. Also the localization of the correct vertebra must be defined to the system by the surgeon. In most times a short fluoroscopy control is necessary.

◨ **Table 67-2.** Data within the literature concerning misplacement rates of pedicle screws placed using a navigation system

Author	Number of screws	Misplacement rate [%]	2–4 mm [%]	>4 mm [%]
Schwarzenbach 1997 [38]	162	2,7	1,3	1,3
Girardi 1999 [17]	330	0	0	0
Kamimura 1999 [23]	169	0	0	0
Merloz 1999 [29]	64	9,4	1,6	1,6
Laine 2000 [28]	219	4,6	1,0	0
Amiot 2000 [2]	294	5,0	0	0

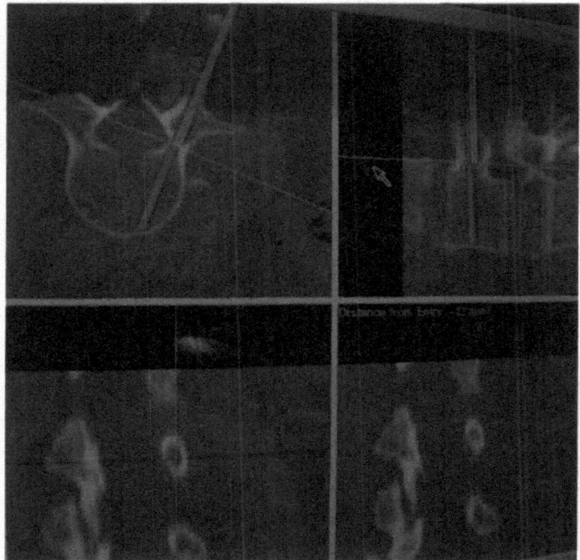

Fig. 67-3. Intraoperative view of the monitor: The navigation is performed at a lumbar vertebra using a peri-operatively planned trajectory (*red*). During surgery the pedicular awl (*green*) should be overlapped with the trajectory

Fluoroscopy-Based Navigation

A definite improvement of the navigation systems within the last past 3 years is the implementation of intraoperative fluoroscopy and to use these images for the navigation (modality-based navigation). The actual images can be used multimodal for navigation (spine, pelvis, extremities). Images can be actualized after reduction or an additional plane can be integrated. Furthermore, the orthopedic surgeon is familiar with the intraoperative use of a fluoroscope.

The principle of fluoroscopy-based navigation in the spine is: The DRB is placed to the spinosus process in the known manner. With the fluoroscope an AP and a lateral view is taken. With small rotation of the fluoroscope out of the AP it is possible to perform oblique views of the vertebra. The images are placed into a »library« at the navigation system. If the image quality is good, the fluoroscope can be removed from the operation situs. The surgeon can choose the images to navigate. There is a maximum of four views displayable simultaneously. Without a paired-point or surface registration it is possible to navigate the instruments within these images. The

images will be stay static on the monitor and the instruments are displayed in real-time.

To date there are just a few results published. Foley [14] reports about an in vitro study of an optoelectronic system controlling the navigated trajectory with additional fluoroscopic control. The accuracy is described within 0.97 ± 0,4 mm and 2.7 ± 0.6°. The advantages of the new technique are described:
- multiplanar visualization in real-time,
- reduction of the radiation exposure.

Due to these results and our own experience [7] it can be expected that fluoroscopy-based techniques will be a major part of navigation in future. The flexible implementation is especially of value in traumatology applications.

References

1. Amiot LP, Labelle H, DeGuise JA, Sati M, Brodeur P, Rivard CH (1995) Computer-assisted pedicle screw fixation – a feasibility study. Spine 20: 1208–1212
2. Amiot LP, Lang K, Putzier M, Zippel H, Labelle H (2000) Comparative results between conventional and computer-assisted pedicle screw installation in the thoracic, lumbar, and sacral spine. Spine 25: 606–614
3. Attar A, Ugur HC, Uz A, Tekdemir I, Egemen N, Genc Y (2001) Lumbar pedicle: surgical anatomic evaluation and relationships. Eur Spine J 10: 10–15
4. Bastian L, Knop C, Lange U, Blauth M (1999) Transpedikuläre Implantation von Schrauben im Bereich der thorakolumbalen Wirbelsäule. Orthopäde 28: 693–702
5. Berlemann U, Monin D, Arm E, Nolte LP, Ozdoba C (1997) Planning and insertion of pedicle screws with computer assistance. J Spinal Disord 10: 117–124
6. Berlemann U, Heini P, Müller U, Stoupis C, Schwarzenbach O (1997) Reliability of pedicle screw assessment utilizing plain radiographs versus CT reconstruction. Eur Spine J 6: 406–410
7. Berlemann U, Heini PF, Nolte LP (2000) Fluoroskopie-basierte Navigation der Pedikelschrauben-Insertion: Systemevaluation und erste klinische Erfahrungen. Akt Traumatol 30: 132–135
8. Bernard TN, Seibert CE (1992) Pedicle diameter determined by computed tomography. Spine 17: S160–S163
9. Brantley AGU, Mayfield JK, Koeneman JB, Clark KR (1994) The effects of pedicle screw fit – an in vitro study. Spine 19: 1752–1758
10. Castro WHM, Halm H, Jerosch J, Malms J, Steinbeck J, Blasius S (1996) Accuracy of pedicle screw placement in lumbar vertebrae. Spine 21: 1320–1324
11. Davne SH, Myers DL (1992) Complications of lumbar spinal fusion with transpedicular instrumentation. Spine 17 (6 Suppl): S 184-189
12. Donovan DJ, Polly DW, Ondra SL (1996) The removal of a transdural pedicle screw placed for thoracolumbar spine fracture. Spine 21: 2495–2499

13. Esses SI, Sachs BL, Dreyzin V (1993) Complications associated with the technique of pedicle screw fixation: a selected survey of ABS members. Spine 18: 2231–2239

14. Foley KT, Simon DA, Rampersaud YR (2001) Virtual fluoroscopy: computer-assisted fluoroscopic navigation. Spine 26: 347–351

15. Gaines RW jr. (2000) The use of pedicle-screw internal fixation for the operative treatment of spinal disorders. J Bone Joint Surg Am 82-A (10): 1485-76

16. Gertzbein SD, Robbins SE (1990) Accuracy of pedicular screw placement in vivo. Spine 15: 11–14

17. Girardi FP, Cammisa FP, Sandhu HS, Alvarez L (1999) The placement of lumbar pedicle screws using computerised stereotactic guidance. J Bone Joint Surg 81-B: 825–829

18. Glossop ND, Hu RW, Randle JA (1996) Computer-aided pedicle screw placement using frameless stereotaxis. Spine 21: 2026–2034

19. Güven O, Yalcin S, Karahan M, Sevinc TT (1994) Postoperative evaluation of transpedicular screws with computed tomography. Orthop Rev 23: 511–516

20. Gwynne Jones DP, Robertson PA, Lunt B, Jackson SA (2000) Radiation exposure during fluoroscopically assisted pedicle screw insertion in the lumbar spine. Spine 25: 1538–1541

21. Haaker RG, Eickhoff U, Schopphoff E, Steffen R, Jergas M, Krämer J (1997) Verification of the position of pedicle screws in lumbar spinal fusion. Eur Spine J 6: 125–128

22. Kalfas IH, Kormos DW, Murphy MA et al. (1995) Application of frameless stereotaxy to pedicle screw fixation of the spine. J Neurosurg 83: 641–647

23. Kamimura M, Ebara S, Itoh H, Tateiwa Y, Kinoshita T, Takaoka K (1999) Accurate pedicle screw insertion under the control of a computer-assisted image guiding system: laboratory test and clinical study. J Orthop Sci 4: 197–206

24. Kim KD, Johnson JP, Bloch O, Masciopinto JE (2001) Computer-assisted thoracic pedicle screw placement – an in vitro feasibility study. Spine 26: 360–364

25. Knop C, Blauth M, Bastian L, Lange U, Kesting J, Tscherne H (1997) Frakturen der thorakolumbalen Wirbelsäule – Spätergebnisse nach dorsaler Instrumentierung und ihre Konsequenzen. Unfallchirurg 100: 630–639

26. Krag MH, Weaver DL, Beynnon BD, Haugh LD (1988) Morphometry of the thoracic and lumbar spine related to transpedicular screw placement for surgical spinal fixation. Spine 13 (1): 27-32

27. Krag MH (1991) Biomechanics of thoracolumbar spinal fixation. A review. Spine 16 (3 Suppl): S. 84-99

28. Laine T, Lund T, Ylikoski M, Lohikoski J, Schlenzka D (2000) Accuracy of pedicle screw insertion with and without computer assistance: a randomised controlled clinical study in 100 consecutive patients. Eur Spine J 9: 235–240

29. Merloz P, Tonetti J, Pittet L et al. (1999) Computer assisted spine surgery: a clinical report. Comput Aided Surg 3: 297–305

30. Moran JM, Berg WS, Berry JL, Geiger JM, Steffee AD (1989) Transpedicular screw fixation. J Orthop Res 7: 107–114

31. Nolte LP, Steffen R, Kramer J, Jergas M (1993) Fixateur interne: a comparative biomechanical study of various systems. Aktuelle Traumatoll 23 (1): 20-6

32. Odgers CJ, Vaccaro AR, Pollack ME, Cotler JM (1996) Accuracy of pedicle screw placement with the assistance of lateral plain radiography. J Spinal Disord 9: 334–338

33. Olsewski JM, Simmons EH, Kallen FC, Mendel FC, Severin CM, Berens DL (1990) Morphometry of the lumbar spine: anatomical perspectives related to transpedicular fixation. J Bone joint Surg AM 72 (4): 541-9

34. Papin P, Arlet V, Marchesi D, Rosenblatt B, Aebi M (1999) Unusual presentation of spinal cord compression related to misplaced pedicle screws in thoracic scoliosis. Eur Spine J 8: 156–159

35. Roy-Camille R (1989) Current trends in surgery of the spine. int Orthop 13 (2): 81-7

36. Schulitz KP (1996) Wird die instrumentierte Pedikelfixation an der Lendenwirbelsäule zu großzügig eingesetzt? – Gedanken zur Indikation. Z Orthop 134: 472–476

37. Schulze CJ, Munzinger E, Weber U (1998) Clinical relevance of accuracy of pedicle screw placement. Spine 23: 2215–2221

38. Schwarzenbach O, Berlemann U, Jost B et al. (1997) Accuracy of computer-assisted pedicle screw placement – an in vivo computed tomography analysis. Spine 22: 452–458

39. Scoles PV, Linton AE, latimer B, Levy ME, Lin LC (1988) Vertebral body and posterior element morphology: the normal spine in middle life. Spin 13 (10): 1082-6

40. Sim E (1993) Location of transpedicular screws for fixation of the lower thoracic and lumbar spine. Acta Orthop Scand 64: 28–32

41. Sjöström L, Jacobsson O, Karlström G, Pech P, Rauschning W (1993) CT analysis of pedicles and screw tracts after implant removal in thoracolumbar fractures. J Spinal Disord 6: 225–231, 1993

42. Vaccaro AR, Rizzolo SJ, Balderston RA, Allardyce TJ, Garfin SR, Dolinskas C, An HS (1995) Placement of pedicle screws in the thoracic spine – part II: an anatomical and radiographic assessment. J Bone Joint Surg 77-A: 1200–1206

43. Weinstein JN, Rydevik BL, Rauschning W (1992) Anatomical and technical considerations of pedicle screw fixation. CORR 284: 34–46

44. Wu SS, liang PL, Pai WM, Au MK, Lin LC (1991) Spinal transpedicular drill guide: design and application. J Spinal Disord 4 (1): 96-103

45. Yoo JU, Ghanayem A, Petersilge C, Lewin J (1997) Accuracy of using computed tomography to identify pedicle screw placement in cadaveric human lumbar spine. Spine 22: 2668–2671

46. Zindrick MR, Wiltse LL, Doornik A, Widell EH, knight GW, Patwardhan AG, Thomas JC, Rothman SL, Fields BT (1987) Analysis of the morphometric charactersistics of the thoracic and lumbar pedicles. Spine 12 (2): 160-6

68 Navigation in Spinal Surgery Using Fluoroscopy

E.W. Fritsch

Introduction

Since popularized by Roy Camille [22], pedicle screws are widely used in combination with rods or plates (internal fixator) for spinal fixation in different conditions because of the biomechanical superiority of this construct [15,27]. Furthermore, higher fusion rates are reported with the use of an internal fixator [3,28].

The main problem with transpedicular screws is the proximity of the spinal cord in the thoracic area [26] and the proximity to the nerve roots at the lumbar spine [4] with the possibility of neurological complications as a consequence of screw mal-placement especially medial-screw mal-placement.

It is reported that between >2 mm [10,26] and >6 mm [11,24] medial mal-placement beyond the pedicle cortex a neurological deficiency becomes predictable. As a consequence, the rate of neurological problems due to screw mal-placement using conventional screw-insertion techniques is up to 7% [5].

With the background of up to 39.9% screw mal-placement overall and a 28.5% rate of medial mal-placement [11] using conventional pedicle screw-insertion techniques, it seems understandable that the first attempt of computer-aided orthopedic surgery (CAOS) or image-guided surgery (IGS) was to improve the accuracy of pedicle screw placement [16,22] which is meanwhile proven in prospective randomized trials at the thoracic and lumbar spine [2,14] for CT-based IGS.

But CT-based navigation still has limits for everyday routine use.

Acknowlegements: I want to thank Dr. Iris Grunwald and Prof. Dr. med Wolfgang Reith, Neuroradiological Institute of the University Hospitals in Homburg for their work to evaluate the screw positions with spiral CT scans.

According to Gebhard et al. [9] the limitations are:

- The limited calculation capacity of the computers used limits the number of available projections and the number of CT-scan slices that are processable.
- The pre-operative planning is influenced by superposing scan protocols and artifacts.
- The CT scan used for navigation reflects the preoperative status of the anatomy-making navigation suitable only with intact vertebral bodies.
- Despite a correct registration process failures in navigation can occur due to mathematical tilting of a vertebral body which is detectable only with intraoperative fluoroscopy.
- The alteration of the preoperative dataset by intraoperative changes of the anatomical situations due to reposition maneuvers are not addressable.

Furthermore, the radiation dose applied with the preoperative CT scan is higher than the radiation dose by intraoperative fluoroscopic control [25] which is of importance especially in scoliosis surgery.

Because of the limitation of CT-based image-guided surgery and with the aim to reduce the radiation dose using the fluoroscope to control every single step during pedicle-screw insertion, fluoroscopic-based navigation [17] (»virtual fluoroscopy« [7,8]) was developed.

The advantages of »virtual fluoroscopy« are [7,8,17]:

- presence of a fluoroscope in an operation where spine surgery is performed,
- automatic registration process without time-consuming matching procedure,
- imaging of the recent anatomical situation,
- updates of the anatomy are possible at any time.

The main problems with the use of fluoroscopic images as a base for navigation are [7,8]:

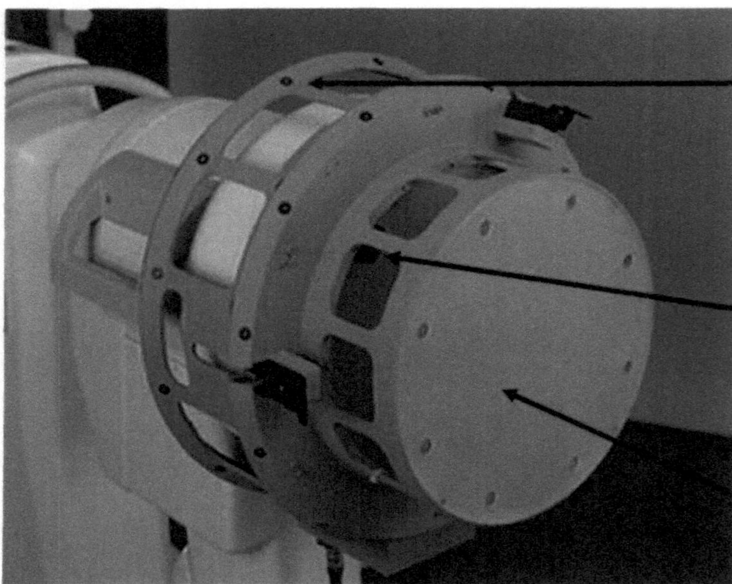

Fig. 68-1a. Calibration target.

- changing of the shape of the radiation cone in different positions of the fluoroscope,
- various distorsions of the fluoroscopic image,
- geometrical errors caused by the reduction of the three-dimensional reality into a two-dimensional image.

Therefore, a genuine fluoroscopic image does not reflect the real anatomy with enough accuracy to be used for image-guided surgery.

This accuracy can only be achieved by calibrating the system, which means an exact calculation of the radiation cone in the different positions of the fluoroscope and an elimination of the distorsions.

This is achieved by a calibration target.

The exact position of the fluoroscopic image intensifier can be determined by active LED trackers and a radiation sensor allows an automatic registration of the position of the fluoroscope whenever an image is obtained (Fig. 68-1a).

With the information of the exact shape of the lead balls in the two planes of the calibration target and their defined position, the shape of the radiation cone is calculable and the image distorsions can be eliminated (Fig. 68-1b).

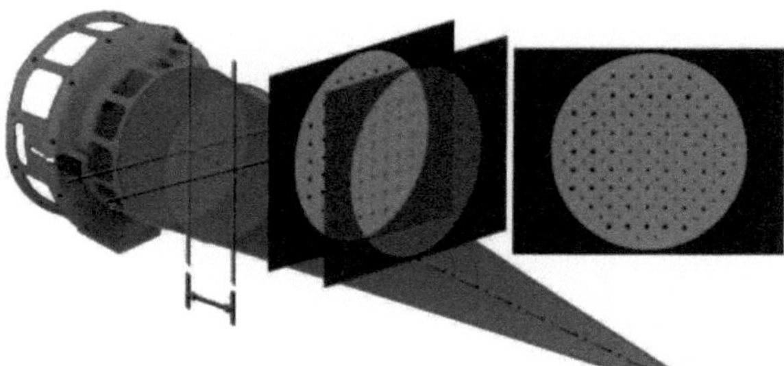

Fig. 68-1b. Using two planes with embedded lead balls of to different diameters in a defined distance the X-ray cone can be calculated and distorsions can be eliminated

Although the in vitro accuracy of the used navigation system and the used software is proven and published [8], a prospective study with a larger number of screws and the aim to evaluate the in-vivo accuracy of pedicle-screw placement at the thoracic and lumbosacral spine was missing.

Therefore, a prospective study was designed using postoperative CT evaluation of the position every single pedicle screw placed with virtual fluoroscopy. An established reconstruction mode [6, 13] was used to avoid the inaccuracy of the determination of the screw position with plain radiographs [6].

Materials and Methods

After being available at the authors institution, a fluoroscopic-based navigation system (ION; Medtronic Surgical Navigation Technology; Louisville, CO) with the software FluoroNAV Ver. 3.0 (Medtronic Surgical Navigation Technology; Louisville, CO) was used to guide the insertion of pedicle screws at the thoracic and lumbar spine in patients undergoing spinal fusion procedures without limitations to certain pathologies.

Patients were positioned on a Wilson frame for surgeries from TH10 to the sacrum. In cases where the higher thoracic levels were addressed, the patients were positioned on two rigid foam cushions, one under the sternum, the second under the pelvis. This resulted in a better image quality otherwise lowered by the superposing aluminia struts of the Wilson frame.

After the surgical approach with preparation of the processi spinosi, the lamina and the capsules of the small vertebral joints, the reference arc was attached to a stable spinous process making the automatic registration of the patient possible (□ Fig. 68-2).

Then the fluoroscopic images were acquired, activated and used for navigation. In multilevel cases the screws were placed in up to 3 vertebral bodies with one registration process. If necessary, a second registration with a new set of images was used.

According to the results of Ebraheim et al. [4] showing that at the thoracic levels a true a.p. and a true lateral fluoroscopic image represents the real anatomical situation, these projections were used at the thoracic spine, whereas at the lumbosacral spine an additional oblique view (»owl's eye-view«) was obtained according to Robertson et al. [21] who found that only with this view

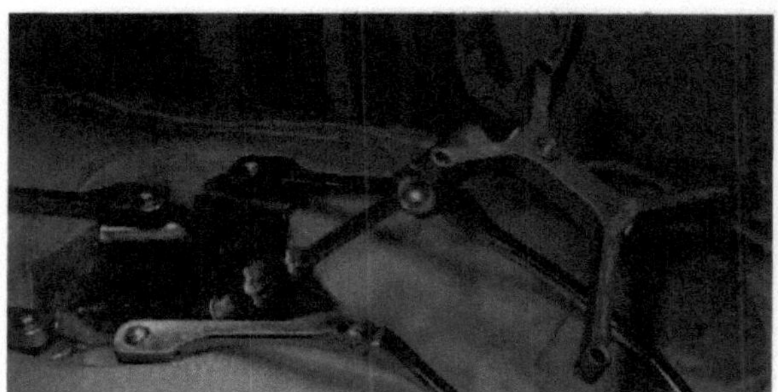

□ **Fig. 68-2.** Intraoperative view: The reference arc is attached to a spinous process

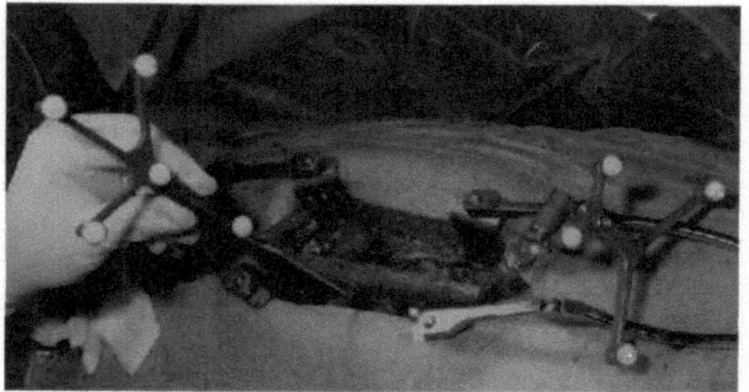

□ **Fig. 68-3.** Intraoperative view: Determination of the screw-entry point with the pointer

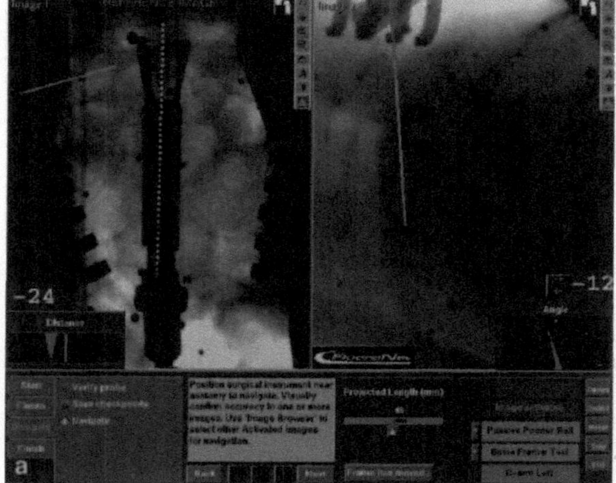

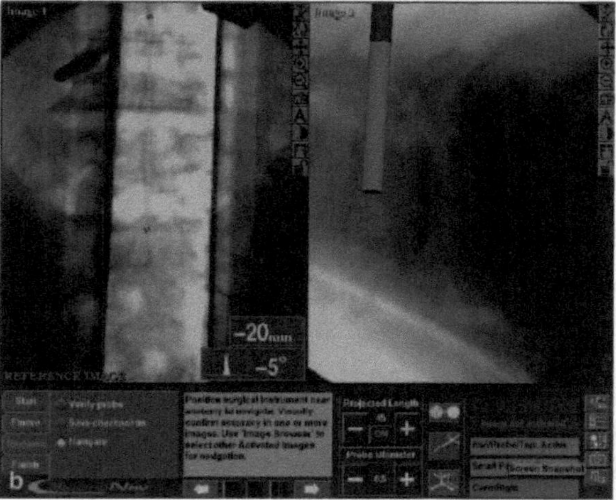

□ **Fig. 68-4a,b.** **a** »Virtual fluoroscopy«: Simulation of the screw lenght; *red:* actual position of the pointer; *green:* simulated screw lenght. **b** »Virtual fluoroscopy«: Simulation of the screw – diameter (6.5 mm in this case); the simulation of the screw-diameter shows that the screw will fit into the pedicle in both dimensions the true center of the pedicle can be properly visualized radiographically.

After determination of the screw entry point with a trackable pointer (■ Fig. 68-3) and simulation of both screw length and diameter (■ Fig. 68-4), the pedicle was opened with a trackable awl/probe/tap instrument. The pedicle was then probed and the thread was cut. Then the screw was inserted with a trackable screw inserter (■ Fig. 68-5).

Every step (opening of the pedicle, probing, thread cutting, screw insertion) was performed with the guidance of the navigation system.

Pedicle screws of the TENOR-system (Medtronic Sofamor Danek, Memphis TN) or M8 (Medtronic Sofamor Danek, Memphis TN) were used in a diameter of 5.5, 6.5 or 7.5 mm according to the simulation of the screw-diameter with the FluoroNAV software.

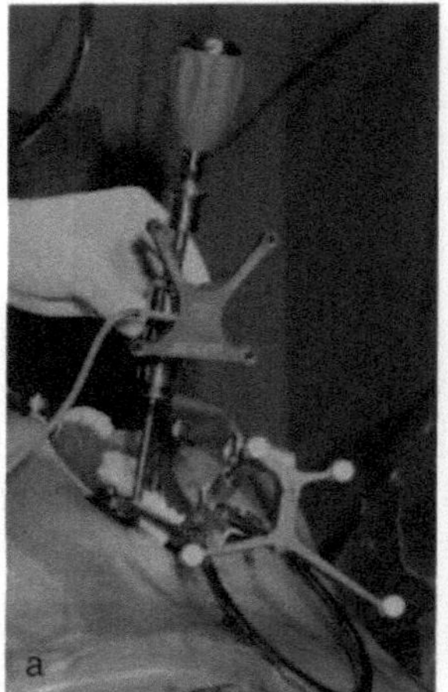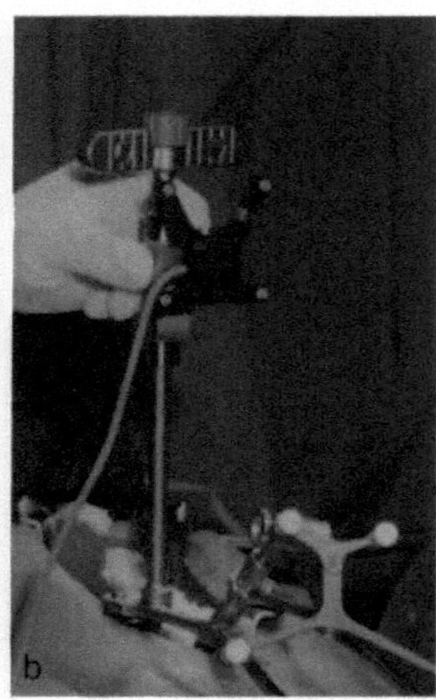

■ **Fig. 68-5a, b. a** Intraoperative view: Preparation of the pedicel with a trackable tool (Awl/Probe/Tap). **b** Intraoperative view: Placement of the screw with a trackable screwdriver

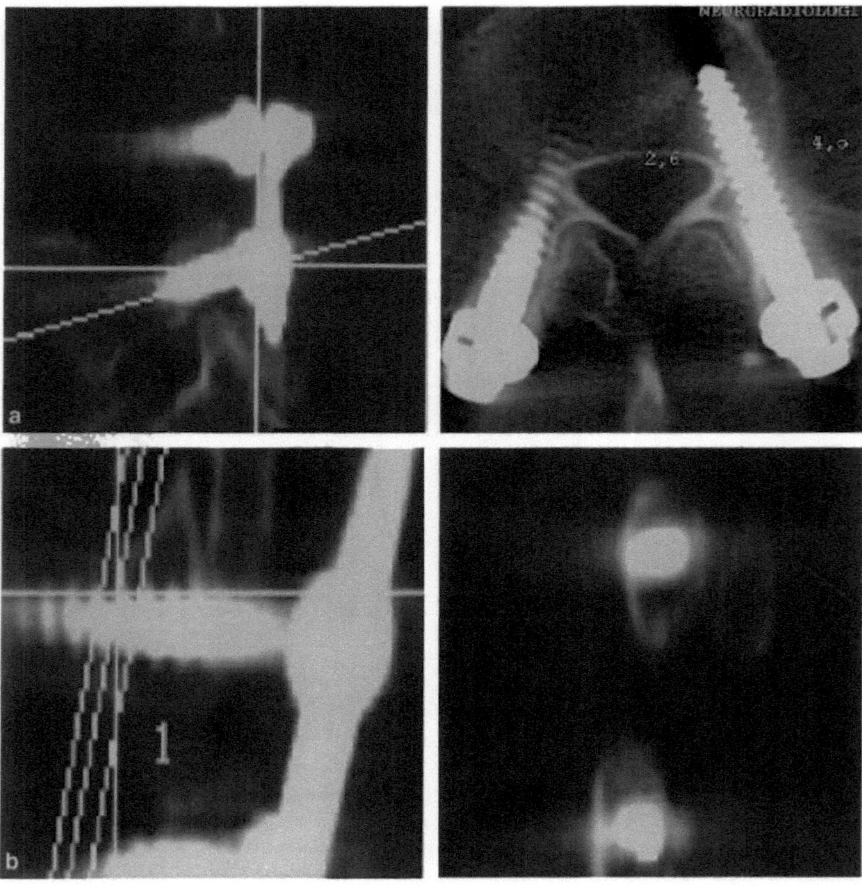

■ **Fig. 68-6a,b.** Scheme of the evaluation of the screw position with a postoperative spiral – CT scan. **a** *Left:* Definition of the reconstruction along the screw axis. *Right:* Resulting CT image. **b** *Left:* Definition of the reconstruction perpendicular to the pedicle. *Right:* Resulting CT-image.

After introducing all screws, a final fluoroscopic view in the a.p. and lateral projection was obtained.

The evaluation of the screw position was prospectively done by 2 independent neuroradiologists in the first consecutive 30 patients with spiral CT scans (1.3 mm slice thickness) and reconstructions along the screw and perpendicular to the pedicles in accordance to Laine et al. [13] for each screw.

A screw was considered ideally placed when it was found to be complete inside the cortical borders of the pedicle. Mal-placement was graded in superior, inferior, lateral or medial and the distance between the thread of the screw and the cortical border was measured for quantification (■ Fig. 68-6).

The postoperative neurological examination was correlated with the findings of the screw-position analysis and thus a possible relation was determined.

The pathologies leading to spinal surgery of the study cohort consisted in 7 patients with failed back surgery syndrome, 8 patients with spinal stenosis often requiring multilevel decompression and stabilization, a degenerative scoliosis with a Cobb angle >40° in 2 cases, a spondylolisthesis (Grade I–III) in 4 cases, a fracture in 3 patients and metastases in 6 patients.

A total of 160 pedicle screws were inserted: 54 screws in 20 patients at the thoracic spine (TH4-TH12) and 106 screws in 27 patients at the lumbosacral area (■ Table 68-1).

The screws were inserted by 4 different surgeons.

Results

All screws could be inserted with guidance of »virtual fluoroscopy«.

A conversion to the conventional insertion technique due to technical problems with the guiding system was never necessary.

All screws could be left in place because the intraoperative fluoroscopic examination after placement of all screws per case did not show a gross screw mal-position.

The CT evaluation showed that 151 (94.4%) of the 160 screws were ideally positioned.

At the thoracic spine 49 of the 54 screws (91%) and at the lumbosacral area 102 of the 106 screws (96.2%) were ideally inserted (■ Fig. 68-7).

A superior or inferior mal-positioning never occurred but 1 (0.6%) medial and 8 (5%) lateral mal-positoned screws were determined.

The only medial mal-placed screw was found at the TH5 level.

4 of the 8 lateral mal-placed screws were noticed at the thoracic spine (4/54=1.8%) and 4 at the lumbar spine (4/106=3.8%; ■ Table 68-2).

In the study cohort screw-related neurologic disorders were not observed.

Since the study showed excellent results and it was observed that using »virtual fluoroscopy« both radiation exposure and operating time can be saved the navigation system was used as a routine procedure in every spinal case with pedicle screws up to the level of TH2.

■ **Table 68-1.** Segmental distribution of the screws placed with »Virtual Fluoroscopy«

	Number of screws
TH 4	6
TH 5	6
TH 6	4
TH 7	10
TH 8	6
TH 9	4
TH 10	4
TH 11	6
TH 12	8
L 1	8
L 2	12
L 3	14
L 4	28
L 5	32
S 1	12

■ **Table 68-2.** Direction and quantity of screw mal-placement

	Overall	Thoracic spine	Lumbosacral spine
Ideally placed [n]	150/160	49/54	101/106
Medial mal-placement [n]	1	1	0
0–2 mm [n]	0	0	0
3–4 mm [n]	1	1	0
5–6 mm [n]	0	0	0
>6 mm [n]	0	0	0
Lateral mal-placement [n]	9	4	5
0–2 mm [n]	0	0	0
3–4 mm [n]	3	1	2
5–6 mm [n]	4	1	3
>6 mm [n]	2	2	0

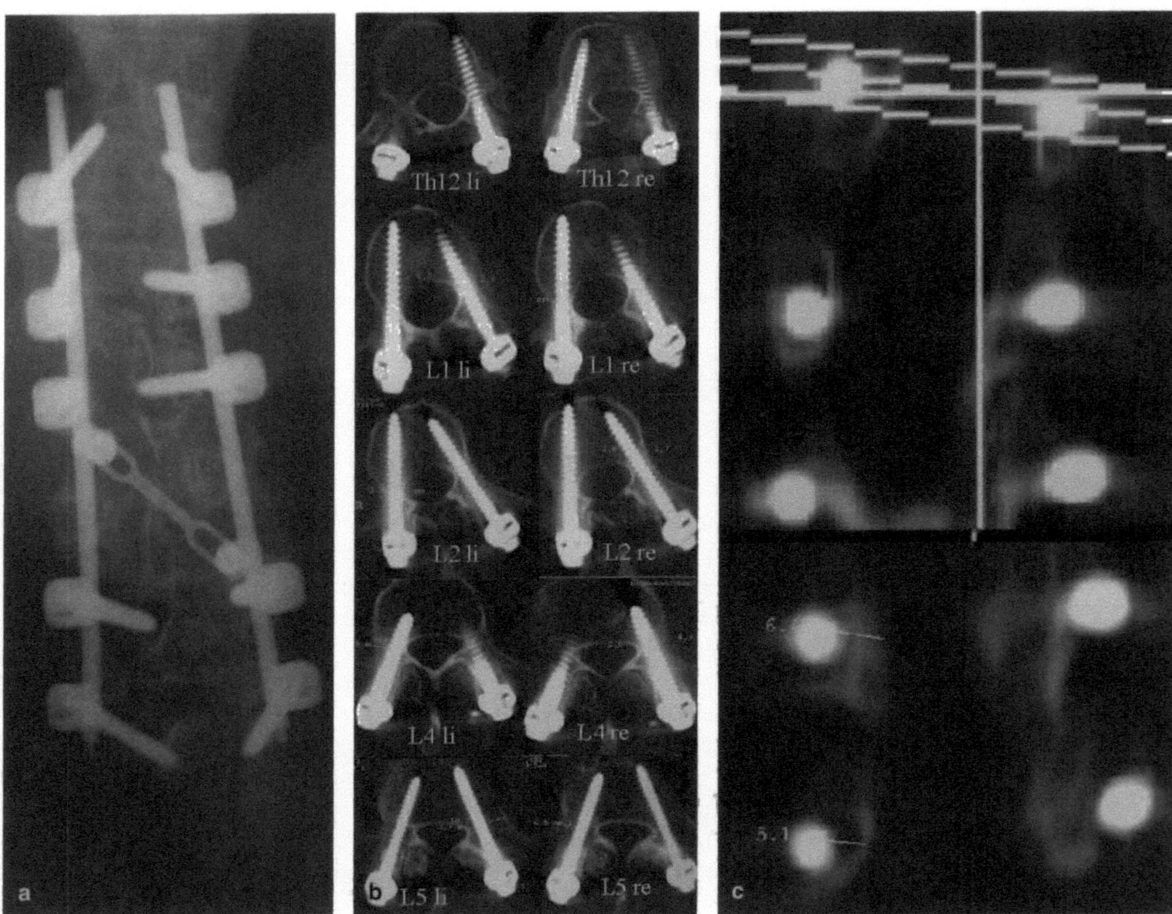

Fig. 68-7a-c. a Standard a.p. X-ray after multisegmental correction of a severe de-novo scoliosis. **b** Reconstruction of all 10 pedicle screws along the screw axis: all screws are ideally placed. **c** Reconstruction of all 10 pedicle screws perpendicular to the pedicle axis: all screws are ideally placed

Since September 2000 up to now a total of approximately 1200 screws were inserted in approximately 220 patients with a distribution of about 800 screws at the lumbosacral spine and 400 screws at the thoracic spine.

Clinically since the use of »virtual fluoroscopy« a screw related neurologic deficiancy was never observed.

Discussion

Data concerning the accuracy of pedicle-screws installed with »virtual fluoroscopy« are rare. Nolte et al. [17] published 30 in vitro placements of aluminum-cylinders in pedicles using virtual fluoroscopy, one series of screw placement in 11 patients and a second series of 25 screws.

Recently Rampersaud et al. [20] reported an accuracy rate of 89% out of 40 pedicle screws inserted with the same software as used in this study from TH3 to L1.

But an evaluation of a larger number of pedicle screws inserted with »virtual fluoroscopy« at the thoracic as well as at the lumbar spine was not available.

Therefore the accuracy rates found in this study can only be compared to data of accuracy rates achieved with CT-based navigation.

Kalfas et al. [12] reported a rate of 91.3% ideally placed pedicle screws (n=150) at the lumbar spine utilizing CT-based navigation. Amiot et al. [1] found 95% of 292 pedicle screws between TH2 and S1 ideally placed with CT guidance and Schlenzka et al. [23] installed 95.7% of 139 screws ideally using CT-based image-guided surgery but pointed out, that in 20.1% of the planned screws the insertion could not be done with navigation due to technical problems with the system.

Recently Amiot et al. [2] and Laine et al. [14] conducted prospective randomized studies comparing the accuracy rated of pedicle screws installed with CT-based navigation vs. screws inserted without navigation.

At the thoracic spine Amiot et al. [2] found a difference of 87.1% vs. 98.3% in advantage for CT-based navigation (TH2-Th12 addressed with CT navigation; TH5-TH12 addressed conventionally). Laine et al. [14] found a difference at the thoracic spine (TH8-TH12) of 73.5% in the conventional group vs. 91% in the CT-navigated group. At the lumbar spine the difference between the two groups was 85.4% vs. 93.2% in the investigation of Amiot et al. [2]; the results of Laine et al. [14] were 88.6% vs. 95.3% ideally placed screws in advantage for the CT-guided group.

The comparison of the presented own results especially with the very differentiated findings of Amiot et al. [2] and Laine et al. [14] reveal no significant differences between the rates of ideally placed screws with »virtual fluoroscopy« and CT-based navigation.

A remarkable increase of the rates of ideally placed screws with reported results for conventional screw placement [11] is also obvious for »virtual fluoroscopy«.

With respect to the not ideally placed screws, in accordance to Schlenzka et al. [23] a shift towards the less dangerous lateral screw mal-placement could also be shown for »Virtual Fluoroscopy«.

But, reviewing literature, a rate of 100% ideally placed screws seems not to be achievable neither with CT-based navigation nor with »virtual fluoroscopy«.

One of the reasons might be seen in the findings of Rampersaud et al. [19] showing that especially at the levels TH4, TH7, TH6, TH3, TH12, L1, TH 11 (descending order) the accuracy requirements for navigation cannot be met neither by CT-based navigation nor by »virtual fluoroscopy«.

Considering the disadvantages of CT-based navigation and the irradiation dose accompanied with the planning CT scan [25], »virtual fluoroscopy« appears to be superior to CT-based navigation at the lumbar and thoracic spine because of the equal accuracy and the minimized irradiation dose.

The easy setup, the automatic registration process and the fact that a planning is not necessary makes »virtual fluoroscopy« suitable for the every day routine use in spinal fusion procedures.

But despite of the help of »virtual fluoroscopy« high surgical skills of the spine surgeon are mandatory.

Furthermore, a profound knowledge of the radiological anatomy [4, 21] which must be properly addressed at all times is essential for the successful use of virtual fluoroscopy.

References

1. Amiot L-P, Labelle H, DeGuise JA, Sati M, Brodeur P, Rivard CH (1995) Computer assisted pedicle screw fixation. Spine 20: 1208–1212
2. Amiot L-P, Lang K, Putzier M, Zippel H, Labelle H (2000) Comparative results between conventional and computer-assisted pedicle screw installation in the thoracic, lumbar and sacral spine. Spine 25: 606–614
3. Dickman CA, Yahiro MA, Lu HTC, Melkerson MN (1994) Surgical treatment alternatives for fixation of unstable fractures of the thoracic and lumbar spine. Spine 19 [Suppl]: 2266–2273
4. Ebraheim NA, Xu R, Ahmad M, Yeasting RA (1997) Projection of the thoracic pedicle and its morphometric analysis. Spine 22: 233–238
5. Esses SI, Sachs BL, Dreyzin V (1993) Complications associated with the technique of pedicle screw fixation. Spine 18: 2231–2239
6. Farber GL, Place HM, Mazur RA, Jones CDE, Damiano TR (1995) Accuracy of pedicle screw placement in lumbar fusions by plain radiographs and computed tomography. Spine 20: 1494–1499
7. Foley KT, Rampersaud YR, Simon DA (2000) Virtual fluoroscopy. Oper Tech Orthop 10: 77–81
8. Foley KT, Rampersaud YR, Simon DA (2001) Virtual Fluoroscopy: computer-assisted fluoroscopic navigation. Spine 26: 341–351
9. Gebhard F, Kinzl L, Arand M (2000) Grenzen der CT basierten Computernavigation an der Wirbelsäule. Unfallchirurg 103: 696–701
10. Gertzbein SD, Robins SE (1990) Accuracy of pedicle screw placement in vivo. Spine 15: 11–14
11. Jerosch J, Malms J, Castro WH, Wagner R, Wiesner L (1992) Lagekontrolle von Pedikelschrauben nach instrumentierter dorsaler Fusion der Lendenwirbelsäule. Z Orthop 130: 479–483
12. Kalfas ICH, Kormos DW, Murphy MA et al. (1995) Application of the frameless stereotaxy to pedicle fixation of the spine. J Neurosurg 83: 641–647
13. Laine T, Mäkilato K, Schlenzka D, Tallroth K, Poussa M, Alho A (1997) Accuracy of pedicle screw insertion: a prospective CT-study in 30 low back patients. Eur Spine J 6: 402–405
14. Laine T, Lund T, Ylikoski M, Lohikoski J, Schlenzka D (2000) Accuracy of pedicle screw insertion with and without computer assistance. A randomised controlled clinical study in 100 consecutive patients. Eur Spine J 9: 235–240
15. Nolte L-P, Steffen R, Kramer J, Jergas M (1993) Fixateur interne; Eine vergleichende biomechanische Studie mit verschiedenen Systemen. Aktuelle Traumatol 23: 20–26
16. Nolte L-P, Zamoranol, Jiang Z, Wang Q, Langlotz F, Berlemann U (1995) Image-guided insertion of transpedicular screws: A laboratory setup. Spine 20: 497–500

17. Nolte L-P, Slomoczykowski MA, Berlemann U et al. (2000) A new approach to computer-aided spine surgery: fluoroscopic based surgical navigation. Eur Spine J 9 [Suppl 1]: 78–88

18. Rampersaud YR, Foley KT, Shen AC, Williams S, Solomito M (2000) Radiation exposure to the spine surgeon during fluoroscopically assisted pedicle screw insertion. Spine 25: 2537–2645

19. Rampersaud YR, Simon DA, Foley KT (2001) Accuracy requirements for image-guided spinal pedicle screw placement. Spine 26: 352–359

20. Rampersaud YR, Montanera W, Salonen D (2001) Computer assisted cervicothoracic (3D) and thoracic (2D) pedicle screw placement: a prospective clinical study. CAOS -USA Pittsburgh, 6.–8. July; Conference Syllabus: 213–215

21. Robertson PA, Stewart NR (2000) The radiologic anatomy of the lumbar and lumbosacral pedicles. Spine 25: 709–715

22. Roy-Camille R (1970) Oseosynthese du rachis dorsal, lombaire et lombo-sacre par plaques metalliques vissees dans les pedicules vertebraux et les apophyses articulaires. Presse Med 78: 1448

23. Schlenzka D, Laine T, Lund T (2000) Computer-assisted spine surgery. Eur Spine J 9 [Suppl 1]: 57–64

24. Schulze CJ, Munzinger E, Weber U (1998) Clinical relevance of accuracy of pedicle screw placement. A computertomographic-supported analysis. Spine 23: 2215–2220

25. Slomoczykowski M, Roberto M, Schneeberger P, Ozdoba C, Vock P (1999) Radiation dose for pedicle screw insertion. Fluoroscopic method vs. computer-assisted surgery. Spine 24: 975–82

26. Vaccaro AR, Rizzolo SJ, Allardyce TJ (1995) Placement of pedicle screws in the thoracic spine: Part 2. An anatomical and radiographic assessment. J Bone Joint Surg [Am] 8: 1200–1206

27. Vahldiek MJ, Panjabi MM (1998) Stability potential of spinal instrumentations in tumor vertebral body replacement surgery. Spine 23: 543–550

28. Yuan HA, Garfin SR, Dickman CA, Mardjetko SM (1994) A historical cohort study of pedicle screw fixation in thoracic, lumbar, and sacral spinal fusions. Spine 19 [Suppl]: 2279–2296

69 Navigation of Tumor and Metastatic Lesions in the Thoracolumbar Spine

F. Gebhard, M. Arand

Introduction

Since the description of transpedicle fixation of posterior spinal implants by Roy-Camille et al. [18], this procedure has gained general acceptance for rigid segmental fixation. Correct implantation of the screws without perforation of the pedicle is difficult and requires detailed anatomic knowledge and good surgical skills. The identification of the correct entry point for the pedicle screw and the correct angle of inclination in the sagittal and transverse planes are crucial. A standard technique for pedicle screw insertion is done with an image intensifier in the lateral and anteroposterior (a.p.) views. In osteolytic tumors identification of anatomical landmarks is difficult and intraoperative imaging can be impossible due to increased radio translucent vertebrae.

Computed-tomography(CT)-controlled studies have had significant rates of incorrect placement of lumbar transpedicle screws [5,8,25] and implant-related and neurologic complications also have been reported [6,26]. The central implant placement in the thoracic pedicle is a more difficult procedure [28], and an increasing rate of misplacement can be expected in this region.

Within the past years, computer-aided systems for CT-based freehand navigation have been introduced [15, 24]. With this technique, a preoperative CT scan (CT dataset) is superimposed onto the intraoperative rigid body (the spinal vertebra). As long as the navigated vertebra is non-deformable, online visualization of the instruments within the preoperative data set is possible. In addition, it is important to have intact posterior structures for stable fixation of the data reference base (DRB).

Using these new techniques, experimental [1, 4, 16] and initial clinical [12, 14] results have shown significantly reduced misplacement rates in the lumbar spine pedicle and a decrease in neurologic complications [2].

Depending on the extent of the disease, the main goals of tumor surgery of the spine are tumor reduction, decompression of the neural structures and stable fixation of a malignancy-induced destabilized spine. As tumor localization in the spine is predominantly in the anterior column, posterior treatment is palliative only, or is done as a first step in a double intervention approach. In corpectomies of tumors of the cervical [17, 23] and thoracic spine [23], initial clinical studies have shown possible applications of image-guided surgery using an anterior approach. No clinical studies have been published regarding posterior treatment of the thoracic spine so far.

Another disadvantage in standard spine tumor surgery is that the extension of the tumor cannot be accurately determined intraoperatively, and therefore, the surgeon cannot do procedures such as neural decompression, hemilaminectomy, or laminectomy in complete safety. However, accurate visualization of the tumor can be obtained preoperatively using CT or magnetic resonance imaging (MRI) scans, which can provide safer surgery for the patient.

The aim of this clinical feasibility study was to investigate the efficacy of a computer-aided visualization technique during neural decompression and transpedicle stabilization in patients who require tumor-related surgery of the spine.

Materials and Methods

Since August 1999, an optoelectronic navigation system (SurgiGATE, Medivision, Oberdorf, Switzerland) has been used by the authors. The navigable data sets have been generated on a four-gantry spiral CT (MX 8000, Marconi, Hofheim-Wallau, Germany).

12 patients with tumors of the spine and acute instability or myelopathy underwent posterior decompression

and stabilization using the navigation system. In 5 patients two or more vertebrae were involved and in 7 patients the tumor was located in one vertebra only. Ten tumors were in the thoracic level, 2 in the lumbar area (see Fig. 69-5). In all patients advanced metastatic disease was diagnosed, therefore, surgical intervention was palliative and no anterior procedure followed the posterior intervention.

In all patients navigated posterior decompression and computer-guided pedicle screw implantations were planned.

After footside installation of the navigation camera and the navigation computer with the screen, correct fluoroscopic identification of the involved spinal region in the lateral and a.p. views were ensured in all patients.

Positioning, covering and the surgical approach corresponded to the standard technique in each patient. To achieve computer guidance, matching of the CT dataset and the patient was done. Having fixed the DRB, the paired point matching procedure was done using four points and a surface matching was added. After achieving an acceptable matching result, verification was done to recheck the accuracy of registration of the CT dataset and the vertebra on the posterior laminar surfaces of the registered vertebra.

Transpedicle instrumentation of the matched vertebra was done with a tracked pedicle awl to have access to the pedicle followed by a tracked pedicle probe to generate the screw hole, in which the 5-mm Schanz screws were implanted with a tracked T handle. After instrumentation of one vertebra, the same procedure was done for the next vertebra.

The second step of the operation consisted of decompression. Therefore, a third matching was done for metastatic vertebrae after fixation of the dynamic reference base to its spinal process, if the latter was intact (n=8). In 4 cases the DRB was fixed at the cranial or caudal neighbor vertebra. Then a small piece of the mediocranial edge of the left or right lamina was resected by an Hayek dissector with intermittent application of the pedicle awl in the guidance or real-time mode of the navigation system. On the screen of the navigation system, the real-time position of the tracked pedicle awl was observed in relation to the tumor on the CT dataset. Complete posterior decompression can be controlled and ensured by the surgeon.

The following data were recorded for each patient:

1. the time required for data transfer and planning the intervention;
2. the time required for intraoperative installation of the computer system;
3. the time required for vertebral matching and instrumentation;
4. the subjective (surgeon) and objective (history mode) performance of the navigation system.

Postoperatively, a CT-based analysis of localization of the pedicle screws and the status of decompression in each patient were confirmed by two independent observers (radiologist and trauma surgeon). Correct pedicle screw insertion was reported in all cases where the patient had a successful intraosseous implant, or where patients experienced perforation less than a screw thread in the case of a pedicle breadth that was smaller than the implant diameter. To evaluate the quality of decompression, in the transverse scans the original vertebral tumor extension was identified in the spinal canal. The rim of the tumor, intruding into the canal was marked and translated posteriorly by graphics software (volume matching, MX-view, Marconi, Hofheim-Wallau, Germany). This was implemented into sagittal and frontal reconstructions and consecutive observation showed if the posterior laminar structures were resected completely, referring to the anterior tumor extension.

Results

Inclusion criteria in this study was palliative posterior tumor treatment of the spine and intraoperative CT-based navigation.

One patient with extensive disease that extended to the posterior spinal structures (not listed above) was excluded from the study before surgery, because a rigid connection between the affected vertebra and the data reference base was not possible due to instability of the spinous process. Six thoracic screws had to be placed in standard technique, because no successful matching procedure could be achieved.

The aim of computer-aided decompression and hemilaminectomy was realized in all patients. The average time of data transfer was 11 min (range, 8–15 min), and the average planning time for the operation was 35 min (range, 13–90 min). intraoperative installation of the system took approximately 5 min and the final matching

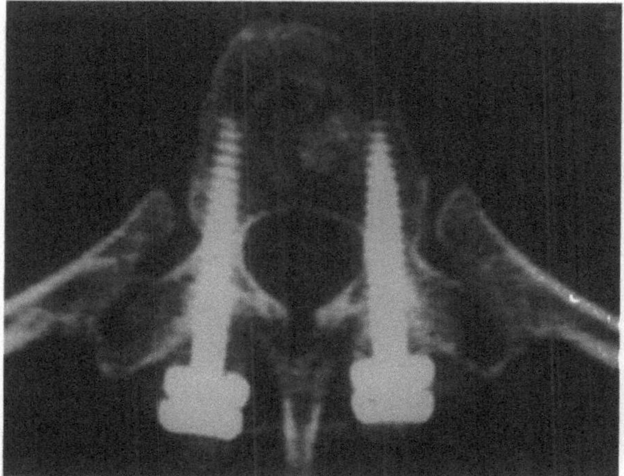

■ **Fig. 69-1.** Central, computer-guided placement of the left pedicle screw, and marginal perforation of the right pedicle screw (less thread depth) can be seen

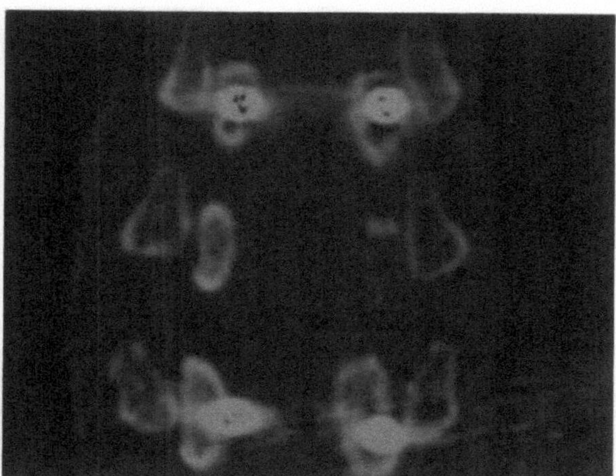

■ **Fig. 69-2.** The postoperative CT scan shows a medial perforation of the left caudal pedicle screw (3 mm)

time per vertebra was 7 min (range, 5–10 min); an average rematching frequency of one procedure with paired point and surface matching was seen. Using computer-guided implantation 86% of pedicle screws were positioned cen-trally as seen on the postoperative CT scan (■ Fig. 69-1). However, three pedicle screws were placed eccentrically (right and left caudal screw, ■ Fig. 69-2), although in all three patients the history mode showed correct matching

■ **Fig. 69-3a-d.** The four figures demonstrate the complete and computer-aided decompression of the posterior structures at different levels of T9 in the postoperative CT scan: **a** A transverse CT scan cranial through Th9 on the level of the pedicles with the most cranial ex-tension of the osteolysis; **b** a trans-verse CT scan of Th9 with the level of the most significant extension of the tumor and **c** a transverse CT scan with the most caudal exten-sion of the tumor. In all transverse CT scans (**a–c**) the posterior ele-ments referring to the tumor exten-sion in the spine were completely removed. Frontal CT reconstruction (**d**) shows the decompression in the plane of the removed posterior ele-ments

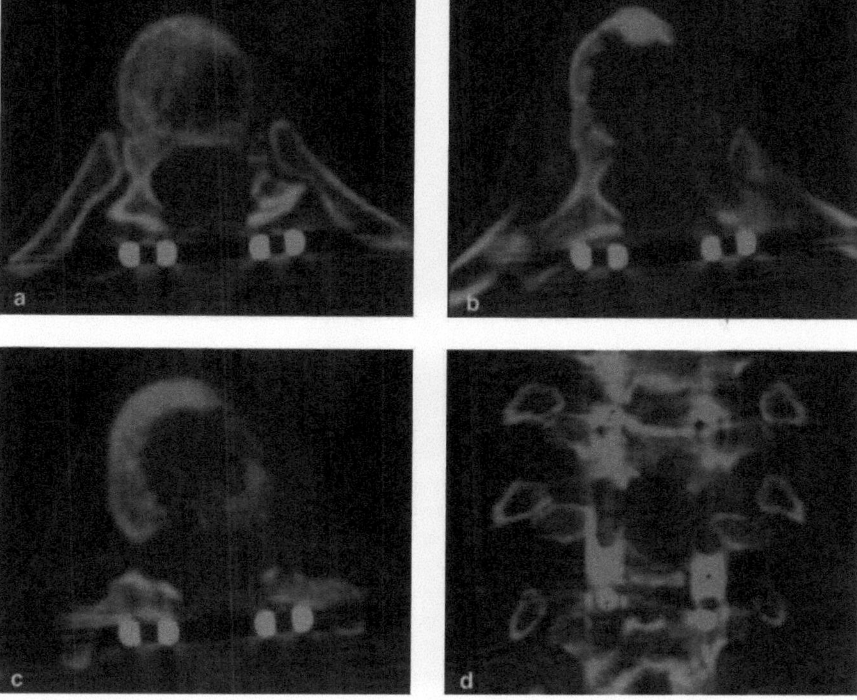

results and no faults in the intraoperative application of the navigation system could be found. It is possible that in these initial two patients, operated on with computer guidance, the DRB loosened during surgery. However, a radicular neurologic disorder of the focal nerve route was not observed in any of the patients with eccentric pedicle screw placement.

In all patients the postoperative CT scan showed accurate decompression of the neural structures (◘ Fig. 69-3). Regarding the preoperative neurologic findings [7], two patients were classified as having Frankel B lesions, three had Frankel C lesions and one patient had a Frankel D lesion. Two patients had no neurologic disorders preoperatively. Postoperatively, one patient with a Frankel B lesion had improvement of the lesion to Frankel C, and two of the three patients with Frankel C lesions and the patient with the Frankel D lesion had no neurologic signs. No neurologic deterioration occurred.

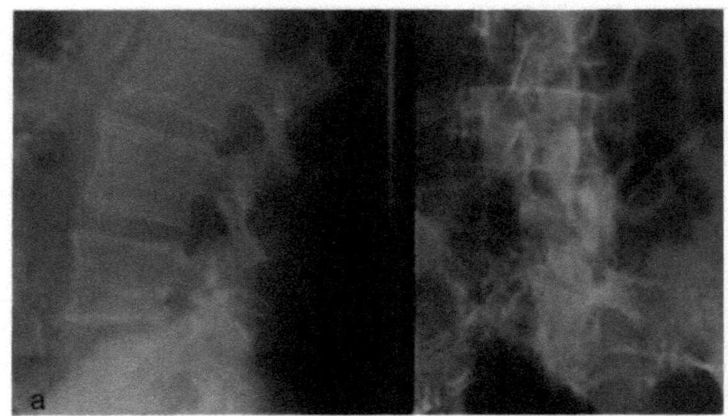

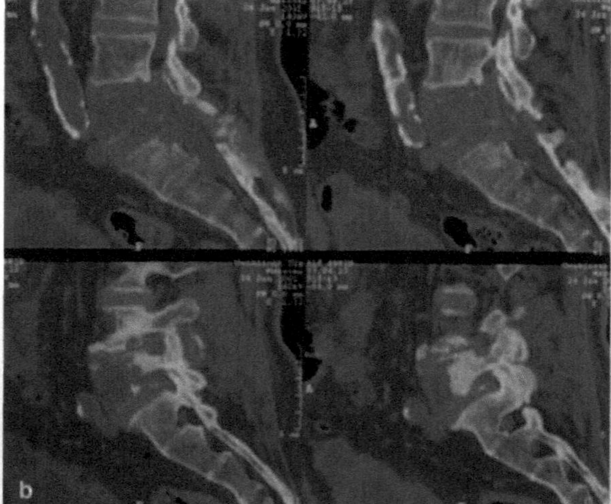

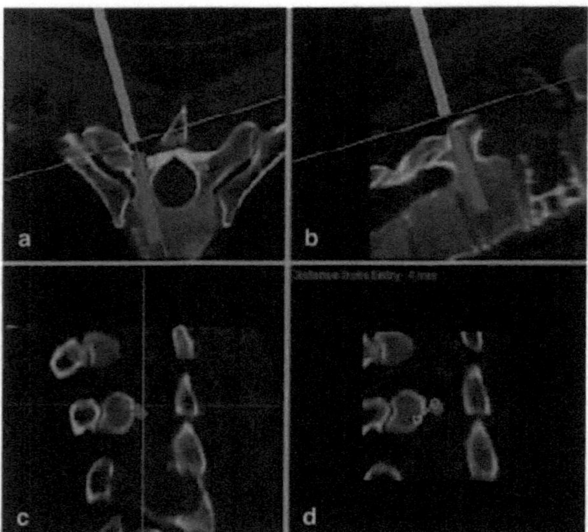

◘ **Fig. 69-4a-d.** The intraoperative screenshot during computer guidance of a patient with a tumor at T11 shows four windows: **a** the left upper window shows the transverse plane, **b** the right upper window shows the sagittal plane and **c** the left and **d** right lower windows show frontal planes in different distances related to the bone surface. In (**d**) the right lower window, in addition, two rings represent the target of the trajectory in case of complete superimposition. The intraoperative relationship between the planned trajectory (large arrow) and the spinal tumor (small arrows) and the instrument (large broken arrow) is clearly seen

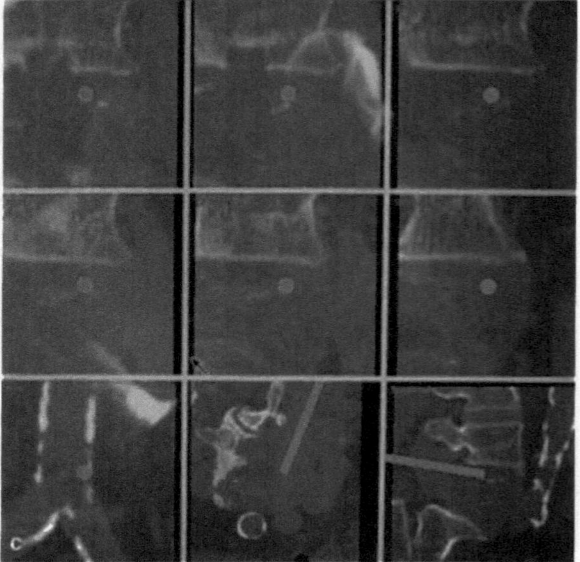

◘ **Fig. 69-5a-c. a, b** Metastasis of an spinocellular tumor in the lumbar spine. **c** Intraoperative position of the biopsy forceps

The illustration of the tumor in relation to the implant allowed exact and stable positioning of the transpedicle screws (◻ Fig. 69-4).

Intra-operativley, biopsies could be taken in the center of tumor lesion (◻ Fig. 69-5).

The main intraoperative pitfalls were the difficulties in thoracic paired-point matching attributable to missing landmarks on the posterior vertebral structures.

Discussion

In this clinical feasibility study, CT-based verification of the efficacy of navigated decompression and pedicle screw placement in patients who had tumor-related posterior surgery has been demonstrated. Eighty-six percent of the pedicle screws were positioned centrally in the bone without perforation; in all patients accurate decompression was seen. The accuracy of transpedicle screw implantation postoperatively has been investigated *in vitro* and *in vivo* with CT-scans [9, 12, 14, 20], plain radiographs [11, 25], MRI [2, 29], and via dissection [16]. In several studies a significant percentage (21% [25], 23% [19], 40% [10], 41% [22], and 42% [13], respectively) of conventional implanted transpedicle screws were inserted incorrectly. However, other reports have indicated that perforation rates of the lumbar pedicle were as low as 10% [21] to 15% [2]. *In vitro* and *in vivo* computer-aided navigation studies have shown an increased accuracy of transpedicle implant fixation with perforation rates from 2.7% to 11.3% [2, 11, 12, 20]. In addition, Zippel et al. [29] achieved in a MRI-controlled study a better reduction of thoracic misplacement rates (11.4%) than for lumbar misplacement rates (16%). Authors with comparable studies [2, 12, 29] have observed higher rates of misplacement in their conventionally treated cohorts (range, 14.3%–42%) as in the navigated groups.

However, the accuracy of the computer-guided insertion of transpedicle screws in this series was higher than in some published reports of studies which used conventional fluoroscopic positioning [10, 19, 22, 25]. Moreover, and unlike other published studies [3, 4, 27], no postoperative neurologic deterioration and non-implant loosening were seen in the patients as a result of using computer-aided surgical procedures. At the same time, we were able to achieve complete decompression of the neural structures for radiologic and neurologic findings.

Because of inaccurate registration, it was not possible to use computer-aided implantation surgery for 15% of the pedicles and, therefore, a conventional fluoroscopic approach was used. These data compare favorably with the findings of other investigators who observed rates of non-navigable pedicles as high as 32% [12, 20].

The average intraoperative time for navigated instrumentation of the spine was 7 min for the matching per vertebra, which is slightly higher than that reported in the literature (5.5 min) [12].

Our initial results indicate that computer-aided frameless navigation of tumor surgery of the spine is a safe technique which improves surgical performance during posterior decompression and transpedicle stabilization. In addition, CAS surgery improved the intraoperative information about the tumor and the current surgical intervention during decompression. In contrast to other authors [9, 20], a learning curve was observed for processing and interpretation of the intraoperative matching, the crucial part of spinal navigation.

The technique should be used only by experienced surgeons who can, if required, continue the operation using conventional techniques. Furthermore, the surgeon should have a complete theoretical understanding of the navigation system to minimize possible misinterpretation of computer guidance information.

References

1. Amiot LP, Bellefleur C, Labelle H (1997) In vitro evaluation of computer-assisted pedicle screw system. Ann Chir 51: 854–860
2. Amiot LP, Lang K, Putzier M, Zippel H, Labelle H (2000) Comparative results between conventional and computer-assisted pedicle screw installation in the thoracic, lumbar, and sacral spine. Spine 25: 606–614
3. Bauer HC (1997) Posterior decompression and stabilization for spinal metastases: Analysis of sixty-seven consecutive patients. J Bone Joint Surg 79A: 514–522
4. Carl AL, Khanuja HS, Sachs BL et al. (1997) In vitro simulation: Early results of stereotaxy for pedicle screw placement. Spine 22: 1160–1164
5. Castro WH, Halm H, Jerosch J et al. (1996) Accuracy of pedicle screw placement in lumbar vertebrae. Spine 21: 1320–1324
6. Esses SI, Sachs BL, Dreyzin V (1993) Complications associated with the technique of pedicle screw fixation: A selected survey of ABS members. Spine 18: 2231–2238
7. Frankel HL, Hancock DO, Hyslop G et al. (1969) The value of postural reduction in the initial management of closed injuries of the spine with paraplegia and tetraplegia. Paraplegia 7: 179–192
8. Gertzbein SD, Robbins SE (1990) Accuracy of pedicular screw placement in vivo. Spine 15: 11–14

9. Girardi FP, Cammisa FP, Sandhu HS, Alvarez L (1999) The placement of lumbar pedicle screws using computerised stereotactic guidance. J Bone Joint Surg 81B: 825–829

10. Jerosch J, Malms J, Castro WH, Wagner R, Wiesner L (1992) Lagekontrolle von Pedikelschrauben nach instrumentierter dorsaler Fusion der Lendenwirbelsäule. Z Orthop 130: 479–483

11. Kamimura M, Ebara S, Itoh H. et al. (1999) Accurate pedicle screw insertion under the control of a computer-assisted image guiding system: Laboratory test and clinical study. J Orthop Sci 4: 197–206

12. Laine T, Schlenzka D, Makitalo K et al. (1997) Improved accuracy of pedicle screw insertion with computer-assisted surgery: A prospective clinical trial of 30 patients. Spine 22: 1254–1258

13. Merloz P, Tonetti J, Pittet L et al. (1998) Pedicle screw placement using image guided techniques. Clin Orthop 354: 39–48

14. Merloz P, Tonetti J, Pittet L, et al: Computer-assisted spine surgery. Comput Aided Surg 3: 297–305, 1998.

15. Nolte LP, Visarius H, Arm E et al. (1995) Computer-aided fixation of spinal implants. J Image Guid Surg 1: 88–93

16. Nolte LP, Zamorano LJ, Jiang Z et al. (1995) Image-guided insertion of transpedicular screws: A laboratory set-up. Spine 20: 497–500

17. Roessler K, Ungersboeck K, Dietrich W et al. (1997) Frameless stereotactic guided neurosurgery: Clinical experience with an infrared based pointer device navigation system. Acta Neurochir 139: 551–559

18. Roy-Camille R, Roy-Camille M, Demeulenaere C (1970) Osteosynthesis of dorsal, lumbar, and lumbosacral spine with metallic plates screwed into vertebral pedicles and articular apophyses. Presse Med 78: 1447–1448

19. Saillant G (1995) Complications de la visee pediculaire, echecs et complications de la chirurgie du rachis. Sauramps, Montpellier

20. Schwarzenbach O, Berlemann U, Jost B et al. (1997) Accuracy of computer-assisted pedicle screw placement: An in vivo computed tomography analysis. Spine 22: 452–458

21. Sim E (1993) Location of transpedicular screws fixation of the lower thoracic and lumbar spine. Acta Orthop Scand 64: 28–32

22. Vaccaro AR, Rizzolo SJ, Balderston RA et al. (1995) Placement of pedicle screws in the thoracic spine. Part II: An anatomical and radiographic assessment. J Bone Joint Surg 77A: 1200–1206

23. Vinas FC, Holdener H, Zamorano L et al. (1998) Use of interactive-intraoperative guidance during vertebrectomy and anterior spinal fusion with instrumental fixation: Technical note. Minim Invasive Neurosurg 41: 166–171

24. Visarius H, Gong J, Scheer C, Haralamb S, Nolte LP (1997) Man-machine interfaces in computer assisted surgery. Comput Aided Surg 2: 102–107

25. Weinstein JN, Spratt KF, Spengler D, Brick C, Reid S (1988) Spinal pedicle fixation: Reliability and validity of roentgenogram- based assessment and surgical factors on successful screw placement. Spine 13: 1012–1018

26. West JL, Bradford DS, Ogilvie JW (1991) Results of spinal arthrodesis with pedicle screw-plate fixation. J Bone Joint Surg 73A: 1179–1184

27. Wise JJ, Fischgrund JS, Herkowitz HN, Montgomery D, Kurz LT (1999) Complication, survival rates, and risk factors of surgery for metastatic disease of the spine. Spine 24: 1943–1951

28. Zindrick MR, Wiltse LL, Doornik A et al. (1987) Analysis of the morphometric characteristics of the thoracic and lumbar pedicles. Spine 12: 160–166

29. Zippel H, Putzier M, Lang K (2000) Computerassistierte Wirbelsäulenchirurgie. In: Reichel H, Zwipp H, Hein W (Hrsg). Wirbelsäulenchirurgie. Standortbestimmung und Trends. Steinkopff, Darmstadt, S 174–201

70 Pedicle Screw Implantation Using the *DISOS* Template System

E. Schkommodau, N. Decker, U. Klapper, K. Birnbaum,

H.-W. Staudte, K. Radermacher

Introduction

In computer-aided pedicle-screw implantation, exactly as in conventional procedures, correct positioning of the screw is only possible based on a precise knowledge of the anatomical structure in question. The choice of screw length and caliber depends to a great extent on detailed knowledge about this structure [6]. Generally, the greater the screw length and caliber, the better the anchoring [4]. In addition, particular attention must be paid to ventral boundaries and the constant danger of perforation in the area of the spinal cord. The proximity of the spinal column means the greatest care is required in introducing the screw in order to avoid damage to surrounding neural and vascular structures. Placement of a pedicle screw is therefore difficult since there is no direct view into the spine. In particular, problems can arise with medial or caudal placement of the screw, possibly resulting in serious neurological dysfunction. In the literature, faulty placements (perforations) using conventional procedures are reported to range from between 8.5% [2], 15.9% [9], 39.9% [3], and 42% [5].

Methods

Radermacher et al. have described investigations into using individual templates (□ Fig. 70-1) in spinal surgery for open door and transcorporal decompression in neck vertebrae, the pedicle screw in relation to scoliosis therapy, repositioning osteotomy and decompression in lumbar vertebrae [7, 8]. A prerequisite for the application of individual templates is generating a computer-tomography (CT) image of the operational area. The CT slices that depending on the anatomic form of the bone are spaced at distances of 2 mm (vertebrae) to 4 mm (pelvis), the region representing the bone is extrapolated using segmentation procedures, then reconstructed and visualized in

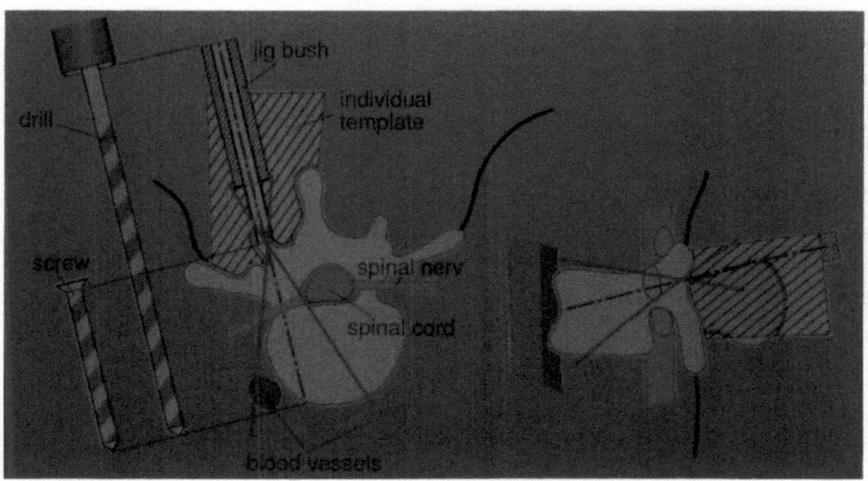

□ **Fig. 70-1.** Principle of the individual template technique be seen

three dimensions. Surgery can then be planned based on these models and positioning of the pedicle screw simulated with the operational planning system DISOS developed at the Helmholtz Institute, Aachen. In addition to using the vertebrae module, it is possible to carry out planning for peri-acetabular osteotomy following the procedure of Tönnis [10] or for endoprothetic treatment in the knee. Osteotomies and drillings are first carried out virtually using the computer model, the operator being led step by step through the program. Starting with the diagnostic dialogue, the operator can assess the entire condition of the spinal column with the aid of artificial X-ray pictures and the pilotscan (topogram). For example, it is possible to determine the Cobb angle. Following the choice of the screw type, the planning dialog continues and defines the entry point as well as the orientation of the drilling. Sectional images vertical to the bore axis help the surgeon (◘ Fig. 70-2). The operational planning concludes with the template positioning step. A virtual template is positioned on the bone model and at the same time marks the intraoperative area of bone that has to be prepared. The contact surface on the bone is automatically milled on a standard polycarbonate block as a negative impression of the bone surface derived from the modeled 3D CT data using a 3D milling device integrated into the planning station. This material is biologically tolerated and can be autoclaved. A typical milling step to create a lumbar vertebrae template takes about eight minutes and proceeds fully automatically.

As a result of the preoperative planning, the polycarbonate template together with a tool guide, in addition to the surgical instruments, are available to the surgeon during the operation. The operation proceeds as normal until presentation of the lamina. The vertebra to be worked on is identified, and the position of the individual template is determined approximately using the 3D planning printouts. Based on this, the template is placed on the bone at the correct position. Due to the shape of the individually milled negative impression, only one position of the template is possible and this is easily found by lightly pressing the template by hand onto the bone structure. When in the predefined position no further free movement of the template should be possible, and therefore the reference situation is identified intuitively [8]. Since instrument orientation is already taken into account in the planning the surgeon can now direct their instrument into the integrated tool guide and carry out the operation (◘ Fig. 70-3). The accompanying fluoroscopy check orthogonal to the pedicle allows the surgeon to directly assess the transpedicular position of their drilling channel.

Results

Development of the template design proved particularly important. Potential contact/positioning surfaces of the

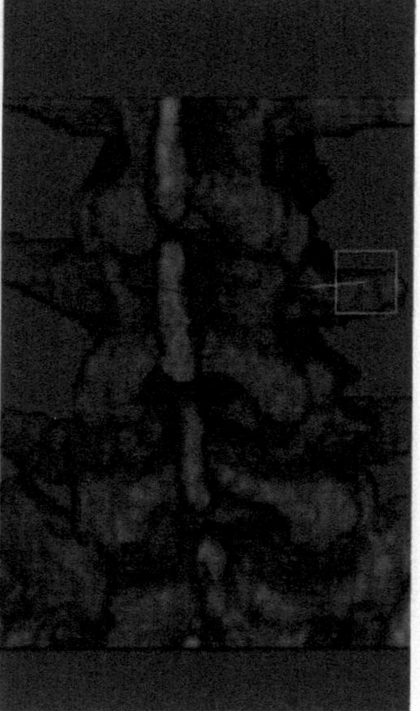
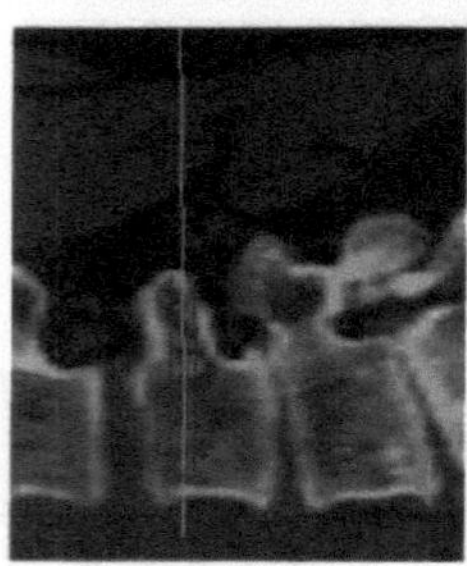

◘ **Fig. 70-2.** CT-based planning of pedicle drilling with the DISOS system

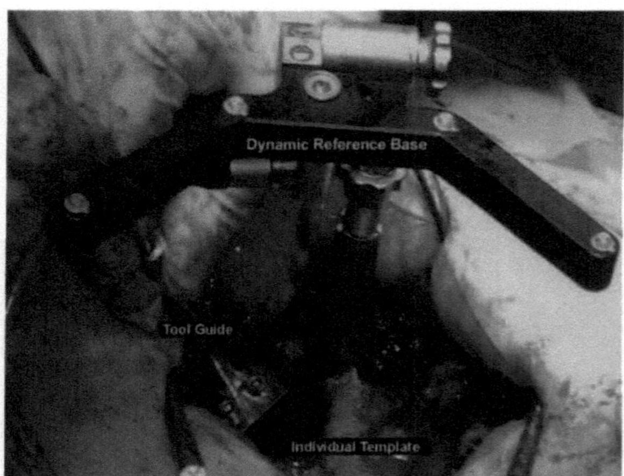

◘ **Fig. 70-3.** Intraoperative use of the template

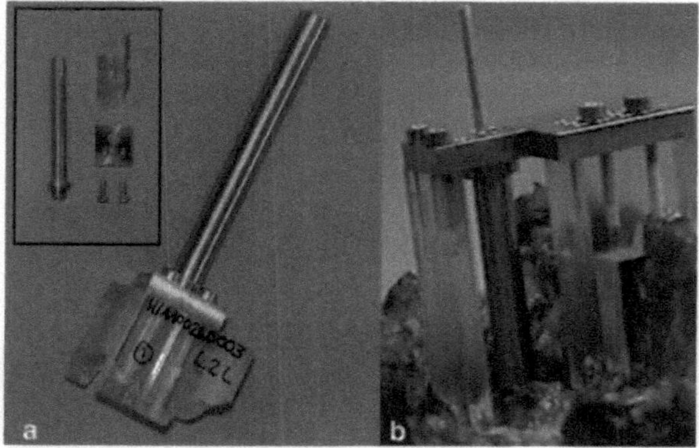

Fig. 70-4a,b. Vertebra templates: **a** unicontact, **b** multicontact

Table 70-1. Results of the anatomical study

Technique	Conventional	Individual templates, experiment series 1	Individual templates, experiment series 2
Number of pedicles	19	17	31
Preparation time [s]	346.6	347.3	338.6
Determining the entry point [s]	133.2	28	14.2
X-ray time for orientation	30.5	0	0
Faulty placement <2 mm	15.8% (n=3)	17.6% (n=3)	12.9% (n=4)
Faulty placement <4 mm	15.8% (n=3)	0	9.6% (n=3)[a]
Faulty placement <6 mm	0	0	12.9% (n=4)[a]
Faulty placement >6 mm	0	0	3.2% (n=1)[a]

[a] 8 faulty templates in one session due to a software problem.

template on the vertebrae were identified. Small contact surfaces tend to lack an unambiguous fit and a small overall design has low tipping stability. These problems led to the development of a design with multiple small contact surfaces. Advantages here included rapid production due to the small total contact surface and good tipping stability due to the long horizontal handle (**Fig. 70-4**). Disadvantages in practical use arise from the large overall form and complex construction. This resulted in the development of a further design with one contact surface on the lamina, the processus mamillaris and the medial part of the processus transversus. The highly structured vertebrae surfaces in these areas promise good referencing points (see Fig. 70-4).

A further evaluation step involved an anatomical study [1] with the goal of obtaining additional results about the precision and usability of the template in spinal surgery. A total of 37 pedicle drillings were carried out on anatomic lumbar vertebrae preparations, on one side using the conventional fluoroscopy technique (n=19), and on the other using the individual template technique (n=17). The duration of the conventional approach as well as the additional time for preparing each pedicle for the template technique and for establishing the template position were determined (**Table 70-1**). Two surgeons evaluated the position of the drilling using data recorded from a second CT. Perforations smaller than 2 mm were considered tolerable. Perforations up to 4 mm were critical, but still scored as acceptable. Five of the six perforations with the conventional technique lay too far in a medial direction. This was definitely atypical since surgeons tend to try and avoid the spinal chord and its structures,

and if in doubt generate a more lateral bias. The reason here is most likely the unusual construction of the experiment, which did not correspond to a normal operation situation. An obvious learning curve in searching for the entry point supports this suggestion. For example, the operator required an average of 245.6 seconds for the first three vertebrae entries but only 32.1 seconds for the last four. The largest perforation size with the template technique was 1.5 mm and was already identified intraoperatively by the only appraisal graded as »inadequate«. A preferential direction for the perforations, as seen with the conventional method, could not be determined here.

Improved orientation was the reason for improvements in the time taken and boring position compared to the conventional method. The results confirmed previous investigations where the positioning accuracy achieved with the individual template procedure was better than 1.5 mm and the angle of deviation less than 1°. For further approaches the unicontact template was favored due to its good fit and, compared to the multicontact model, its reduced tendency to collide with surrounding soft tissue.

Statistical analysis was not possible due to the small number of cases, therefore a second study followed. 31 pedicles were drilled using computer-generated individual templates. Initially, 6 planned drillings were terminated because in one case visual inspection revealed a faulty template relief, in another case the 3D model was interpreted falsely, in two cases template labeling was incorrect, in one preparation the CT image of the processus transversus was missing and in one case the contact surface was too small and therefore the template fit was ambiguous. The results of the second series of experiments are also presented in Table 70-1. Of note here is the high number of perforations larger than 2 mm. All these perforations arose in one experimental session and lay too far in a lateral direction. This was concluded to arise from a one-off system failure: the spread was not larger; rather the entry point was always biased in the same direction with reference to the template design. At that time the planning and milling software were still under development and were possibly the source of the error. Another source of error could have been the clamping device for milling the template. In connection with these experiments a mounting especially designed for vertebrae templates was subsequently used. After working on these possible sources of error such problems did not reoccur in subsequent studies.

During the clinical studies attention was paid to the operation time and improved radiological exposure. As an example here, the results of a comparative study of positioning the pedicle drilling using the individual template technique and an optical navigation system similarly based on CT data should be discussed. In 2 operations and 10 planned pedicle drillings the navigation system to be used as a control was cancelled at the registration stage or could not be used. In total the template technique was used 14 times. No problems arose in eight cases, while in six cases placement of the template was not possible:

- In four cases the expected preparation efforts turned out to be too high for the surgeon (L5 left/right and sacrum left/right). The positioning surface on the processus transversus of L5 was planned too far in a lateral direction. With the available template design for positioning on the sacrum the problem of soft tissue was compounded by the additional danger of the drill housing colliding with the spina iliaca posterior superior.
- During one operation the correct sequence of instruments to be used was not observed. Previously implanted pedicle screws (L4 left and right) were located in the positioning contact surface area of the template for the right and left L5 screws.

The average additional preparation time for the template contact surface amounted to 2 min 26.7 s. An average of 32 s was required for positioning the template. In comparison, installation of the navigation system demanded the surgeon's attention for 7 min on average, the referencing of a vertebral body for 11 min. The duration of X-ray exposure was the same with both systems and served only as a control.

- The control comparison of the screws positioned with the template as opposed to the navigation system revealed no significant differences. The template positioning corresponded in each case to an optimal location in the pedicle.
- No cases of neurological dysfunction were observed.
- These initial investigations showed that achieving placement of the template in the sacral region (sacrum and L5) was unsatisfactory. The soft tissue component pressed against the drill housing. A modified template design is required here. Support in the form of a second contact surface or a rod on the other side of the proc. spinosus could increase stability against tipping and reduce the preparation efforts required.

Discussion

The individual template technique is generally applicable in spinal surgery. Specifically, it promises advantages where spatial orientation is complicated by pathological deformities, where prothetic treatment of several segments is required or where direct access to the bone surface is anyway indicated (e. g. scoliosis). In comparison to the navigation system, it is simpler to use intraoperatively as well as more time- and cost-effective. In contrast to the intraoperative computer-supported navigation process, use of the template technique requires no additional equipment during surgery.

A preoperative CT-image is however unavoidable, and therefore with the individual template technique as with the CT-based navigation systems, an intraoperative fluoroscopic monitoring using the C arm is recommended.

In comparison to conventional radiological-based approaches, exposure time to X-rays is greatly reduced. Disadvantages in comparison to X-ray-based navigation systems are clearly that neither percutaneous minimally invasive applications nor intraoperative situation-dependent corrections in the direction of pedicle drilling are possible, since the preoperative planning results are statically saved in the template. With trauma patients in particular it is therefore recommended that radiological navigation is used rather than the template technique.

References

1. Birnbaum K, Schkommodau E, Decker N, Prescher A, Klapper U, Radermacher K (2001) Computer-assisted orthopedic surgery with individual templates an comparison to conventional operation method. Spine 26: 365–370

2. Haaker RG, Eickhoff U, Schopphoff E et al. (1997) Verification of the position of pedicle screws in lumbar spinal fusion. Eur Spine J 6: 125–128

3. Jerosch J, Malms J, Castro WHM et al. (1992) Lagekontrolle von Pedikelschrauben nach instrumentierter dorsaler Fusion der Lendenwirbelsäule. Z Orthop 130: 479–483

4. Krag MH (1988) Depth of insertion of transpedicular vertebral screws into human vertebrae: effect upon screw-vertebra interface strength. J Spinal Disorders 1: 287–294

5. Merloz P, Tonetti J, Pittet L et al. (1998) Pedicle screw placement using image guided techniques. Clin Orthop 354: 39–48

6. Olsewski JM, Simmons EH, Kallen FC et al. (1990) Morphometry of the lumbar spine: anatomical perspectives related to transpedicular fixation. J Bone Joint Surg 72: 541–549

7. Radermacher K, Portheine F, Anton M et al. (1998) Computer assisted orthopaedic surgery with image-based individual templates. Clin Orthop 354: 28–38

8. Radermacher K (1999) Computerunterstützte Operationsplanung und -ausführung mittels individueller Bearbeitungsschablonen in der Orthopädie. Berichte aus der Biomedizinischen Technik, Bd 7. Shaker, Aachen

9. Schlenzka D, Laine T, Lund T (2000) Computer-assisted spine surgery. Eur Spine J 9 [Suppl 1]: S57–64

10. D, Arning A, Bloch M, Heinecke A, Kalchschmidt K (1994) Triple pelvic osteotomy. J Pediatr Orthop 3: 54–67

71 Navigation – Where do we go from here?

F. Langlotz

Introduction

Trying to predict the future of a quickly developing domain such as navigational surgery always bares a certain risk. One easily faces the danger of wrongly estimating current trends and developments, and within in a few years being proven as wrong as Thomas Watson, the former chairman of IBM. In 1943, Mr. Watson was convinced that »there is a potential for maybe five computers worldwide«. Nevertheless, we can look back at almost 10 years of computer-assisted orthopaedic surgery and identify a number of weak points which still exist. We can observe numerous concepts and ideas that have recently been developed for, or are currently being introduced into CAOS. These observations surely suggest certain directions for speculation about what the future of CAOS may be. Conjuring up science fiction will definitely not be the goal of this chapter, since such forecasts often turn out to remain »visions« even after 10 or 20 years, but rather an overview shall be provided that estimates which developments may become reality within the next years and will be usable in the OR on a routine basis.

Novel Tracking Technology

A navigator is the central element of each surgical navigation system (see chapter 3). It enables measuring of the position of instruments in relation to the operated anatomy. Certain limitations are set by the laws of physics and the boundary conditions within an operating room. In the past, any feasible measurement technology has been implemented by research groups or the developers of tracking technology. Navigators based on the principle of direct mechanical contact [25] as well as contact-less trackers using optical [3], acoustic [23], or electromagnetic [2]

signals have been or are still being used in surgical navigation systems. However, it seems to be a commonly accepted fact now that only optical tracking of surgical instruments combines the required accuracy [16] with an acceptable intraoperative handling to guarantee ergonomic navigation system design. Stryker-Leibinger is currently the only company using active wireless LED equipped instruments in their navigation system (see chapter 44, 46). This concept will surely be used more widely in the future and will become the third option complementing passive tracking and active instruments with wired LEDs. The power supply for this type of tracked rigid bodies is still a problem today, and there seems to be no elegant solution available in the near future. None of today's single use or rechargeable batteries is autoclavable, and at the same time possesses sufficient capacity in small dimensions to allow for the construction of compact and handy instruments. Batteries that are separately sterilizable, e. g., by means of plasma sterilization, may be used in surgical instruments and are actually employed in Stryker-Leibinger's system. However, they require an easily accessible battery compartment and will add considerably to the per-case costs if they are not reusable. One could also think of unsterile batteries that are fed into sterile instruments with the help of a capsulated loading device, but such a construction will most likely lead to heavier and bulkier instruments than those available with today's wired tracking probes.

The line-of-sight problem is another disadvantage that is common to all optical navigators. To enable uninterrupted tracking, there must not be any objects in between the camera and LED or reflecting sphere, respectively. Logistic difficulties may be an immediate result, in particular in small operating theaters. There have been attempts with electromagnetic trackers, but they failed due to the unavoidable presence of metallic objects and their adverse and non-predictable effects on measuring accuracy. One alternative could be the development of a rather small camera system that could be mounted right above the operating table like an OR lamp. Surgical staff would not interfere that easily with the camera's line-of-sight to the instruments to be tracked. It is the manufacturers' turn now to bring into play new measurement solutions that can be employed by the developers of surgical navigation systems.

Imaging

Not only will novel tracking devices enable better navigation systems in the future, but also additional imaging modalities will be adapted to navigation. During the advent of computer-assisted orthopaedic surgery, CT scans were used exclusively for virtual objects. The advantages were obvious: computed tomography represents bony structures in a geometrically correct and three-dimensional way. On top of that, scans are available in digital format making them ideal candidates for further digital processing in a computer system. Disadvantages are the (often additional) logistical and financial efforts and the radiation exposure to the patient. Consequently, researchers started searching for alternatives rather soon. Although the advantages of preoperatively computed tomography will justify their usage as virtual objects for a number of indications in the future, several intraoperative imaging techniques become increasingly relevant.

Parallel employment of several image data sets originating from different sources is common during neurosurgical navigation [10]. A similar trend may be foreseen for orthopaedic surgery in the years to come. It will open new fields of application of CAOS.

Intraoperative Imaging

Interventional CT [12] or MRI scanners [20] were the first devices that were used for the intraoperative generation of image data for navigation systems. However, these devices require high investment costs and often even reconstruction work within the clinic [19]. Therefore, they have not become a standard in orthopaedic navigation so far.

In contrast, the introduction of the fluoroscope [11] into computer-assisted surgery represented a milestone. For the first time, it became possible with an acceptable effort to update the virtual object based on intraoperative changes applied to the therapeutic object, e. g., during the reduction of a fracture. The calibrated C-arm was observed by the tracking camera during image acquisition. As an immediate result, the spatial relationship between generated image and the visualized anatomy could be measured automatically without the need for an error-prone manual registration. As outlined in chapter 1, virtual fluoroscopy also comes with a number of disadvantages. For that reason, it should be seen as complementary to CT-based navigation, not as its replacement. Fluoro-CT as presented in chapter 3 by the description of Siemens's SIREMOBIL ISO-C^{3D} has surely the strongest potential. At present, neither image quality nor size of the scanned volume can compete with the possibilities of CT scanning, but it can be foreseen that improvements of hardware and software will yield better results in the future. In addition, market introduction of the Siemens device demonstrated that the potential of novel imaging technology in the context of navigation systems is nowadays analyzed at a very early state.

Fusion of Modalities

The simultaneous usage of different image data sets opens the door for a variety of new opportunities. For instance, during computer-assisted planning and realization of pelvic osteotomies, bony structures could be visualized by means of CT while, at the same time, MRI data would let the surgeon respect joint cartilage. Co-registration of both images is a pre-requisite for such fused virtual objects. In order to minimize planning efforts, this step should be automated. As an output, a merged tomogram should be made, which in turn would be used as the navigational basis of the intraoperative system. At this point in time, such a procedure is impossible. In particular, the automatic manipulation of MRI scans is an extremely challenging image processing task.

However, 3D-3D fusion of preoperative scans represents just one possibility of the simultaneous usage of two sets of images. Matching a preoperative CT scan with an intraoperatively acquired, calibrated C-arm image could be a means to automate registration of virtual and therapeutic objects. One group of researchers has already presented this approach on an experimental basis [8], but additional research is necessary before such a 2D-3D fusion can be used routinely. Once CT-C-arm registration has become reality, there will be a wide field of application for this technology. On the one hand, it would be an easily applicable, method of registering preoperative CTs in a minimally invasive manner (see below). On the other hand, when the intraoperative treatment has altered sections of the bony topology, the new configuration could be scanned with a fluoroscope and section by section be registered with the original 3D data set. Ultimately, it might then be possible to modify the initial preoperative data to reflect the intraoperative changes.

Minimally Invasive Approaches

Many of the articles that were published on computer-assisted orthopaedic surgery in the 1990's pointed out that the new technology would have a large potential to allow for fantastic and never expected minimally invasive operations in the future [13, 18, 21]. Reality has proven that this hope unfortunately remained a wish, except for a small number of cases in which invasiveness could be reduced slightly by the application of CAOS technology [5]. In some applications of robots [9] or navigation systems [14], surgical trauma was even increased, which turned out to be too high a price for the achieved gain in accuracy. When looking at orthopaedic interventions from an abstract point of view, three reasons become evident why they have to be invasive in the first place: Firstly, instruments have to have access to their place of application, the bone. Secondly, the surgeon has to have visual contact to this place of action in order to carry out the intervention with the required accuracy. Last but not least, devices such as screws, plates, or endoprostheses have to be attached to the bone in many cases. The delivery of these implants can only be performed in an invasive manner. Navigational surgery is aiming at the second problem. It tries to replace direct visual contact to the situs by a virtual representation of the scene on a computer monitor. To do so, referencing and – for preoperative images – registration of the operated anatomy are necessary as has been explained in detail in chapter 1 of this book. Today's

techniques require both steps to have direct physical contact to the bone and are therefore incompatible with the minimally invasive use of a navigation system. However, it can be expected that current trends in research may overcome this dilemma.

Minimally Invasive Registration

The above-mentioned automatic fusion of fluoroscopic images and CT scans is only one way to achieve registration between virtual and therapeutic object in a minimally invasive manner. Two other alternatives shall be discussed now. Both of them attempt to acquire bony surface points for point-based registration algorithms non-invasively.

Ultrasonic devices allow the transcutaneous scanning of bone surfaces. First approaches incorporating calibrated A- [17] or B-mode [1] ultrasound probes are very promising and will make their way into surgical navigation systems within due time. However, their application will be successful only if existing problems [22] are solved that are related to the automatic processing of the noisy images and signals. Alternatively, a navigated fluoroscope may be employed to digitize points. Several authors pointed out that coordinates inside a patient's body may be calculated from two C-arm images that had been acquired from different angulations [11, 15]. At this point in time, it cannot be stated which of these alternative technologies for the acquisition of matching points will prove to be more accurate and reliable.

Minimally Invasive Referencing

Minimally invasive referencing represents an even more demanding challenge than minimally invasive registration. Its aim is the constant measurement and mathematical compensation of potential relative movements between operated anatomy and tracking system. This problem is reduced to the detection of bone inside the body of a patient. Precise observation of the skin surface and a derived prediction of the underlying bone structures do not appear to be an acceptable approach as long as the biomechanical influence of soft tissue layers is not fully understood. The generalization of any minimally invasive registration procedure could turn out to be a fruitful methodology. If such a registration could be performed fully automatically and in real-time, an additional referencing would become obsolete and instead the (varying) matching transformation would be calculated constantly. Fluoroscopy exposes patient and surgical staff to radiation and thus does not qualify for a continuous application. This leaves only ultrasonic solutions as future methods of choice. Though, as long as ultrasound-based registration has not become state-of-the-art, ideas about analogous referencing approaches remain an ambitious vision.

Virtual Reality and Augmented Reality

Implementing elements of virtual or augmented reality (AR/VR) as parts of a CAOS system may appear equally futuristic.

Thinking of virtual reality, one might imagine surgeons wearing data gloves and head mounted displays while standing at the OR table. However, the use of the term »virtual reality« may not appear that exotic any more if its meaning is expanded to also describe a realistic computer representation of a selected aspect of reality. Many of today's navigation systems represent quite abstractly the operational target, instruments, implants, or even bony anatomy reconstructed from CT data. There is an ongoing discussion about whether abstract or photorealistic rendering of the operation scene is more appropriate. Nonetheless, it might be hypothesized that at least a number of navigation applications of future generations will continuously increase the realism of their representations.

The field of augmented reality is different in that AR applications present to the user real views that are enhanced by overlaid computer graphics. This principle was first developed for the military domain. Aiming and navigational information was projected into fighter jet windshields or the helmet visors of pilots. In an equivalent way preoperative planning data or anatomical structures that are hidden below the visible tissue surface may be presented to the surgeon. When optical viewing aids such as endoscopes or microscopes [7] are employed, the fusion of real and artificial views is relatively easy from a technical point of view. The computer-generated overlay can be fed directly into the optics of the device. Most modern microscopes offer this option even as a standard feature. It becomes much more difficult if artificial information must be »smuggled« into the view of the surgeon's naked eye. This type of manipulation may be carried out at three locations between the eye and the real object: Using a laser or video projector, information can be written directly onto the object's surface [24]. To achieve a realistic representation, the projected image has to be distorted dynamically according to the possibly varying topology of the »projection screen«. Alternatively, a semi-transparent mirror [4] placed in between eye and real object or a pair of semi-transparent glasses can be used. Since the projection surface is planar in these cases, there is no need for distorting the projected image. Last but not least, retina projectors are available now. They »overwrite« parts of the natural image that the eye sees by projecting information directly onto the retina. With any of these possibilities, two aspects have to be taken into account: a) the virtual image has to appear at the correct spatial position and b) both real environment and augmenting information have to be seen focused. The first requirement calls for a matching between real and virtual world incorporating also the surgeon's eye or head position if the projection is not directly on the patient. The requirement for simultaneous focus of real and virtual image can be fulfilled only partially. If additional information is presented by a mirror or a pair of glasses, the eye will focus on one of the two images, making the other one appear more or less blurry. Retina-based projectors are calibrated for a dedicated eye-object distance, so a clear presentation can be achieved only when a constant distance between object and surgeon's eye can be guaranteed.

All these difficulties have been solved only partially in the available prototype setups, or even not at all. On top of that, the special hardware required is still quite expensive and more or less bulky. Consequently, one can foresee that augmented reality outside optical devices such as endoscopes or microscopes will not play a major role in the near future.

Quality Assurance and Surgical Education and Training

There are two emerging fields in the application of surgical navigation: Quality assurance, which is being paid more and more attention in all aspects of medical treatment, and surgical education and training. There is no doubt that the usage of CAS systems increases procedural accuracy, in many cases yielding an increased repeatability. It cannot be foreseen today if, and to what extend, this will make surgical navigation the state-of-the-art for selected interventions. However, such a process would automatically turn this technique into an obligatory method. Each of today's available systems already allows the documentation of the steps preformed, e.g., by means of screenshots. It is just a question of time until this particular documentation method will become legally admissible in the United States, which – in this case– is lagging behind Europe. The application of CAOS technology for documentation purposes could thus become mandatory.

But even for clinical research, navigation systems offer a large and up to now only partially explored potential. They may be used as precise measurement tools to question established opinions [6] or to evaluate new surgical techniques.

Despite all this euphoria, one should not forget that the successful application of navigational technologies requires an amount of extra knowledge and skills that must not be underestimated. Without them, the computer can easily turn out to prolong operations and cause frustration. The responsibility for continuing education cannot be passed on to one particular person within the operating team. Everyone is involved who is in contact with the new system and the associated instruments: surgeons and assistants, nurses and OR technicians, even the departments of sterilization and radiology. »Classical« forms of education and training should be questioned and new pedagogical concepts have to be elaborated. For instance, perfect control over the machine may require regular »refreshing sessions« in dedicated simulators, as is common for professional pilots.

The combination of the above-mentioned VR/AR techniques and so-called force-feedback devices may even enable the development of special navigation systems dedicated exclusively to education and training; even for conventional, i.e., non-CAS-based surgical techniques. Such devices might feature perfect visual and tactile simulation of tissue structures, instruments, and even pathologies or possible complications. At the end of the day, they may even complement surgical education using cadavers and patients.

Wherever the future may lead us to in the innovative field of surgical navigation, one thing will be certain: technology will remain an assistant to the human surgeon. It cannot copy or replace his experience and skills, nor compete with them, but it will perfectly complement them.

References

1. Amin DV, Kanade T, DiGioia AM, Jaramaz B, Nikou C, Labarca RS (2001) Ultrasound-based registration of the pelvic bone surface for surgical navigation. Comput Aided Surg 6(1):48, 2001.
2. Amiot LP, Labelle H, DeGuise JA, Sati M, Brodeur P, Rivard CH (1995) Computer-assisted pedicle screw fixation – a feasibility study. Spine 20: 1208–1212
3. Berlemann U, Langlotz F, Langlotz U, Nolte L-P (1997) Computerassistierte Orthopädische Chirurgie (CAOS) – Von der Pedikelschraubeninsertion zu weiteren Applikationen. Orthopäde 26: 463–469
4. Blackwell M, Morgan F, DiGioia AM III (1998) Augmented reality and its future in orthopaedics. Clin Orthop 354: 111–122
5. DiGioia AM III, Jaramaz B, Nikou C, LaBarca RS, Moody JE, Colgan BD (2000) Surgical navigation for total hip replacement with the use of Hip-Nav. Oper Tech Orthop 10: 3–8
6. Digioia AM III, Jaramaz B, Plakseychuk AY et al. (2002) Comparison of a mechanical acetabular alignment guide with computer placement of the socket. J Arthroplasty 17: 359–364
7. Friets EM, Strohbehn JW, Roberts DW (1995) Curvature-based nonfiducial registration for the stereotactic operating microscope. IEEE Trans Biomed End 42: 867–878
8. Hamadeh A, Lavallée S, Cinquin P (1998) Automated 3-dimensional computed tomographic and fluoroscopic image registration. Comput Aided Surg 3: 11–19
9. Heeckt R, Rühl M, Buchhorn G et al. (1999) Computer Assisted Surgical Planning and Robotics mit dem CASPAR-System. In: Jerosch J, Nicol K, Peikenkamp K (Hrsg) Rechnergestützte Verfahren in Orthopädie und Unfallchirurgie. Steinkopff, Darmstadt, S 414–433
10. Hill DL, Hawkes DJ, Crossman JE et al. (1991) Registration of MR and CT images for skull base surgery using point-like anatomical features. Br J Radiol 64: 1030–1035
11. Hofstetter R, Slomczykowski M, Sati M, Nolte L-P (1999) Fluoroscopy as an imaging means for computer-assisted surgical navigation. Comput Aided Surg 4: 65–76
12. Jacob AL, Messmer P, Kaim A, Suhm N, Regazzoni P, Baumann B (2000) A whole-body registration-free navigation system for image-guided surgery and interventional radiology. Invest Radiol May 35: 279–288
13. Kalfas IH, Kormos DW, Murphy MA et al. (1995) Application of frameless stereotaxy to pedicle screw fixation of the spine. J Neurosurg 83: 641–647
14. Langlotz F, Stucki M, Bächler R, Scheer C, Ganz R, Berlemann U, Nolte L-P (1997) The first twelve cases of computer assisted periacetabular osteotomy. Comput Aided Surg 2: 317–326
15. Langlotz U, Grützner PA, Bernsmann K et al. (2003) A hybrid CT-free navigation system for acetabular cup placement. J Arthroplasty (submitted)

16. Li Q, Zamorano L, Jiang Z, Gong JX, Pandya A, Perez R, Diaz F (1999) Effect of optical digitizer selection on the application accuracy of a surgical localization system – a quantitative comparison between the OPTOTRAK and flashpoint tracking systems. Comput Aided Surg 4: 314–321

17. Maurer CR, Gaston RP, Hill DLG et al. (1999) AcouStick: A tracked A-mode ultrasonography system for registration in image-guided surgery. In: Taylor C, Colchester A (eds) Medical image computing and computer-assisted intervention – MICCAI'99. Springer, Berlin Heidelberg New York Tokyo, pp 953–962

18. Merloz P, Tonetti J, Pittet L et al. (1999) Computer-assisted spine surgery. Comput Aided Surg 3: 297–305

19. Messmer P, Jacob AL, Fries E et al. (2001) Technologieintegration und Prozessmanagement – Konzept und Implementierung einer neuartigen Plattform für einzeitige Diagnostik und Therapie des akut Kranken und Verletzten sowie für elektive computerassistierte Chirurgie (CAS). Unfallchirurg 104: 1025–1030

20. Moche M, Busse H, Dannenberg C et al. (2001) Fusion von MRT-, fMRT- und intraoperativen MRT-Daten – Methode und klinische Bedeutung am Beispiel neurochirurgischer Interventionen. Radiologe 41: 993–1000

21. Nolte L-P, Visarius H, Langlotz F, Schwarzenbach O, Berlemann U, Rohrer U (1996) Computer assisted spine surgery – a generalized concept and early clinical experiences. Int Soc Comput Aided Surg 3: 1–6

22. Tonetti J, Carrat L, Blendea S, Merloz P, Troccaz J, Lavallée S, Chirossel J-P (2001) Clinical results of percutaneous pelvic surgery – computer assisted surgery using ultrasound compared to standard fluoroscopy. Comput Aided Surg 6: 204–211

23. Wallny T, Klose J, Steffny G, Schulze-Bertelsbeck D, Perlick L, Schumpe G (1999) Dreidimensionaler Ultraschall und intraoperative Navigation: Ein neuer Einsatz des Ultraschalltopometers bei Umstellungsosteotomie des proximalen Femurs. Ultraschall Med 20: 158–160

24. Wörn H, Hoppe H (2001) Augmented reality in the operating theatre of the future. In: Niessen WJ, Viergever MA (eds) Medical image computing and computer-assisted intervention – MICCAI 2001. Springer, Berlin Heidelberg New York Tokyo, pp 1195–1196

25. Zamorano L, Jiang Z, Kadi AM (1994) Computer-assisted neurosurgery system: Wayne State University hardware and software configuration. Comp Med Imaging Graph 18: 257–271

72 The Asian Knee – Is Navigation Possible?

K.Y. Chiu

Introduction

While primary osteoarthritis of the hip is rare, primary osteoarthritis of the knee is relatively common in the Asian populations [4]. The exact reason remains unclear, but it could be due to different mechanical environment in the Asian knees [12, 13]. Despite knee osteoarthritis is common, the Asian patients did not like surgery. They preferred to live with the pain, frequently at the expense of the daily activities. The view points have changed in the past 5 to 10 years, and more patients now demand for active lives despite of old age. In many Asian countries, the frequency of total knee arthroplasties (TKAs) has been rising constantly. In some places, TKAs have become significantly more common than total hip arthroplasties in the ratio of 2 or 3 knees to 1 hip, or even higher.

Although most TKAs in Asians are successful, problems such as aseptic loosening and polyethylene wear still occur. While it is easy to attribute these failures to patient and prosthetic factors, it is possible that the surgeon did not do a perfect job at time of the operation. It has been well documented that TKAs with varus alignment fail substantially earlier than those with neutral or valgus alignment [9]. Mal-rotation of the femoral or tibial components could lead to increased polyethylene wear and also suboptimal patellar tracking. Some Asian patients may not be happy about their TKAs, since they cannot flex the replaced knees adequately to perform activities specific to the Asian cultures. Apart from component malalignment, it may be due to suboptimal ligament balance and stability that result in abnormal kinematics.

Such flaws in surgical techniques are likely to be a bit more common when the Asian knees are replaced. First, the Asian knee is technically more difficult to replace. Asian patients are often stoical, and very reluctant to have surgery. By the time they agree for TKAs, the articular surfaces are severely damaged, and the capsule and ligaments are grossly contracted. The surgical landmarks are less distinct because of the bone defects, and the soft tissues become more difficult to balance. Furthermore, the patients may continue to ambulate despite advanced knee deformities; it is possible that in this situation the bone may remodel in the presence of abnormal stress to produce secondary bone deformities such as bowing or torsion of the diaphyses. Second, with the exception of a few places, most Asian surgeons who perform TKAs are not high volume joint replacement surgeons. As a result, accurate and precise bone cuts and perfect balancing of the soft tissues are not always achievable. Third, the Asian

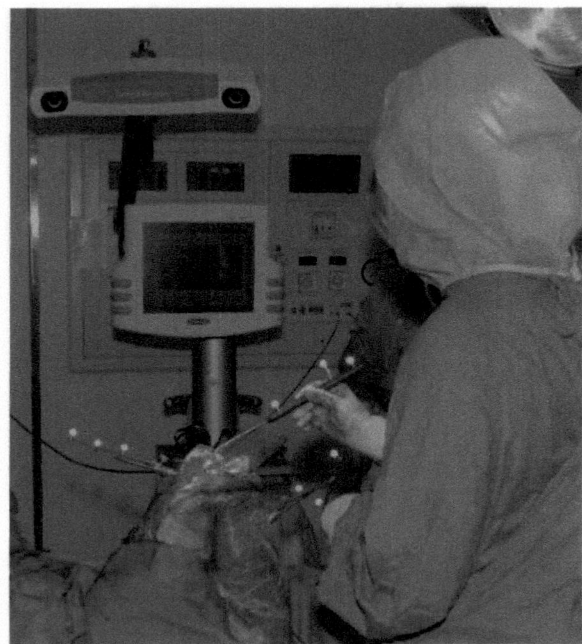

Fig. 72-1. Image-guided total knee replacement is performed in a Chinese patient

knees are not just miniature of the Western knees; they are different [2]. It may be inaccurate if the instruments that are designed for average Western anatomy are used to do TKA in Asian patients.

Is navigation the solution to the above problems? The intention of this chapter is not to discuss whether it is possible to use the navigation system when replacing the Asian knees; the answer is affirmative (◘ Fig. 72-1). The point is whether navigation can possibly address the specific issues related to the Asian knees. In the following sections, the need of navigation to deal with the different knee anatomy and specific needs for high knee flexion in Asians will be discussed.

Asian Knees are Different

To get the mechanical axis right, the distal femoral bone cut is usually made perpendicular to the line joining the centre of the hip joint and the centre of the distal femur. Since the center of the hip joint is notoriously difficult to locate without imaging, most knee-system manufacturers will recommend the use of an intra-medullary alignment rod to guide the distal femoral bone cut. However, it is not that straight forward for the Asian knees. In Japanese patients, it was shown that the femoral medullary canal was often not straight, and the central line of the proximal femoral diaphysis formed an angle of 2 degrees with the central line of the distal diaphysis [8]. Such lateral femoral bowing is not uncommon in the Chinese population (◘ Fig. 72-2). The use of an intra-medullary guide could result in erroneous distal femoral cut. This is especially so if the preoperative anteroposterior radiograph of the whole femur is not available and the distal femoral cutting angle suggested in the surgical technique brochure is blindly followed. Even if the surgeon is aware of such lateral bowing, it is still hard to handle if the lateral bowing is excessive – the valgus angle of distal femoral cutting jig in most convention knee systems cannot exceed a certain limit; the entry hole may need to be translated sideway but this adds the risk of being even less exact in the final alignment. With the navigation system, the center of the hip joint can be located either by CT-based or CT-free navigation algorithm (◘ Fig. 72-3). There is no need to insert an alignment into the medullary canal, which is not a straight forward situation and reliable thing to do in the Asian knees.

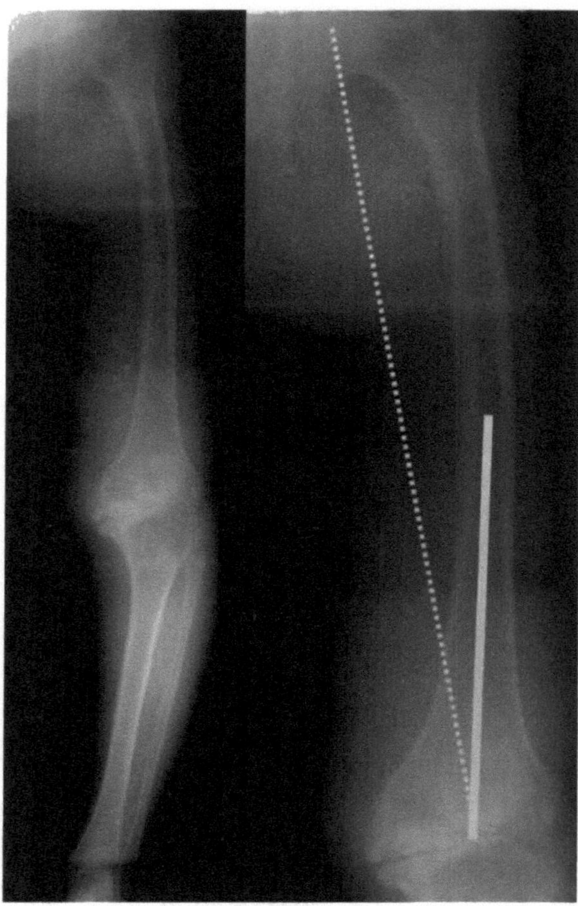

◘ **Fig. 72-2.** The femur in this Chinese women showed obvious lateral bowing. If an intra-medullary alignment guide was used with the entry hole made over the inter-condylar fossa (*solid thick line*), it formed an angle of 12° with the mechanical axis (*dotted thin line*). If such long anteroposterior radiograph was not available and the surgeon followed the usual distal femoral cutting angle such as 5°, it could result in a 7° varus alignment. It is possible that the use of an intra-medullary guide could result in erroneous distal femoral cut

The same problem also exists in the tibial side. In Chinese patients, over 20% of varus knees showed tibial bowing to the degree that the intra-medullary alignment guide could result in an unacceptable cut of the proximal tibia [6]. Many surgeons choose to use extra-medullary alignment guide. However, the latter relies a lot on »eyeballing« and the experience of the surgeon, and an accurate tibial cut is not always reproducible.

While it is important to get the varus-valgus alignment correct, attention to the flexion-extension alignment of

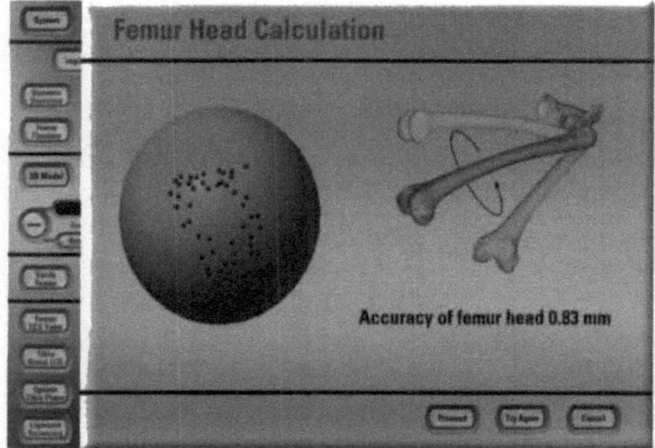

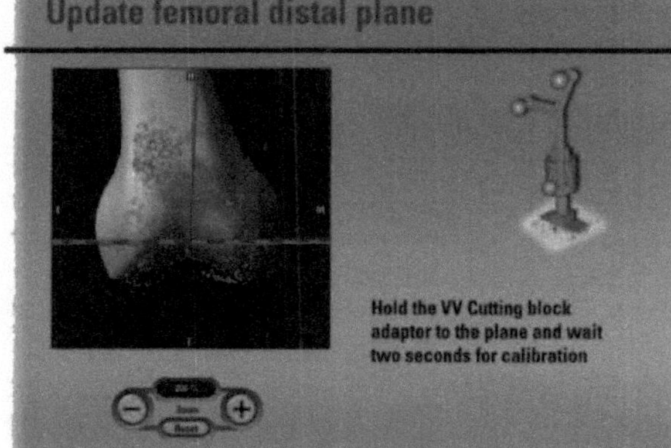

Fig. 72-3. The center of the hip joint can be located in a three-dimensional manner with the use of CT-free hip pivoting algorithm (*upper*). The distal femoral cutting jig can then be positioned with reference to hip center to obtain the correct varus-valgus alignment (*lower*)

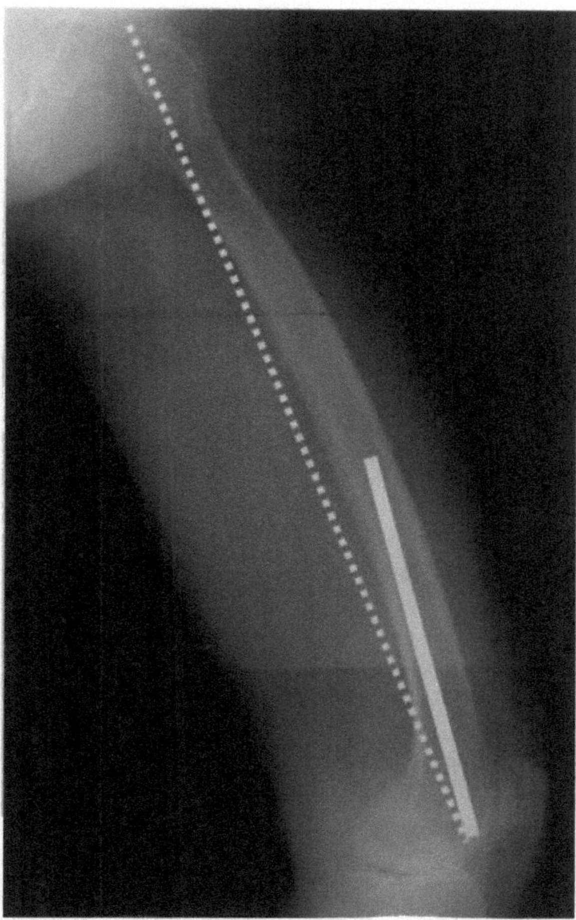

Fig. 72-4. The medullary canal of the Asian femur is often not straight, but bowed in the lateral view. The intra-medullary alignment guide rod (*solid thick line*) will follow the curvature of the distal femur. In this radiograph, it forms an angle of 7° with the lateral mechanical axis (*dotted thin line*). If the distal femur is cut with reference to the lateral mechanical axis, it will be 7° »extended« with reference to the intra-medullary guide rod. If the distal femur is cut with reference to the intra-medullary guide rod, it will be 7° »flexed« with reference to the lateral mechanical axis

the femoral component is also important but often neglected. The latter can adversely affect the knee kinematics and the functional outcome, and can lead to problems such as anterior notching. Since intra-medullary alignment guide is commonly used in the femoral side, the sagittal alignment of the femoral component will usually follow the direction of the distal femoral medullary canal. If the medullary canal is straight in the lateral view, the femoral component should be properly aligned relatively to the lateral mechanical axis. However, the medullary canal of the Asian femur is not straight, but it often shows anteroposterior bowing that increases progressively from the proximal to the distal end (**Fig. 72-4**). We studied the radii of curvature of the femoral medullary canal in 100 lateral radiographs of the entire lower limbs of 86 Chinese patients admitted for total knee replacements. The radii

of curvature of the proximal, middle and distal one-thirds of the femora were about 1100 mm, 900 mm and 730 mm, respectively. The distal one-third of the femora was significantly curvier than the other parts of the femora. Since the intra-medullary guide rod follows the curvature of the distal femoral medullary canal, it is likely that the femoral component will be placed in a »flexed« position relative to the lateral mechanical axis. On the other hand, if it is desirable to place the femoral component perpendicular to the lateral mechanical axis, then the component will appear to be too much »extended« relative to the distal part of the femur; this may end up in anterior notching. With the use of conventional TKA instruments, there is very little leeway, and the control of the bone cut is rather crude. With the help of navigation, the surgeon can decide on the best position to place the jig so that the desirable flexion-extension alignment of the femoral component relative the centre of hip joint can be achieved. The jig can then be translated anteroposteriorly according to the anatomical landmarks captured, so that anterior notching will not occur.

The next issue is on rotational alignment of the distal femur. When we do TKAs, we first balance the collateral ligaments, and cut the proximal tibia perpendicular to the tibial axis. If the femur is then distracted from the tibia with the knee in 90° of flexion, the proximal tibia cut surface and the transepicondylar axis will be parallel. Normally this results in slightly more bone being removed from the posterior medial femoral condyle than the lateral. However, in our Chinese population we found that the amount resected from the posterior medial condyle was relatively much bigger than the lateral. This discrepancy led us to hypothesize that the usual relationship between the posterior condylar line and the trans-

epicondylar axis was not 3° as reported in Western patients, but was more in Asian knees. This is in line with what we found in a study that looked at the axial alignment of the lower extremity [12]. Using anteroposterior weight-bearing radiographs of the entire lower limb in 50 young, normal Chinese subjects, the knee joint line was found to be more oblique, averaging 5° compared with 3° in Western studies. Similar findings were reported in a group of Japanese patients with medial osteoarthritis [8]. With the joint line in 5° of varus, the posterior condylar line should also form a 5° angle with the transepicondylar axis that is perpendicular to the tibial axis. This postulation correlated very well with what we found in another study using 25 pairs of Chinese cadaveric femora [13]. The rotational alignment was such that the transepicondylar axis was externally rotated by more than 5° relative to the posterior condylar line. In other words, one may not get the necessary external rotation if the jig that usually produces only 3° of external rotation relative to the posterior condylar line is used in the Asian knees. This could result in a trapezoidal flexion gap and a problem with patellofemoral tracking. Unfortunately, most TKA systems only provide 3° external rotation cutting jig. With the use of navigation system, the cuts are guided by the transepi-

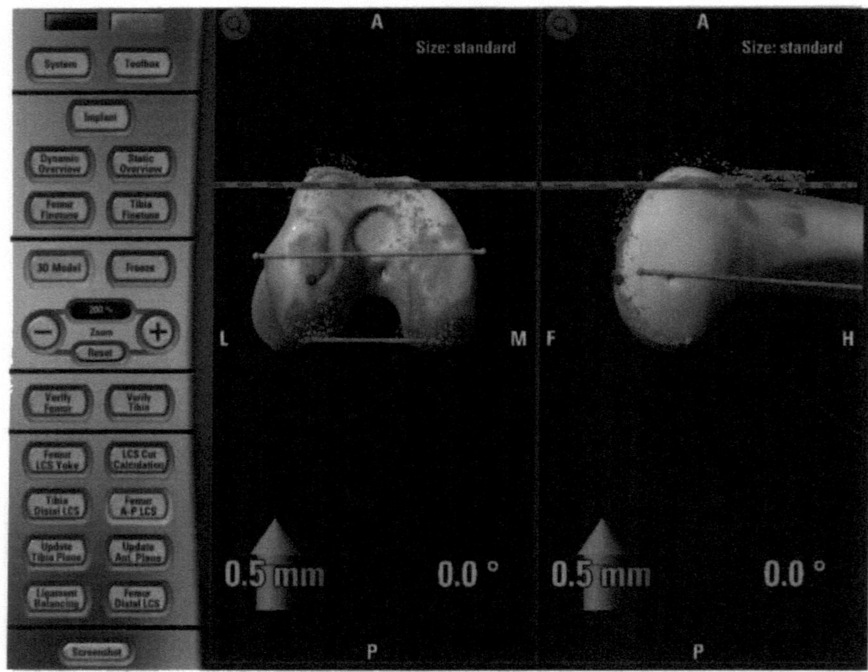

Fig. 72-5. With navigation, the cuts that set the femoral component rotation are guided by the transepicondylar axis. The surgeon can do fine-tuning according to the feedbacks from the system to achieve the desirable femoral rotation

condylar axis, while the surgeon can do fine-tuning according to the feedbacks from the system to achieve the desirable femoral rotation (■ Fig. 72-5).

Range of Motion After TKA

It has been demonstrated that 67° of knee flexion is needed for the swing phase of gait, 83° are needed to climb stairs, 90° are needed to descend stairs, and 93° are needed to rise from a chair [5]. Most recent published series reported that final flexion was between 100° and 115° after TKA. While this may be enough according to the criteria above, some Asian patients may need knee flexion from 120° to 150°. For example, full squatting with the knees to the floor is commonly practiced every day because of the sitting environment in Japan. Similar positions are required for prayers in many religions, such as Buddhism and Islam. Many factors affect range of motion after TKAs [3]. There is no doubt that one must pay attention to every detail at the time of the surgery. Navigation may be helpful to achieve higher flexion by providing the surgeons with more precise information on soft tissue balancing and the bone cuts.

The need to appropriately balance the ligaments cannot be over-emphasized. If any of the ligaments are tight, the range of motion will be limited. Laskin [7] studied the effect of a trapezoidal flexion gap. In the first group (92 knees), equal resection of the posterior femoral condyles combined with 90° tibial resection resulted in a trapezoidal flexion gap – the average preoperative flexion was 120°, and it was 100° after surgery. In the second group (96 knees), the femoral resections were externally rotated by an average of 3° to give a rectangular flexion gap – the average preoperative flexion was 115°, and it was 112° after surgery. The navigation system permits accurate evaluation of the flexion and extension gaps, and guides the femoral bone cuts such that the rotational alignment of the distal femur is correct. While the gaps are tested with spacer blocks inserted to tense up the ligaments **after** the bone cuts in many conventional knee replacement system, the navigation system will let the surgeon knows about the status of the gaps **before** the actual bone cuts are made.

Excessive elevation of joint line has also been shown to lead to poor knee flexion. Shoji et al. [11] studied 231 primary TKAs. If the joint line was elevated by 10 mm or less, 32% of knees could flex beyond 120°. Only 7% of knees could do so if the joint line was elevated by more than 10 mm. Ryu et al. [10] reviewed 90 TKAs in 60 patients. They reported that the joint line was elevated by an average of only 2.1 mm in the good flexion group. In the poor flexion group, the joint line elevation averaged 5.7 mm. With the use of navigation system, the surgeon can gather information about any possible change of the joint line, and adjust the level of the bone cuts accordingly.

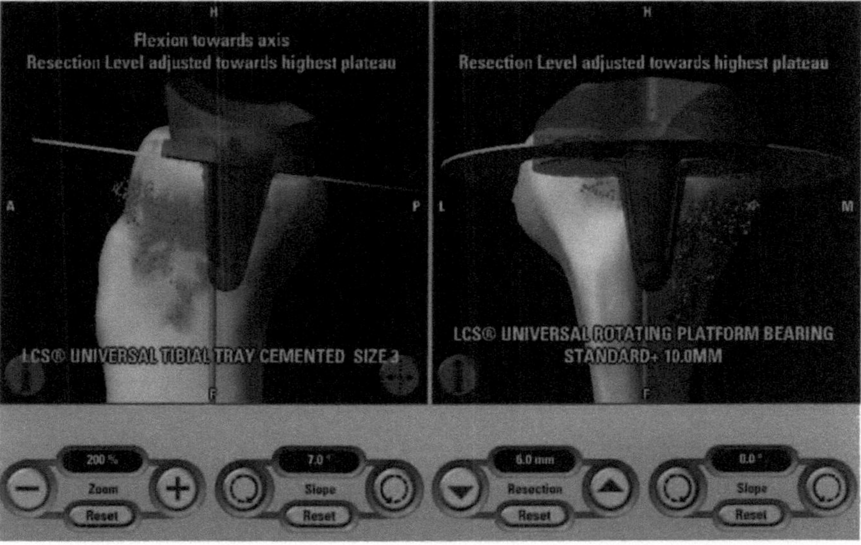

■ **Fig. 72-6.** The plane of the tibial cut is determined. The degree of posterior slope, which may affect the postoperative knee flexion, is accurately showed. There is no need to estimate from the »eye-balling« with the use of conventional knee instrumentation

The posterior tibial slope may affect the knee flexion range. Many surgeons use extra-medullary alignment guide and apply the cutting jig as recommended in the surgical technique brochure to cut the proximal tibia, but little attention is paid to the exact alignment of the guide rod in the sagittal plane. Some surgeons place the alignment parallel to the anterior tibial crest, but this may end up in a slope less than what is expected. We evaluated the posterior tibial slope in 25 pairs of Chinese cadaveric tibia [1], and found that the anterior tibial crest is not parallel to the intra-medullary axis. Using the same cutting jig, the extra-medullary alignment method will result in 3° less posterior slope if its rod is placed parallel to the anterior tibial crest rather than the intra-medullary axis. If posterior slope is desired, one must put the extra-medullary guide rod parallel to the intra-medullary axis by pulling it away from the ankle distally. Just referring to the degrees of slope inscribed on the cutting jig is meaningless. With the navigation system, the posterior slope refers to well defined anatomical landmarks in the ankle joint (◻ Fig. 72-6). This eliminates the problem of possible sagittal curvature of the medullary canal if the intra-medullary alignment system is used, and the imprecision when the slope is estimated crudely with the use of the extra-medullary alignment system.

Summary and Future Perspective

Even an experienced pilot needs navigation to assist the landing of the aircraft, especially if the weather is bad. It is possible that navigation will help the Asian surgeons to attain optimal bone cuts and good soft tissue balancing in a reliable manner, despite the Asian knees are tough to replace. Clinical evidence that the use of navigation will result in better knee function and less failures due to aseptic loosening and polyethylene wear after TKA is not available yet. Because the benefits of navigation may not be as apparent if the knees are not too severely deformed, the chance that a difference can be found between navigated knees and control knees is higher in Asian patients.

In addition to old patients with tricompartmental knee osteoarthritis, the Asian surgeons see an increasing number of younger patients with knee osteoarthritis who will benefit from unicompartmental knee replacements and are more receptive to surgical intervention. Navigation will permit this procedure to be properly done by an average surgeon using a minimal invasive approach. This will become a big point to include navigation in the armamentarium for the surgical treatment of Asian knees.

References

1. Chiu KY, Zhang SD, Zhang GH (2000) Posterior slope of tibial plateau in Chinese. J Arthroplasty 15: 224–227
2. Chiu KY (2002) Approaching the Asian knee. In: Hamelynck KJ, Stiehl JB (eds) LCS mobile bearing knee arthroplasty – 25 years of worldwide experience. Springer, Berlin Heidelberg New York Tokoy, pp 195–200
3. Chiu KY, Ng TP, Tang WM, Yau WP (2002) Knee flexion after total knee arthroplasty. J Orthop Surg 10: 194–202
4. Hoaglund FT, Yau ACM, Wong WL (1973) Osteoarthritis of the hip and other joints in southern Chinese in Hong Kong. Incidence and related factors. J Bone Joint Surg 55-A: 545–557
5. Kettelkamp DB, Johnson RJ, Smidt GL, Chao EYS, Walter M (1970) An electrogoniometric study of knee motion in normal gait. J Bone Joint Surg 52-A: 775–790
6. Ko PS, Tio MK, Ban CM, Mak YK, Ip FK, Lam JJ (2001) Radiologic analysis of the tibial intramedullary canal in Chinese varus knees. Implications in total knee arthroplasty. J Arthroplasty 16: 212–215
7. Laskin RS (1995) Flexion space configuration in total knee arthroplasty. J Arthroplasty 10: 657–660
8. Nagamine R, Miura H, Bravo CV et al. (2000) Anatomic variations should be considered in total knee arthroplasty. J Orthop Sci 5: 232–237
9. Ritter MA, Faris PM, Keating EM, Meding JB (1994) Postoperative alignment of total knee replacements. Its effect on survival. Clin Orthop 199: 153–156
10. Ryu J, Saito S, Yamamoto K, Sano S (1993) Factors influencing the postoperative range of motion in total knee arthroplasty. Bull Hosp Joint Dis 53: 35–40
11. Shoji H, Solomonow M, Yoshino S, D'Ambrosia R, Dabezies E (1990) Factors affecting postoperative flexion in total knee arthroplasty. Orthopedics 13: 643–546
12. Tang WM, Chiu KY, Zhu YH (2000) Lower limb alignment in Chinese adults. J Bone Joint Surg 82-A: 1603–1608
13. Yip DKH, Chiu KY, Zhu YH, Ng TP (2003) Distal rotational alignment of the Chinese femur and its relevance in TKA. Another reason why Chinese females need more knee arthroplasty? J Arthroplasty (in press)

73 Status Quo and Options in Medical Robotics

M. Börner, W. Ditzen

Introduction

»Where humans can't go, they build robots.« This principle is common practice in space science and nuclear power engineering as demonstrated i.e. with remote cars on planet Mars or robots working on nuclear substances steered by humans located behind protecting glass.

»ROBODOC, the new star in the operating room works precisely within a tenth of a millimeter« and »Future robotic cardiac surgeons will be precision mechanics working for hours without tiring or trembling.« These are two of many news headings indicating the possibilities of robots that may increase both accuracy and optimal technique during anatomically difficult surgery. Robotics is a new field in orthopaedic and trauma surgery and many questions remain to be answered including efficacy, security, as well as economical aspects. The number of robots used in practice is marginal, although manufactures provide broad clinical experiences. Whereas the use of robots within industry increased exponentially since the 1970s their surgical application is limited due to medical staff rejection.

There are different evolving robot systems within the medical field, five of which were classified by Taylor according to different techniques:

1. Internet Application
2. Tele-Surgery
3. Navigation Tool
4. Precision Positioning
5. Path and Search Systems

Howe and Matsuoka [31] as well as Caddedu [15] further classified different systems and application in both the orthopaedic and neurosurgical field. A widely accepted classification of robots was published by Troccaz et al. [49] and DiGioia [22], who subspecified passive, semiactive and active systems.

- Passive systems are limited for preoperative planning, surgical simulation, and intraoperative navigation.
- Semiactive systems include preoperatively planned robotic surgery, supervised by the surgeon.
- Active systems become relatively autonomic during surgery, but are closely supervised by the surgeon.

History

Medical robotics is a relatively new field with first applications in neurosurgery in 1985. These were passive navigation systems for positioning biopsy needles and other tools within the cranium [34]. CT data allowed exact guidance of the tool by a robot arm. Unaltered industrial robots evolved to medical tools for all kind of applications in Europe, Asia and the US. In the early 1990s the Imperial College in London, UK, developed a robot capable of performing prostate surgery [20]. The Medical University in Grenoble, France, took cranial biopsies using a robot. This scientific innovation led to commercially available NeuroMate systems (Integrated Surgical Systems, France). Meanwhile the medical university in Tokyo, Japan developed a robot that was able to place needles using CT data [51]. The first semiactive robot that could mill bone resections emerged in the US in the early 1990s [47]. It is called ROBODOC and is now used worldwide.

Clinical Applications: Orthopaedic Surgery

Since the structure of bone is relatively rigid, bone resections (milling) are ideal indications in orthopaedic surgery. Preoperative planning and intraoperative anatomy varies little with bone compared with soft tissues. Therefore, robotics adopted early within orthopaedics. The ROBODOC system was developed by Integrated Surgical Systems, IBM Research and successfully implanted a total hip arthroplasty in dogs in 1992, milling the femoral shaft for component implantation. After successful results were obtained, this system was first applied worldwide for human THA in 1994 at the Trauma Clinic of Trade Associations (BGU) in Frankfurt, Germany [10].

There are three main components: Orthodoc planning station calculating the proximal femur with high precision via CT data for perfect milling and prosthetic fit. Transfer of collected CT data from the central computer, which runs the actual robot. In 1994 shaft milling required insertion of three pins into the femur, which could be abandoned in 1996. A further system improvement led to a pin-less surface matching procedure with sizing and milling of the femoral canal in 1998 [9] (◘ Fig. 73.1). Milling time averages between 10 to 20 min, continuously supervised by the surgeon via a monitor. The remaining THA operation is continued manually. At the Trauma Clinic of Trade Associations (BGU) in Frankfurt, Germany, over 4000 stems were implanted with the ROBODOC system so far and counts for the largest series worldwide [10]. There are further European centers using this technique as well.

Since 2000 three ROBODOC centers gain experience in robotic total knee arthroplasty (TKA) [11]. Two pins are

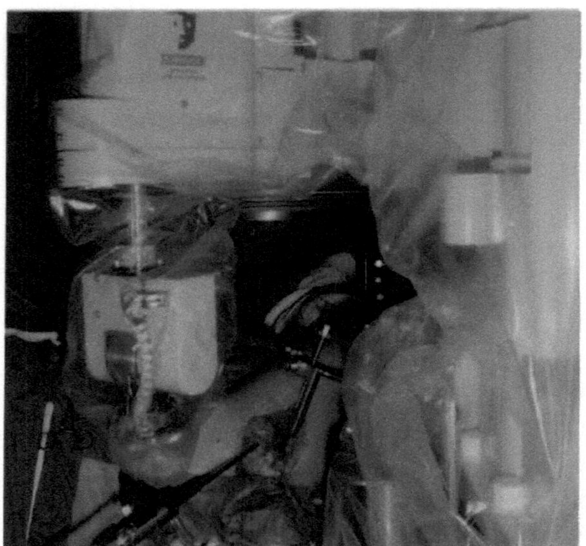

◘ **Fig. 73-1.** THA Robodoc during milling process

required in both tibia and femur for referencing all CT data. Preoperative planning includes CT data of femoral head and femur, tibia and ankle joint in order to calculating mechanical axes and optimal rotational alignment of both prosthetic components. Cementless components are used because of highly accurate milling resection planes and complete preservation of the PCL and other soft tissues [50].

The CASPAR robot (Ortho Maquet, Town, Country) is a competitive system, which was first used in 2000 after the introduction of ROBODOC. CT data and one reference screw at both femur and tibia are required for correct planning of the knee prosthesis. Intraoperative supervision is realized via two rigid bodies and LED navigation. First robotic clinical data showed perfect 3D alignment of all implanted knee components.

At the Imperial College in London a new TKA robot was developed by Jakopec and Harris [30] named AKROBOT with pinless femoral and tibial 20 to 30 points surface matching referencing. Resection milling is similar compared with both CASPAR and ROBODOC systems according to preoperative CT data. First successful clinical application took place in 2001.

ACL reconstruction (tibial and femoral tunnel placement) is another field of robotics as introduced by Petermann et al. [43] in 1999 using the CASPAR system. Preceding anatomical studies and healthy contralateral ACL fed CT data to the workstation for calculation of individual and physiological isometric graft position. Femoral insertion was defined 25% anterior to the posterior edge of the lateral condyle and 25% distal of posterosuperior Blumensaat line (according to quadrant method). Reference pins are required in tibia and femur. This technique resurrected discussion about optimal isometric positioning of the ACL graft. Comparative studies between robotic and conventional technique failed to showing significant advantages in optimal graft position depending on the surgeons experience [13], which questions the importance of optimal graft implantation.

Neurosurgery

From the historical point of view neurosurgeons were the first applying computer navigation and robotics as an operating tool. There are considerable public resonance and understanding that neurosurgeons claim highest accuracy in stereotactical orientation in brain surgery in order to minimize potential damages. There are a number of neurosurgical robots available including:

- Minerva, University of Lausanne, Switzerland [27],
- NeuroMate, Integrated Surgical System, ISS, USA,
- MRI compatible robot, University of Tokio, Japan [38].

The eldest robot for stereotacting a biopsy needle is the Minerva system, in which the robot is integrated in the CT scanner and supervised during CT investigation. The precision warrants five degrees of freedom, however, only two procedures were performed in September 1993, none after.

NeuroMate

The NeuroMate is a robot defined over six axes of freedom for neurosurgical applications, developed due to basic science by Benabid [4], Lavallée et al. [35] at the University of Grenoble, France. The original system was developed for specific stereotactic application and recently improved quality of digital imaging led to FDA approval of this technology. Over 1600 implementations were performed since 1989 (◘ Fig. 73-2). Predominant indication include tumor biopsies, stereoelectro encephalographic investigations in epileptic patients, as well as midline oriented stereotactic neurosurgery and functional basal ganglion surgery. This technology was applied at the Trauma Clinic of Trade Associations (BGU) in Frankfurt, Germany in September 2001 in cases including intracranial hematoma decompression, functional neurosurgery in Parkinson disease, brain tumor surgery, and spine surgery such as disc prolaps or bilateral kyphoplasty procedures, latter of which allows percutaneous minimally invasive robotic due to physiologic dorsal tension.

Robotic guidance is generally executed from skin to region of interest using a specific software application fed by digital DSA, CT or MRI data. A patient marker module matches patients anatomy with the robot arm localized at the skull. Robotic electrode or drill intrusion is performed after adjustment of CT data and patient calibration markers.

MRI Compatible Robots

Whereas most robotic neurosurgical system use CT data, more accurate MRI data become increasingly available today. The problem with MRI data is the requirement of non-magnetic instruments. At the University of Tokyo, Japan, a MRI compatible polyethyltereftalat (PET) robot was developed for stereotactic operations [38]. All assembling screws, gear parts, and poles had to be made of non-magnetic material. Trials on melons resulted in a 3.3 mm accuracy. The robot needle itself is embedded within the MRI scanner with a bow mechanism on top of the MRI base and connected via cables to a shielded control unit outside the MRI room, which also carries the robotic drive motor. A similar robot was developed at Brighams and Women Hospital, Boston, Massachusetts [17]. It consist of two open »polo mint« spools with the robot on top in between both spools (◘ Fig. 73-3). First applications of this experimental system include needle positioning in prostrate brachytherapy. German engineers developed a MRI compatible robot biopsy system for mamma tumors, which was preliminary tested with a 1.5 megatessla magnets on pig liver gaining an accuracy of 4 mm [32].

Other non-neurosurgical robot applications include interventional needle placement as demonstrated by different co-operations i. e. Georgetown University, Washington DC, USA [18, 19], and John Hopkins University, Baltimore, Maryland, USA, as well as intercontinental

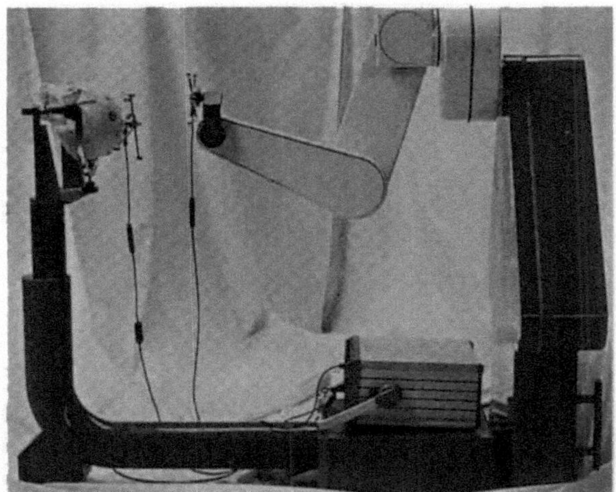

◘ **Fig. 73-2.** Neurosurgical robot system NeuroMate

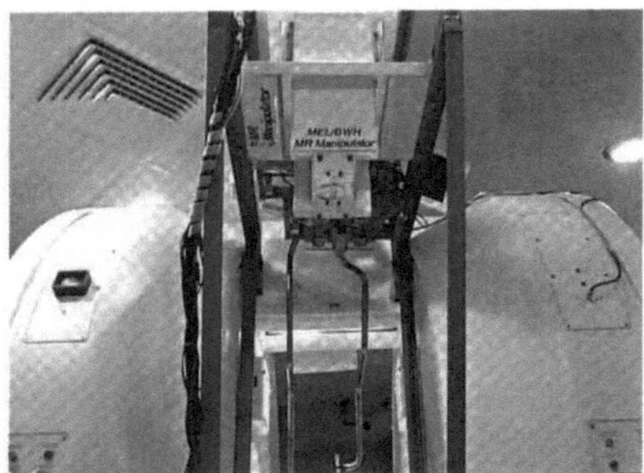

Fig. 73-3. MRI compatible robot with interventional MRI system

projects between John Hopkins University and Tokyo University, Japan. There are fluoroscopic and CT-guided system with an accuracy of 0.6 degrees and 1.04 mm as shown in cadaver studies [39]. Clinical trials for placing a 22-gauge needle for facet joint blockade are currently run with the PAKI/RCM robot system at the John Hopkins University and preliminary result are expected in late 2002.

Urology

In 1988 Davies et al. [20] developed a robot system Probot that was capable performing transurethral prostate resections in London, UK. Initial trials with a 6 degrees industrial Puma robot proved to be impractical and led to development of a medical robot, which was used in 1991 reflecting the first machine ever removing substantial human tissue in history. The frame itself had three axes plus a rectoscope for tissue removal. The geometry allows excavitation due to spatial restriction of the measured prostate. The system includes four security margins: 1) calculation; 2) imaging; 3) determination of the cavity; and 4) excavation. Internal anatomy is monitored via a video camera with the rectoscope. An ultrasound head is placed at the bladder neck through the rectoscope feeding 5 mm interval 3D information of the prostate to the robot. The surgeon defines all resection margins with a light pointer. Final excavation is performed within those margins.

The urological department at John Hopkins University in Baltimore developed a specific robot capable of

percutaneous access to a kidney (PAKI) via a remote center of motion (RCM) for minimally invasive kidney surgery [44].

Cardiac Surgery

Cardiothoracic surgeons joined relatively late the technology of robotics and minimally invasive operations in order to reduce the surgical trauma. Starting point for numerous endoscopic cardiothoracic procedures was the possibility of cardioplegic heart arrest in closed chests. The portal access technology includes transfemoral endovasal balloon occlusion of the ascending aorta and with the femorofemoral bypass technique arrested heart surgery becomes available without canulating and occluding the aorta. Same time development of complex robot systems progressed to telemanipulating surgery, a technology that led to a paradigm change in surgical applications. Whereas other field use robots for execution of preoperatively planned resections (i. e. bone milling) cardiac surgeons use a so-called online system that is continuously in the control by the surgeon.

The DaVinci telemanipulation system has two instrument grips, which are controlled by a master board. A high resolution 3D video is presented on a monitor. Movements on the instrument grips are transferred by motion sensors onto manipulators without delay. A central arm carries the videoscope and two side arms allow endoscopic instruments, so-called end effector (Fig. 73-4), which appears like a mechanical hand and has six degrees of freedom for complex motions such as coronary

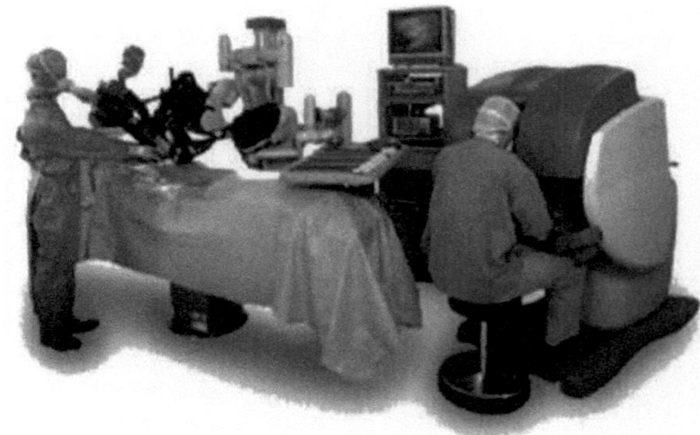

Fig. 73-4. Complex DaVinci telemanipulation system

anastomosis suturing within the thorax. The motion is transmitted 1:3, but can be programmed individually. Motion scaling allows up to 10 times magnification for optimal endoscopic quality. Tremor motions with a frequency of 6 to 10 Hz can be filtered [25]. The master board may be placed in a different room and the videoscope has optional speech control via a robot that allows for continuous two-arm endoscopy (automated endoscope system for optimal positioning = AESOP). This technology reduced misunderstanding in communication with an operating colleague, who usually has a reversed image. This technology may be described as a single surgeon procedure and was first executed at the cardiac center in Leipzig, Germany [26].

Zeus is a similar surgical system developed by Computer Motion Inc., CA, USA, that has three manipulators with one camera arm and two instrumentation ports (◘ Fig. 73-5). In comparison with the DaVinci system, the effectors have four degrees of freedom only. Both systems represent early stages in cardiothoracic robotics with first successes in coronary bypass surgery and aortic valve replacement, however, minimally invasive techniques and shorter hospital stay are important aspects in these kind of technology. With further improvements endoscopic

bypass surgery could be performed on beating hearts in the future [7]. Troccaz et al. at the University in Grenoble, France, developed a synergistic robot in cooperation with the surgeon that is capable performing pericardiac aspirations [49].

Since October 1999, 500 DaVinci procedures were performed, not only in cardiac surgery but also in abdominal surgery such as Nissen fundoplication [16], robot-assisted laparoscopic cholecystectomies [28], urological nephrectomies and adrenalectomies [45], and gynecological robot-assisted tubar anastomoses [24]. In experimental animal studies an intrauterine myelomeningocele defect was closed using robot navigated telemanipulators (DaVinci) [1].

Maxillofacial Indications

Maxillofacial indications include a broad spectrum of procedures that require accurate surgery of relatively small bones and aesthetic aspects such as
1. guiding non-flexible catheter implantations;
2. navigation of electronic drills, screw drivers for fixing bone and implants;
3. navigation of electronic saws and retracting hooks.

At the Charité Medical University, in Berlin, Germany, a special operating room with the SurgiScope robotic was set up (◘ Fig. 73.6) navigating three basic parallel lined arms with one moveable end effector. The parallel kinematic structures allow a very stable construct for precise procedures. First animal studies implant radioactive substrates into bones for local brachytherapy [36].

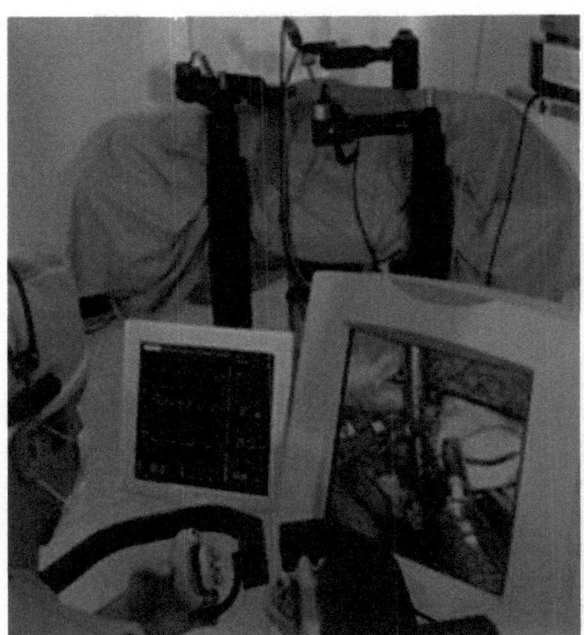

◘ **Fig. 73-5.** ZEUS manipulation robot system

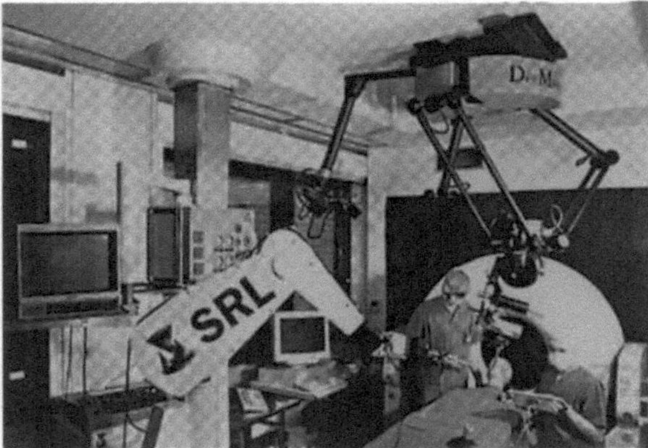

◘ **Fig. 73-6.** Interactive robot system Surgi-Scope

Craniofacial Osteotomies

Another maxillofacial robotic system was developed at University Maxillo Facial Institute for Processor Control and Robotics in Heidelberg, Germany. A RX90 robot navigates a surgical saw according to a surface model marked with 12 titanium screws. A haptical interface was created for marking the skull cross section [14].

Radiosurgery

Local radiation therapy is common management for malignant tumors. Radiosurgery inserts radioactive agents into the tumor with maximal protection of adjacent tissues. Radiosurgery in the brain is navigated via a stereotactic frame, which is firmly attached to the skull. Adler et al. at the Stanford University in CA, USA developed Image Guided Radiosurgery using a light weight linear accelerator, a Kuka robot, and orthogonal twined radiographs [2] (◘ Fig. 73-7). The radioactive agent insertion is navigated

by the robot arm according to the coordinates using radiographs of the lesion.

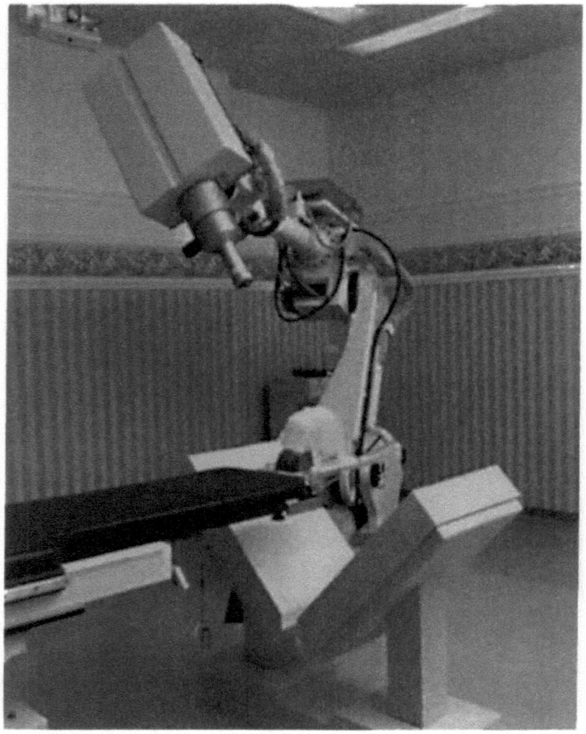

Ophtalmology

Applications of robots in ophthalmology increase the requirement of highly precise positioning and manipulation of surgical tools and instruments [48]. The main difference between so-called steady hand robots and other systems is that steady-hands robots still require manual actions from the surgeon, who guides the instruments via robot arms in a way that manual pressure is translated without tremor into smooth actions accordingly (◘ Fig. 73-8). Various studies comparing 1) surgery without assistance, 2) manually guided steady-state robots; and 3) entirely autonomous surgery without manual cooperation confirmed a significant superiority of needle action. The success rate increased from 43% in free hand surgery to over 79% steady state robots to 96% with fully automated robots [33].

Future Applications and Options

Despite increasing possibilities and applications of medical robots the number of users is limited and a handful of commercial providers struggle because of the complexity of this technology and its difficulties of introduction. A closer teamwork and cooperation between clinicians and engineers has to be established. Technological

◘ **Fig. 73-7.** CyberKnife radio surgical robot system

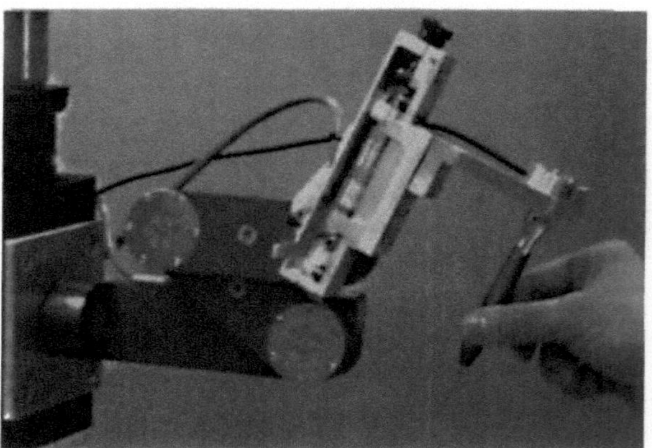

◘ **Fig. 73-8.** Steady Hand robot for microsurgical instrument guidance

challenges for medical robotics include components as well as hole component systems. Improvements of future system components include newer hardware architecture, software and imaging design with regards to user interface and security. The system hardware should allow better modularity of the electronic control equipment. This is realized i. e. with the steady hand robot PAKY-RCM, where a number of mechanical modules were developed for precise interventions. The compact Crigos robot system shows similar features [12].

Commercially available software design applications for surgical procedures face competition with inexpensive availability of this software. Standardized software configurations should be adapted to different surgical procedures in order to facilitate future software development and costs. The equipment design is developed from relatively affordable industrial robots, but individual medical applications are rarely profitable. This demands less specialized base module with different end effectors for all sorts of surgical applications. Robots should also benefit from the increasing popularity of imaging interventions such as CT and MRI.

With regards to user-friendly interfaces, the questions remain whether robots should proceed autonomically, are joysticks or keyboards better, should the surgeon himself manipulate the instrument directly, and should there be power feedback with the robotic manipulators. The answers will be everything but uniform, however, medical robotics will certainly gain acceptance when the surgeon has the potential of final control over the procedure. Medical robots certainly differ from industrial robots particularly because of individual user terms. This goes along with additional safety features that are yet to be defined and include redundant sensors, safety features for errors that allow manual continuation, as well as the necessity of sterilization and infection control within the operating room.

With the goal of universal platforms available for different radiographic, navigational and robotics optimal intraoperative applications will have to enhance visualization, control, and technical integration process, factors causing developmental challenges. Medicolegal aspects will almost certainly focus on basic principles, patient's claims, and the search for culprits [37]. Further problems may be expected from forensic physicians, who are inexperienced or contraire with this technology. When tele-surgery is performed the question arises whether the executing surgeon should be as experienced as the surgeon on front of the monitor and whether he should be located within the operating room able to execute all complications manually finishing the operation at any time himself.

Due to medicolegal concerns, there is so far no realistic hope that all robot centers are connected via internet in order to perform operations on patients in different places by more experienced surgeons comfortable with this technique. Fact is that robotic surgery must produce as good or better results when compared with conventional technique [48]. Therefore, training and learning centers for robotics are a requirement for innovative progress. An assignment of the faculty would be in depth communication between clinicians and engineers. A recent survey in the USA [23] showed that only 14% of surgical training centers offer robotics within the teaching program. Limited clinical resources pose the question whether industrial suppliers should increase financial support for medical robotic training centers.

Despite significantly increased precision and noval complex procedures with minimally invasive techniques robotic surgery is still at the beginning of its possibilities. In the field of joint replacement femoral stem preparation has clear advantages with regards to precision and prosthetic fit. There is significantly less aseptic loosening and earlier postoperative mobility due to optimal anatomical stem position, decreased stress shielding, and better muscle function. Local forces at the stem bone interface are better orientated and will further improve longevity in combination with optimal bone ingrowth (■Fig. 73-9a,b). The cancellous lamellar microstructure remains uninjured allowing optimal microcirculation at the bone prosthesis interface [42]. These factors suggests a significantly increased stem longevity, however, comparative long-term studies will have to confirm this hypothesis.

An unsolved problem is still the ideal cup position, which has considerable influence on bone ingrowth and prosthetic longevity. There are no hard data for best placement of the cup in the current literature, but there is uniform disagreement on extreme steep and horizontal cup positions. Traditional measuring instruments rely on the patient's body without focus on pelvis and relative body movements. Robotics and preoperative planning represents significant potential for improvements. Cup

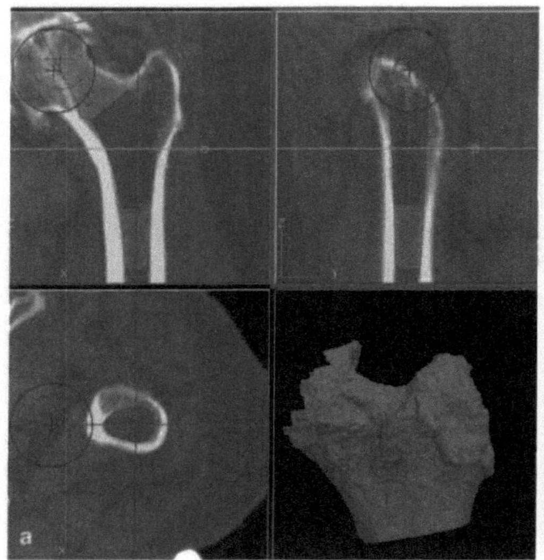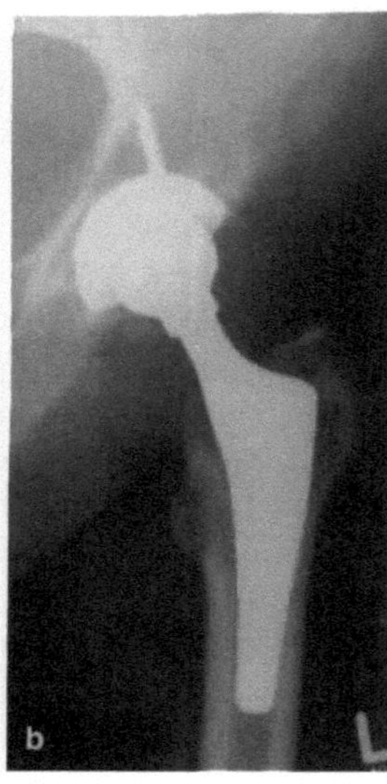

Fig. 73-9. a Orthodoc planning of a short press-fit stem. **b** Postoperative radiograph showing an implanted press-fit life-quality prosthetic stem

navigation is advantageous over robotics because of reasons including interactive instrument position and difficult anatomical reach for robots. Therefore, robotics and navigation complement one another instead of competition. Such combinations will be shortly available for clinical use (i. e. RoboNav, Integrated Surgical System, CA, USA).

Robotics has proven its use in total knee arthroplasty (TKA) because of optimized mechanical axes. Due to lack of precise anatomical landmarks of the lower extremity during surgery, a combination of robotics and navigation is likely. This increases the potential of both systems and allows perfect implant positioning in addition with correct soft tissue and ligament balancing.

Rapid and parallel development of telesurgical concepts and robot-guided endoscopic surgery will attract cardiac and abdominal surgeons as well as complex minimally invasive gynecological and urological application. Complex coronary revascularization via an alternative endoscopic approach as successfully demonstrated on beating animal hearts are possible. Minimally invasive techniques and navigation will certainly increase neurosurgical indications. The possibilities of robotics, navigation, telemanipulation systems and its integrative capabilities will eventually decide whether surgeons may successfully begin treating diseases that are today only subject to diagnosis.

References

1. Aaronson OS, Tulipan NB, Cywes R, Sundell HW, Davis GH, Bruner JP, Richards WO (2002) Robot-assisted endoscoric intrauterine myelomeninocale repair: A feasibility study. Pediatr Neurosurg 36: 85–89
2. Adler JR Jr, Murphy MJ, Chang SI, Hancock SL (1999) Image-guided robotic radiosurgery. Neurosurgery 44: 1299–1306, discussion 1306–1307
3. Bauer A, Börner M, Lahmer A (1999) Clinical experience with a medical robotic system for total hip replacement. In: Nolte LP, Ganz R (eds) Computer assisted orthopedic surgery. Hogrefe & Huber, Bern, pp 128–133
4. Benabid AL, Cinquin P, Lavallée S, Le Bas JF, Demongeot J, de Rougemont J (1987) Computer-driven robot for stereotactic surgery connected to CT scan and magnetic resonance imaging. Technological design and preliminary results. Appl Neurophysiol 50: 153–154
5. Benabid AL, Hoffmann D, Ashraff A, Koudsie A, Bas JFL (1999) Robotic guidance in advanced imaging environments. In: Alexander E III, Maciunas RJ (eds) Advanced neurosurgical navigation. Thieme, New York, pp 571–583
6. Bernsmann K, Langlotz U, Ansari B, Wiese M (2000) Computerassistierte navigierte Pfannenplazierung in der Hüftendoprothetik – Anwendungsstudie im klinischen Routinealltag. Z Orthop 138: 515–521
7. Boehm DH, Reichenspurner H, Detter C, Arnold M, Gulbins H, Meiser B, Reichart B (2000) Clinical use of a computer–enhanced surgical robotic system for endoscopic coronary artery bypass grafting on the beating heart. Thorac Cardiovasc Surg 48: 198–202
8. Börner M, Bauer A, Lahmer A (1997) Rechnerunterstützter Robotereinsatz in der Hüftendoprothetik. Orthopäde 26: 251–257
9. Börner M, Lahmer A, Bauer A, Stier U (1998) Experiences with the ROBODOC system in more than 1000 cases. In: Lemke HU, Vannier MW, Inamura K, Farman AG (eds) Computer aided radiology and surgery. Proceedings of the 12th International Symposium and Exhibition (CARS '98), Tokyo, Japan, June 1998. Elsevier, Amsterdam, pp 689–693
10. Börner M, Wiesel U (2002) Rechnerunterstützter Robotereinsatz in der Hüftendoprothetik – Erfahrungen bei über 4000 Patienten, 50. Jahrestagung der Vereinigung Süddeutscher Orthopäden 01.–05.05.2002
11. Börner M, Wiesel U (2001) Erste Ergebnisse der roboterassisierten Kniegelenkendoprothetik mit dem ROBODOC(r)-System. Trauma Berufskrankh 3: 355–359

12. Brandt G, Radermacher K, Zimolong A et al. (2000) CRIGOS – Entwicklung eines Kompaktrobotersystems für die bildgeführte orthopädische Chirurgie. Orthopäde 29: 645–649

13. Burkart A, Debski RE, McMahon PJ et al. (2001) Precision of ACL tunnel placement using traditional and robotic techniques. Comp Aided Surg 6: 270–278

14. Burghart C, Krempien R, Redlich T et al. (1999) Robot assisted craniofacial surgery: first clinical evaluation. In: Lemke HU, Vannier MW, Inamura K, Farman AG (eds) Computer assisted radiology and surgery. Proceedings of the 13th International Congress and Exhibition (CARS '99), Paris, France, June 1999. Elsevier, Amsterdam, pp 828–833

15. Cadeddu JA, Stoianovici D, Kavoussi LR (1998) Robotic surgery in urology. Urol Clin North Am 25: 75–85

16. Cadière GB, Himpens J, Vertruyen M, Bruyns J, Germay O, Leman G, Izizaw R (2001) Evalutation of telesurgical (robotic) Nissenfundoplication 2001. Surg Endosc 15: 918–923

17. Chinzei K, Hata N, Jolesz FA, Kikinis R (2000) MR compatible surgical assist robot: system integration and preliminary feasibility study. In: Delp SL, DiGioia AM, Jaramaz B (eds) Proceedings of Third International Conference on Medical Image Computing and Computer-Assisted Intervention (MICCAI 2000), Pittsburgh, PA, October 2000. Lecture Notes in Computer Science 1935. Springer, Berlin Heidelberg New York Tokyo, pp 921–930

18. Cleary K, Banovac F, Lindisch D, Watson V (2001) Robotically assisted spine needle placement: program plan and cadaver study. Computer Based Medical Systems (CBMS), 14th IEEE International Symposium. IEEE, pp 339–342

19. Cleary K, Stoianovici D, Watson V, Cody R, Hum B, Lindisch D (2000) Robotics for percutaneous spinal procedures: initial report. In: Lemke HU, Vannier MW, Inamura K, Farman AG, Doi K (eds) Computer assisted radiology and surgery. Proceedings of the 14th International Congress and Exhibition (CARS 2000), San Francisco, CA, 28 June–1 July 2000. Elsevier, Amsterdam, pp 128–133

20. Davies BL, Hibberd RD, Ng WS, Timoney AG, Wickham JEA (1991) A surgeon robot for prostatectomies. Presentation at Fifth International Conference on Advanced Robotics (ICAR '91), z

21. Diegeler A, Falk V, Walther T, Mohr FW (1997) Minimally invasive coronary-artery bypass surgery without extracorporeal circulation. N Eng J Med 336: 1454

22. DiGioia AM (1998) What is computer assisted orthopaedic surgery? Clin Orthop Rel Res 354: 2–4

23. Donias HW, Karamandoukian RL, Glick PL, Bergsland J, Karmandoukian HL (2002) Survey of resident training in robotic surgery. Am Surg 68: 177–181

24. Falcone T, Goldberg J, Garcia-Ruiz A, Margossian H, Stevens L (1999) Full robotic assistance for laparoscopic tubal anastomosis: a case report. J Laparoendosc Adv Surg Tech 9: z–z

25. Falk V, Gummert JF, Walther T, Hayase M, Berry GJ, Mohr FW (1999) Quality of computer enhanced totally endoscopic coronary bypass graft anastomosis–comparison to conventional technique. Eur J Cardiothorac Surg 15: 260–264, discussion 264–265

26. Falk V, Walther T, Diegeler A et al. (1996) Echocardiographic Monitoring of minimally invasive mitral valve surgery using an endoaortic clamp. J Heart Valve Dis 5: 630–637

27. Glauser D, Flury P, Villotte N, Burckhardt C (1993) Mechanical concept of the neurosurgical robot Minerva. Robotica 11: 567–575

28. Goh PMY, Lomanto D, So JBY (2002) Robotic-assisted laparoscopic cholecystectomy. The first in Asia. Surg Endoscopy 16: 216–217

29. Guthart GS, Salisbury JJK (2000) The intuitive telesurgery system: overview and application. Proceedings of IEEE International Conference on Robotics and Automation, pp 618–621

30. Jakopec M, Harris S, Baena FRy, Gomes P, Cobb J, Davies B (2001) The first clinical application of a »hands-on« robotic knee surgery system. Comp Aid Surg 6: 329–339

31. Howe RD, Matsuoka Y (1999) Robotics for surgery. Annu Rev Blomed Eng 1: 211–240

32. Kaiser WA, Fischer H, Vagner J, Selig M (2000) Robotic system for biopsy and therapy of breast lesions in a high–field whole–body magnetic resonance tomography unit. Invest Radiol 35: 513–519

33. Kumar R, Gordia TM, Barnes AC et al. (1999) Performance of robotic augmentation in microsurgeryscale motions. In: Taylor C, Colchester A (eds) Proceedings of Second International Symposium on Medical Image Computing and Computer-Assisted Intervention (MICCAI '99), Cambridge, England, September 1999. Lecture Notes in Computer Science 1679. Springer, Berlin Heidelberg New York Tokyo, pp 1108–1115

34. Kwoh YS, Hou J, Jonckheere EA, Hayati S (1988) A robot with improved absolute positioning accuracy for CT guided stereotactic brain surgery. IEEE Trans Biomed Eng 5: 153–160

35. Lavallée S (1989) A new system for computer assisted neurosurgery. Proceedings of the Eleventh IEEE Engineering in Medicine and Biology Conference, pp 926–927

36. Lueth TC, Hein A, Albrecht J et al. (1998) A surgical robotic system for maxillofacial surgery. Proceedings of the 24th Annual Conference of the IEEE Industrial Electronics Society (IECON), pp 2470–2475

37. Mächler H, Bergmann P, Mächler E, Anelli-Monti M, Rigler B (2001) Forensische Aspekte eines Anfängers in der Roboterchirurgie am Herzen; Kongressband d. Jahres Dt. Ges. f. Chirurgie 2001, S 689–691

38. Masamune K, Kobayashi E, Masutani Y, Suzuki M, Dohi T, Iseki H, Takakura K (1995) Development of an MRI-compatible needle insertion manipulator for stereotactic neurosurgery. J Image Guid Surg 1: 242–248

39. Masamune K, Fichtinger G, Patriciu A et al. (2001) System for robotically assisted percutaneous procedures with computed tomography guidance. Comp Aid Surg 6: 370–383

40. Mai S, Lörke C, Siebert W (2000) Implantation von Knieendoprothesen mit dem neuen Operationsroboter-System CASPAR. Orthopädische Praxis 36: 792–800

41. Olk A, Franck WM, Hennig FF (2001) Stand und Perspektiven der Robotronik in der Unfall- und Wiederherstellungschirurgie. Trauma Berufskrankh 2 [Suppl]: 286–291

42. Okoniewski M, Birke A, Schietsch U, Thoma M, Hein W (2000) Frühergebnisse einer prospektiven Studie bei Patienten mit computergestützter Femurschaftpräparation bei Hüft-TEP-Implantationen (System ROBODOC) – Indikation, Ergebnisse, Komplikationen. Z Orthop 138: 510–514

43. Petermann H, Kober, R. Heinze P (2000) Computer assisted planning and robot-assisted surgery in anterior cruciate ligament reconstruction. Operat Tech Orthoped 10: 50

44. Stoianovici D (2001) URobotics – urology robotics at Johns Hopkins. Comp Aid Surg 6: 360–369

45. Tak Sung G, Gill IS (2001) Robotic laparoscopic surgery: A Comparison of the da VINCI and ZEUS systems. Urology 58: 893–898

46. Taylor RH (1997) Robots as surgical assistants: where we are, whither we are tending, and how to get there. Proceedings of the 6th Conference on Artificial Intelligence in Medicine Europe (AIME 97). Grenoble, France, pp 3–11

47. Taylor RH, Mittelstadt BD, Paul HA et al. (1994) An image-directed robotic system for precise orthopaedic surgery. IEEE Trans Robotics Automat 10: 261–273

48. Taylor RH, Jenson P, Whitcomb L (1999) A steady–hand robotic system for microsurgical augmentation. Int J Roboties Res 18: 1201–1210

49. Troccaz J, Delnondedieu Y (1996) Robots in Surgery. IARP Workshop on Medical Robots, Vienna, Austria

50. Wiesel U, Boerner M (2001) First experiences using a surgical robot for total knee replacement. Proc. CAOS/USA, Pittsburgh, USA 6–8 July 2001, pp 143–146

51. Yamauchi Y, Dohi T et al. (1993) A needle insertion manipulator for X–ray CT image–guided neurosurgery. Proc LST 5: 814–821

52. Yanof J, Haaga J, Klahr P, Bauer C, Nakamoto D, Chaturvedi A, Bruce R (2001) CT integrated robot for interventional procedures: preliminary experiment and computer–human interfaces. Comp Aid Surg 6: 352–359

VIII   Visions of the Industry

tion system and for the transfer of data from these instruments to the application computer in the non-sterile area. The actual detectors for the optical-electromagnetic position transmitters are situated in the lights of the operating theatre. Here too is mounted a digital camera which records the course of the operation and transmits it to the central documentation computer, either by a voice command or directly through the application software accompanying the operation. The data stamps date, time and patient ID and later forms part of the patient's medical file.

The procedure kits ordered lie opened and ready for use on the nurse's instrument cart. Some instruments are equipped with sensors so that they can be used under navigation. Apart from the implant, there is also a sterile-packed memory chip containing the latest OrthoPilot application software to accompany this operation. The cordless reading station on the operating table receives the program and transfers it so that it starts automatically on the central, permanently installed application computer of the operating theater. The hip program guides the surgeon and the support team through the procedure on several 45" flat screens: firstly, 1 cm long electromagnetic position sensors in glass capsules are fixed onto the pelvis, femur and tibia by means of stab incisions and drilling into the bone. These sensors remain in place postoperatively as an implant. Therefore, an objective assessment of the range of mobility of the joint, the leg axis and the position of the hip prostheses can be made at any time after the operation.

After this, 3D data on the hip joint is required. Thanks to digital technology, the 3D fluoroscope is compact and mobile. A measuring volume of max. 50×50×50 cm with a resolution of 0.2 mm permits an exact intraoperative 3D representation of the site within one minute. Each piece of data recorded is distortion free and location specific, i.e. directly suitable for navigation.

The 3D images taken are transferred »cable free« to both the central documentation computer and the application system, where they are matched with the preoperative images (complete leg X-ray under weight-bearing, lateral femur X-ray). Images of the prosthesis selected in the preoperative planning and its position are also displayed as an overlay.

The surgeon performs the referencing to the pelvic entry plane on a semi-transparent touch screen which is set up between the surgeon and the supine patient. Simultaneously with the large screen monitors, it shows the 3D fluoroscope data in the correct position with respect to the patient. Referencing to the pelvis is done automatically through recognizing the referencing transmitter on the pelvis.

A 3 cm long incision is then made in the skin and the muscle and tissue carefully prepared. To dissect the neck of the femur a navigated, battery operated saw is used, which the surgeon orientates and guides using the intraoperative 3D model. The site of the acetabular cup is also prepared with a navigated reamer which can be adjusted to size in situ. During this procedure the 3D model is modified online, since the geometry of the reamer is known and its position is determined by the position transmitter. After the acetabular cup site has been prepared, the cup is implanted under navigation without cement and fixed securely into place with a press-fit. Comparison with the planning data can be called up by a foot switch and is automatically transferred to the documentation computer.

The stem, a modular Aesculap short stem prosthesis, is designed to be implanted under navigation with the assistance of imaging. The medullary cavity is carefully opened and the preparation of the implant bed should be very precise. To do this the surgeon uses a special instrument with a position sensor on it, so that the reaming of the medullary cavity can be followed on the intraoperative 3D model in an optimal position. This means that information on the anteversion and anterotation of the femoral stem can already be taken into account while preparing the implant site. The geometry of the preoperatively selected implant, i.e. the midpoint of the press-fit cup, the relative position of the pelvis and femur before the opening of the joint capsule, as well as the target values for the range of motion to be achieved are all important to help navigate the implantation of the hip stem. Graphics, figures and the 3D model on the large screen monitor assist the surgeon carry out the operation. The tension in the ligaments is subsequently checked and if necessary corrected by selecting a different neck length.

The result of the hip operation is assessed objectively according to the range of motion, the difference in leg lengths, the angle of inclination/anteversion, the anterotation angle etc. and is documented in the procedure file. The surgeon subsequently performs a navigated varus correction osteotomy on the patient.

The mechanical leg axis is established intraoperatively according to the OrthoPilot principle (kinematic determination of the femoral head and the midpoint of the knee and ankle joints) and the preoperatively defined correction angle is read into the software.

After preparing a minimally invasive approach to the tibia, the first plane is cut with a navigated CO_2 hand laser, optimally adapted to the treatment of bone. First the hand laser is roughly positioned in a holding mechanism and then finely adjusted via sterilisable servomotors according to the actual/target values given by the software. The servomotors are controlled manually by the surgeon, in order to be able to react quickly to any critical situation that might arise.

The surgeon also adjusts the second plane of the wedge section with the servomotors and performs the section using the CO_2 laser. After the bone wedge has been removed, intraoperative 3D fluoroscopy is once more carried out. The automatic recognition of the bone structures, the known geometry of the wedge and the position of the tibia established by the position sensor permit navigated alignment of the pieces of bone. Before the sectioned area is fixed and stabilized with bio-inert synthetic clamps, the result of the corrective osteotomy is checked and compared with the planning data. Transfer of the data to the documentation computer and wound closure with resorbable tissue adhesive complete the operation.

After 75 min the patient has received the optimum treatment and can expect to enjoy unrestricted mobility of the right femur.

Summary

Aspects such as time and cost become increasingly important with regard to the introduction of DRGs and the associated cost limitations per operation. CAS systems must be closely investigated to see what cost/benefit relationship they offer the patient and the surgeon. Only computer-assisted systems which justify their investment and usage costs by clear improvements in patient treatment will be used as a matter of routine, since only these will be affordable. OrthoPilot already represents the start of this development, which now needs to be built upon. More economical, easier to use, semi-automatic systems are the goal of further development. Integration of intraoperative imaging such as ultrasound, endoscopy, 3D fluoroscopy will become just as much a matter of course as instruments and implants optimized for navigation.

74 Evolution of Navigation: The Operating Room in the Year 2012

H.-P. Tümmler, *Aesculap*

There are many visions of what the operating theater will be like in a decade's time. Key words such as robotics, tele-manipulation, multimodality, or intraoperative imaging are terms which crop up again and again in this connection. The patient appears to retreat into the background as more and more complex technology moves into the operating theatre.

Visions should relate as closely as possible to reality. The following factors should therefore be taken into consideration:

- Patients' quality of life and life expectancy will increase. Patients are becoming older and demanding »optimum« treatment into advanced age. Operations will be minimally invasive with the aim of achieving natural, pain-free mobility. In addition, bone-preserving revision surgery is also gaining in importance.
- Costs pressure on the hospital is growing stronger. DRGs (diagnostic related groups), standard charges per case and patient-related accounting are the beginning of greater cost consciousness and cost transparency in the hospital. »Procedure kits«, reprocessed and sterilized ready for use by external hospital service centers for a fixed cost will be one avenue leading in this direction.
- Legal aspects will become more important. Doctors, surgeons, hospital administrators are forced to pay more and more attention to the quality of their services and to document them. The threat of criminal proceedings in serious cases of failure will not only have an effect on the hospital's reputation, but also be a burden on its financial budget.

Taking these points into consideration, the following is an attempt to describe the course of a hip operation and a simultaneous varus correction in the year 2012.

A 45-year old patient complains of severe pain in the right hip.

On his cheque-card-sized personal medical file a 10 year old complete left and right leg X-rays taken under weight beating conditions as well as data about the range of mobility of his hip have been stored. As a prophylactic measure, the determination of the mobility range of the hip and knee joints began to be recorded regularly 10 years previously. This data can be referred to today and serve as the target values for the postoperative result.

A new complete leg X-ray of the weight-bearing right extremity is taken preoperatively using digital X-ray equipment, and a digital lateral radiological image of the right femur is also made.

This data is conveyed to the surgeon for preoperative preparation. The surgeon receives the data from the hospital's in-house intranet and selects the matching short stem prosthesis and cup from a database. From the previous flexion/extension data the software used swiftly calculates that the original range of mobility can in theory be restored with this stem/cup combination.

The correction angle for the high tibial osteotomy to be performed on the patient in the same operation is also defined. As a reference, the surgeon uses both the new and the 10 year old complete leg X-rays.

The results of this 10 min planning are used in the consequent preparations for surgery. An order for the sterile procedure kits required to perform the operation is automatically placed with the hospital service center, which delivers the appropriate instruments and implants just in time.

The preparation for primary hip arthroplasty with simultaneous varus correction is complete. The patient lies on an X-ray transparent, speech-controlled operating table which contains magnetic coils. These provide the power for the cordless instruments of the hybrid naviga-

75 Joint and Spinal Surgery 2005

A. Steiner, J. Hey, *Siemens*

In our capacity as a solutions provider, Siemens Medical Solutions analyzes the workflow of our customers and seeks to optimize it to achieve greater quality, efficiency and cost effectiveness. We provide our customers with the information and tools needed to obtain an economical solution from diagnosis to treatment planning, to the treatment itself and aftercare.

In the field of joint and spinal surgery, we achieve improved quality of care and higher productivity by developing and providing innovating technologies. These new technologies support the trend towards minimally invasive surgery and enable the patient to recover more quickly. At the same time workflow within the hospital improves and the duration of treatment is shortened.

3D Imaging and Navigation

An example of one such innovation is SIREMOBIL Iso-C3D, a mobile C arm from Siemens which generates three-dimensional image data during surgical procedures whenever three-dimensional information is required but has previously not been available. An interface to the navigation systems enables the surgeon to pinpoint the position of the image data record generated by the C-arm system while still in the operating theater, without relaying on complicated and invasive procedures to register pre-operative 3D data. (Until now corresponding points had to be found both on the object, e. g. on the joint surface, and in the image.) Automating this process avoids mistakes being made and reduces the duration of surgical procedures. SIREMOBIL Iso-C3D provides surgeons with an instrument that enables them to immediately check the result of a surgical intervention, for example the reconstruction of a joint surface, and to react accordingly during the course of the operation (□ Fig. 75-1). This guar-

antees an optimum result and reduces the need for further treatment and the likelihood of future complications, and thus ultimately saves costs.

In addition, SIREMOBIL Iso-C3D, together with its navigation interface, also allows you to carry out planning on the 3D image data. This can be very helpful, for example, in the positioning of a pedicle screw, as the structures involved are very delicate and the potential risks for the patient from incorrect positioning are substantial. During the operation, the surgeon can monitor his or her actions on the screen and synchronize them with the planning data which is displayed simultaneously. This automati-

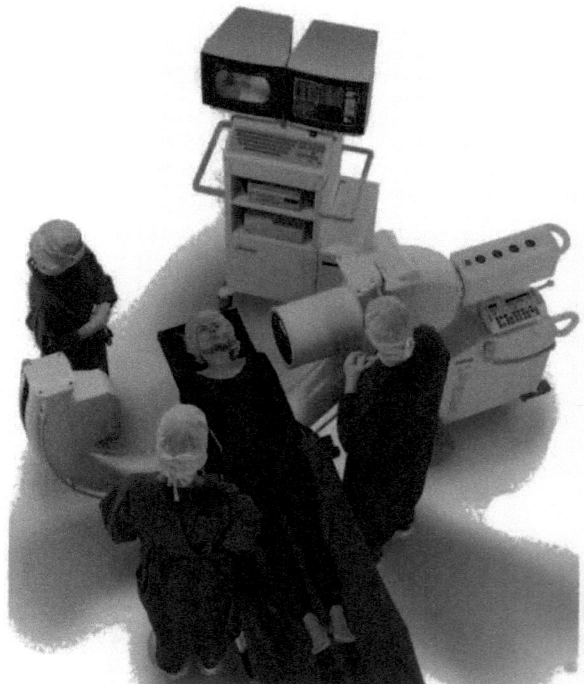

□ **Fig. 75-1.** Intraoperative 3D imaging with the Siemens SIREMOBIL Iso-C3D

cally reduces the dose since surgery itself no longer takes place under continuous fluoroscopy which until now had made online imaging possible.

In the future, new detector technologies could open up the possibility of an intraoperative 3D display of soft parts, such as cartilage in joint surgery or intervertebral disks in spinal surgery.

With intraoperative data on the image position available in the OR, it is possible to generate larger volumes by merging individual 3D data records because the exact position of the 3D image data is known.

Integration

The availability of relevant information in a surgical OR during therapy procedure as well as the integration of surgical modalities and components require a system solution which allows you to integrate application-oriented software and hardware from various vendors while at the same time ensuring user-friendly control of all OR equipment. Therefore Siemens and KARL STORZ bundled their competencies and developed a common OR system solution which meets all these requirements.

This system solution consists of the syngoOR system of Siemens and the OR1 system of STORZ.

The syngo software platform from Siemens is just such an architecture. All Siemens systems are already equipped with a uniform user interface and operating philosophy and are also equipped with an interface for accessing the digital hospital intranet. Patient management can be carried out on the spot and all patient data relevant

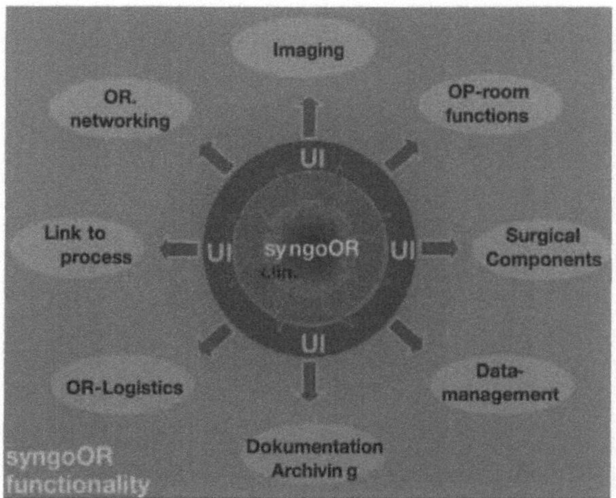

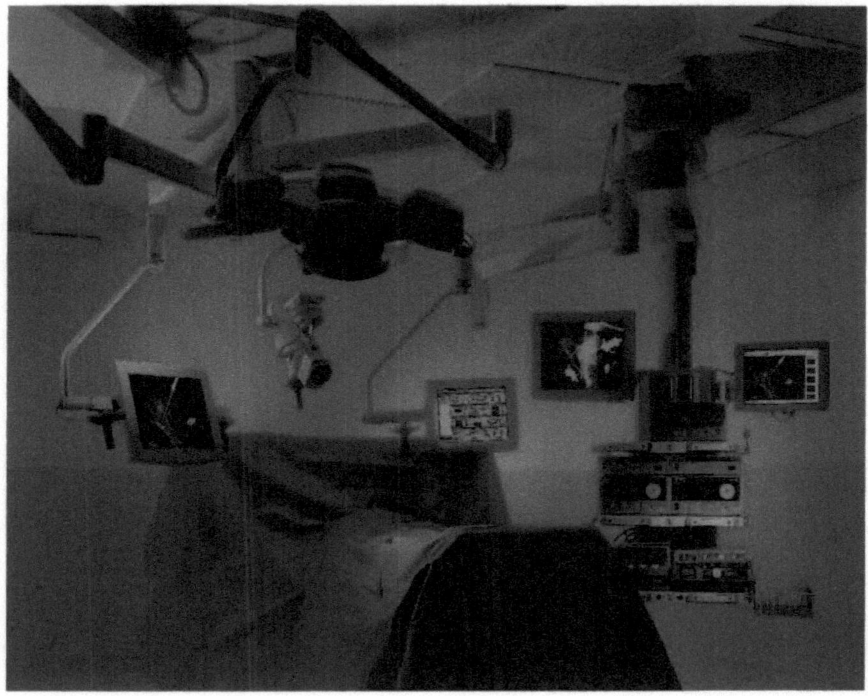

◘ Fig. 75-2. Siemens Integrated OR syngoOR.

to the surgical procedure can be displayed where they are needed. It is not only possible to display image data from other modalities, for example a preoperative MR image of the spine showing the intervertebral disks and the nerve structures, but to superimpose or merge this data with the current image data. This provides surgeons with additional information that benefits the treatment of patients. The Siemens syngoOR system and the STORZ OR1 system use a common centralized system control based on a touchscreen in the sterile area to control endoscopy systems, operating tables, RF units and intraoperative imaging systems like ultrasound and X-ray C-arms. In addition this system solution offers the opportunity to integrate the OR into hospital IT-systems (PACS, HIS). In the future, units such as navigation systems which currently have to be operated separately in the OR will also become part of the integrated solution. In addition to the integration of hardware components, the syngo platform allows you to integrate software planning tools, such as three-dimensional planning for selecting and positioning implants. Compared to standalone systems, integrated solutions offer many advantages. They not only take up less space in the operating theater, but are very user-friendly and substantially reduce training times due to the standard user interfaces (◘ Fig. 75-2).

Robotic and Virtual/Augmented Reality

In the future, further improvement of surgical procedures will be achieved in a number of ways: a C arm controlled by a navigation system will independently acquire images of those areas for which further surgical treatment is planned. In addition, new software will integrate the various two-dimensional or three-dimensional image data into a surgical planning program. The image data currently generated will be displayed via 3D lenses worn by the surgeon and will be superimposed with the planning data and other information relevant to the surgical procedure. Via a headset, the surgeon will be able to control the instruments and equipment required for the surgical procedure. If, for example, a joint surface reduction requires implants shaped to fit the bone surface, individual implants are prepared based on the intraoperatively generated 3D image data and are implanted using a minimally invasive procedure.

If, for example, during spinal surgery a surgeon requires the help or advice of other specialists in the same field, he or she can simply contact them via the central OR control center and discuss all the available information including the current image data and the planning data with the specialist in a video conference. To this end, the surgical procedure is filmed by a video camera that is integrated in the navigation system.

In the future, surgeons will be assisted by robots controlled by a navigation system which will be able to guide the instruments or perform the surgical action independently. The map needed to perform the action will be produced from the previously generated 3D image data and the surgeon's planning data.

It is also possible to perform the surgical procedure virtually, before the actual intervention takes place. This is helpful in very complex operations, but can also be used for educational purposes. 3D image data records and instruments which provide the surgeon with haptical feedback during surgery form the basis for these virtual procedures. This enables the surgeon to realistically plan and perform, for example, the positioning of a pedicle screw with the aid of a computer. These new technologies relieve the surgeon of many minor and supplementary tasks, thus allowing him or her to concentrate on the more critical issues that arise during the surgical procedure.

76 Computer-Guided Navigation in Orthopaedic Surgery

S. Christmann, *BrainLAB*

Software-guided medical technology has conquered the modern operating room, and many fields of medicine are hard to imagine without it today. Innovative medical technology makes it possible to perform complex surgical operations with a higher degree of safety and lower risks for patients. Modern computer systems, for instance, allow precision radiation of tumors and blood clots. BrainLAB AG develops and distributes software-based medical solutions to ease the work of doctors around the world. The company first made a name for itself in the fields of neurosurgery and the radio therapeutic treatment of brain tumors – as the name suggests – and has become the international market leader in these fields. Now, with the close cooperation of doctors specializing in different fields, BrainLAB has expanded its product range to include solutions in the field of ENT, where it supports, among other things, sinus surgery, and in orthopaedics, where it is used especially for hip and knee replacement surgery. Describing the company's future plans, Stefan Vilsmeier, founder and CEO of BrainLAB AG, explains, »Cooperating with doctors and implant manufacturers, we will continue to push the development and establishment of minimally invasive technologies, such as computer-assisted surgery, to offer patients new treatment options that improve medical outcome and entail lower risks and side effects.«

What is Navigated or Computer-Assisted Surgery?

In computer-assisted surgery, the VectorVision navigation system developed by BrainLAB provides a link between diagnostic data, such as computed tomography or MRI data, and the patient anatomy as seen during the operation. The system computes the three-dimensional model of the patient's anatomy from the diagnostic data obtained before the operation and displays them on the monitor. The surgeon can see the target area preoperatively and precisely plan the best route for accessing it. During the surgery, the surgeon can follow the location and movement of the instruments on the system's screen in real time, thus »navigating« accurately to the target. The system provides the surgeon with the important information needed to help get oriented in areas such as the brain or sinuses, but also around bone structures, such as the spine, the hip, or the knee. To do this, the system uses infrared cameras to track the position of the patient in the operating room and the position of the surgical instruments, constantly comparing these with the diagnostic image data.

The patient benefits from this method of minor incisions, reduced risks, and minimized recovery times.

BrainLAB Provides Minimally Invasive Solutions for Hip and Knee Surgery

The VectorVision navigation system from BrainLAB now automatically allows surgeons to select the optimal implant size and type for total knee and hip replacement surgery using the integrated database and then to intraoperatively precisely place the selected implant. »In the future this advanced navigation technology will allow patients to leave the hospital after only a short hospital stay, which is truly progressive when compared with the invasive operations common in orthopedic surgery today«, explains Wolfgang Steinle, Director of the Orthopedics Department at BrainLAB. Stefan Vilsmeier, BrainLAB AG CEO, sees the greatest growth potential for his company in this market segment at the moment. As Vilsmeier points out, »Just about any hospital would want to offer this technology – and the demands of informed patients will also play a role – and increase the competition among cli-nics. Educating patients is an important part of our work.«

Image-Guided total Hip and Knee Replacement Surgery

It is already common practice in conventional surgery to take diagnostic images, such as X-ray or computed tomography images, to help plan the procedure preoperatively. Yet the surgeon is left without any navigation during the operation itself, having to rely on what the naked eye can see in the operating room. Image-guided navigation with the VectorVision system is a new technology where the navigation system supports the surgeon pre- and intraoperatively with essential visual information.

The diagnostic image data of the patient's hip are transferred to a computer integrated with the navigation system. The computer uses this data to create into a three-dimensional model for the surgeon displayed on the touch screen monitor of the navigation system. During the planning process, the surgeon can select the ideal implant needed for the individual operation from the system's integrated database and position it virtually on the three-dimensional model of the patient's anatomy. All the while, the system takes into consideration the existing bone structures and mechanical axes not only of the leg to be treated, but also of the healthy leg. The software also performs a range-of-motion analysis. Based on this information, the navigation system guides the surgeon by tracking his instruments, when implanting the selected prosthesis, and indicates the correct positioning of the implant on the monitor screen (◘ Fig. 76-1).

During the surgery, the instruments are shown in the 3D model of the patient's anatomy so that the surgeon can watch the computer screen to see where he is placing his instruments. The navigation system's cameras constantly tracks the movements of the patient and of the surgical instruments used in the operation. This allows the surgeon to keep an exact overview of the effects at each step of the surgical procedure. The navigation system supports the surgeon during knee operations in the same manner.

CT-Based and CT-Free navigation

Based on the preoperative CT data of the patient, VectorVision knee enables three-dimensional planning of implants from different manufacturers (◘ Fig. 76-2). An

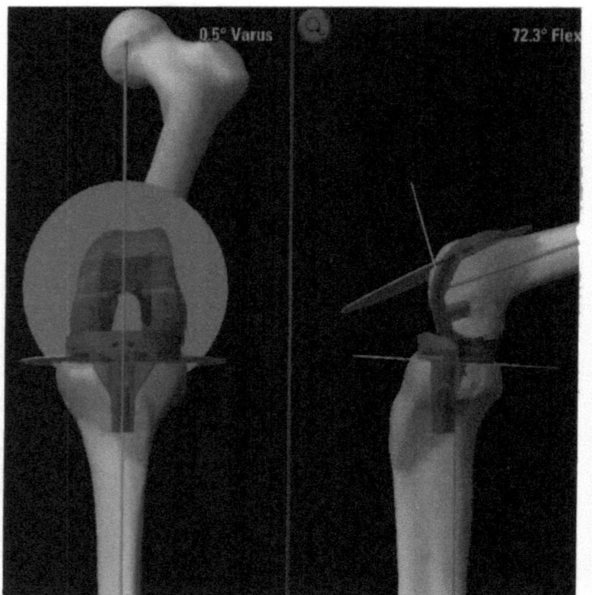

◘ **Fig. 76-1.** The VectorVision CT-free knee software intraoperatively visualizes the bone movements with the planned implant

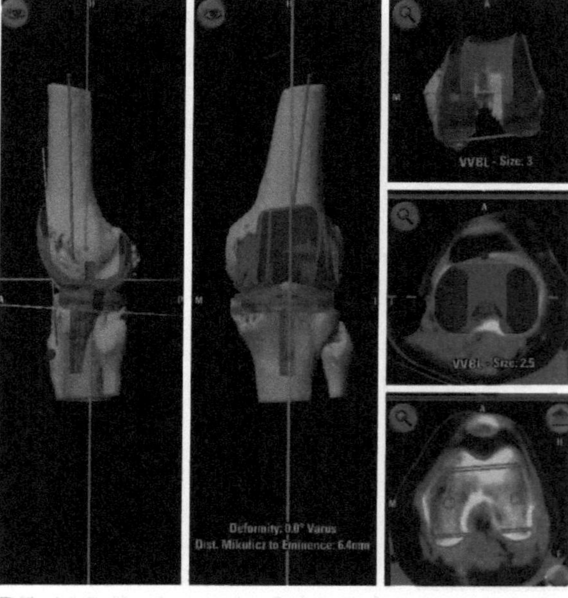

◘ **Fig. 76-2.** Planning overview for knee replacement surgery using VectorVision knee from BrainLAB

automatic planning algorithm calculates the optimum implant position while considering all the medically relevant anatomical landmarks. BrainLAB also offers the »VectorVision CT-free knee« software for CT-free navigation. Using this software, the surgeon acquires a series of landmarks and surface points in just a few seconds during the surgery. Using this data, the system calculates a generic three-dimensional bone model that corresponds to the individual patient anatomy at relevant points. In both cases, the system then suggests the optimum implant in terms of size and position. A comprehensive treatment plan shows the implant and its position in the knee simultaneously from different views. The surgeon can fine-adjust the knee prosthesis quickly in three dimensions as needed. Since the navigation system uses an innovative simulation technology to test the success of the implantation before it actually occurs, the surgeon can make changes to optimize the implant position during the surgery. This reduces the risks of implant misplacement and reduces the need for early revision surgery.

On the Relevance of Correct Implant Positioning

Biomechanical simulation models allow to predict the loads on the surfaces of prostheses as well as the ligament balancing situation that can arise from suboptimum placement (A.C. Godest, University of Southampton and PSI Group Paris). These simulations show that comparatively minor deviations from the original rotational axis (between 3° and 5°) can result in substantial changes in the natural force distribution and ligament tension (Andrew New, University of Southampton). Using navigation, implants can be precisely placed and as a result, improved ligament balancing and force distribution can be achieved.

Added Benefits of Image-Guided Surgery

Image-guided surgery allows the rapid advancements in diagnostic imaging to be optimally utilized in therapy. With the aid of navigation systems, surgeons can above all handle complex cases much more confidently. Since exact 3D planning occurs prior to the navigated surgery, the results can be more closely controlled, and the surgical data can be collected and evaluated. Based on this data, the potential risks, complications, and level of patient trauma related to surgery can all potentially be reduced, and the hospital stay can be shortened. The documentation and collection of scientific data allow more exact prognoses for the symptoms and the anticipated course of an illness, and these data can help reduce medical mal-practice liability risks.

Pressure from competitors is forcing medical institutions to continuously improve the quality of their treatments while at the same time keeping down costs. As with doctors, patients as well are increasingly educating themselves about innovative methods and selecting hospitals and clinics based on the equipment and the related treatment options. Computer-assisted surgery is thus becoming an important competitive factor with a significant influence on the number of patients and the profitability of individual clinics.

77 Planning, Navigation and Robotics in Orthopaedic Surgery

R. Nassutt, *ESKA Implants*

Introduction

Computer-aided surgery techniques are successfully applied in neuro- and spinal surgery for several years. Now, there is a tendency for digital planning software and navigation systems to become standard clinical equipment for endoprosthetic surgery, too. But for further establishment of these new electronic devices, it is strongly required that existing and proved clinical practice in the OR has to be considered. Not everything technically possible is clinically useful.

Digital Planning

Today's quality management activities in hospitals require basic adaptive changes in internal organization structures. Documentation is the key word and includes collecting documents (digital or paper) describing all surgical preparations and inventions taking place. Preoperative planning and its documentation prove the surgeon's care for the invention and the patient.

The hip and knee products from ESKA Implants are available in two different planning systems. The mediCAD software is based on digital X-ray pictures (digital or scanned). The mediCAD system supports all common file formats and can be connected to all clinically used data management systems. The Cappa software package allows to perform 3D planning on CT data. Both systems support data storage and documentation (◘ Fig. 77-1).

Navigation

Long-term success of an endoprosthetic intervention is strongly influenced by the right implant positioning and

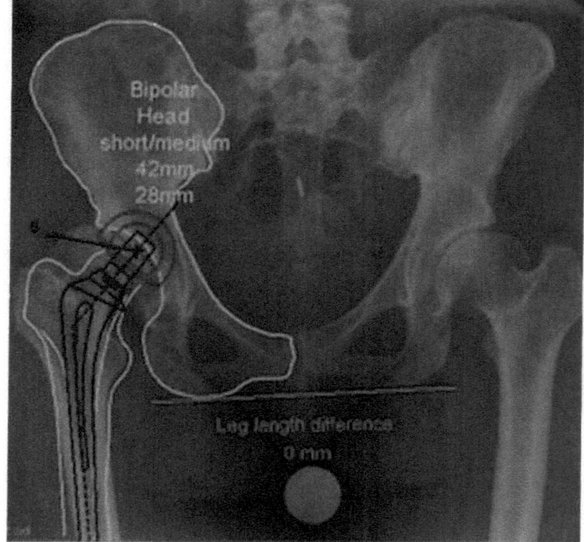

◘ **Fig. 77-1.** Digital planning system mediCAD, based on standard X-rays. Based on a few landmarks, several biomechanical factors are calculated automatically to support the surgeon in choosing the perfect size and position of the implant components

fixation. Well-prepared bone resections support the biomechanical performance, minimize tribological and mechanical load, and therefore, increase longevity and function of the artificial joint.

Navigation has already scientifically proved its positive influence on the precision of joint implant positioning and an increased reliability and reproducibility. For navigated applications the choice of the type of data base is essential and has to be adapted to the surgical requirements. Due to the common political and economic considerations, especially in health care, effective costs, necessary time, and expected personnel qualification are taken into account to value the clinical benefit of navigation. For

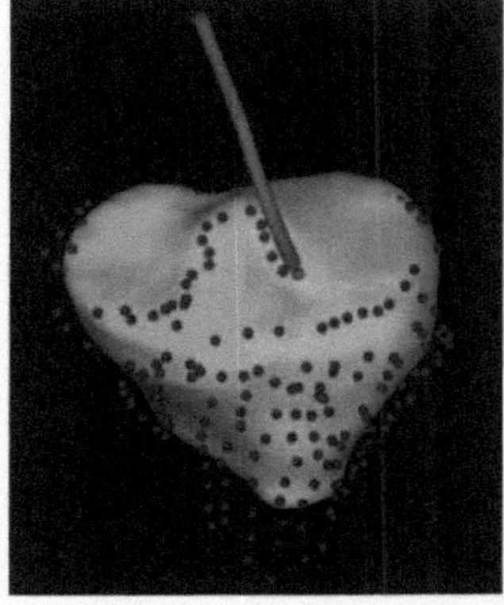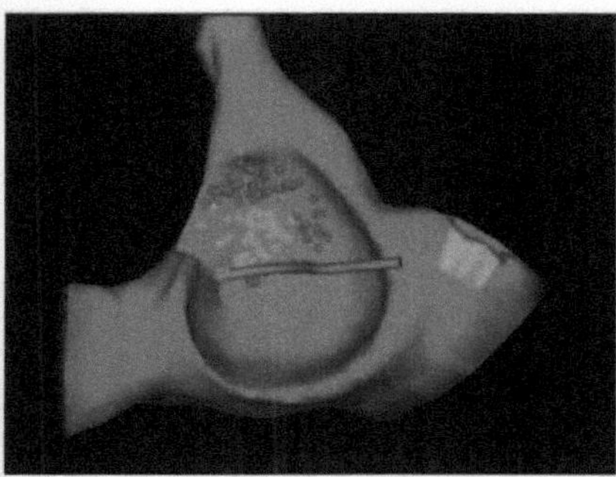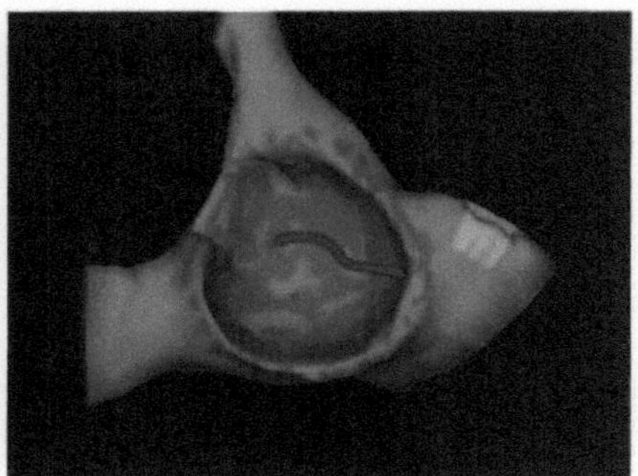

▫ Fig. 77-2. Bone Morphing steps during knee (*left*) and hip (*right*) navigation with SURGETICS. This simple procedure allows to create a precise 3D model of the individual patient intra-operatively

neuro-, ENT or spinal surgery three-dimensional CT data is necessary to have all important information. But for joint surgery we expect the CT-less navigation as the most reasonable and effective way to assist the surgeon. The SURGETICS system together with CT-less ESKA applications allow to navigate TKA and THA with maximum handling comfort. This is achieved by perfect adaptation of hard- and software and the patented Bone Morphing procedure. Our partner in navigation, PRAXIM Corp./ France, represents one of the origins of this technology and continuously works on new and easy-to-handle image sources for navigation (▫ Fig. 77-2).

Robotics

Robotics represents the highest level of automation in today's orthopaedic field. There are several examples for successful use of computer-controlled manipulators in medical environment such as micro- or heart surgery. Here, these machines allow to perform operations which were manually not possible. But in orthopaedics the robot does substitute the surgeon in some way, it performs work steps originally done by the surgeon. Highest precision was the only argument but precision in that range was never proved to be relevant for the clinical outcome of joint replacement. So the effort/benefit ration was never really satisfying.

Due to this controversy, ESKA Implants together with its users was one of the first examine and to consider the robot technology for clinical practice. At the orthopaedic section of the St. Franziskus-Hospital in Münster (head: CA Dr. Decking) a 2-year follow-up study was performed including a migration RSA analysis. Manually and robot-supported implanted ESKA-G2 hip stems were compared. In addition, the first 300 robot-implanted (system CASPAR) implants were analyzed. Results will be published soon.

In summary, the new PC-based technologies like planning and navigation systems will be the future of orthopaedics and also robotics might see a revival within the next years. Image data processing and tracking systems might open the way to revolutionary developments, but how fascinating these new achievements might be, the cost/benefit ratio always has to be taken into account.

There are still several details to improve which always have one background: to increase clinical acceptance and benefit. Digital planning systems as the initial stage of computer-aided surgery have to be easy to use with no loss of time compared to the basic planning procedure with pencil and pattern on the X-ray. Navigation technology still requires additional invasions and non-comfortable and time-consuming work steps. Robotics has to turn to be an universal assistant to the surgeon. The medical robots of the future have to be smaller, faster, and easier to handle than today's machines. So, there is still much to do but there are many reasons to let us be anxious for what the next years bring.

78 Computer-Assisted Operational Techniques from the Perspective of a System and Implant Manufacturer

W. Moser, *Pi Systems, PLUS Endoprothetik*

No other technology in the field of orthopaedics and traumatology can match the success of computer-assisted operational procedures over the last ten years. This has been achieved thanks to advances in industrial measurement techniques and robot technology. The obvious potential of these technologies for increasing safety and accuracy in surgery has yielded a range of products for the active and passive support of orthopaedic and traumatology surgery. For example, the implant manufacturer Precision Implants AG/PI Systems, the development and production centre of the companies PLUS Endoprothetik and Intraplant, exploited its existing know-how and developed the PiGalileo navigation and robot system using industrial measurement technology. A small robot, the PiGalileo CAS, was the first product developed. It was a two-axis system for knee endoprostheses controlled by a laptop computer and was based on the large robots used in industry, with adaptation for a sterile environment. The cost of this equipment, without navigational support, was about the same as the equipment and instruments used to carry out conventional knee prosthesis and allowed the technology to be accessible to a large area of application (◘ Fig. 78-1).

The state of present technical development in the area of navigation-assisted orthopaedic surgery is for systems to be equipped with infrared measurement technology and active or passive optical elements for tracking the object. Systems differ according to the software and instruments used for specific applications. The high capital investment means that it is desirable to find a variety of uses. Since the operating theatre is not a high technology environment, user-friendly solutions with good cost-benefit advantages are favored.

Only a small percentage of conventional endoprosthesis operations are now performed with CT-based plan-

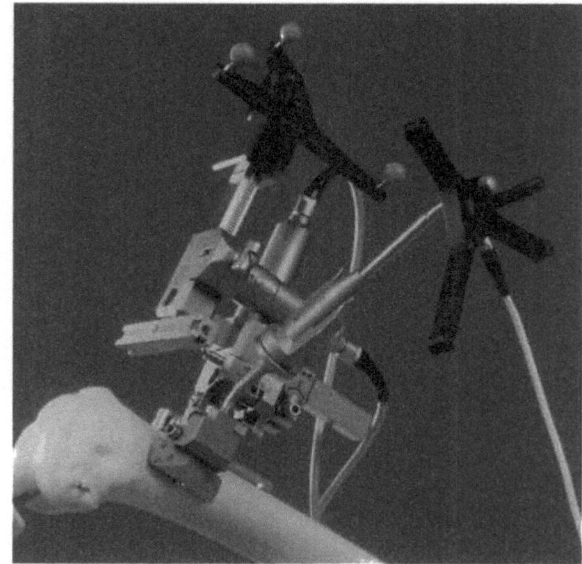

◘ **Fig. 78-1.** PiGalileo CAS small robot system, controlled by laptop computer or integrated into a navigation system

ning. There is a noticeable trend for systems using navigated endoprosthesis to be non-CT-based. More complex operations such as pronounced dysplasia require CT planning and are not performed in all surgical centers.

PiGalileo navigation modules have been designed to be used without preoperative CT data preparation. In the area of knee endoprosthesis the system was developed as a product that combines navigation and a robot.

Apart from combining navigation and robot, a special feature of the system is its high accuracy in determining axes without it being necessary to record the relative movement of the patient on the operating table, with a separate invasive application of a marker field (◘ Fig. 78-2). Whether it will be necessary to develop a CT-based mod-

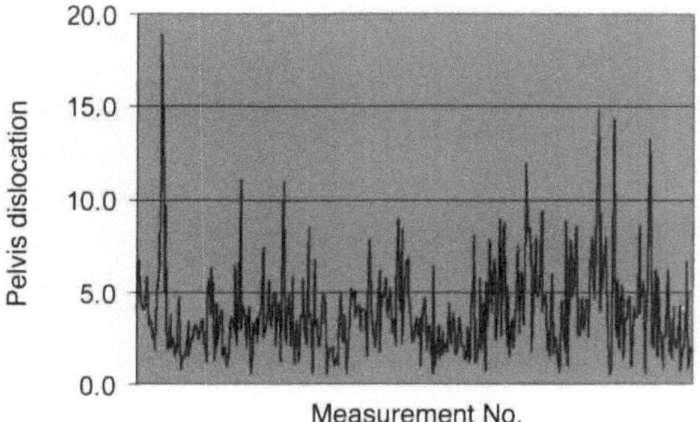

◘ Fig. 78-2. Pelvic movement during determination of mechanical axis by navigation (X axis: measurement no.; Y axis: pelvic movement)

ule depends on how widely the non-CT based navigational techniques can be applied in the next few years.

There is a high success rate for modern joint replacement methods but it will be difficult, if not impossible, to obtain statistically certain proof of better long-term clinical outcomes due to the number of cases and long monitoring periods required. For this reason, known factors affecting successful outcomes, such as maintenance of positional accuracy and axial alignment, are used as assessable parameters. It is essential for both the patients and the doctor that the systems used in computer-assisted operations can meet recognized standards, such as those relating to leg length or axial alignment. As part of this quality assurance process, the techniques can also provide documentation regarding the course of the operation.

Industrial suppliers of joint prostheses have recognized the advantages of computer-assisted surgical techniques in safely using their products and thus securing commercial benefits. In collaboration with system manufacturers, they can supply conventional implants together with computer-assisted surgical techniques. The operational procedure used is similar to that used in a conventional approach but has higher achievable accuracy for the required goals. In order to fully exploit the real potential that these new technologies can offer in terms of quality, new operational procedures are required.

There are two main aims for using these systems in joint replacement operations:

- to extend their use to all standard orthopaedic operations, with greatly simplified procedures.
- to develop combinations of surgical systems and suitable implants which can help realize the potential of the technology when used with new surgical techniques (e.g. MIS).

Suppliers having a high level of competence in both system and implant development will have an advantage in achieving these aims.

79 How Much Technology is Needed in the Operating Room?

J.L. Moctezuma de la Barrera, *Stryker Navigation*

D. Malackowski, *Stryker Navigation Instruments*

It is not long ago that personal digital assistants replaced organizers of the traveling businessman. Not just the recently added functionality like telephony, wireless communication, etc. but its seamless integration into powerful applications is what truly enabled the mobile warrior to enhance his productivity. Typical multi-tasking activities involve now for instance voice activation through a wireless headset, instant messaging and data processing on web-supported applications on one and the same handheld device.

A Decade of Surgical Navigation

During the first decade of surgical navigation the basic enabling technology was able to mature to a now de facto standard. Not only were the different components that make up a navigation system submitted to a series of development loops, but also the required surgical protocols. At the beginning, as the protocols were not in place, the impact that surgical navigation had on surgery could only be measured in terms of attained accuracy or difficulty of the procedure. Meanwhile dedicated surgical navigation packages with streamlined workflow enable the surgeon to sustain outcome performance in a well constrained operating time. Over the past few years, Stryker has played a key role in surgical technology innovation. The combination of Stryker's Flashpoint 5000 localization system with the largest working volume in the industry together with the wireless remote control capabilities fused into ergonomically designed surgical instruments have contributed to set a new standard for ergonomics. Also pioneering the dedicated workflow concept that seamlessly integrates navigation guidance with the specific operative technique, Stryker's focus has been to provide simplistic powerful solutions rather than cumbersome ad-hoc enhancements.

Current Developments

The established surgical navigation techniques propel these days surgical protocols to the next level, where less invasive techniques are being explored. These techniques have the potential to diminish morbidity and sometimes accelerate recovery thus impacting short term outcome and rehabilitation as well as the involved care costs. Hip and knee arthroplasty are among the most notorious examples where not only long ago explored surgical approaches but also less conventional therapy forms as e.g. unicondylar knee replacement gain on momentum. These newly rediscovered areas have both in common that they will certainly benefit the most through consequent exploitation of surgical navigation and will most probably proof superior to their non-navigated variations which will eventually be considered fallbacks.

A New Decade

As in the described commodity of the mobile warrior, high integration and interconnectivity of already available technologies will play a decisive role in the operating room of the future and modern management of health care institutions. The goal and motivation will be effectiveness increase across all structures.

The ability to handle a patient analogously to the industry's dream of an order of magnitude one will enable hospital management to track and relate all of the cost involved with a patient's treatment.

Innovation will manifest in the operating theater to the surgeon as the integration of multiple devices. Up to now, the focus of technological innovation has been around the functionality of the specific devices, as e. g. better performance of power tools, better imaging from postoperative diagnostic devices. Through integration surgical navigation will abandon its pedestal as a powerful stand-alone system and will become a mere embedded technological feature of surgical devices.

The most dramatic impact of connectivity and integration on surgery will be the ability to better monitor and control process parameters of a given procedure. The surgeon will be able to streamline procedures on a case-by-case basis where partly automated control or tasks as turning on and off accessory devices will take place. Not only surgical tools enhancements will be the result but also the ability to store and retrieve procedure related information. With on the fly access to hospital information services, picture archiving and retrieval systems as well as world wide web data bases and services the surgeon will be able to pre-, intra- and postoperatively manage procedural information.

The surgeon, as with today's navigation, will learn how to use and exploit these technical advancements which in turn will kick off a new wave of paradigm shifts.

These will bring a new generation of smart surgical instruments and their corresponding devices which will inherently demand a technically sophisticated procedure and in contrast to current therapy forms will not be able to be carried out manually or conventionally.

Stryker's Answer to the Future

Stryker's commitment to continuously improve patient outcome leads to excel in the arena of enabling technologies such as localization, visualization, imaging, cutting, etc. as well as in bringing these technologies to the surgeon's hands. A glance at the company's take on tomorrow's technology offers the **Stryker Total Suite, the OR of the Future**. Its consolidated OR equipment with full integration and connectivity capabilities delivers functionality that surgeons will demand once they unleash their creativity. The **Total Suite** through its ability to master complexity with **Reactive Workflow**, ergonomic user interfaces as e. g. voice activation, heads-up displays etc. frees up the surgeon from unwanted device interaction. Unburdened to master the technology himself, the surgeon can now concentrate on what he does best: surgery.

Subject Index

If you have any concerns about our products,
you can contact us on
ProductSafety@springernature.com

In case Publisher is established outside the EU,
the EU authorized representative is:
**Springer Nature Customer Service Center GmbH
Europaplatz 3, 69115 Heidelberg, Germany**

Printed by Libri Plureos GmbH
in Hamburg, Germany